Clinical Chemistry

Commissioning Editor: Timothy Horne
Project Development Manager: Siân Jarman
Project Manager: Nancy Arnott
Designer: Judith Wright
Illustrator: Cactus Design and Illustration Ltd

Clinical Chemistry

Fifth edition

William J Marshall
MA PhD MSc MB BS FRCP FRCPath FRCPEdin FIBiol

Reader in Clinical Biochemistry
Guy's, King's and St Thomas' School of Medicine
King's College, London
University of London
London, UK

Honorary Consultant in Clinical Biochemistry
King's College Hospital NHS Trust
London, UK

Stephen K Bangert
MA MB BChir MSc MBA FRCPath

Consultant Chemical Pathologist
East Sussex Hospitals NHS Trust
Eastbourne, UK

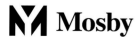

Edinburgh   London   New York   Oxford   Philadelphia   St Louis   Sydney   Toronto   2004

MOSBY
An imprint of Elsevier Limited

First published 1988 by Gower Medical Publishing
Second edition 1992 by Gower Medical Publishing
Third edition 1995 by Mosby
Fourth edition 2000 by Harcourt Publishers Limited
Fifth edition 2004

ISBN 0-7234-3328-3

British Library Cataloguing in Publication Data
A catalogue record for this book is available from the British Library

Library of Congress Cataloging in Publication Data
A catalog record for this book is available from the Library of Congress

Notice
Medical knowledge is constantly changing. Standard safety precautions must be followed, but as new research and clinical experience broaden our knowledge, changes in treatment and drug therapy may become necessary or appropriate. Readers are advised to check the most current product information provided by the manufacturer of each drug to be administered to verify the recommended dose, the method and duration of administration, and contraindications. It is the responsibility of the practitioner, relying on experience and knowledge of the patient, to determine dosages and the best treatment for each individual patient. Neither the Publisher nor the authors assumes any liability for any injury and/or damage to persons or property arising from this publication.
The Publisher

Cover photograph courtesy of
Bill Longscore/Science Photo Library.
False-colour transmission electron micrograph
(TEM) of a mitochondrion in a cell.

ELSEVIER your source for books, journals and multimedia in the health sciences
www.elsevierhealth.com

The publisher's policy is to use **paper manufactured from sustainable forests**

Printed in China

Preface to the fifth edition

Since the first edition of this book appeared, in 1988, cumulative English language sales have exceeded 50,000, and the publication of a fifth edition only four years after the fourth confirms its continuing popularity. In addition to thorough revision, this edition introduces two major changes: first, the introduction of full colour and second, the recruitment of a second author. By the time work needs to begin on a sixth edition, WJM will be nearing retirement; to ensure that the book retains its youth and appeal he invited his friend and colleague SKB to join him in preparing this edition, with a view to his taking over as lead author in the future.

As in our previous collaborations, this has been stimulating for both of us, and we believe that the book has benefited from both the constructive criticism and the discussion that the partnership has engendered.

The overall aims have remained the same and are essentially twofold: to discuss the use of biochemical investigations in the investigation and management of disease, and to discuss the many conditions that have a metabolic aetiology. It does not seek to be a comprehensive textbook of metabolic medicine, although we have included more details of clinical presentation and management than are conventionally included in textbooks of clinical biochemistry in order to better place the subject in the context of clinical practice. For this reason, we have alluded to other techniques for investigating patients where appropriate, recognizing that, in recent years, the expanding scope of imaging, for example, has altered the way in which many conditions are investigated and the contribution that biochemical tests make to this process. And while neither does it seek to be a textbook of physiology or biochemistry, we have continued to emphasize the basic science underlying the application of biochemical principles in clinical medicine.

By extending the scope of the book towards both basic science and clinical practice, we believe that it maps well against the integrated curricula that are now widespread in undergraduate medical training. It should also continue to prove appropriate for two other major groups of readers: clinical and biomedical scientists in clinical biochemistry, and junior doctors preparing for postgraduate examinations.

With examinations in mind, we have expanded the scope of the self-assessment section, including extended matching and single best response questions as well as traditional multiple choice questions.

The text has been thoroughly revised: obsolete matter has been deleted (though appreciating that what is obsolete in the UK may not yet be so in some supposedly less developed countries) and new material has been introduced to reflect current practice and new knowledge. Various colleagues have kindly advised on areas of their own particular expertise: in alphabetical order, they are Ruth Ayling, Susan Chambers and Beverley Harris. But while we gratefully acknowledge their help, and the constructive comments made by many of our own students as well as correspondents worldwide, the responsibility for the text is ours alone.

It is a pleasure to thank Timothy Horne and Siân Jarman and their colleagues at Elsevier for their encouragement in transforming two floppy disks into this volume.

And at home, we have been sustained by our beloved wives, Lorraine (Bangert) and Wendy (Marshall), whose own busy jobs as head teachers have not prevented them giving us their unstinting support throughout this project. We dedicate this book to them.

2004   W.J.M.
                                                                                         S.K.B.

Further reading

Cited references quickly become outdated. Readers seeking the most up to date information on a topic are recommended to use one of the bibliographic databases specializing in medical and scientific journals, for example Medline (the database of the National Library of Medicine in the United States of America, which encompasses over nine million references to reviews and papers published in nearly 4000 journals).

Journals which publish articles and reviews relating to clinical chemistry include *Annals of Clinical Biochemistry* and *Clinical Chemistry*. Each issue of *Endocrine and Metabolism Clinics of North America* comprises sets of reviews on related topics, most of which are of direct relevance to clinical chemistry. General medical journals such as the *British Medical Journal*, *Lancet* and *New England Journal of Medicine* carry editorials and reviews of topics related to clinical chemistry from time to time. The monthly issues of *Medicine* together comprise a textbook of medicine, which is updated on a three-year cycle and are highly recommended.

Contents

1 Biochemical tests in clinical medicine

INTRODUCTION

A central function of the chemical pathology or clinical chemistry laboratory is to provide biochemical information for the management of patients. Such information will be of value only if it is accurate and relevant, and if its significance is appreciated by the clinician so that it can be used appropriately to guide clinical decision-making. This chapter examines how biochemical data are acquired and how they should be used.

USE OF BIOCHEMICAL TESTS

Biochemical tests are used extensively in medicine, both in relation to diseases that have an obvious metabolic basis (e.g. diabetes mellitus, hypothyroidism) and those in which biochemical changes are a consequence of the disease (e.g. renal failure, malabsorption). Biochemical tests are used in diagnosis, prognosis, monitoring and screening (*Fig. 1.1*).

Diagnosis

Medical diagnosis is based on the patient's history, if available, the clinical signs found on examination, the

Screening	Diagnosis
detection of subclinical disease	confirmation or rejection of clinical diagnosis
Monitoring	Prognosis
monitoring progression or response to treatment	information regarding the likely outcome of disease

Fig. 1.1 The principal functions of biochemical tests.

results of investigations and sometimes, retrospectively, on the response to treatment. Frequently, a confident diagnosis can be made on the basis of the history combined with the findings on examination. Failing this, it is usually possible to formulate a differential diagnosis, in effect a short-list of possible diagnoses. Biochemical and other investigations may then be used to distinguish between them.

Investigations may be selected to help either confirm or refute a diagnosis, and it is important that the clinician appreciates how useful the chosen test is for these purposes. Making a diagnosis, even if incomplete, such as a diagnosis of hypoglycaemia without knowing its cause, may allow treatment to be initiated.

Prognosis

Tests used primarily for diagnosis may also provide prognostic information and some are used specifically for this purpose; for example, serial measurements of plasma creatinine concentration in progressive renal disease are used to indicate when dialysis may be required. Tests can also indicate the risk of developing a particular condition; for example, the risk of coronary artery disease increases with increasing plasma cholesterol concentration. However, such risks are calculated from epidemiological data and cannot give a precise prediction for a particular individual.

Monitoring

A major use of biochemical tests is to follow the course of an illness and to monitor the effects of treatment. To do this, there must be a suitable analyte, for instance glycated haemoglobin in patients with diabetes mellitus. Biochemical tests can also be used to detect complications of treatment, such as hypokalaemia during treatment with diuretics, and are extensively used to screen for possible drug toxicity, particularly in trials, but also in some cases when a drug is in established use.

Screening

Biochemical tests are widely used to determine whether a condition is present subclinically. The best-known example is the mass screening of all newborn babies for phenylketonuria (PKU), which is carried out in many countries, including the UK and the USA. The use of the 'biochemical profile', a battery of biochemical tests usually performed on a multichannel auto-analyzer, is discussed later in this chapter.

SAMPLING

Test request

The sample for analysis must be collected and transported to the laboratory according to a specified procedure if the data are to be of clinical value. This procedure begins with the test request form, which should include:

- patient's name, sex and date of birth
- hospital number (if appropriate)
- ward/clinic/address
- name of requesting doctor (telephone/page number for urgent requests)
- clinical diagnosis/problem
- test(s) requested
- type of specimen
- date and time of sampling
- relevant treatment (e.g. drugs).

It is essential that sufficient information be provided to identify the patient. In practice, vital information is often omitted and this may either cause delay in analysis and reporting or make it impossible to interpret the results.

Relevant clinical information and details of treatment, especially with drugs, are necessary to allow laboratory staff to assess the results in their clinical context. Drugs may interfere with analytical methods *in vitro* or may cause changes *in vivo* that suggest a pathological process; for instance, oestrogens increase thyroxine-binding globulin and thus total thyroxine concentration.

Patient

Some analytes are affected by variables such as posture, time of day, etc. (*Fig. 1.2*), and it may be necessary to standardize the conditions under which the sample is

Factor	Example of variable affected
age	alkaline phosphatase
sex	gonadal steroids
pregnancy	thyroxine (total)
posture	proteins
exercise	creatine kinase
stress	prolactin
nutritional status	glucose
time	cortisol

Fig. 1.2 Important factors which influence biochemical variables.

obtained. Factors of importance in this respect are listed in *Fig. 1.2* and are discussed further in subsequent chapters.

Even when standardized conditions are used for sampling, the results of repeated quantitative tests (e.g. daily measurements of fasting blood glucose concentration) will themselves show a Gaussian distribution, clustering about the 'usual' value for the individual. Typically, the scatter, which can be assessed by determining the standard deviation (SD), is less for analytes subject to strict regulation (e.g. fasting blood glucose and plasma calcium concentrations) than for others (e.g. plasma enzyme activities). Biological variation can be expressed as the coefficient of variation (CV) for repeated tests where CV = SD × 100/mean value.

Sample

The sample provided must be appropriate for the test requested. Most biochemical analyses are made on serum or plasma, but occasionally whole blood is required (e.g. for 'blood gases'), and analyses of urine, cerebrospinal fluid, pleural fluid, etc. can also be valuable. For most analyses on serum or plasma, either fluid is acceptable but in some instances it is of critical importance which of these is used; for example, serum is necessary for protein electrophoresis and plasma for measurement of renin activity. Haemolysis must be avoided when blood is drawn and, if the patient is receiving intravenous therapy, blood must be drawn from a remote site (e.g. the opposite arm) to avoid contamination. Haemolysis causes increases in plasma potassium and phosphate concentrations and aspartate aminotransferase activity, owing to leakage from red cells. If haemolysis is a consequence of a delay in centrifugation to separate blood cells from plasma, glucose concentration can fall. Other analytes may also be affected by haemolysis, depending on the analytical method used. The laboratory should always draw attention to potentially spurious results. It should be noted that leakage from cells *in vitro* can cause increases in plasma potassium and phosphate concentrations even in the absence of obvious haemolysis, particularly in patients with high white blood cell or platelet counts.

Collecting a blood sample into the wrong container can lead to (usually obviously) erroneous results (*see Case History 1.1*): oxalate and EDTA, which are used as anticoagulants in containers used for some haematological tests, combine with calcium and cause low measured concentrations in the plasma; so does citrate (the anticoagulant in containers for blood glucose measurement, which also contain fluoride to inhibit glycolysis), and it is clearly inappropriate to collect blood for lithium measurement into a container with lithium heparin as an anticoagulant. Laboratory handbooks should provide clear guidance on the types of sample, and, where appropriate, the sampling conditions, for all laboratory tests.

All samples must be correctly labelled and transported to the laboratory without delay. The serum or plasma is then separated from blood cells and analyzed. When analysis is delayed, or when samples are sent to distant laboratories for analysis, degradation of labile analytes must be prevented by refrigerating or freezing the serum or plasma.

Equal care is needed with the collection and transportation of other samples, such as urine and spinal fluid. All samples should be regarded as potentially infectious; great care is required with 'high-risk' samples, for example from patients infected with hepatitis B or C, or human immunodeficiency virus (HIV).

SAMPLE ANALYSIS AND REPORTING OF RESULTS

Analysis

The ideal analytical method is accurate, precise, sensitive and specific. It gives a correct result (accurate: *Fig. 1.3*) that is the same if repeated (precise: *Fig.1.3*). It measures low concentrations of the analyte (sensitive) and is not subject to interference by other substances (specific). In addition, it should preferably be cheap, simple and quick to perform. In practice, no test is ideal, but the pathologist must ensure that the results are sufficiently reliable to be clinically useful. Laboratory staff make considerable efforts to achieve this and analytical methods are subject to rigorous quality control and quality assurance procedures.

Nevertheless, there will always be a potential for some degree of imprecision or analytical variation in a result. The extent of this can be assessed by making repeated analyses (using exactly the same method) on the same sample (cf. biological variation, above). The results will cluster about a mean for which the SD can be calculated. The imprecision of the analysis can be

---

 Case history 1.1

The laboratory staff were concerned when a serum sample from an outpatient due to attend the diabetic clinic was analyzed and the following results were found:

Investigations

serum:	potassium	12.2 mmol/L
	sodium	140 mmol/L
	creatinine	84 µmol/L
	calcium	0.34 mmol/L
	phosphate	1.22 mmol/L

Comment

The potassium and calcium concentrations are not compatible with life. Investigation disclosed that the locum phlebotomist, who had taken the blood, had collected the original sample into a tube containing (potassium) fluoride and citrate, the correct container for an accurate blood glucose measurement, but then compounded his error by transferring the sample to a plain tube. Citrate acts as an anticoagulant by binding to calcium ions to form insoluble calcium citrate.

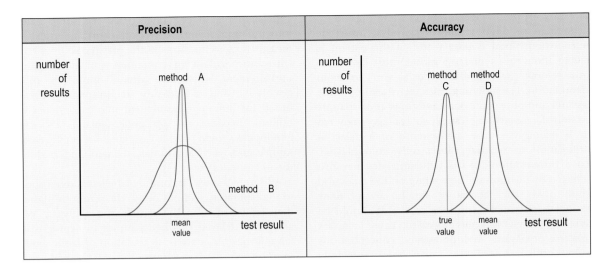

Fig. 1.3 Precision and accuracy of biochemical tests. Both graphs show the distribution of results for repeated analysis of the same sample by different methods.
Precision: the mean value is the same in each case, but the scatter about the mean is less in method A than in method B. Method A is, therefore, more precise.
Accuracy: both are equally precise, but in method D the mean value differs from the true value. The mean for method C is equal to the true value. Both methods are equally precise, but method C is more accurate.

expressed as the CV where $CV = SD \times 100/mean$ result. An understanding of the concepts of both analytical and biological variation is essential to the informed interpretation of laboratory data.

It is important to appreciate that results obtained using different methods may not be interchangeable. When a comparison between two results is being made, the same analytical method should be used on both occasions.

It is often appropriate to perform a group of related tests on a sample. For example, plasma calcium and phosphate concentrations and alkaline phosphatase activity all provide information that may be useful in the diagnosis of bone disease; several liver 'function' tests may usefully be grouped together. Such groupings are sometimes referred to as 'biochemical profiles'. Labour-saving multichannel auto-analyzers and similar instruments can perform more than 20 assays simultaneously on a single serum sample. However, although it may be tempting to perform all the assays on every sample, this approach generates an enormous amount of information, much of which may be unwanted, ignored or misinterpreted; worst of all, it may actually prevent the clinician from discerning the important

results. Discrete analysis, that is performing only the necessary tests, is to be preferred.

Reporting results

Once analysis has been completed and the necessary quality control checks made and found to be satisfactory, a report can be issued. Computers are widely used for data processing in laboratory medicine. The ability of the computer to store and process data facilitates the production of cumulative reports, allowing trends in the data to be picked out at a glance.

Near-patient testing

Not all analyses need to be performed in a central laboratory. Reagent sticks for testing urine at the bedside or in the clinic have long been available. Various substances, including glucose, protein, bilirubin, ketones and nitrites (indicative of urinary tract infection), can be tested for using such sticks.

Near-patient testing of blood for analytes such as glucose, and hydrogen ion and 'blood gases' has also been available for some time. Indeed, the development of instruments to allow patients with diabetes to monitor their blood glucose concentrations at home has revolutionized the management of this condition. Increasingly, manufacturers are developing instruments that can perform a wide range of tests suitable for near-patient use. Such instruments may allow the more rapid provision of analytical results for patients (e.g. in intensive therapy units) than if samples have to be transported to a central laboratory. It is clearly desirable that such instruments should be capable of providing results that are as robust with regard to accuracy and precision as those provided by the main laboratory. These instruments are designed to be very simple to operate but it is nevertheless essential that individuals using them, who may include nurses and doctors, are properly trained in their use, and adhere to protocols designed to ensure quality. Both the training and quality issues should be supervised by trained laboratory staff.

SOURCES OF ERROR

Erroneous results are at best a nuisance; at worst, they have potential for causing considerable harm. Errors can be minimized by scrupulous adherence to robust, agreed protocols at every stage of the testing process: this means a lot more than ensuring that the analysis is performed correctly. Errors can occur at various stages in the process:

- pre-analytical, occurring outside the laboratory, e.g. the wrong specimen being collected, mislabelling, incorrect preservation, etc.
- analytical, occurring within the laboratory, e.g. human or instrumental error
- post-analytical, whereby a correct result is generated but is incorrectly recorded in the patient's record, e.g. because of a transcription error.

Many of the few errors that do occur even in good laboratories are detected by quality control procedures, including data-handling software or personal scrutiny of reports by laboratory staff. Many are so bizarre that they are easily recognized for what they are. More subtle ones are more likely to go undetected. Unfortunately, the risk of errors occurring can never be entirely eliminated.

INTERPRETATION OF RESULTS

When the result of a biochemical test is obtained, the following points must be taken into consideration:

- is it normal?
- is it significantly different from previous results?
- is it consistent with the clinical findings?

Is it normal?

The use of the word 'normal' is fraught with difficulty. Statistically, it refers to a distribution of values from repeated measurement of the same quantity and is described by the bell-shaped Gaussian curve (*Fig. 1.4*). Many biological variables show a Gaussian distribution: the majority of individuals within a population will have a value approximating to the mean for the whole, and the frequency with which any value occurs decreases with increasing distance from the mean.

Skewed distributions are also often found, for example that of plasma bilirubin concentration, but can often be mathematically transformed to a normal distribution: data distributed with a skew to the right of the mean can often be transformed to a normal distribution if replotted on a semi-logarithmic scale.

If the variable being measured has a normal (Gaussian) distribution in a population, statistical theory predicts that approximately 95% of the values in the

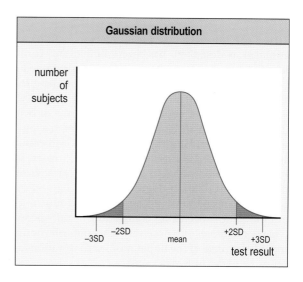

Fig. 1.4 Gaussian distribution. The range of the mean ± 2 standard deviations (SDs) encompasses 95.5% of the total number of test results. The range of the mean ± 3 standard deviations encompasses 99.7% of the total number.

population will lie within the range given by the mean ± two SDs (*Fig. 1.4*); of the remaining 5%, half the values will be higher and half will be lower than the limits of this range.

When establishing the range of values for a particular variable in healthy people, it is conventional to first examine a representative sample of sufficient size to determine whether or not the values fall into a Gaussian distribution. The range (mean ± two SDs) can then be calculated; this is, in statistical terms, the 'normal range'. Several important points arise from this.

- Although it is assumed that the population is healthy, values from 5% of individuals by definition lie outside the normal range. This suggests that, if the measurement were to be made in a group of comparable individuals, 1 in 20 would have a value outside this range.
- The specialized statistical use of the word 'normal' does not equate with what is generally meant by the word, that is, 'habitual' or 'usually encountered'.
- The statistical 'normal' may not be related to another common use of the word, which is to imply freedom from risk. For example, there is an association between increased risk of coronary heart disease and plasma cholesterol concentrations even within the normal range as derived from measurements on apparently healthy men.

Thus, the normal range for an analyte, defined and calculated as described, has severe limitations. It only identifies the range of values that can be expected to occur most often in individuals who are comparable to those in the population for whom the range was derived. It is not necessarily normal in terms of being 'ideal', nor is it associated with no risk of having or developing disease. Further, by definition, it will exclude values from some healthy individuals. In all cases, like must be compared with like. When physiological factors affect the concentration of an analyte (*see Fig. 1.2*), an individual's result must be assessed by comparing it with the value expected for comparable healthy people. It may, therefore, be necessary to establish normal ranges for subsets of the population, such as various age groups, or males or females only.

To alleviate the problems associated with the use of the word 'normal', the term 'reference interval' (RI) (often colloquially called the reference range) has been widely adopted by laboratory staff, using numerical values (reference limits) generally based on the mean ± two SDs. Results can be compared with the RI without assumptions being made about the meaning of normal. In practice, the term 'normal range' is still in general use outside laboratories. It is used synonymously with 'reference interval' in this book. Reference intervals for some common analytes are given in the Appendix: these are as used in one of the authors' laboratory, and are appropriate for the Case Histories, but may not apply to other laboratories, because of differences in methodology and in the characteristics of the population on which the data are based.

In using RIs to assess the significance of a particular result, the individual is being compared with a population. Some analytes show considerable biological variation, but the combined analytical and biological variations will usually be less for an individual than for a population. For example, although the reference interval for plasma creatinine concentration is 60–120 μmol/L, the day-to-day variation in an individual is less than this. Thus it is possible for a test result to be abnormal for an individual, yet still be within the accepted 'normal range'.

An abnormal result does not always indicate the presence of a pathological process, nor a normal result its absence. However, the more abnormal a result, that is the greater its difference from the limits of the reference interval, the greater is the probability that it is related to a pathological process.

In practice, there is rarely an absolute demarcation between normal values and those seen in disease; equivocal results must be supported by further investigation. If an important decision in the management of a patient is to be based upon a single result, it is vital that the cut-off point, or 'decision level', is chosen to ensure that the test functions efficiently. In screening for PKU, for example, the blood concentration of phenylalanine selected to indicate a positive result must include all infants with the condition; in other words, there must be no false negatives. This means that some normal children will be test positive (false positives) and will be subjected to further investigation. Generally, it is unusual to have to determine a patient's management on the basis of one result alone.

It has been explained that 5% of healthy people will, by definition, have a value for a given variable that is outside the reference interval. If a second and independent variable is measured, the probability that this result will be 'abnormal' is also 0.05 (5%). However, the abnormal results may not arise in the same individuals and the overall probability of an abnormal result from at least one test will be higher than 5%. It follows that the more tests that are performed on an individual, the greater the probability that the result of one of them will be abnormal; for ten independent variables the probability is 0.4; in other words, at least one abnormal result would be expected in 40% of healthy people. For 20 variables, the probability is 0.64.

Although biochemical parameters are frequently, to some extent, interdependent (e.g. albumin and total protein), the use of multichannel auto-analyzers to produce biochemical profiles inevitably generates a number of spuriously 'abnormal' results. Before any decision can be made on the basis of such results, some information is required about the probability that they are indicative of a pathological process. This topic is discussed on *p. 10.*

Is it different?

If the result of a previous test is available, the clinician will be able to compare the results and decide whether any difference between them is significant. This will depend upon the precision of the assay itself (a measure of its reproducibility) and the natural biological variation. Some examples of variation in common analytes are given in *Fig. 1.5.*

The probability that the difference between two results is *analytically* significant at a level of $p < 0.05$ is 2.8 times the *analytical* SD. Thus for plasma calcium concentration, with an analytical SD of 0.04 mmol/L, an apparent increase in calcium concentration from 2.54 mmol/L to 2.62 mmol/L ($2 \times$ SD) is within the limits of expected analytical variation, whereas an increase from 2.54 to 2.70 ($4 \times$ SD) is not. However, to decide whether an analytical change is *clinically* significant it is necessary to consider the extent of natural biological variation. The effects of analytical and biological variation can be assessed by calculating the overall standard deviation of the test given by:

$$SD = \sqrt{SD_A^2 + SD_B^2}$$

where SD_A and SD_B are the SDs for the analytical and biological variation, respectively. If the difference between two test results exceeds 2.8 times the SD of the test, the difference can be regarded as of potential clinical significance: the probability of this difference being a result of analytical and biological variation is <0.05. (*See Case History 1.2.*)

Analyte	Analytical variation	Biological variation
sodium	1.1 mmol/L	2.0 mmol/L
potassium	0.1 mmol/L	0.19 mmol/L
bicarbonate	0.5 mmol/L	1.3 mmol/L
urea	0.4 mmol/L	0.85 mmol/L
creatinine	5.0 µmol/L	4.1 µmol/L
calcium	0.04 mmol/L	0.04 mmol/L
phosphate	0.04 mmol/L	0.11 mmol/L
total protein	1.0 g/L	1.66 g/L
albumin	1.0 g/L	1.44 g/L
aspartate transaminase	6.0 U/L	8.0 U/L
alkaline phosphatase	4.0 U/L	15.0 U/L

Fig 1.5 Analytical and biological variation.
Analytical variation: typical standard deviations for repeated measurements made using a multichannel auto-analyzer on a single quality control serum with concentrations in the normal range.
Biological variation: means of standard deviations for repeated measurements made at weekly intervals in a group of healthy subjects over a period of 10 weeks, corrected for analytical variation.

Is it consistent with clinical findings?

If the result is consistent with clinical findings, it is evidence in favour of the clinical diagnosis. If it is not consistent, the explanation must be sought. There may have been a mistake in the collection, labelling or analysis of the sample, or in the reporting of the result. In practice, it may be simplest to request a further sample and to repeat the test. If the result is confirmed, the utility of the test in the clinical context should be considered and the clinical diagnosis itself may have to be reviewed.

Case history 1.2

A GP measured the serum creatinine concentration of a 41-year-old man newly diagnosed as having diabetes mellitus and hypertension. The result was 105 μmol/L. Six months later, both conditions were well controlled and the test was repeated.

Investigation

serum creatinine 118 μmol/L

The patient was alarmed at the apparent increase, but the GP was uncertain as to whether this was a significant change.

Comment

The analytical variation for creatinine is 5.0 μmol/L, the biological variation 4.1 μmol/L (*Fig. 1.5*). The critical difference is thus:

$$2.8 \times \sqrt{4.1^2 + 5.0^2}$$

that is, 18 μmol/L. Thus the apparent increase in creatinine is not significant at a level of $p = 0.05$.

THE CLINICAL UTILITY OF LABORATORY TESTS

In using the result of a test, it is important to know how reliable the test is and how suitable it is for its intended purpose. Thus, the laboratory personnel must ensure, as far as is practicable, that the data are accurate and precise, and the clinician should appreciate how useful the test is in the context in which it is used. Various properties of a test can be calculated to provide this information.

Specificity and sensitivity

Earlier in the chapter, the terms 'sensitivity' and 'specificity' were used to describe characteristics of analytical methods. The terms are also widely used in the context of the utility of laboratory tests. The specificity of a test is a measure of the incidence of negative results in persons known to be free of a disease, that is 'true negative' (TN). Sensitivity is a measure of

the incidence of positive results in patients known to have a condition, that is 'true positive' (TP). A specificity of 90% implies that 10% of disease-free people would be classified as having the disease on the basis of the test result: they would have a 'false positive' (FP) result. A sensitivity of 90% implies that only 90% of people known to have the disease would be diagnosed as having it on the basis of that test alone: 10% would be 'false negatives' (FN).

Specificity and sensitivity are calculated as follows:

$$\text{Specificity} = \frac{\text{TN}}{\text{all without disease (FP + TN)}} \times 100$$

$$\text{Sensitivity} = \frac{\text{TP}}{\text{all with disease (TP + FN)}} \times 100$$

An ideal diagnostic test would be 100% sensitive, giving positive results in all diseased subjects, and also 100% specific, giving negative results in all subjects free of disease. Because the ranges of results in quantitative tests that can occur in health and in disease almost always show some overlap, individual tests do not achieve such high standards. Factors that increase the specificity of a test tend to decrease the sensitivity and vice versa. To take an extreme example, if it were decided to diagnose thyrotoxicosis only if the plasma free thyroxine concentration were at least 32 pmol/L (the upper limit of the reference range is 26 pmol/L), the test would have 100% specificity; positive results (greater than 32 pmol/L) would only be seen in thyrotoxicosis. On the other hand, the test would have a low sensitivity in that many patients with mild thyrotoxicosis would be misdiagnosed. If a concentration of 20 pmol/L were used, the test would be very sensitive (all those with thyrotoxicosis would be correctly assigned) but have low specificity, because many normal people would also be diagnosed as having thyrotoxicosis. These concepts are illustrated in *Fig. 1.6*.

Whether it is desirable to maximize specificity or sensitivity depends on the nature of the condition that the test is used to diagnose and the consequences of making an incorrect diagnosis. For example, sensitivity is paramount in a screening test for a harmful condition, but the inevitable false positive results will have to be investigated further. However, in selecting patients for a trial of a new treatment, a highly specific test is more appropriate to ensure that the treatment is being given only to patients who have a particular

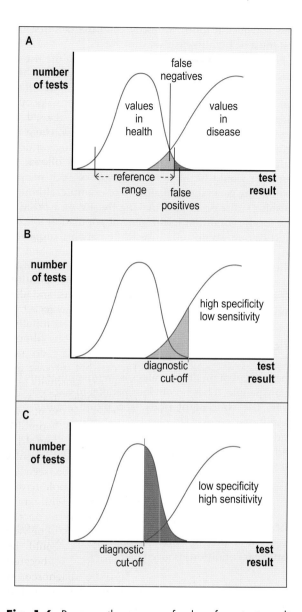

Fig. 1.6 Because the ranges of values for a test result in health and disease overlap (A), some patients with disease will have results within the reference range (false negatives) while some individuals free of disease will have results outside this range (false positives). If the diagnostic cut-off value for a test is set too high (B), there will be no false positives, but many false negatives; specificity is increased but sensitivity decreases. If the diagnostic cut-off value is set too low (C), the number of false positives, and sensitivity, increases, at the expense of a decrease in specificity.

condition. In some cases, this decision may not be straightforward, for example in the context of chest pain and suspected acute myocardial infarction where the possible options are to identify all those who have had a myocardial infarction ('rule in') or to identify all those who have definitely not ('rule out'). The preferred option should depend on the relative outcomes of treatment and non-treatment for patients in the two groups.

One way of comparing the sensitivity and specificity of different tests is to construct 'receiver operating characteristic curves' (ROC curves). Each test is performed in each of a series of appropriate individuals. The specificity and sensitivity are calculated using different cut-off values to determine whether a given result is positive or negative (*see Fig. 1.7*). The curves can then be assessed to determine which test performs best in the specific circumstances for which it is required.

The specialized use of the terms 'sensitivity' and 'specificity' that has been discussed here in the context of the *utility* of laboratory tests sometimes causes confusion, since these terms are also used to describe purely *analytical* properties of tests. Readers should appreciate that, in this latter context, 'sensitivity' relates to the ability of a test to detect low concentrations of an

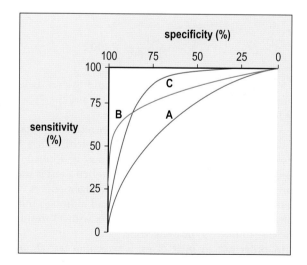

Fig. 1.7 ROC curves for three hypothetical tests, A, B and C. Examination of the curves shows that test A performs less well in terms of both sensitivity and specificity than tests B and C. Test B has better specificity than C, but C has better sensitivity.

analyte and 'specificity' to its ability to measure the analyte of interest and not some other (usually similar) substance.

Efficiency

The efficiency of a test is the number of correct results divided by the total number of tests. Thus efficiency is given by:

$$\frac{TP + TN}{\text{total number of tests}} \times 100$$

When sensitivity and specificity are equally important, the test with the greatest efficiency should be used.

Predictive values

A highly specific and sensitive test does not necessarily perform well in a clinical context. This is because the ability of a test to diagnose disease depends on the prevalence of the condition in the population being studied (prevalence is the number of people with the condition in relation to the population). This ability is given by the 'predictive value' (PV). PV_{+ve}, the PV for a positive result, is the percentage of all positive results that are TPs, that is:

$$PV_{+ve} = \frac{TP}{TP + FP} \times 100$$

If a condition has a low prevalence and the test is less than 100% specific, many FPs will result and the PV will be low.

A high predictive value for a positive test is important if the appropriate management of a patient with a TP result would be potentially dangerous if applied to someone with an FP result. However, when a test is used for screening, the appropriate management is to perform further confirmatory tests, and although these may cause inconvenience for subjects with FP results, they are unlikely to be dangerous.

In order not to miss cases, a screening test should have a very high PV_{-ve}, the PV for a negative result, this being the percentage of all negative results that are TNs, that is:

$$PV_{-ve} = \frac{TN}{TN + FN} \times 100$$

This conclusion follows directly from the fact that the test must be highly sensitive.

For clarity, this discussion has centred on the use of single tests for diagnostic purposes but, in practice, the clinician will combine clinical information and, often, the results of several investigations to make the diagnosis. If the tests are used rationally, the PV of positive results will be higher since the tests will be used only in patients who have other features suggesting a particular diagnosis (the prevalence of the disease in question would be higher in a group of such people than in the general population). For example, although Cushing's disease is rare, making the PV of a positive test for the condition in the general population low, in practice one would only investigate patients suspected on clinical grounds of having the condition and in whom the prevalence will therefore be higher. This may be self-evident, but doctors frequently order tests on flimsy clinical grounds and fail to appreciate how unhelpful, or even misleading, the results may be.

Likelihood ratios

The concept of predictive values is an unfamiliar one for many people: it has no obvious parallel in our everyday lives. The concept of odds is a more familiar one. 'Likelihood ratios' (LRs) express the odds that a given finding (e.g. a particular result) would occur in a person with, as opposed to without, a particular condition. The LR for a positive result is given by:

$$LR_{+ve} = \text{sensitivity}/(1 - \text{specificity})$$

The LR_{-ve} (the odds that a negative test result would occur in a person with, as opposed to without, a particular condition) is given by:

$$LR_{-ve} = (1 - \text{sensitivity})/\text{specificity}$$

LRs can be used to convert the probability of a condition being present before the test was done (in the case of a screening test, this is the prevalence) to the post-test probability of its being present. The greater the value of the LR, the more useful the test will have been.

Discriminant functions

Another approach, useful when several tests are performed, is to combine the results mathematically, usually after each result has been weighted by a multiplier, to produce one or more figures called 'discriminant functions' (DFs) or 'indices'. These can then be compared with the range of values calculated for a group of patients shown, by an independent, definitive technique, to have a particular condition. If the DF for an individual falls within this range, there is a high probability that he or she has the condition in question. This approach has been applied, for example, to the differential diagnosis of both hypercalcaemia and obstructive jaundice, but has yet to gain wide acceptance in clinical biochemistry.

Evidence-based clinical biochemistry

Most clinicians and pathologists use laboratory tests primarily on the basis of their own clinical expertise and interpret results intuitively. Ideally, tests should be chosen on the basis of evidence of their utility, and their results used on the basis of outcome measures. Such an approach is now advocated as part of the practice of evidence-based medicine, and could be facilitated by the use of test characteristics such as have been discussed above. However, it remains the case that many well-established tests have been introduced into clinical practice without being properly evaluated, and few systematic reviews of existing tests have been performed.

AUDIT

Audit is part of the process of ensuring quality – in this context, of ensuring the provision of a high quality laboratory service. In this respect, it is complementary to the other techniques of quality assurance, which in the main concentrate on the analytical aspects of the service, that is, the provision of precise and accurate results. Audit is the process of systematically examining practice in order to ensure that it is efficient and beneficial to patients. It involves identifying an area of practice, setting standards or guidelines (e.g. a protocol for investigation of patients suspected of having a particular condition), implementing changes designed to achieve these and then examining compliance with them and the effects on patient care. The cycle is completed by revision of the standards in the light of this analysis and their modification as required. It should be followed by re-audit after an appropriate interval.

SCREENING

Screening tests are used to detect disease in groups of apparently healthy individuals. Such tests may be applied to whole populations (e.g. the detection of PKU in the newborn), to groups known to be at risk (the detection of hypercholesterolaemia in the relatives of people with premature coronary heart disease), or to groups of people selected for other reasons (biochemical profiling of pre-operative patients, health screening for business executives and screening for common conditions in the elderly).

As previously discussed, high sensitivity is essential for screening tests and, to avoid unnecessary further tests of normal people, high specificity is desirable. Screening tests for PKU are designed to maximize sensitivity but are also highly specific. However, PKU has a low incidence so that even with a sensitivity of 100% and specificity of 99.9%, the predictive value of a positive test is only 10%, that is, nine out of ten positive tests will be shown on further investigation to be false positives. These calculations are made as follows:

1. incidence of PKU = 1 in 10,000 live births

2. sensitivity = 100% or $\dfrac{1\ TP}{1\ case\ of\ PKU}$

3. specificity = 99.9% or $\dfrac{9990\ TN}{9999\ without\ PKU}$

4. number of positive tests per 10,000 infants tested =
$\dfrac{(100 - 99.9)}{100} \times 10,000 = 10$

5. numbers of TP and FP results:
$$TP = 1,\ FP = 9$$

6. predictive value of a positive test =
$$\dfrac{1}{10} \times 100 = 10\%$$

On the other hand, the predictive value of a negative test will be 100%, confirming that no cases will be missed using the screening test.

Screening for specific conditions is discussed in other chapters of this book. Such screening is often based on the use of considerably less specific or sensitive tests and therefore has a low efficiency for detecting disease. Indiscriminate biochemical profiling is also inefficient. The more tests that are performed, the greater is the probability that an 'abnormal' result will arise, which is not the result of a pathological process.

When multichannel auto-analyzers are used to generate biochemical data and an unexpected abnormality is found, a decision must be made as to what action to take. The abnormality may be considered insignificant in some clinical circumstances but if it is not, further investigations must be made. Although these may be of ultimate benefit to the patient, their cost and economic consequences may be considerable. At the very least, the tests should be repeated to ensure that the abnormality was not due to analytical error.

The ready availability of an investigation often leads to it being used unnecessarily or inappropriately. Doctors should be encouraged to be selective in making test requests. They should also join with laboratory staff in critically examining all current tests and investigative techniques to ensure that they are using these tests to their best advantage in medical practice.

SUMMARY

- **Biochemical tests** are used for **diagnosis, monitoring, screening** and in **prognosis.**

- **Samples for analysis** must be collected and transported to the laboratory under appropriate conditions.

- Analytical results are affected by both **analytical and biological variation.**

- Results can be compared either with **reference values** or with the results of previous tests.

- **The utility of test results** depends on many factors: an 'abnormal' result should not be assumed to indicate a pathological process, nor a 'normal' one to exclude disease or potential disease.

- The utility of tests can be measured and described mathematically: applying this information can considerably enhance the value of laboratory test results in clinical practice.

i Plasma and serum

Plasma is the aqueous phase of blood and can be obtained by removal of blood cells from blood to which an anticoagulant has been added. Serum is the aqueous phase of blood that has been allowed to clot. For technical reasons, many biochemical measurements are more conveniently made on serum, but the concentrations of most analytes are effectively the same in both fluids. In this book, the term 'serum' is used only where actual measurements made in serum are referred to (e.g. in the Case Histories) and in the few instances where serum must be used for analysis.

2 Water, sodium and potassium

INTRODUCTION

Water distribution

Water accounts for approximately 60% of body weight in men and 55% in women, reflecting the greater body fat content in women. Approximately 66% of this water is in the intracellular fluid (ICF) and 33% in the extracellular fluid (ECF); only 8% of body water is in the plasma (*Fig. 2.1*). Water is not actively transported in the body. It is, in general, freely permeable through the ICF and ECF and its distribution is determined by the osmotic contents of these compartments. Except in the kidney, the osmotic concentrations, or osmolalities, of these compartments are always equal: they are isotonic. Any change in the solute content of a compartment engenders a shift of water, which restores isotonicity.

The major contributors to the osmolality of the ECF are sodium and its associated anions, mainly chloride and bicarbonate; in the ICF, the predominant cation is potassium. Other determinants of ECF osmolality include glucose and urea. Protein makes a numerically small contribution of approximately 0.5%. This is because osmolality is dependent on the molar concentrations of solutes: although the total concentration of plasma proteins is approximately 70 g/L, their high molecular weight results in their combined molar concentrations being less than 1 mmol/L. However, since the capillary endothelium is relatively impermeable to protein and since the protein concentration of interstitial fluid is much less than that of plasma, the osmotic effect of proteins is an important factor in determining water distribution between these two compartments. The contribution of proteins to the osmotic pressure of plasma is known as the colloid osmotic pressure or oncotic pressure (*see Chapter 13*).

Under normal circumstances, the amounts of water taken into the body and lost from it are equal over a period of time. Water is obtained from the diet and oxidative metabolism and is lost through the kidneys, skin, lungs and gut (*Fig. 2.2*). The minimum volume of urine necessary for normal excretion of waste products is about 500 mL/24 h but, as a result of obligatory losses by other routes, the minimum daily water intake necessary for the maintenance of water balance is approximately 1100 mL. This increases if losses are abnormally large, for example with excessive sweating or diarrhoea. Water intake is usually considerably greater than this minimum requirement but the excess is easily excreted through the kidneys.

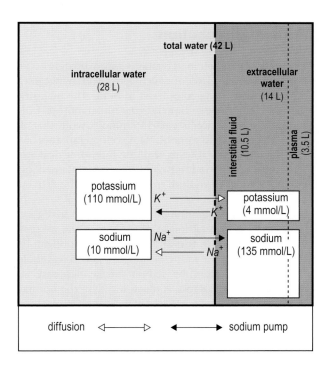

Fig. 2.1 Distribution of water, sodium and potassium in the body of a 70 kg man. The distribution is similar in women although the amount of water as a percentage of body weight is less. In children and infants, total body water is 75–80% of body weight, with a higher ECF:ICF volume ratio than in adults, but the proportion of the total body water contained in the plasma is the same. Note that, although plasma volume is approximately 3.5 L, blood volume in a 70 kg man is approximately 5.5 L.

Obligatory losses		Sources	
skin	500 mL		
lungs	400 mL		
		water from	
gut	100 mL	oxidative metabolism	400 mL
kidneys	500 mL	minimum in diet	1100 mL
total	1500 mL	total	1500 mL

Fig. 2.2 Daily water balance in an adult. The minimum intake necessary to maintain balance is approximately 1100 mL. Actual water intake in food and drink is usually greater than this, and the excess over requirements is excreted in the urine.

Sodium distribution

The body of an adult man contains approximately 4000 mmol of sodium, 70% of which is freely exchangeable, the remainder being complexed in bone. The majority of the exchangeable sodium is extracellular: normal ECF sodium concentration is 135–145 mmol/L while that of the ICF is only 4–10 mmol/L. Most cell membranes are relatively impermeable to sodium but some leakage into cells occurs and the gradient is maintained by active pumping of sodium from the ICF to the ECF by Na^+,K^+-ATPase.

As with water, sodium input and output normally are balanced. The normal intake of sodium in the western world is 100–200 mmol/24 h but the obligatory sodium loss, via the kidneys, skin and gut, is less than 10 mmol/24 h. Thus the sodium intake necessary to maintain sodium balance is much less than the normal intake; excess sodium is excreted in the urine. Despite this, excessive sodium intake may be harmful: there is evidence that it may be a contributory factor in hypertension.

It is important to appreciate that there is a massive internal turnover of sodium. Sodium is secreted into the gut at a rate of approximately 1000 mmol/24 h and filtered by the kidneys at a rate of 25,000 mmol/24 h, the vast majority being regained by reabsorption in the gut and renal tubules, respectively. If there is even a partial failure of this reabsorption, sodium homoeostasis will be compromised.

Potassium distribution

Potassium is the predominant intracellular cation.

Ninety per cent of the total body potassium is free and therefore exchangeable, whilst the remainder is bound in red blood cells, bone and brain tissue. However, only approximately 2% (50–60 mmol) of the total is located in the extracellular compartment (*see Fig. 2.1*), where it is readily accessible for measurement. Plasma potassium concentration is not, therefore, an accurate index of total body potassium status, but, because of the effect of potassium on membrane excitability, is important in its own right. The potassium concentration of serum is 0.2–0.3 mmol/L higher than that of plasma, owing to the release of potassium from platelets during clot formation, but this difference is not usually of practical significance.

There is a constant tendency for potassium to diffuse down its concentration gradient from the ICF to the ECF, opposed by the action of Na^+,K^+-ATPase (the sodium pump), which transports potassium into cells.

Potassium homoeostasis and its disorders are described later in this chapter.

WATER AND SODIUM HOMOEOSTASIS

Water and ECF osmolality

Changes in body water content independent of the amount of solute will alter the osmolality (*Fig. 2.3*). The osmolality of the ECF is normally maintained in the range 282–295 mmol/kg of water. Any loss of water from the ECF, such as occurs with water deprivation, will increase its osmolality and result in movement of water from the ICF to the ECF. However, a slight increase in ECF osmolality will still occur, stimulating the hypothalamic thirst centre, which promotes a desire to drink, and the hypothalamic osmoreceptors, which causes the release of vasopressin (antidiuretic hormone or ADH).

Vasopressin renders the renal collecting ducts permeable to water, permitting water reabsorption and concentration of the urine; the maximum urine concentration that can be achieved in humans is about 1200 mmol/kg. The osmoreceptors are highly sensitive to osmolality, responding to a change of as little as 1%. Vasopressin is undetectable in the plasma at a plasma osmolality of 282 mmol/kg, but its concentration rises sharply if plasma osmolality increases above this level (*Fig. 2.4a*).

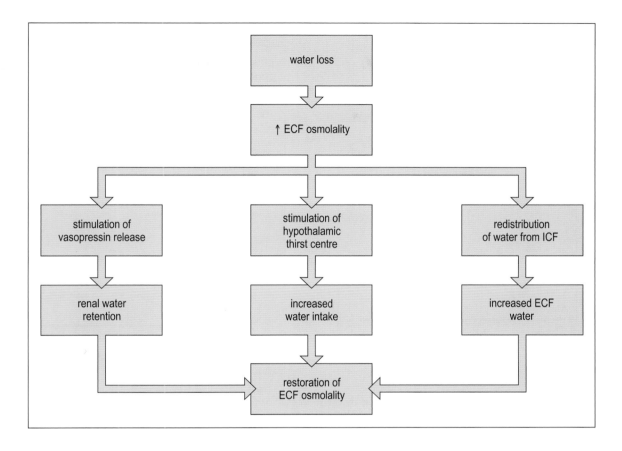

Fig. 2.3 Physiological responses to water loss.

If ECF osmolality falls, there is no sensation of thirst and vasopressin secretion is inhibited. A dilute urine is produced, allowing water loss and restoration of ECF osmolality to normal. If an increase in ECF osmolality occurs as a result of the presence of a solute such as urea that diffuses readily across cell membranes, ICF osmolality is also increased and osmoreceptors are not stimulated.

Other stimuli affecting vasopressin secretion (*Fig. 2.5*) include angiotensin II, arterial and venous baroreceptors and volume receptors (which sense blood pressure and volume, respectively). Hypovolaemia and hypotension increase the slope of the vasopressin response to an increase in osmolality (*see Fig. 2.4a*) and lower the threshold osmolality for vasopressin secretion. The vasopressin response to a fall in blood pressure is exponential: it is relatively small with small decreases in plasma volume, but greater falls cause a massive increase in vasopressin secretion (*Fig 2.4b*). Osmolar controls are overridden, tending to defend ECF volume (by stimulating water retention) at the expense of a decrease in osmolality.

Sodium and ECF volume

The volume of the ECF is directly dependent upon the total body sodium content since water intake and loss are regulated to maintain a constant ECF osmolality, and hence sodium concentration, and because sodium is virtually confined to the ECF.

Sodium balance is maintained by regulation of its renal excretion. Sodium excretion is dependent upon glomerular filtration, but the glomerular filtration rate (GFR) appears to become an important limiting factor in sodium excretion only at extremely low rates of filtration (sodium retention is a late feature of chronic

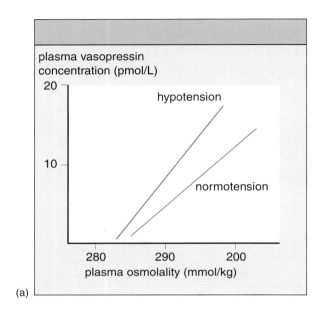

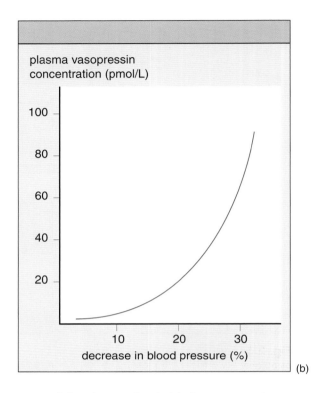

Fig. 2.4 (a) Vasopressin secretion is stimulated by a rise in ECF osmolality above a threshold of approximately 282 mmol/kg; in hypotension (blue line), this threshold is reduced and the response is greater. (b) Vasopressin secretion is stimulated exponentially by hypotension. Note the difference in the scales of the vertical axes.

renal failure). Normally, approximately 70% of filtered sodium is actively reabsorbed in the proximal convoluted tubules, with further reabsorption in the loops of Henle. Less than 5% of filtered sodium reaches the distal convoluted tubules. Aldosterone, released from the adrenal cortex in response to activation of the renin–angiotensin system, stimulates sodium reabsorption in the distal convoluted tubules and collecting ducts and is the major factor controlling renal sodium excretion.

Other factors must, however, be involved in the control of sodium reabsorption since patients with adrenal insufficiency, on a fixed replacement dose of mineralo-corticoids, maintain sodium balance even though their plasma mineralocorticoid concentrations are not controlled by sodium status. In such subjects, chronic loading with mineralocorticoids causes sodium retention only for a short period; thereafter sodium balance is regained, albeit with an increased ECF volume.

This response may be mediated by atrial natriuretic peptide (ANP). This is a 28 amino acid peptide, one of a family of similar peptides secreted by the cardiac atria in response to atrial stretch following a rise in atrial pressure (e.g. due to ECF volume expansion). ANP acts both directly by inhibiting distal tubular sodium reabsorption and through decreasing renin (and hence aldosterone) secretion. It also antagonizes the pressor effects of noradrenaline and angiotensin II and has a systemic vasodilatory effect. It appears to provide 'fine tuning' of sodium homoeostasis.

Two other structurally similar peptides have been identified: one (BNP) is secreted by the cardiac ventricles and has similar properties to ANP; the other (CNP) is present in high concentrations in vascular endothelium and is a vasodilator. Measurement of BNP is proving to be of value in the management of patients with cardiac failure (*see Chapter 14*). Increased secretion of natriuretic peptides has been postulated to be the

Control of vasopressin secretion	
Stimulating factors	**Inhibiting factors**
increased ECF osmolality	decreased ECF osmolality
severe hypovolaemia (via angiotensin II and arterial and venous receptors)	hypervolaemia
	alcohol
stress, including pain	
nausea	
exercise	
drugs: narcotic analgesics, nicotine, some sulphonylureas, carbamazepine, clofibrate, vincristine	

Fig. 2.5 Factors affecting vasopressin secretion. ECF osmolality is normally the most important of these.

mechanism responsible for the natriuresis seen in cerebral salt-wasting (*see p. 25*).

In general, the control mechanisms for ECF volume respond less rapidly and are less precise than the control mechanisms for ECF osmolality. Unless hypovolaemia is severe, maintenance of osmolality takes precedence.

WATER AND SODIUM DEPLETION

Water depletion or combined water and sodium depletion will occur if losses are greater than intake. Pure water depletion is seen much less frequently than depletion of both water and sodium. As sodium cannot be excreted from the body without water, sodium loss never occurs alone but is always accompanied by some loss of water. The fluid may be isotonic or hypotonic with respect to the plasma.

The clinical and biochemical features of pure water depletion and of isotonic sodium and water loss are quite different, as are the physiological responses. In clinical practice, however, states of fluid depletion encompass the whole spectrum between these two

extremes and the clinical and biochemical features will reflect this. Furthermore, it should be appreciated that they may have been modified by treatment.

Water depletion

Water depletion will occur if water intake is inadequate or if losses are excessive (*Fig. 2.6*). Excessive loss of water without any sodium loss is unusual, except in diabetes insipidus, but, provided that the sodium loss is small, the clinical consequences will be related primarily to the water depletion (*Fig. 2.6*).

Loss of water from the ECF causes an increase in osmolality, which in turn causes movement of water from the ICF to the ECF, thus lessening the increase. Nevertheless, the increase in ECF osmolality will be sufficient to stimulate the thirst centre and vasopressin secretion. Plasma sodium concentration is increased; plasma protein concentration and the haematocrit are usually only slightly elevated. Unless water depletion is due to uncontrolled loss through the kidneys, the urine becomes highly concentrated and there is a rapid decrease in its volume (*see Fig. 2.9*). Because water loss is borne by the total body water pool, and not just the ECF (*Fig. 2.7*), signs of a reduced ECF volume are not usually present. Furthermore, the increased colloid osmotic pressure of the plasma tends to hold extracellular water in the vascular compartment. Circulatory failure may be a very late feature of water depletion: it is much more likely to occur if sodium depletion is also present.

Severe water depletion induces cerebral dehydration, which may cause cerebral haemorrhage through tearing of blood vessels. Cerebral damage can also occur if rehydration is too rapid. If dehydration persists, brain cells synthesize osmotically active organic compounds ('osmolytes') and cerebral oedema may then follow rapid fluid replacement.

The management of water depletion involves treatment of the underlying cause and replacement of the fluid deficit. Water should preferably be given either orally or via a nasogastric tube. If this is not possible, either 5% dextrose or, if there is also some sodium depletion, 'dextrose–saline' (4% dextrose, 0.18% sodium chloride) should be given intravenously. The aim should be to correct approximately two-thirds of the deficit in the first 24 h and the remainder in the next 24 h, but plasma osmolality should not be allowed to fall too rapidly.

Water depletion	
Causes	**Clinical features**
Increased loss	**Symptoms**
from kidneys:	thirst
renal tubular disorders	dryness of mouth
diabetes insipidus	difficulty in swallowing
increased osmotic load due to diabetes mellitus,	weakness
osmotic diuretics or high protein intake	confusion
from skin:	
sweating	**Signs**
from lungs:	weight loss
hyperventilation	dryness of mucous membranes
from gut:	decreased saliva secretion
diarrhoea (in infants)	decreased urine volume (early)
Decreased intake	
infancy dysphagia	
old age restriction of	
unconsciousness oral intake	

Fig. 2.6 Causes and clinical features of predominant water depletion. In infantile gastroenteritis and in acclimatization to high temperatures, some sodium is lost from the gut and skin, respectively, but the effects of water loss may predominate.

Sodium depletion

Sodium depletion is seldom due to inadequate oral intake alone, but sometimes inadequate parenteral input is responsible. More often, sodium depletion is a consequence of excessive sodium loss (*Fig. 2.8*). Sodium can be lost from the body either isotonically (e.g. in plasma) or hypotonically (e.g. in sweat or dilute urine). In each case, there will be a decrease in ECF volume (*see Fig. 2.7*), but this will be less with hypotonic loss since some of the water loss will then be shared with the ICF. The clinical features of sodium depletion (*Fig. 2.8*) are primarily a result of the decrease in ECF volume.

The normal responses to hypovolaemia are an increase in aldosterone secretion, stimulating renal sodium reabsorption in the distal convoluted tubules, and a fall in urine volume as a consequence of a decreased GFR. Significantly increased vasopressin secretion, which stimulates the production of a highly concentrated urine, only occurs with more severe ECF volume depletion (*see Fig. 2.4*).

The decrease in GFR may lead to prerenal uraemia (*see Case History 4.1*). In contrast to the effects of pure

water depletion, plasma protein concentration and the haematocrit are usually clearly increased in sodium depletion, unless this is a result of the loss of plasma or blood. Furthermore, because the fluid loss is borne mainly by the ECF, signs of a reduced ECF volume are usually present and peripheral circulatory failure is more likely to occur than in water depletion. The features of sodium and water depletion are compared in *Fig. 2.9*.

The plasma sodium concentration can give an indication of the relative amounts of water and sodium that have been lost: plasma sodium will be normal if fluid is lost isotonically and increased if it is lost hypotonically. With severe sodium depletion, increased vasopressin secretion secondary to the resulting hypovolaemia may cause water retention; plasma volume is then maintained at the expense of osmolality and hyponatraemia develops. Thus the plasma sodium concentration in a sodium-depleted patient may be low, normal or high (*Fig. 2.10*).

The management of sodium depletion involves treatment of the underlying cause and, if necessary, restoration of the intravascular volume by giving isotonic fluid ['normal saline' (0.9% sodium chloride) or colloid

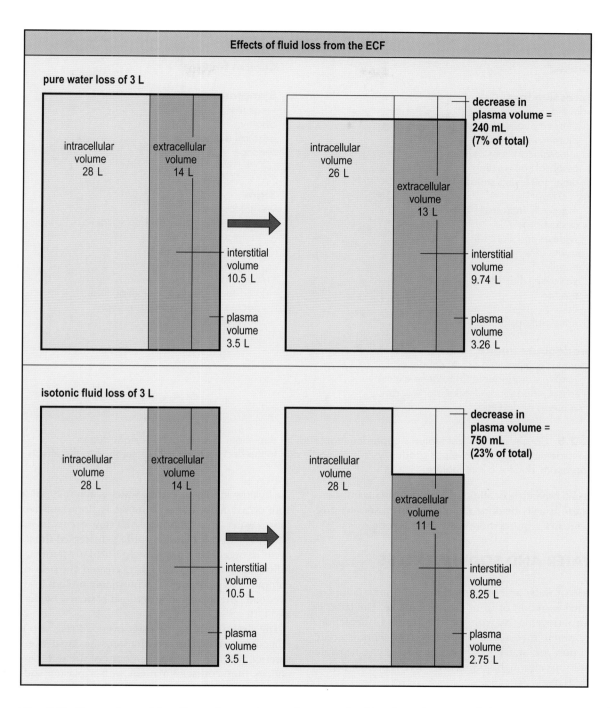

Fig. 2.7 Comparison of the effects of water loss and isotonic fluid loss from the extracellular compartment. When only water is lost from the ECF, the increase in osmolality causes water to move from the ICF, which minimizes the decrease in plasma volume. When isotonic fluid is lost from the ECF, no osmotic imbalance is produced, there is no movement of water from the ICF and the effect on plasma volume is, therefore, much greater. Similarly, excess isotonic fluid is confined to the ECF, but an excess of water is shared by the whole body water compartment and the effect on the ECF is thus much less.

Sodium depletion	
Causes	**Clinical features**
Excessive loss	**Symptoms**
from kidneys:	weakness
diuretic phase of 'acute tubular necrosis'	apathy
diuretic therapy	postural dizziness
mineralocorticoid deficiency	syncope
cerebral salt-wasting	
other salt-losing states	
from skin:	**Signs**
massively increased sweating	weight loss
cystic fibrosis	related to decreased plasma volume:
widespread dermatitis	tachycardia
burns	hypotension
from gut:	peripheral circulatory failure
vomiting, diarrhoea	oliguria
fistulae	related to decreased interstitial fluid:
ileus	decreased intraocular pressure
intestinal obstruction	decreased skin turgor
Inadequate intake	
sodium depletion will occur whenever	
intake is inadequate to balance excessive	
losses; inadequate intake alone is rarely	
a cause of depletion	

Fig. 2.8 Causes and clinical features of predominant sodium depletion. The clinical signs are due to hypovolaemia. Oliguria develops gradually: it is primarily due to the decrease in GFR, rather than to the effects of vasopressin. Thirst is a late feature.

(plasma expanders or albumin)] by intravenous infusion. This can usually be done rapidly, but any associated free water deficit requires more cautious correction.

WATER AND SODIUM EXCESS

Excess of water and sodium can result from a failure of normal excretion or from excessive intake. The latter is often iatrogenic. As with the syndromes of depletion, pure water excess and sodium excess with isotonic retention of water can be considered as separate conditions although, in practice, there is often a degree of overlap.

Water excess

This is usually related to an impairment of water excretion (*Fig. 2.11*). However, the limit to the ability of

the healthy kidney to excrete water is about 20 mL/min and, occasionally, excessive intake is alone sufficient to cause water intoxication. This can occur in some patients with psychiatric disorders. Increased thirst can occur in organic brain disease (particularly trauma, and following surgery), although decreased thirst is more common. Hyponatraemia is invariably present in water overload. The increased water load is shared by the ICF and ECF.

The clinical features of water overload (*Fig. 2.11*) are related to cerebral over-hydration, the incidence and severity depending upon the extent of the water excess and its time course. A patient with a plasma sodium concentration of 120 mmol/L, in whom water retention has occurred gradually over several days, may be asymptomatic, while one in whom this is an acute phenomenon may show signs of severe water intoxication.

The management of water overload is discussed with that of hyponatraemia on *p. 27*.

Clinical and laboratory findings in sodium and water depletion		
	Sodium depletion	**Water depletion**
plasma [Na⁺]	normal or ↓	↑
haematocrit	↑↑↑*	normal or slightly ↑
ECF volume	↓↓↓	usually normal
plasma [urea]	↑	high normal
urine volume	↓	↓↓↓
urine concentration	↑	↑↑↑
thirst	late	early
tachycardia hypotension	early	late

Fig. 2.9 Clinical and laboratory findings in sodium and water depletion.
*Unless due to loss of blood.

Mechanism of sodium depletion	Plasma sodium concentration
sodium and water loss, water loss predominating, e.g. excessive sweating	increased
isotonic sodium and water loss, e.g. burns, haemorrhage	normal
sodium loss with water retention, e.g. treatment of isotonic sodium depletion with low sodium fluids	decreased

Fig. 2.10 Plasma sodium concentration with various causes of sodium depletion. The plasma sodium concentration alone is a poor guide to ECF sodium status.

Excess body water	
Causes	**Clinical features**

Increased intake
compulsive water drinking
excessive parenteral fluid administration
water absorption during bladder irrigation
 	
Decreased excretion
renal failure (severe)
cortisol deficiency
inappropriate or ectopic secretion of vasopressin
drugs:
    stimulating vasopressin release (see Fig. 2.5)
    potentiating the action of vasopressin,
      e.g. chlorpropamide
    agonists of vasopressin,
      e.g. oxytocin
    interfering with renal diluting capacity,
      e.g. diuretics
	behavioural disturbances
	confusion
	headache
	convulsions
	coma
	muscle twitching
	extensor plantar responses

Fig. 2.11 Causes and clinical features of excess body water.

Sodium excess

Sodium excess can be due to increased intake or decreased excretion. The clinical features are related primarily to expansion of ECF volume. When related to excessive intake (e.g. the inappropriate use of hypertonic saline), a rapid shift of water from the intracellular compartment may also cause cerebral dehydration. When sodium overload is due to excessive intake, hypernatraemia is usual (*see Case History 2.5*).

Sodium overload is more usually due to impaired excretion than to excessive intake. Renal disease is a relatively uncommon cause (*Fig. 2.12*). Increased mineralocorticoid secretion due to primary adrenal disease is also uncommon. Sodium overload is most frequently due to secondary aldosteronism. This is seen in patients who, despite clinical evidence of increased ECF volume (e.g. peripheral oedema), appear to have a decreased effective plasma volume, due, for example, to venous pooling or a disturbance in the normal distribution of ECF between the vascular and extravascular compartments. Many such patients with sodium excess are, paradoxically, hyponatraemic, implying the coexistence of a defect in free water excretion. This is probably in part due to an increase in vasopressin secretion as a result of the decreased effective plasma volume. Also, the decrease in GFR and consequent increase in proximal tubular sodium reabsorption decreases the delivery of sodium and chloride to the loops of Henle and distal convoluted tubules. This reduces the kidneys' diluting capacity, thereby compromising water excretion.

The management of sodium excess should be directed towards the cause, where possible. In addition, diuretics may be used to promote sodium excretion, and sodium intake must be controlled. Dialysis may be necessary if renal function is poor and is occasionally necessary in acute sodium overload associated with the use of hypertonic fluids.

LABORATORY ASSESSMENT OF WATER AND SODIUM STATUS

The plasma sodium concentration is dependent upon the relative amounts of sodium and water in the plasma. In isolation, therefore, plasma sodium concentration provides no information about the sodium content of the ECF. It may be raised, normal or low, in states of sodium excess or depletion, according to the amount of water in the ECF.

Sodium excess	
Causes	**Clinical features**
Increased intake excessive parenteral administration absorption from saline emetics	peripheral oedema dyspnoea pulmonary oedema venous congestion hypertension effusions weight gain

Decreased excretion
decreased glomerular filtration:
   acute and chronic renal failure
increased tubular reabsorption:
   primary mineralocorticoid excess:
      Cushing's syndrome
      Conn's syndrome
   secondary mineralocorticoid excess:
      congestive cardiac failure
      nephrotic syndrome
      hepatic cirrhosis with ascites
      renal artery stenosis	

Fig. 2.12 Causes and clinical features of predominant sodium excess.

The plasma sodium concentration is one of the most frequent measurements made in clinical chemistry laboratories (largely for historical reasons) but definite indications for its measurement are few and results are often misinterpreted. Plasma sodium concentration should be measured in the following:

- patients with dehydration or excessive fluid loss, as a guide to appropriate replacement
- patients on parenteral fluid replacement who are unable to indicate or respond to thirst (e.g. the comatose, infants and the elderly)
- patients with unexplained confusion, abnormal behaviour or signs of CNS irritability.

In the assessment of a patient's water and sodium status, clinical observations, such as measurements of central venous pressure, fluid balance and body weight, may all provide vital information. An increase in the concentration of plasma proteins or in the haematocrit suggests haemoconcentration. Other abnormal results may suggest specific conditions; for example, hyperkalaemia in a hyponatraemic patient with clinical evidence of sodium depletion suggests adrenal failure.

Analysis of urine can provide valuable information but results may be misleading. It should be established whether the urine volume and composition are physiologically appropriate for the patient's water and sodium status. If they are not, the reason should be sought. For example, a low urinary sodium excretion is an appropriate response in a patient with hyponatraemia who is sodium depleted. Natriuresis in such a patient would imply either a failure of aldosterone secretion or a failure of the kidney to respond to the hormone (*see Case History 2.1*).

Sodium measurement

Sodium concentration has traditionally been measured by flame photometry, which determines the number of sodium atoms in a defined volume of solution. Sodium is now usually measured by ion-selective electrodes, which determine the activity of sodium, that is the number of atoms that act as true ions in a defined volume of water.

Under most circumstances, the two techniques give results that are, for practical clinical purposes, the same. However, as activity is a measure of sodium in the water fraction of plasma (normally 93% by volume), significant discrepancies between activity and concentration may arise if the fractional plasma water content is decreased, such as in severe hyperlipidaemia and hyperproteinaemia. The sodium concentration, measured by flame photometry in millimoles per litre of plasma, will be less than the concentration inferred from the activity. This is because, although the concentration of sodium in plasma water is unchanged, there is less water and thus less sodium in a given volume of plasma. Analyzers employing electrodes for which the plasma is diluted before measurement also give a spuriously low result. This effect, known as pseudohyponatraemia, is only seen with severe hyperlipidaemia when the plasma will usually appear turbid to the naked eye (*see Case History 14.2*) and with large increases in total protein due to paraproteinaemia. If it is suspected, plasma osmolality should be measured: it is osmolality that is regulated by the hypothalamus through the release of vasopressin. Plasma osmolality should be normal in a patient with pseudohyponatraemia.

Osmolality measurement

Given that it is osmolality, rather than sodium concentration, that is controlled by the hypothalamus, it might appear logical to measure plasma osmolality rather than sodium concentration. The measurement of osmolality is, however, less precise than that of sodium and is not easily automated. It is nevertheless useful under certain circumstances.

Measurement of osmolality may help in the interpretation of a low plasma sodium concentration and is necessary in water deprivation tests. It can also be useful in the investigation of patients suspected of having ingested substances such as ethanol or ethylene glycol (*see Case History 19.3*) since, if present, these increase the osmolality. This can be revealed by comparing the measured osmolality with the approximate expected value calculated from the formula:

$$\text{osmolarity} = 2 \times [\text{Na}^+] + [\text{urea}] + [\text{glucose}]$$

where all concentrations are measured in mmol/L.

Measured osmolality and calculated osmolarity are normally numerically very similar. Significant discrepancies (an 'osmolar gap') occur when abnormal osmotically active species are present in plasma (as may occur in poisoning) and when the fractional water content of plasma is reduced, as in severe hyperlipidaemia or hyperproteinaemia.

Anion measurement

A change in plasma sodium concentration must be matched by a change in anion concentration. The major anions of the ECF are chloride and bicarbonate. Bicarbonate (strictly, total carbon dioxide) is frequently measured since it reflects the extracellular buffering capacity (note that the measurement must be made on a fresh sample to obtain an accurate result, owing to the loss of carbon dioxide to the atmosphere on standing), but the measurement of plasma chloride rarely adds to the information that can be derived from knowledge of the sodium concentration alone, and few laboratories in the UK measure plasma chloride concentration routinely. However, it may occasionally be helpful in the diagnosis of patients with non-respiratory acidosis and with rare chloride-losing states.

HYPONATRAEMIA

A slightly low plasma sodium concentration is a frequent finding. The mean plasma sodium concentration of hospital inpatients is 5 mmol/L lower than in healthy controls. Mild hyponatraemia is seen with a wide variety of illnesses and may be multifactorial in origin (*see the 'sick cell syndrome', p. 28*). It is essentially a secondary phenomenon that merely reflects the presence of disease; treatment should be directed at the underlying cause and not at the hyponatraemia. Severe hyponatraemia does sometimes warrant primary treatment, but usually only when it is associated with clinical features of water intoxication (*see Fig. 2.11*).

Causes

It has been emphasized that plasma sodium concentration depends upon the amounts of both sodium and water in the plasma, and so a low sodium concentration does not necessarily imply sodium depletion. Indeed, it is more frequently a defect in water homoeostasis that causes water retention and hence dilution of sodium. One of three mechanisms is usually primarily responsible for the development and maintenance of hyponatraemia, although in individual patients more than one factor may be involved. These are:

- depletion of sodium (hypovolaemic hyponatraemia)
- excess of water (euvolaemic hyponatraemia)

 Case history 2.1

A 50-year-old woman with a long history of rheumatoid disease complained of fainting episodes following an attack of gastroenteritis and, on examination, was found to have postural hypotension.

Investigations

serum:	sodium	118 mmol/L
	potassium	3.9 mmol/L
	urea	9.1 mmol/L

short Synacthen test: normal cortisol response to ACTH

| plasma aldosterone (recumbent) | 720 pmol/L |
| 24 h urinary sodium excretion | 118 mmol |

Comment

Postural hypotension may be due to hypovolaemia, autonomic neuropathy or hypotensive drugs. This patient was not taking such medication and there was no other evidence of neuropathy. The hyponatraemia with a slightly raised urea is consistent with sodium depletion producing hypovolaemia. The Synacthen test is normal, excluding adrenal failure, and indeed the aldosterone is appropriately raised. The patient's urinary sodium excretion is excessive: although the input was not assessed, normal kidneys should retain sodium in a sodium-depleted patient with hypovolaemia.

It was concluded that the patient had a renal salt-losing state such that the kidneys could not respond to the normal physiological stimuli to retain sodium. She only became symptomatic when diarrhoea and vomiting caused further fluid loss. This was later confirmed by sodium balance studies and the patient was found to have renal papillary necrosis, an occasional complication of the use of certain analgesic drugs, which principally affects renal tubular function.

- excess of water and sodium (hypervolaemic hyponatraemia).

Depletion of sodium

Sodium is never lost without water, and isotonic or hypotonic loss would not be expected to cause a fall in plasma sodium concentration. However, hyponatraemia can occur in sodium-depleted patients, and is due either to inappropriate replacement of fluid (e.g. containing insufficient sodium) or, in severe sodium depletion, to the hypotonic stimulus to vasopressin secretion, which overrides the osmotic control and permits water retention at the expense of a decrease in osmolality. A case of adrenal failure with hyponatraemia as a result of sodium depletion is presented in *Case History 8.1*.

 Case history 2.2

Blood was taken for biochemical tests from a man who had undergone major abdominal surgery 36 hours earlier.

Investigations

serum: sodium   127 mmol/L
      urea   4.0 mmol/L

Serum potassium and bicarbonate were normal. The patient was alert and appeared neither under- nor over-hydrated.

Comment

Hyponatraemia is a very common finding in postoperative patients on intravenous fluid infusions. It is usually a reflection of excessive administration of hypotonic fluids (5% dextrose or 'dextrose–saline') at a time when the ability of the body to excrete water is depressed as part of the normal metabolic response to trauma. It may also be due, in part, to the sick cell syndrome. If, as is usually the case, there are no clinical features of water intoxication, the only action necessary is adjustment of the fluid input. This patient had been given a total of 3.5 L of dextrose–saline since his operation and examination of the fluid balance chart showed that he had a positive balance of 2 L.

It should be noted that, in patients with hyponatraemia due to sodium depletion, clinical signs of sodium depletion (*see Fig. 2.8*) may be expected. Unless the sodium loss is occurring through the kidneys, increased aldosterone secretion should cause maximal renal sodium retention and the urinary sodium concentration will be low (usually <20 mmol/L). This finding is a valuable aid to the diagnosis of sodium depletion as a cause of hyponatraemia.

The management of hyponatraemia associated with sodium depletion involves correction of the underlying cause, and appropriate fluid replacement (e.g. physiological saline or plasma expanders).

Plasma sodium concentration is usually normal in patients treated with diuretics, but these drugs have complex effects on sodium and water homoeostasis. Although primarily tending to cause sodium depletion, the blocking of sodium reabsorption in the cortical diluting segment of the nephron may impair free water excretion. This, perhaps exacerbated by the effect of vasopressin secretion secondary to hypovolaemia and an increase in water intake due to thirst, can result in (usually mild) hyponatraemia. Except in hospitals, treatment with diuretics is the most frequent cause of hypovolaemic hyponatraemia.

Cerebral salt-wasting is a relatively recently recognized cause of sodium loss and hyponatraemia. Because it typically occurs in patients following brain injury or cranial surgery, the hyponatraemia may be misdiagnosed as being caused by the syndrome of inappropriate antidiuretic hormone secretion (SIADH, *see p. 27*). However, unlike in SIADH, in cerebral salt-wasting, clinical and biochemical features of hypovolaemia are typically present and there is often marked diuresis. The distinction is vital, as the management of the two conditions is quite different: patients with cerebral salt-wasting require intravenous isotonic saline, often in large volumes. SIADH is treated by water restriction or, in severe cases, hypertonic saline (*see p. 27*). The cause of the salt loss is postulated to be the release of natriuretic peptides from the brain.

Water excess

This gives rise to a dilutional hyponatraemia with reduced plasma osmolality. It can occur acutely purely due to excessive water intake, but this is rare. Normal kidneys are capable of excreting 1 L of water per hour; water intoxication and hyponatraemia will thus be seen only when very large quantities of fluid are ingested

Case history 2.3

An elderly man was admitted to hospital in an acute confusional state. No history was available but the nicotine stains on his fingers indicated that he was a heavy smoker. Physical examination revealed he had digital clubbing and signs of a right-sided pleural effusion, but no other obvious abnormality was detected. He was neither dehydrated nor oedematous.

Investigations

serum:	sodium	114 mmol/L
	potassium	3.6 mmol/L
	bicarbonate	22 mmol/L
	urea	2.5 mmol/L
	glucose	4.0 mmol/L
	total protein	48 g/L
	osmolality	236 mmol/kg
urine:	osmolality	350 mmol/kg
	sodium	50 mmol/L

A chest radiograph confirmed the presence of the effusion and showed a mass in the right lower zone with an appearance typical of a carcinoma.

Comment

There is severe hyponatraemia. The patient is not clinically dehydrated and the low serum protein and urea concentrations suggest that the hyponatraemia is dilutional. The serum osmolality is equal to the calculated osmolarity, militating against the presence of additional solute in the plasma. The normal response should be for vasopressin secretion to be inhibited, resulting in the production of a dilute urine. However, in this case, the urine is inappropriately concentrated in relation to the serum, indicating continuing vasopressin secretion. The chest radiograph indicates the likely source: ectopic secretion of vasopressin by a bronchial carcinoma, an example of the syndrome of inappropriate antidiuretic hormone secretion (SIADH). The diagnostic features of SIADH are:

- hyponatraemia
- decreased plasma osmolality
- inappropriately concentrated urine
- continued natriuresis (>20 mmol/L)
- no clinical evidence of fluid depletion or overload
- normal renal function
- normal adrenal function
- clinical and biochemical response to fluid restriction.

In SIADH, there is continued natriuresis despite the low plasma sodium concentration because plasma volume is maintained by water retention and there is therefore no hypovolaemic stimulus to aldosterone secretion. Hyponatraemia with natriuresis can also occur in adrenal failure and in renal disorders and these must be excluded before a diagnosis of SIADH can be made.

Water intoxication should always be considered as a possible cause of a confusional state, especially in the elderly, and this is one of the few situations in which urgent measurement of plasma sodium concentration is genuinely indicated.

rapidly, as in some psychotics and heavy beer drinkers. More frequently, the acute development of water excess and hyponatraemia is due to a combination of excessive hypotonic fluid intake and impairment of diuresis.

Since osmolality is normally precisely controlled, the persistence of dilutional hyponatraemia implies either a failure of diuresis, which must be due to either continued (and inappropriate) production of vasopressin or an impairment of the renal diluting mechanism.

A diagnosis of SIADH is frequently made on insufficient evidence without regard to other possible causes of hyponatraemia. The diagnosis is usually made on the basis of clinical and other laboratory data. It is essential to measure urine and plasma osmolalities: the urine may not be more concentrated than the plasma but must be less than maximally dilute (osmolality >50 mmol/kg). Oedema is not a feature of SIADH: the excess of water is shared by the ICF and the ECF and the effect on ECF volume is insufficient to cause oedema. Measurement of vasopressin concentration is seldom helpful in differential diagnosis: raised values are present in the majority of patients with hyponatraemia, irrespective of the cause.

There is undoubtedly more than one type of SIADH. Tumours may produce the hormone (ectopic production), but patients with many other conditions (*Fig. 2.13*) can also fulfil the criteria for SIADH. In some of these, there may be an inappropriate stimulus to vasopressin release, such as stimulation of volume receptors during artificial ventilation, and in others the 'osmostat' appears to be reset, so that osmolality is still controlled but at a lower level. Decreased intracellular organic solute ('osmolyte') content may be one mechanism whereby the osmostat can be reset.

Patients have been described in whom suppression of vasopressin release when osmolality falls is incomplete (a 'vasopressin leak'), while in others the production of vasopressin is entirely normal and antidiuresis must be presumed to reflect an abnormal response to the hormone. Finally, certain drugs either stimulate vasopressin release (*see Fig. 2.5*) or have a vasopressin-like action on the kidneys. Clearly, inappropriate secretion of the hormone is not always present in patients satisfying the criteria for the diagnosis of SIADH, and because of this the term 'syndrome of inappropriate antidiuresis' may be preferable.

The logical treatment of dilutional hyponatraemia is to restrict the patient's water intake to less than that required to maintain normal water balance, for example

Conditions associated with SIADH

Ectopic secretion
bronchial carcinomas
other tumours, e.g. thymus and prostate

Inappropriate secretion
pulmonary diseases:
   pneumonia
   tuberculosis
   positive pressure mechanical ventilation

cerebral diseases:
   head injury
   encephalitis
   tumours
   aneurysms

miscellaneous:
   pain, e.g. postoperative
   intermittent acute porphyria
   Guillain–Barré syndrome
   hypothyroidism
   drugs, e.g. narcotics,
      chlorpropamide, carbamazepine,
      oxytocin and vinca alkaloids

Fig. 2.13 Conditions associated with the syndrome of inappropriate antidiuretic hormone secretion (SIADH).

to 400 mL/24 h. In mild ([Na$^+$] 125–130 mmol/L) chronic dilutional hyponatraemia, patients are usually asymptomatic, and such reduction of water intake is usually sufficient treatment; if patients have clinical features of water intoxication (*see Fig. 2.11*), as is more likely if the hyponatraemia is severe, or the sodium concentration has fallen rapidly, urgent correction may be necessary. Water restriction is unpleasant and may be impractical in chronic cases. Demeclocycline, a drug that antagonizes the action of vasopressin on the renal collecting ducts, has been widely used for this purpose, but it can cause photosensitivity and is potentially nephrotoxic. Peptide vasopressin antagonists are being investigated.

If patients are symptomatic, urgent correction of the hyponatraemia is required. Hypertonic saline (3%) is infused at a rate sufficient to increase the plasma sodium concentration initially by 1 mmol/L/h but not by more than 12 mmol/L over 24 h. Paradoxically, giving a loop diuretic at the same time can be beneficial:

this reduces the slight increase in ECF volume that is present and stimulates distal renal tubular sodium retention. Regular clinical assessment and measurement of plasma sodium concentration are essential. The infusion should be stopped if patients become asymptomatic, irrespective of sodium concentration. In chronic dilutional hyponatraemia, correcting the sodium concentration too rapidly risks causing central pontine myelinolysis, a brain syndrome characterized by spastic quadriplegia, pseudobulbar palsy and cognitive changes. This condition has a poor prognosis.

Combined water and sodium excess

This is a frequent cause of hyponatraemia. It underlies the hyponatraemia of congestive cardiac failure, hypoproteinaemic states and some patients with renal failure. The mechanism is discussed on *p. 22*.

The fact that there is sodium excess is indicated by signs of increased ECF volume (e.g. peripheral oedema). The logical treatment in these patients involves measures to treat the underlying cause and remove the excess sodium and water (e.g. with diuretics). Despite the hyponatraemia, saline should not be given as they are already sodium overloaded.

Other causes of hyponatraemia

Decreased fractional water content of plasma can occur with severe hyperproteinaemia and hyperlipidaemia, *see p. 23*.

Addition of a solute to the plasma that is confined to the ECF will tend to increase ECF osmolality. Acutely, this will cause a shift of water from the ICF to the ECF, lowering the ECF sodium concentration, and stimulation of vasopressin secretion, leading to water retention. The resulting increase in ECF volume inhibits aldosterone secretion, leading to natriuresis.

Movement of water from the ICF to the ECF does not occur in uraemia. In renal failure, the rate of increase in plasma urea concentration is slow, allowing time for urea to equilibrate between the ECF and the ICF, and thus preventing an osmotic imbalance.

A decrease in the total negative charge on plasma proteins, which contributes to the anion gap, can displace sodium from the plasma. This is unusual, but it may contribute to hyponatraemia in severe hypoalbuminaemia and in paraproteinaemias if the paraprotein is positively charged.

 Case history 2.4

An insulin-dependent diabetic patient woke up feeling hypoglycaemic and drank two glasses of a sugar-rich drink, which abolished the symptoms. She had a hospital appointment that morning and, worried that she might become hypoglycaemic while driving, decided to omit her usual injection of insulin. She felt quite well on arrival at the hospital. Blood was taken for biochemical tests.

Investigations

blood:	glucose	28 mmol/L
serum:	sodium	126 mmol/L
	osmolality	290 mmol/kg

serum urea, potassium and bicarbonate concentrations were normal.

Comment

The hyponatraemia is dilutional. It is the result of a movement of water from the ICF to the ECF to maintain isotonicity as the plasma glucose concentration rose. In that short time, there was no significant osmotic diuresis and thus no dehydration.

Hyponatraemia can occur for the same reason when glucose is administered intravenously at a rate greater than it can be metabolized, as may happen during parenteral nutrition. It can also occur following mannitol infusion. Mannitol may be given to patients with cerebral oedema, to reduce intracellular water content, and is also used as an osmotic diuretic.

The 'sick cell syndrome'

Hyponatraemia is frequently observed in patients with either acute or chronic illness, without any obvious cause. The term 'sick cell syndrome' has been used to describe this phenomenon, which used to be attributed to an increase in the permeability of cell membranes to sodium with or without a decrease in the activity of the sodium pump. However, any transmembrane shift of sodium would be expected to be accompanied by an iso-osmotic movement of water, which should not affect plasma sodium concentration, although it is possible that sodium could become bound to intracellular macromolecules, thus nullifying its effect on osmolality.

Many sick patients may have a degree of stress-related increased vasopressin secretion or another cause of SIADH. Resetting of the osmostat, for example due to depletion of intracellular organic solutes, may also be contributory.

In practice, however, the mechanism of the hyponatraemia of the 'sick cell syndrome' is relatively unimportant. The hyponatraemia reflects the presence of the underlying disease, and it is this that should be treated, not the hyponatraemia.

Investigation of hyponatraemia

It should be apparent from the previous section that, in many instances, the cause of hyponatraemia can often be recognized clinically and that additional investigation may add nothing to the management of the patient. Even in apparently obscure cases, careful clinical evaluation and study of fluid balance charts (if reliable) will often indicate the underlying mechanism or mechanisms, and thus point the way to a diagnosis.

As has been indicated, hyponatraemia due to sodium depletion may be accompanied by physical signs of a decrease in ECF volume whereas this is normal in patients with water excess, and in combined water and sodium excess, the signs will be of ECF expansion.

An algorithm for the diagnosis of hyponatraemia is given in *Fig. 2.14*. Some of the commoner causes of hyponatraemia are indicated in *Fig. 2.15* and some investigations that may help in elucidating its cause in *Fig. 2.16*. It must be emphasized that an appreciation of the underlying principles is vital for correct interpretation of their results.

Management of hyponatraemia

Hyponatraemia is essentially a sign of a disorder involving water or sodium homoeostasis or both. As has been discussed, measures to treat the causative condition may need be supplemented by direct measures to correct the imbalance of sodium and water. These will vary according to the mechanism of the hyponatraemia and it is therefore essential to both diagnose the cause and understand the pathogenesis. If symptoms of water

intoxication are present, urgent (though cautious) correction will be required.

HYPERNATRAEMIA

Hypernatraemia is much less common than hyponatraemia, but is much more frequently of clinical significance. The causes include pure water depletion, combined sodium and water depletion, with water loss

 Case history 2.5

A male infant aged 15 weeks was admitted to hospital for the investigation of recurrent diarrhoea. He had been well until 8 weeks of age, when the first episode had occurred. Since then, there had been several further attacks, he had lost weight and on admission was dehydrated.

Investigations

serum:	sodium	167 mmol/L
	potassium	4.9 mmol/L
	urea	2.6 mmol/L
urine:	sodium	310 mmol/L

Comment

Hypernatraemia is a feature of hypotonic fluid loss such as can occur with diarrhoea, but with chronic diarrhoea hyponatraemia is more usual, due to the loss of sodium. In dehydration, however, the kidneys should conserve sodium. The combination of high urine sodium excretion together with hypernatraemia in this case suggests salt overload. Stool chromatography revealed the presence of an abnormal sugar, which was identified as lactulose. Lactulose is a non-absorbed osmotic laxative. Careful observation confirmed the suspicion that the child's mother was adding salt and lactulose to his feeds. She was not allowed to stay with him unattended and the diarrhoea and electrolyte abnormalities resolved rapidly. This was a case of Munchausen's syndrome by proxy.

Case history 2.6

Following surgery for major abdominal injuries sustained in a knife fight, a young man was fed parenterally and artificially ventilated. On the fifth day after his operation, serum biochemical results, which had been normal the day before, were as follows:

Investigations

serum: sodium   150 mmol/L
       potassium   4.2 mmol/L
       urea   10.2 mmol/L
       glucose   25 mmol/L

During the previous 24 h he had become pyrexial and positive blood cultures were subsequently obtained. His fluid intake had been 3000 mL, urine output had been steady at 90–100 mL/h and 300 mL of fluid had been aspirated via a nasogastric tube. The sodium intake had been 70 mmol.

Comment

Sodium input is not excessive; water depletion is the more likely cause of the hypernatraemia. His measured *net* fluid intake is only 400 mL. This is insufficient to balance insensible losses, which will have been increased by the pyrexia and possibly by ventilation. The urine output has not decreased and there has therefore also been an excessive renal water loss. This was due to an osmotic diuresis as a result of glycosuria and a high urea output.

Glucose intolerance may be a problem in patients receiving parenteral nutrition and can be exacerbated by sepsis, which causes insulin resistance. Parenteral administration of excessive nitrogen will result in increased formation of urea, which will also contribute to an osmotic diuresis: this patient was receiving amino acids equivalent to over 100 g of protein per day, more than his probable requirements. Inadequate humidification of inspired air may also be a causative factor in water depletion in such circumstances.

predominating, or sodium excess; of these, excess sodium is the least common.

In most cases of hypernatraemia, the cause is obvious from the history and clinical observations. Diabetes insipidus is an important cause and the investigation of patients suspected of having this condition is considered in *Chapter 7*.

Regardless of its cause, hypernatraemia should be treated by administration of hypotonic fluids such as water (orally) or 5% dextrose (parenterally). In patients with sodium overload, measures to remove excess sodium may have to be considered. As already emphasized, it is important not to correct too rapidly hypernatraemia due to water depletion.

POTASSIUM HOMOEOSTASIS

Extracellular potassium balance is controlled primarily by the kidneys and, to a lesser extent, by the gastro-intestinal tract. In the kidneys, filtered potassium is almost completely reabsorbed in the proximal tubules. Some active potassium secretion takes place in the most distal part of the distal convoluted tubules but potassium excretion is primarily a passive process. The active reabsorption of sodium generates a membrane potential that is neutralized by the movement of potassium and hydrogen ions from tubular cells into the lumen. Thus, urinary potassium excretion depends upon several factors:

- the amount of sodium available for reabsorption in the distal convoluted tubules and the collecting ducts
- the relative availability of hydrogen and potassium ions in the cells of the distal convoluted tubules and the collecting ducts
- the ability of these cells to secrete hydrogen ions
- the circulating concentration of aldosterone
- the rate of flow of tubular fluid: a high flow rate (e.g. osmotic diuresis, treatment with diuretics) favours the transfer of potassium into the tubular lumen.

Aldosterone stimulates potassium excretion both indirectly, by increasing the active reabsorption of sodium in the distal convoluted tubules and the collecting ducts, and directly, by increasing active potassium secretion in the distal part of the distal convoluted tubules. Aldosterone secretion from the adrenal cortex is stimulated indirectly by activation of the renin–angiotensin system in response to hypovolaemia (*see p. 144*), and directly by hyperkalaemia.

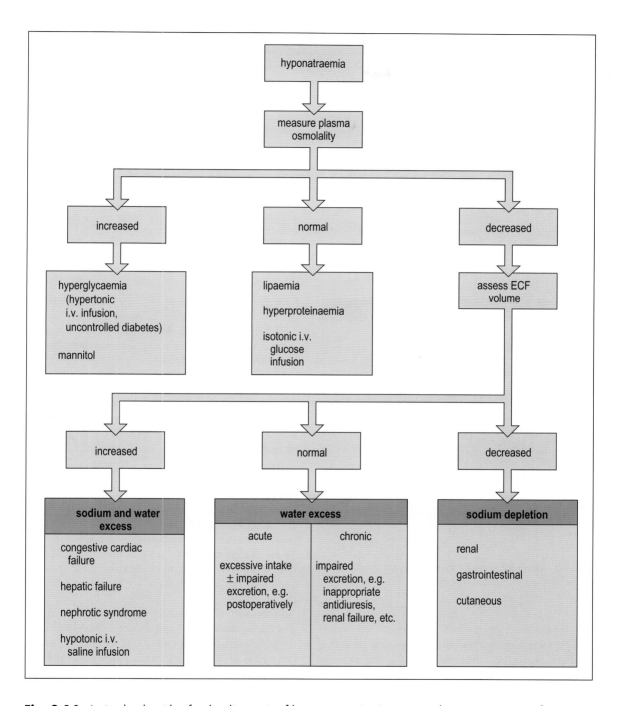

Fig. 2.14 A simple algorithm for the diagnosis of hyponatraemia. In practice, hyponatraemia is often multifactorial, but one cause may predominate and determine the clinical features.

Some common causes of hyponatraemia		
Cause	**Mechanism**	**ECF volume**
inappropriate i.v. fluids	water excess	normal or increased
diuretic therapy	sodium depletion and water retention (*see text*)	decreased
non-specific ('sick cell syndrome')	*see text*	normal
congestive cardiac failure and hypoproteinaemic states	sodium and water retention	increased
carcinoma of bronchus	water excess	normal
hyperglycaemia, parenteral feeding	isotonic redistribution	normal

Fig. 2.15 Some common causes of hyponatraemia.

Investigations for hyponatraemia
inspection of serum for lipaemia
serum: osmolality   potassium   urea   creatinine   total protein   TSH and free T4
haematocrit
Synacthen test
urine: sodium   osmolality

Fig. 2.16 Some laboratory investigations of value in the investigation of hyponatraemia.

Since both hydrogen and potassium ions can neutralize the membrane potential generated by active sodium reabsorption, there is a close relationship between potassium and hydrogen ion homoeostasis. In a state of acidosis, hydrogen ions will tend to be secreted in preference to potassium; in alkalosis, fewer hydrogen ions will be available for excretion and there will be an increase in potassium excretion. Thus, there is a tendency to hyperkalaemia in acidosis and to hypokalaemia in alkalosis. An exception to this tendency is renal tubular acidosis caused by defective renal hydrogen ion excretion (*see p. 81*). In this condition, because of the decrease in hydrogen ion excretion, potassium secretion must increase to balance sodium reabsorption. The result is the unusual combination of hypokalaemia with acidosis.

The relationship between the excretion of hydrogen and potassium ions also explains why potassium depletion tends to produce alkalosis. If there is insufficient potassium available for excretion as sodium is reabsorbed, then the excretion of hydrogen ions will be increased.

Healthy kidneys are less efficient at conserving potassium than sodium: even on a potassium-free intake, urinary excretion remains at 10–20 mmol/24 h. Since there is also an obligatory loss from the skin and gut of approximately 15–20 mmol/24 h, the kidneys cannot compensate if intake falls much below 40 mmol/ 24 h. The average diet contains more potassium than this. However, even on a normal diet, potassium depletion can occur if there are increased losses from the body.

Potassium is secreted in gastric juice and much of this, along with dietary potassium, is reabsorbed in the small intestine. In the colon and rectum, potassium is secreted in exchange for sodium, partly under the control of aldosterone. Stools normally contain some potassium, but considerable amounts can be lost in patients with fistulae or chronic diarrhoea, or in patients who are losing gastric secretions through persistent vomiting or nasogastric aspiration.

Movement of potassium between the intracellular and extracellular compartments can have a profound effect on plasma potassium concentration. The cellular uptake of potassium is stimulated by insulin. Potassium ions move passively into cells from the ECF in exchange for sodium, which is actively excluded by a membrane-bound, energy-dependent sodium pump. Hyperkalaemia can result if the activity of this sodium pump is impaired or if there is damage to cell membranes.

Transcellular shifts of hydrogen ions can cause reciprocal shifts in potassium. In a systemic acidosis, intracellular buffering of hydrogen ions results in the displacement of potassium into the ECF. In alkalosis, there is a shift of hydrogen ions from the ICF to the ECF, and a net movement of potassium ions in the opposite direction, which tends to produce hypokalaemia.

POTASSIUM DEPLETION AND HYPOKALAEMIA

Potassium depletion occurs when output exceeds intake. Potassium is available in many foods (normal dietary intake is 60–200 mmol/24 h) and, except in patients who are fasting, inadequate intake is rarely the sole cause of potassium depletion. However, increased loss of potassium is a frequent occurrence. Such loss can be from the gut or through the kidneys. If renal potassium excretion is <40 mmol/L in a patient with hypokalaemia, excessive renal excretion is unlikely to be the cause. Drug therapy is often implicated in the pathogenesis of potassium depletion.

The causes of hypokalaemia are shown in *Fig. 2.17*. When hypokalaemia is a result of potassium depletion, it usually develops slowly and is only corrected slowly when the cause is effectively treated. In contrast, hypokalaemia as a result of redistribution of potassium from the extra- to the intracellular compartment usually develops acutely, and can normalize rapidly.

Clinical features

Even severe hypokalaemia may be asymptomatic. Hypokalaemia causes hyperpolarization of excitable membranes, thus decreasing their excitability; when symptoms are present, they are related primarily to disturbances of neuromuscular function (*Fig. 2.18*): muscular weakness, constipation and paralytic ileus are common problems.

Management

Although the plasma potassium concentration is a poor guide to total body potassium, a plasma concentration

Cause of hypokalaemia
Decreased K⁺ intake

Cause of hypokalaemia

Decreased K$^+$ intake
oral (rare)
parenteral

Transcellular K$^+$ movement
alkalosis
insulin administration
β-adrenergic agonists
rapid cellular proliferation

Increased K$^+$ excretion
renal:
   diuretics
   diuretic phase of acute renal failure
   mineralocorticoid excess:
     primary aldosteronism
     secondary aldosteronism
     Cushing's syndrome
     carbenoxolone, liquorice (*see p. 153*)
     renal tubular acidosis (types 1 and 2)
extrarenal:
   diarrhoea
   purgative abuse
   villous adenoma of the rectum
   vomiting, gastric aspiration
   enterocutaneous fistulae
   excessive sweating

Fig. 2.17 Causes of hypokalaemia.

of 3.0 mmol/L generally implies a deficit of the order of 300 mmol. However, since this deficit is almost entirely from the ICF and since administered potassium first enters the ECF, replacement must be undertaken with care, particularly when the intravenous route is used.

As a guide, the following potassium dosages should not be exceeded without good reason: a rate of 20 mmol/h, a concentration of 40 mmol/L in intravenous fluid or a total of 140 mmol/24 h. Thorough mixing with the bulk of the fluid to be infused is vital. Plasma concentrations should be monitored during treatment. If unusually large amounts of potassium are necessary and particularly if there is impaired renal function, electrocardiographic (ECG) monitoring is useful since characteristic changes in the waveform occur with changing plasma potassium concentrations (*Fig. 2.19*).

Case history 2.7

A 67-year-old woman presented with severe muscular weakness. She had been in the habit of taking large amounts of purgatives and recently had been prescribed a thiazide diuretic for mild heart failure.

Investigations

serum: potassium   2.4 mmol/L
       bicarbonate   36 mmol/L

Comment

The patient is severely hypokalaemic and the high serum bicarbonate concentration reflects the associated extracellular alkalosis.

Purgative abuse can cause considerable potassium loss from the gut. Thiazides act by decreasing chloride reabsorption, and thus sodium reabsorption, in the distal part of the ascending limbs of the loops of Henle and in the first part of the distal convoluted tubules. As a result, there is an increase in the amount of sodium delivered to and available for reabsorption from the distal tubules: this will tend to increase potassium excretion from the kidneys. Loop diuretics similarly increase renal potassium excretion, although to a lesser extent. With either type of diuretic, however, plasma potassium concentrations tend to stabilize unless, as in this case, other causes of hypokalaemia are present.

Potassium supplements are often prescribed at the same time as diuretics; combined preparations are available but are generally expensive and typically provide less than 10 mmol of potassium per tablet. Hypokalaemia potentiates digoxin toxicity. This is an important practical consideration since diuretics and digoxin are often prescribed together. However, in general, the routine use of potassium supplements should not be encouraged. They are probably unnecessary unless the plasma concentration is below 3.0 mmol/L and they are potentially dangerous in patients with renal impairment since hyperkalaemia may result.

 Case history 2.8

A 60-year-old man underwent total gastrectomy for a carcinoma. He was malnourished prior to surgery and it was decided to provide parenteral nutrition postoperatively. On the fifth day, his serum potassium concentration was 3.0 mmol/L despite the provision of 60 mmol potassium per 24 h in the intravenous feed.

Comment

The patient is hypokalaemic in spite of the provision of sufficient potassium to cover normal obligatory losses.

Potassium excretion increases during the metabolic response to trauma but, once a patient becomes anabolic, the body's requirements increase as potassium is taken up into cells. Furthermore, during total parenteral nutrition, glucose is often the predominant energy source and thus provides a considerable stimulus to insulin release. Potassium requirements may, therefore, be much greater than normal because insulin stimulates its uptake into cells.

This patient had recently undergone abdominal surgery and an ileus is usual in these circumstances. This will result in decreased reabsorption of any potassium secreted into the gut and can also contribute to the loss of potassium from the ECF.

Clinical features of hypokalaemia	
Disorder	**Feature**
neuromuscular	weakness constipation, ileus hypotonia depression confusion

cardiac	arrhythmias
	potentiation of digoxin toxicity
	ECG changes (ST depression,
	   T depression/inversion,
	   prolonged P-R interval,
	   prominent U wave)

renal	impaired concentrating ability
	   leading to polyuria and
	   polydipsia

metabolic	alkalosis

Fig. 2.18 Clinical features of hypokalaemia. Excitable membranes become hyperpolarized in hypokalaemia, decreasing their excitability. The effect on the kidneys is due to increased synthesis of prostaglandins, which antagonize the action of ADH.

POTASSIUM EXCESS AND HYPERKALAEMIA

Potassium excess can be due to excessive intake or decreased excretion. A normal intake may be excessive if excretion is decreased (e.g. in renal failure). Excessive intake is otherwise virtually always iatrogenic and parenteral.

Hyperkalaemia (*Fig. 2.20*) may result from potassium excess but can also be a result of redistribution of potassium from the intra- to the extracellular compartment. This mechanism can sometimes give rise to hyperkalaemia even in a patient who is potassium depleted (e.g. in diabetic ketoacidosis). As with hypokalaemia, more than one cause of hyperkalaemia is often present. Spurious hyperkalaemia, due to the leakage of potassium from blood cells *in vitro*, often occurs. If hyperkalaemia is found unexpectedly, the possibility that it is spurious should be explored by repeating the measurement on a fresh sample. Spurious hyperkalaemia may be present in the absence of frank haemolysis. Loss of potassium from cells into plasma

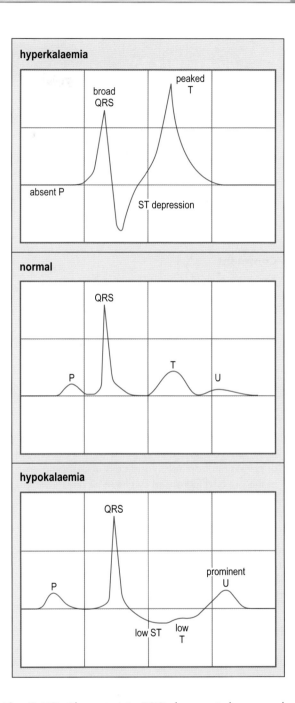

Fig. 2.19 Characteristic ECG changes in hyper- and hypokalaemia. Each sinus discharge produces atrial depolarization (P wave) followed by ventricular depolarization (QRS complex) and ventricular repolarization (T wave). A shallow U wave, of unknown cause, is present in many normal ECGs.

Case history 2.9

A young man was admitted to hospital after sustaining a fractured femur and ruptured spleen in a motorcycle accident. He underwent splenectomy and was put in traction. Twenty-four hours after admission, he had passed only 300 mL of urine.

Investigations

serum: urea   21.5 mmol/L
         potassium   6.5 mmol/L

Comment

Since the patient is oliguric with a high serum urea, he is by definition in renal failure; this might be reversible, i.e. prerenal (*see p. 70*). The hyperkalaemia is due to a combination of decreased renal perfusion (hypovolaemic shock), and the loss of potassium either from cells damaged directly by trauma or from cells whose membrane integrity is impaired by hypoxia.

Similar results may be seen in patients who have sustained a gastrointestinal haemorrhage. This may itself cause hypovolaemic shock, affecting renal function. In addition, there will be absorption of potassium from red blood cells undergoing lysis in the gut and increased synthesis of urea from the amino acids released.

Case history 2.10

Blood from an outpatient being treated with diuretics was received in the laboratory for biochemical analysis. The serum potassium concentration was 6.7 mmol/L. There was no visible haemolysis and the blood was freshly drawn.

Comment

The patient was recalled and asked to bring all her tablets with her. It transpired that she had initially been prescribed a loop diuretic and potassium supplements for congestive cardiac failure. However, at an outpatient attendance she had been prescribed spironolactone, an antagonist of aldosterone used as a potassium-sparing diuretic, instead of the potassium supplements. She had misunderstood the instructions given to her and continued to take both the supplements and the diuretic.

She surrendered the potassium supplements and her serum potassium concentration was normal when checked one week later.

---

can occur rapidly in patients with high white blood cell or platelet counts (e.g. in patients with leukaemia).

Clinical features

Hyperkalaemia is less common than hypokalaemia but is more dangerous: through its effect on the heart, it can kill without warning. It lowers the resting membrane potential, shortens the cardiac action potential and increases the speed of repolarization. Cardiac arrest in asystole or slow ventricular fibrillation may be the first sign of hyperkalaemia. It is therefore necessary to be alert for this disorder in appropriate circumstances, for instance in acute renal failure, to ensure that effective early management is instituted. Characteristic ECG changes may precede cardiac arrest (*Fig. 2.19*). Peaking of T waves occurs first, followed by loss of P waves and, finally, the development of abnormal QRS complexes.

Management

Intravenous calcium gluconate (10 mL of a 10% solution given over 1 minute and repeated as necessary) affords some degree of immediate protection to the myocardium by antagonizing the effect of hyperkalaemia on myocardial excitability. Intravenous glucose and insulin, for example 500 mL of 20% dextrose with 20 units of soluble insulin given over 30 minutes, promotes intracellular potassium uptake. Salbutamol, which activates Na^+,K^+-ATPase, has a similar effect. In an acidotic patient, hyperkalaemia can be controlled temporarily by bicarbonate infusion.

In acute renal failure and in other circumstances where the hyperkalaemia is uncontrollable, dialysis or haemofiltration will be required. In chronic renal failure, restriction of potassium intake and the administration of oral ion-exchange resins are often successful in preventing dangerous hyperkalaemia until such time as dialysis becomes necessary for other reasons.

ECG monitoring can be valuable in patients with hyperkalaemia. Changes in the plasma potassium concentration are reflected by changes in the ECG waveform more rapidly than could be determined by biochemical measurement.

Cause of hyperkalaemia

Spurious
haemolysis
delayed separation of serum
contamination

Excessive K⁺ intake
oral (rare except with K^+-sparing diuretics taken
  simultaneously)
parenteral infusion
transfusion of stored blood

Transcellular K⁺ movement
tissue damage

catabolic states
systemic acidosis
insulin lack

Decreased K⁺ excretion
acute renal failure
chronic renal failure (late)
K^+-sparing diuretics
angiotensin-converting enzyme (ACE) inhibitors

mineralocorticoid deficiency:
  Addison's disease
  adrenalectomy

Fig. 2.20 Causes of hyperkalaemia.

ℹ Perioperative intravenous fluid therapy

The provision of appropriate fluids to patients before, during and following surgery is, in the authors' opinion, best learned at the bedside, but must be informed by a thorough understanding of the underlying physiological and pathological principles. Accurate measurement of fluid losses is important. Biochemical measurements can provide valuable information but are frequently misinterpreted (e.g. that hyponatraemia necessarily indicates sodium depletion).

Body water, sodium and potassium status should be normal prior to surgery. In emergencies, this may require rapid resuscitation with intravenous fluids, plasma expanders or blood. Considerable quantities of water can be lost from exposed mucosal surfaces during surgery, in addition to any loss of blood and other continuing insensible losses.

Postoperatively, the metabolic response to trauma causes relative water retention due to increased secretion of vasopressin. Stress also decreases sodium excretion and there is loss of potassium from damaged cells into the ECF. In the first 24 h following surgery a total of 1500 mL of intravenous fluid ('dextrose–saline', i.e. 4% dextrose, 0.18% sodium chloride) is often sufficient if overload is to be avoided, and potassium is not usually required. As the metabolic response to trauma resolves, fluid input can be increased to maintain an adequate urine output. A typical intravenous postoperative fluid regimen after the first 24 h would be 2.5 L of water, 70 mmol sodium and 60 mmol potassium, but account must also be taken of urine output, any additional losses (e.g. from fistulae) and, if the patient is unable to take fluid orally after a couple of days, the results of measurements of plasma concentrations of sodium, potassium, urea and creatinine.

The composition of some more frequently used intravenous fluids is shown in *Fig. 2.21*.

The composition of some intravenous fluids		
Fluid	**Composition**	**Use**
0.9% sodium chloride (physiological saline)*	sodium 150 mmol/L chloride 150 mmol/L	isotonic fluid replacement
dextrose–saline	sodium 30 mmol/L chloride 30 mmol/L dextrose 222 mmol/L	hypotonic fluid replacement**
5% dextrose	dextrose 278 mmol/L	water replacement**
1.26% sodium bicarbonate	sodium 150 mmol/L bicarbonate 150 mmol/L	treatment of acidosis
Ringer's solution	sodium 147 mmol/L potassium 4.0 mmol/L calcium 2.2 mmol/L chloride 156 mmol/L	isotonic fluid replacement, especially during surgery
Hartman's solution ('Ringer–lactate', compound sodium lactate)	sodium 131 mmol/L potassium 4.0 mmol/L calcium 2.0 mmol/L chloride 111 mmol/L lactate 29 mmol/L	isotonic fluid replacement, especially during surgery

Fig. 2.21 The composition of some intravenous fluids.
*Sometimes referred to as normal saline. This is incorrect: a normal solution is defined as having a concentration of 1 mol/L.
**These solutions are isotonic with plasma, but metabolism rapidly removes the glucose so they are effectively hypotonic.

SUMMARY

- **Sodium, potassium and water homoeostasis are closely linked.** Sodium is the principal extracellular cation and the amount of sodium in the body is the major determinant of ECF volume. Potassium is the major intracellular cation.

- **Sodium and potassium are transported actively** in the body; **water moves passively** in response to changes in the solute contents of the body's fluid compartments.

- **Sodium excretion** is primarily controlled by **aldosterone**, a hormone secreted in response to a decrease in ECF volume that causes sodium retention and loss of potassium.

- **Water excretion** is controlled by **vasopressin** (antidiuretic hormone). This promotes water retention and is secreted in response to an increase in ECF osmolality and a decrease in ECF volume.

- **Potassium excretion** is regulated in part by aldosterone, but also depends on extracellular hydrogen ion concentration and sodium and water excretion.

- Disturbances of either water or sodium homoeostasis can produce characteristic clinical and biochemical features, but combined disturbances are common and the features may then be less clear-cut.

SUMMARY (cont'd)

- Changes in plasma sodium concentration can be due to changes in the amounts of extracellular sodium or water or both. **Hyponatraemia is common**; it is sometimes an appropriate physiological response to disease. **Hypernatraemia is less common** than hyponatraemia and usually is related to a decrease in body water.

- **Plasma potassium concentration** is a poor guide to the body's overall potassium status. Depletion is not always associated with hypokalaemia, nor is hypokalaemia always due to potassium depletion; similar considerations apply to potassium excess and hyperkalaemia.

- **Hypokalaemia** is most frequently a result of excessive gastrointestinal or renal loss of potassium and may be exacerbated by a poor intake. It can also be a consequence of increased cellular uptake of potassium from the plasma. It can cause skeletal and smooth muscle weakness and impairment of myocardial contractility and renal concentrating ability. It also potentiates digoxin toxicity.

- **Hyperkalaemia** is most frequently due to decreased renal excretion or to loss of potassium from cells; excessive intake should be avoidable, since it is usually iatrogenic. Spurious hyperkalaemia, due to release of potassium from cells *in vitro*, is common. Hyperkalaemia can cause cardiac arrest: this can occur in the absence of any warning clinical symptoms or signs.

3 Hydrogen ion homoeostasis and blood gases

INTRODUCTION

The normal processes of metabolism result in the net formation of 40–80 mmol of hydrogen ions per 24 h, principally from the oxidation of sulphur-containing amino acids. This burden of hydrogen ions is excreted by the kidneys, in the urine. In addition, there is a considerable endogenous turnover of hydrogen ions as a result of normal metabolic processes. Incomplete oxidation of energy substrates generates acid [e.g. lactic acid by glycolysis, ketoacids from triacylglycerols (triglycerides)], while further metabolism of these intermediates consumes it (e.g. gluconeogenesis from lactate, oxidation of ketones). Temporary imbalances between the rates of production and consumption may arise in health (e.g. the accumulation of lactic acid during anaerobic exercise), but in general they are in balance and so make no contribution to net hydrogen ion excretion.

Potentially far more acid is generated as carbon dioxide during energy-yielding oxidative metabolism. In excess of 15,000 mmol per 24 h of carbon dioxide is produced in this way, and is normally excreted by the lungs. Although carbon dioxide itself is not an acid, in the presence of water it can undergo hydration to form a weak acid, carbonic acid (*Equation 3.1*).

(3.1) $$CO_2 + H_2O \rightleftharpoons H_2CO_3$$

Carbon dioxide is removed from the body in expired air. Since hydrogen ions can be generated stoichiometrically from carbon dioxide, the normal daily production of carbon dioxide is potentially equivalent to at least 15 mol of hydrogen ions. In health, pulmonary ventilation is controlled so that carbon dioxide excretion exactly matches the rate of formation.

The homoeostatic mechanisms for hydrogen ions and carbon dioxide are very efficient. Temporary imbalances can be absorbed by buffering and, as a result, the hydrogen ion concentration of the body is maintained within narrow limits [35–45 nmol/L (pH 7.35–7.46) in extracellular fluid (ECF)]. The intracellular hydrogen ion concentration is slightly higher but is also rigorously controlled. In disease, however, imbalances between the rates of acid formation and excretion can occur and persist, resulting in acidosis or alkalosis.

Buffering of hydrogen ions

As hydrogen ions are generated they are buffered, thus limiting the rise in hydrogen ion concentration that would otherwise occur. A buffer system consists of a weak acid, that is, one that is incompletely dissociated, and its conjugate base. If hydrogen ions are added to a buffer, some will combine with the conjugate base and convert it to the undissociated acid. Thus, the addition of hydrogen ions to the bicarbonate–carbonic acid system (*Equation 3.2*) drives the reaction to the right, increasing the amount of carbonic acid and consuming bicarbonate ions.

(3.2) $$H^+ + HCO_3^- \rightleftharpoons H_2CO_3$$

Conversely, if the hydrogen ion concentration falls, carbonic acid dissociates, thereby generating hydrogen ions.

The efficacy of any buffer is limited by its concentration and by the position of the equilibrium. A buffer operates most efficiently at hydrogen ion concentrations that result in approximately equal concentrations of undissociated acid and conjugate base. The bicarbonate buffer system is the most important in the ECF, yet at normal ECF hydrogen ion concentrations the concentration of carbonic acid is about 1.2 mmol/L, while that of bicarbonate is 20 times greater. However, the capacity of the bicarbonate system in the body is greatly enhanced by the fact that carbonic acid can readily be formed from carbon dioxide or disposed of by conversion into carbon dioxide and water (*Equation 3.1*).

For every hydrogen ion buffered by bicarbonate, a bicarbonate ion is consumed (*Equation 3.2*). To maintain the capacity of the buffer system, the bicarbonate must be regenerated. Yet, when bicarbonate is formed from carbonic acid (indirectly from carbon dioxide and water), equimolar amounts of hydrogen ions are formed simultaneously (*Equation 3.2*). Bicarbonate formation can only continue if these hydrogen ions are removed. This process occurs in the cells of the renal tubules, where hydrogen ions are secreted into the urine, while bicarbonate is generated and retained in the body.

Proteins, including intracellular proteins, are also involved in buffering. The proteinaceous matrix of bone is an important buffer in chronic acidosis. Phosphate is a minor buffer in the ECF but is of fundamental importance in the urine. The special role of haemoglobin is considered on *p. 43*.

Bicarbonate reabsorption and hydrogen ion excretion

The glomerular filtrate contains the same concentration of bicarbonate ions as the plasma. If this bicarbonate were not reabsorbed, copious amounts would be excreted in the urine, depleting the body's buffering capacity and causing an acidosis. In health, at normal plasma bicarbonate concentrations, virtually all the filtered bicarbonate is reabsorbed.

The luminal surface of renal tubular cells is impermeable to bicarbonate and, therefore, direct reabsorption cannot occur. Within the renal tubular cells, carbonic acid is formed from carbon dioxide and water (*Fig. 3.1*). This otherwise rather slow reaction (*Equation 3.1*) is catalyzed in the kidney by the enzyme carbonate dehydratase (carbonic anhydrase). The carbonic acid thus formed dissociates into hydrogen and bicarbonate ions. The bicarbonate ions pass across the basolateral borders of the cells into the interstitial fluid. The hydrogen ions are secreted across the luminal membrane in exchange for sodium ions, which accompany

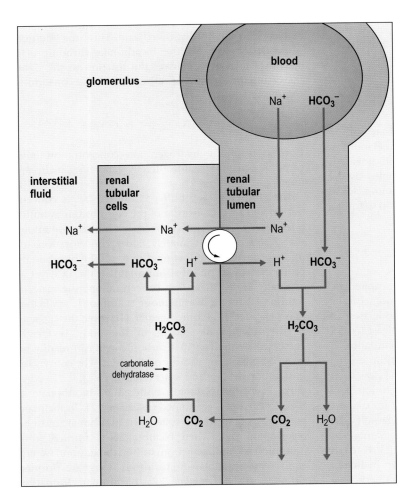

Fig. 3.1 Reabsorption of filtered bicarbonate by renal tubular cells. Bicarbonate cannot be reabsorbed directly. Hydrogen and bicarbonate ions are generated in renal tubular cells and the hydrogen ions are secreted in exchange for sodium into the tubular lumen where they combine with filtered bicarbonate to form carbon dioxide and water. Bicarbonate ions diffuse with sodium from the tubular cells into the interstitial fluid and thence into the plasma.

bicarbonate into the interstitial fluid (*Fig. 3.1*). The formation of bicarbonate and hydrogen ions is promoted by their continuous removal and by the presence of carbonate dehydratase.

In the tubular fluid, hydrogen ions combine with bicarbonate to form carbonic acid, most of which dissociates into carbon dioxide and water. Some of the carbon dioxide diffuses back into the renal tubular cells while the remainder is excreted in the urine. This whole process effectively results in the reabsorption of filtered bicarbonate.

Although hydrogen ions are secreted into the tubular fluid during bicarbonate reabsorption, there is no net acid excretion. The formation of these hydrogen ions merely provides the means for the reabsorption of bicarbonate. Net acid excretion depends upon the same reactions occurring in the renal tubular cells but, in addition, requires the presence of a suitable buffer system in the urine. This is because the minimum urinary pH that can be generated, 4.6, is equivalent to a hydrogen ion concentration of approximately 25 µmol/L. Given a normal urine volume of 1.5 L/24 h, free hydrogen ion excretion can account for less than a thousandth of the total amount that has to be excreted. The principal urinary buffer is phosphate. This is present in the glomerular filtrate, approximately 80% being in the form of the divalent anion, HPO_4^{2-}. This combines with hydrogen ions and is converted to $H_2PO_4^-$ (*Equation 3.3*).

$$(3.3) \qquad HPO_4^{2-} + H^+ \rightleftharpoons H_2PO_4^-$$

At the minimum urinary pH, virtually all the phosphate is in the $H_2PO_4^-$ form. About 30–40 mmol of hydrogen ions are normally excreted in this way every 24 h.

Ammonia, produced by the deamination of glutamine in renal tubular cells, is also an important urinary buffer. The enzyme that catalyzes this reaction, glutaminase, is induced in states of chronic acidosis, allowing increased ammonia production and hence increased hydrogen ion excretion via ammonium ions. Ammonia can readily diffuse across cell membranes, but ammonium ions, formed when ammonia buffers hydrogen ions (*Equation 3.4*), cannot. Passive reabsorption of ammonium ions is therefore prevented.

$$(3.4) \qquad NH_3 + H^+ \rightleftharpoons NH_4^+$$

At normal intracellular hydrogen ion concentrations, most ammonia is present as ammonium ions. Diffusion of ammonia out of the cell disturbs the equilibrium,

causing more ammonia to be formed. The simultaneous production of hydrogen ions would seem to negate the process. However, these ions are used up in gluconeogenesis, when they combine with glutamate formed by the deamination of glutamine. Urinary hydrogen ion excretion is summarized in *Fig. 3.2*.

It will be apparent that hydrogen and bicarbonate ions are generated in equimolar amounts in renal tubular cells. This is essential for the reabsorption of filtered bicarbonate but also means that, when a hydrogen ion is excreted in the urine, a bicarbonate ion is produced and retained. This process effectively regenerates the bicarbonate ions consumed when hydrogen ions are buffered.

Transport of carbon dioxide

Carbon dioxide, produced by aerobic metabolism, diffuses out of cells and into the ECF. A small amount combines with water to form carbonic acid, thereby increasing the hydrogen ion concentration of the ECF.

In red blood cells, metabolism is anaerobic and little carbon dioxide is produced. Carbon dioxide thus diffuses into red cells down a concentration gradient and carbonic acid is formed, facilitated by carbonate dehydratase (*Fig. 3.3*). Haemoglobin buffers the hydrogen ions formed when the carbonic acid dissociates. Haemoglobin is a more powerful buffer when in the deoxygenated state and the proportion in this state increases during the passage of blood through capillary beds, as oxygen is lost to the tissues.

The overall effect of this process is that carbon dioxide is converted to bicarbonate in red blood cells. This bicarbonate diffuses out of the red cells because a concentration gradient develops: electrochemical neutrality is maintained by inward diffusion of chloride ions (the chloride shift). In the lungs, the reverse process occurs: oxygenation of haemoglobin reduces its buffering capacity, liberating hydrogen ions; these combine with bicarbonate to form carbon dioxide, which diffuses into the alveoli to be excreted in the expired air while bicarbonate diffuses into the cells from the plasma.

Most of the carbon dioxide in the blood is present in the form of bicarbonate. Dissolved carbon dioxide, carbonic acid and carbamino compounds (compounds of carbon dioxide and protein) account for less than 2.0 mmol/L in a total carbon dioxide concentration of approximately 26 mmol/L. The terms 'bicarbonate' and 'total carbon dioxide' are frequently used synonymously. They are not strictly the same but may be considered to

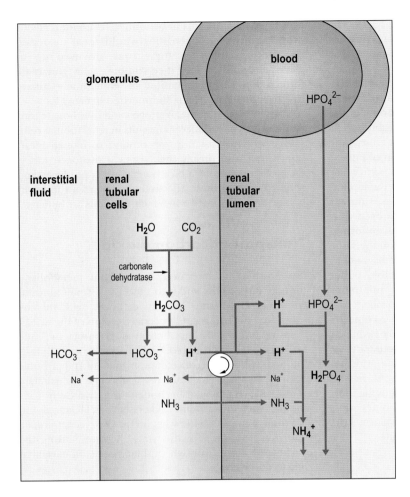

Fig. 3.2 Renal hydrogen ion excretion. Hydrogen and bicarbonate ions are generated in renal tubular cells from carbon dioxide and water by the reversal of the buffering reaction. The hydrogen ions are excreted in the urine buffered by phosphate and ammonia while the bicarbonate enters the ECF, replacing that which was consumed in buffering.

be, for most practical clinical purposes. It is technically difficult to measure bicarbonate concentration alone: most analytical techniques for bicarbonate actually measure total carbon dioxide.

CLINICAL AND LABORATORY ASSESSMENT OF HYDROGEN ION STATUS

As will be seen, many conditions are associated with abnormalities of blood hydrogen ion concentration and partial pressure of carbon dioxide (P_{CO_2}). The clinical features associated with these abnormalities and those with an altered partial pressure of oxygen (P_{O_2}) are shown in *Fig. 3.4*.

It is usual to measure hydrogen ion concentration

[H⁺] in arterial blood, anticoagulated with heparin. The arteriovenous difference for [H⁺] is small (<2 nmol/L), but the difference is significant for P_{CO_2} [approximately 1.1 kPa (8 mmHg) higher in venous blood] and P_{O_2} [approximately 7.5 kPa (56 mmHg) lower in venous blood].

It is vital that air is excluded from the syringe, both before and after drawing blood, and that, if possible, analysis is performed immediately. If the blood sample has to be transported, the syringe, capped with a blind hub and enclosed in a plastic bag, should be chilled in ice–water. Analytical instruments measure [H⁺] (strictly, activity), P_{CO_2} and P_{O_2} using specific electrodes; these measurements are together known colloquially as 'blood gases'.

By the law of mass action it follows, from the equations describing the dissociation of carbonic acid

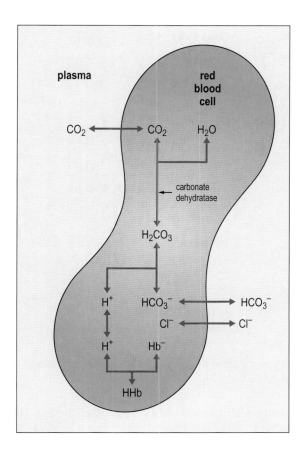

Fig. 3.3 Transport of carbon dioxide in the blood. In capillary beds, carbon dioxide diffuses into red blood cells and combines with water to form carbonic acid; the reaction is catalyzed by carbonate dehydratase. The carbonic acid dissociates to form hydrogen ions, which are buffered by haemoglobin, and bicarbonate, which diffuses out of the cell; chloride diffuses in to maintain electrochemical neutrality. In the alveoli, the process reverses; carbon dioxide is produced from bicarbonate and is excreted in the expired air.

(*Equations 3.1 and 3.2*), that $[H^+]$ is directly proportional to P_{CO_2} and inversely proportional to bicarbonate concentration; that is, it is determined by the ratio of P_{CO_2} to bicarbonate (*Equation 3.5*).

$$(3.5) \qquad [H^+] = K \frac{P_{CO_2}}{[HCO_3^-]}$$

The constant, K, embraces the dissociation constants for *Equations 3.1 and 3.2* and the solubility coefficient of carbon dioxide, which governs the concentration of the gas in solution at a given partial pressure. When $[H^+]$ is measured in nmol/L, bicarbonate in mmol/L and P_{CO_2} in kilopascals (kPa), the value of K is approximately 180 at $37°C$; if P_{CO_2} is measured in mmHg, the value of K is 24.

It follows that it is possible to calculate the bicarbonate concentration from the $[H^+]$ and P_{CO_2} alone. In blood gas analyzers, the bicarbonate concentration is *derived* by calculation and not measured. It is not the same as the bicarbonate (strictly, total carbon dioxide) *measured* by auto-analyzers. There has been considerable argument over whether it is valid to derive a bicarbonate concentration in this way, given that the values of the constants involved are based upon observations in supposedly ideal solutions, which biological fluids are not. However, for most practical purposes the derivation is an acceptable one.

An appreciation of the relationship between $[H^+]$, bicarbonate concentration and P_{CO_2} is of fundamental importance to an understanding of the pathophysiology of hydrogen ion homoeostasis. It will be apparent from *Equation 3.5* that the relationships between $[H^+]$ and P_{CO_2} and between bicarbonate concentration and P_{CO_2} are linear. These relationships have been quantified by measurements made *in vivo* and it is therefore possible to predict the effect of a change in one variable on another, for example the effect of an acute rise in P_{CO_2} on $[H^+]$. This information is an important aid in the interpretation of acid–base data.

The relationships between $[H^+]$, P_{CO_2} and bicarbonate concentration are plotted in *Fig. 3.5*. This diagram may be useful as an *aide-mémoire* to the interpretation of acid–base data but should not be used as a substitute for a full understanding of the underlying principles.

Many instruments for blood gas analysis generate other data such as standard bicarbonate and base excess. The meanings, uses and misuses of these terms are described later.

DISORDERS OF HYDROGEN ION HOMOEOSTASIS

Four components can be identified in the patho-physiology of hydrogen ion disorders (acid–base disorders):

- generation
- buffering
- compensation
- correction.

	Increase		**Decrease**
P_{CO_2}	peripheral vasodilation headache bounding pulse papilloedema flapping tremor drowsiness, coma	} late signs	paraesthesiae dizziness muscle cramps headache tetany

P_{O_2}	pulmonary and retinal
	  fibrosis (only with
	  prolonged use of high
	  inspiratory P_{O_2},
	  particularly in infants)
			breathlessness
			cyanosis
			drowsiness, confusion and coma
			pulmonary hypotension (in chronic
			  hypoxaemia)

$[H^+]$	hyperventilation increased catecholamine release hyperkalaemia decreased myocardial contractility CNS depression	} severe acidosis only	hypoventilation paraesthesiae muscle cramps dizziness headache tetany drowsiness, confusion and coma

Fig. 3.4 Effects of increased or decreased values of P_{CO_2}, P_{O_2} and $[H^+]$ in the blood. Paraesthesiae, dizziness, muscle cramps and tetany are related to a decrease in ionized calcium.

It is helpful to consider these separately, although in reality they occur concurrently, albeit with different time courses.

Acid–base disorders are classified as either respiratory or non-respiratory (metabolic) according to whether or not there is a primary (causative) change in P_{CO_2}. The term 'acidosis' signifies a tendency for the $[H^+]$ to be above normal and 'alkalosis' for it to be below normal.

Primary mixed acid–base disorders, that is disorders of combined respiratory and non-respiratory origin, are common. However, the secondary, or compensatory, responses to a primary disorder of hydrogen ion homoeostasis may produce changes indistinguishable from those seen in primary mixed disorders.

Non-respiratory (metabolic) acidosis

The primary abnormality in non-respiratory acidosis is either increased production or decreased excretion of hydrogen ions. In some cases, both may contribute. Loss of bicarbonate from the body can also, indirectly, cause an acidosis. Causes of non-respiratory acidosis are given in *Fig. 3.6*. Excess hydrogen ions are buffered by

bicarbonate (*Equation 3.2*) and other buffers. The carbonic acid thus formed dissociates (*Equation 3.1*) and the carbon dioxide is lost in the expired air. This buffering limits the potential rise in hydrogen ion concentration at the expense of a reduction in bicarbonate concentration.

Compensation is effected by hyperventilation, which increases the removal of carbon dioxide and lowers the P_{CO_2}. The $P_{CO_2}/[HCO_3^-]$ ratio falls, thus tending to reduce the $[H^+]$ (*Equation 3.5*). Hyperventilation is a direct result of the increased $[H^+]$ stimulating the respiratory centre. Respiratory compensation cannot completely normalize the $[H^+]$ since it is the high concentration itself that stimulates the compensatory hyperventilation. Furthermore, the increased work of the respiratory muscles produces carbon dioxide, thereby limiting the extent to which the P_{CO_2} can be lowered.

If the cause of the acidosis is not corrected, a new steady state may be attained, with a raised $[H^+]$, low bicarbonate and low P_{CO_2}. In the steady state, the decrease in P_{CO_2} attributable to respiratory compensation is approximately 0.17 kPa (1.3 mmHg) for each 1 mmol/L decrement in bicarbonate concentration. The

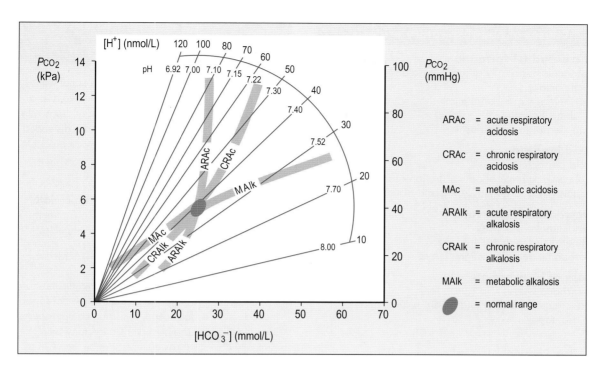

Fig. 3.5 The relationship between P_{CO_2}, hydrogen ion concentration and bicarbonate concentration. The shaded areas represent the ranges of values found in simple disturbances of acid–base homoeostasis. Data falling outside these areas indicate mixed disturbances.

extent to which compensation can take place will be limited if respiratory function is compromised. Even with normal respiratory function, it is exceptional for a P_{CO_2} of less than 1.5 kPa (11.3 mmHg) to be recorded, however severe the non-respiratory acidosis.

In a healthy person, hyperventilation would produce a respiratory alkalosis. In general, the compensatory mechanism for any acid–base disturbance involves the generation of a second, opposing disturbance. In the case of a metabolic acidosis, compensation is through the generation of a respiratory alkalosis (although this only limits the severity of the acidosis: the patient does not become alkalotic). In a respiratory acidosis, compensation is through the generation of a metabolic alkalosis (*see below*).

If renal function is normal in a patient with non-respiratory acidosis, excess hydrogen ions can be excreted by the kidneys. However, in many cases there is impairment of renal function, although this may not be the primary cause of the acidosis.

The complete correction of a non-respiratory acidosis requires reversal of the underlying cause, for example,

rehydration and insulin for diabetic ketoacidosis (*see Case History 11.2*) and removal of salicylate in salicylate overdose. It is important to maintain adequate renal perfusion to maximize renal hydrogen ion excretion. The use of exogenous bicarbonate to buffer hydrogen ions is discussed below and on *p. 203*.

Increased production of hydrogen ions

This is the cause of the acidosis in ketoacidosis (diabetic, alcoholic), lactic acidosis and acidosis seen in poisoning, for example with salicylate and ethylene glycol.

Decreased excretion of hydrogen ions

Acidosis occurs in renal glomerular failure (*see Case History 4.2*), when the decreased glomerular filtration causes a reduction in the amount of sodium that is filtered and, therefore, available for exchange with hydrogen ions. The amount of phosphate filtered and available for buffering also decreases. Renal tubular acidosis is discussed in *Chapter 4*.

Causes of non-respiratory acidosis

Increased H⁺ formation
ketoacidosis (usually diabetic, also alcoholic)
lactic acidosis
poisoning, e.g. ethanol, methanol, ethylene glycol
   and salicylate
inherited organic acidoses

Acid ingestion
acid poisoning
excessive parenteral administration of amino
   acids, e.g. arginine, lysine and histidine

Decreased H⁺ excretion
renal tubular acidoses
generalized renal failure
carbonate dehydratase inhibitors

Loss of bicarbonate
diarrhoea
pancreatic, intestinal and biliary fistulae or
   drainage

Fig. 3.6 Principal causes of non-respiratory (metabolic) acidosis.

Causes of lactic acidosis

tissue hypoxia:
   decreased perfusion
   reduced arterial PO_2

drugs, etc.:
   ethanol, methanol
   phenformin
   fructose, sorbitol

congenital:
   glucose 6-phosphatase deficiency
   other inherited diseases with defective
      gluconeogenesis or pyruvate oxidation

Fig. 3.7 Causes of lactic acidosis. Lactic acidosis is sometimes classified as type A (tissue hypoxia) and type B (all other causes).

Case history 3.1

A 60-year-old man was admitted to hospital with severe abdominal pain that had begun two and a half hours earlier. He was not taking any drugs. On examination, he was shocked and had a distended, rigid abdomen; neither femoral pulse was palpable.

Investigations
arterial blood:
   hydrogen ion   90 nmol/L (pH 7.05)
   PCO_2 3.5 kPa (26.3 mmHg)
   PO_2 12 kPa (90 mmHg)
bicarbonate (derived)   7 mmol/L

Comment
The patient is acidotic (raised [H⁺]) and this must be non-respiratory in origin since the PCO_2 is not raised. Indeed, PCO_2 is decreased, reflecting compensatory hyperventilation. The hyperventilation may be clinically obvious (Kussmaul respiration, *see Case History 11.2*). An even lower PCO_2 might have been expected as a result of respiratory compensation, but, in this case, splinting of the abdominal muscles (the abdomen is rigid) has restricted respiratory movements. The low bicarbonate concentration reflects the primary abnormality: bicarbonate is consumed as hydrogen ions are buffered. If there is no respiratory component to the acidosis, the plasma bicarbonate concentration is a good guide to the severity of a metabolic acidosis.

The clinical diagnosis (confirmed at laparotomy) is a ruptured abdominal aortic aneurysm. The patient is severely shocked following extravasation of blood from the aneurysm. Impaired tissue perfusion has led to inadequate oxygenation, despite the normal arterial PO_2, with consequently increased anaerobic metabolism of glucose to lactic acid.

Lactic acid is a normal metabolite of muscle and is converted back to glucose in the liver (the Cori cycle). However, with greatly increased production and possible impairment of hepatic metabolism due to poor perfusion, lactic acid accumulates. If renal function is compromised, for instance by hypoperfusion, the ability of the kidneys to excrete excess hydrogen ions may also be impaired.

Other causes of lactic acidosis are given in *Fig. 3.7*.

Loss of bicarbonate

Loss of bicarbonate and retention of hydrogen ions may result in acidosis in patients losing alkaline secretions from the small intestine (e.g. through fistulae). In the stomach, bicarbonate generated from carbon dioxide and water is retained and hydrogen ions are secreted into the lumen (*Fig. 3.8*). In the pancreas and small intestine, the movements of bicarbonate and hydrogen ions occur in the opposite directions (*Fig. 3.8*); therefore, hydrogen ions that are secreted into the stomach lumen are neutralized by bicarbonate in the small intestine.

Under normal circumstances, since most of the fluid and ions secreted into the gut are reabsorbed, the gut is effectively a closed system with regard to acid–base balance. If, however, alkaline secretions are lost, the patient is at risk of becoming acidotic. Increased renal hydrogen ion excretion (with generation and retention of bicarbonate) may prevent this, but excessive fluid loss from the gut may deplete the ECF to such an extent that the glomerular filtration rate falls and the kidneys are no longer able to compensate.

The anion gap

When bicarbonate concentration falls in a non-respiratory acidosis, electrochemical neutrality must be maintained by other anions. In many cases, anions are produced simultaneously and equally with hydrogen ions, for example acetoacetate and β-hydroxybutyrate in diabetic ketoacidosis, and lactate in lactic acidosis. When this does not occur, the deficit is met by chloride ions.

The difference between the sums of the concentrations of the principal cations (sodium and potassium) and of the principal anions (chloride and bicarbonate) is known as the 'anion gap', *Equation 3.6*.

(3.6) Anion gap = $([Na^+] + [K^+]) - ([Cl^-] + [HCO_3^-])$

In health, the anion gap has a value of 14–18 mmol/L and mainly represents the unmeasured net negative charge on plasma proteins.

In an acidosis in which anions other than chloride are increased, the anion gap is increased. In contrast, in an acidosis due to loss of bicarbonate, for example renal tubular acidosis, the plasma chloride concentration is

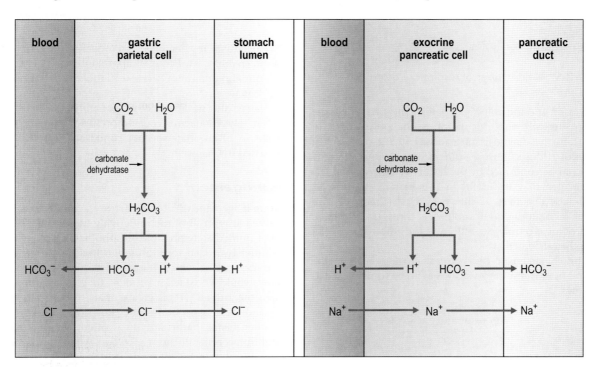

Fig. 3.8 Generation of acidic gastric and alkaline pancreatic secretions. Hydrogen and bicarbonate ions are generated from carbon dioxide and water, catalyzed by carbonate dehydratase. In the stomach, the hydrogen ions are secreted while bicarbonate is retained. The reverse process occurs in the pancreas.

Causes of respiratory acidosis

Airway obstruction
chronic obstructive airway disease,
    e.g. bronchitis, emphysema
bronchospasm, e.g. in asthma
aspiration

Depression of respiratory centre
anaesthetics
sedatives
cerebral trauma
tumours

Neuromuscular disease
poliomyelitis
Guillain–Barré syndrome
motor neuron disease
tetanus, botulism
neurotoxins, curare

Pulmonary disease
pulmonary fibrosis
severe pneumonia
respiratory distress syndrome

Extrapulmonary thoracic disease
flail chest
severe kyphoscoliosis

Fig. 3.9 Major causes of respiratory acidosis.

Case history 3.2

A young man sustained injury to the chest in a road traffic accident. Effective ventilation was compromised by a large flail segment.

Investigations
arterial blood:

Po_2	8 kPa (60 mmHg)
Pco_2	8 kPa (60 mmHg)
hydrogen ion	58 nmol/L (pH 7.24)
bicarbonate (derived)	25 mmol/L

Comment
There is a severe acidosis and the raised Pco_2 indicates that it is respiratory in origin. The magnitude of the increase in [H+] suggests that no renal compensation has occurred. Such compensation can take several days to become fully effective, in contrast to the rapid respiratory compensation in non-respiratory disorders.

increased and the anion gap is normal. It has therefore been suggested that calculation of the anion gap is of value in the diagnosis of acidosis. In the majority of cases of acidosis, however, the cause is obvious clinically and can be confirmed by the results of simple tests. The anion gap may be useful in the analysis of complex acid–base disorders, as shown by *Case History 3.7*, but some laboratories do not routinely measure chloride as part of an 'electrolyte profile' and the anion gap cannot then be calculated.

The characteristic biochemical changes seen in the blood in non-respiratory acidosis can be summarized as follows:

Non-respiratory acidosis	
[H+]	↑
pH	↓
P_{CO_2}	↓
[HCO_3^-]	↓↓

The decrease in Pco_2 is a compensatory change; the decrement in Pco_2 is approximately 0.17 kPa (1.3 mmHg) per mmol decrease in the concentration of bicarbonate.

Changes due to the underlying condition will also be present. Hyperkalaemia is common in acidotic patients, except in bicarbonate-wasting conditions, for reasons discussed in *Chapter 2*.

Management

The management of non-respiratory acidosis must be directed at reversal of the underlying cause. Where this is not immediately possible, bicarbonate may be given to buffer hydrogen ions, although there is no general agreement as to when bicarbonate should be used. Many would consider it prudent to give bicarbonate when the arterial [H+] is greater than 100 nmol/L (pH <7) and there is no immediate prospect of lowering it by other means, particularly in a patient whose clinical condition is generally poor. However, when bicarbonate is used it should be given in small quantities and the effect on the arterial [H+] measured. Large amounts of bicarbonate, given rapidly in an attempt to correct an acidosis, can be dangerous.

Case history 3.3

A 70-year-old man, known to suffer from chronic obstructive airways disease, was admitted to hospital with an acute exacerbation of his illness. Arterial blood analysis was carried out on admission (results A). In spite of vigorous physiotherapy and medical treatment his condition deteriorated (results B) and it was decided to start artificial ventilation. Analysis was repeated after 6 h (results C). After 12 h he had a generalized fit (results D).

Investigations

arterial blood:	A	B	C	D
P_{CO_2} (kPa)	9.5	11.0	7.7	5.7
(mmHg)	71.3	82.5	58.5	42.8
hydrogen ion (nmol/L)	50	58	40	29
pH	7.30	7.24	7.40	7.54
bicarbonate (mmol/L) (derived)	35	35	34	35

Comment

The results on admission (A) indicate an acidosis. This is of respiratory origin since the P_{CO_2} is raised. However, the $[H^+]$ is only slightly elevated, indicating that renal compensation is occurring as would be expected in a case of chronic carbon dioxide retention. The raised bicarbonate, which suggests a non-respiratory alkalosis, is the result of the compensatory increase in renal hydrogen ion excretion. Indeed, the commonest causes of raised plasma bicarbonate concentration in the elderly are chronic carbon dioxide retention and diuretic-induced potassium depletion (*see p. 33*).

A more severe acidosis (B) subsequently develops, commensurate with the rise in P_{CO_2}. This is a result of further carbon dioxide retention with no corresponding increase in renal hydrogen ion excretion.

Artificial ventilation lowers the P_{CO_2} rapidly (C); the $[H^+]$ is now normal although the P_{CO_2} is still elevated. This represents this patient's normal steady state, in which there is an almost complete renal compensation of the acidosis.

Continued ventilation reduces the P_{CO_2} (D) to within the normal range for a healthy subject but to below this patient's normal. He has become alkalotic and suffers a fit as a consequence. The alkalosis is due to the continued high rate of renal hydrogen ion excretion in response to the chronically raised P_{CO_2}. Adaptation of renal hydrogen ion excretion in response to a change in P_{CO_2} takes several days. Thus, rapid reduction of the P_{CO_2} exposes the compensatory, secondary response, which then appears to be the sole acid–base abnormality. The compensatory mechanism in respiratory acidosis involves the generation of a metabolic alkalosis.

Respiratory acidosis

Some of the many conditions associated with the development of respiratory acidosis are shown in *Fig. 3.9*. They are all characterized by an increase in P_{CO_2}. For every hydrogen ion that is produced, a bicarbonate ion is generated. The majority of the hydrogen ions are buffered by intracellular buffers, particularly haemoglobin (*see Fig. 3.5*). With an acute rise in P_{CO_2}, every 1 kPa (7.5 mmHg) increase is associated with a concomitant increase in bicarbonate concentration of less than 1 mmol/L and $[H^+]$ of approximately 5.5 nmol/L. In chronic carbon dioxide retention, when renal compensation is maximal, the $[H^+]$ is increased by only 2.5 nmol/L for each 1 kPa (7.5 mmHg) rise in

P_{CO_2} whereas bicarbonate concentration increases by 2–3 mmol/L.

A respiratory acidosis can only be corrected by means that restore the P_{CO_2} to normal but, if a high P_{CO_2} persists, compensation occurs through increased renal hydrogen ion excretion.

In acute respiratory acidosis, unless very severe, the bicarbonate concentration, although increased, is usually within the reference range. If the bicarbonate concentration is clearly elevated in a respiratory acidosis, either a more chronic course with renal compensation (*see Case History 3.3*) or a coexisting non-respiratory alkalosis is suggested. A low bicarbonate would suggest a coexisting non-respiratory acidosis.

Management

The aim when treating respiratory acidosis is to improve alveolar ventilation and lower the P_{CO_2}. In acute alveolar hypoventilation, however, it is usually hypoxaemia rather than hypercapnia that poses the main threat to life, unless the P_{O_2} is being maintained by the supply of additional oxygen. If ventilation ceases abruptly, death from hypoxaemia will occur in approximately four minutes; the P_{CO_2} by comparison rises at such a rate that it would take more than ten minutes for it to reach a lethal level.

In chronic respiratory acidosis, it is seldom possible to correct the underlying cause and treatment is directed at maximizing alveolar ventilation by, for example, utilizing physiotherapy, bronchodilators and antibiotics. If artificial ventilation becomes necessary, it is vital to monitor the patient's arterial blood gases and hydrogen ion in order to avoid over-correction of the respiratory acidosis.

Oxygen may safely be used at high concentrations in patients with acute respiratory failure. In many patients with chronic carbon dioxide retention, however, the respiratory centre becomes insensitive to carbon dioxide and hypoxaemia provides the main stimulus to respiration. Oxygen administration in such patients must be carefully controlled to prevent abolition of this stimulus.

It is important to appreciate that, on the basis of the data alone, it would not be possible to tell whether results 'C' in *Case History 3.3* represent a state of either compensated chronic carbon dioxide retention or acute carbon dioxide retention developing in a patient with a pre-existing metabolic alkalosis. The management of these two states would not be the same.

The characteristic biochemical changes in arterial blood in acute and chronic respiratory acidosis can be summarized as follows:

Respiratory acidosis

	acute	chronic
[H$^+$]	↑	slight ↑ or high–normal
pH	↓	slight ↓ or low–normal
P_{CO_2}	↑	↑
[HCO$_3^-$]	slight ↑	↑

Non-respiratory (metabolic) alkalosis

Non-respiratory alkalosis is characterized by a primary increase in the ECF bicarbonate concentration, with a consequent reduction in [H$^+$] (*see Equation 3.5*). In a normal subject, an increase in plasma bicarbonate concentration leads to incomplete renal tubular bicarbonate reabsorption and excretion of bicarbonate in the urine. Massive quantities of bicarbonate must be ingested to produce a sustained alkalosis.

Since the body is a net producer of acid, it might be supposed that non-respiratory alkalosis should be corrected by normal acid production. In practice, and in contrast to non-respiratory acidosis and to respiratory disorders of acid–base balance, a non-respiratory alkalosis may persist even after the primary cause has been corrected. It is thus necessary to consider both the mechanisms that can cause non-respiratory alkalosis and those that can perpetuate it.

Causes of non-respiratory alkalosis are shown in *Fig. 3.10*. Alkali loading causes only a transient alkalosis unless there are additional factors operating to sustain it. Disproportionate loss of chloride, for example during diuretic-induced mobilization of oedema fluid, when little bicarbonate is excreted in the urine, can cause a non-respiratory alkalosis but, if this is the sole mechanism, the disturbance is always mild.

The maintenance of a non-respiratory alkalosis requires inappropriately high (as far as hydrogen ion homoeostasis is concerned) renal bicarbonate reabsorption. Factors which may be responsible for this include a decrease in ECF volume, mineralocorticoid excess and potassium depletion.

In hypovolaemia, there is an increased stimulus to renal sodium reabsorption (*see p. 18*). Sodium reabsorption is dependent upon the availability of adequate

Causes of non-respiratory alkalosis

Loss of unbuffered hydrogen ion
gastrointestinal:
    gastric aspiration
    vomiting with pyloric stenosis
    congenital chloride-losing diarrhoea
renal:
    mineralocorticoid excess:
        Cushing's syndrome
        Conn's syndrome
    drugs with mineralocorticoid activity,
      e.g. carbenoxolone
    diuretic therapy (not K^+-sparing)
    rapid correction of chronically raised $P\text{CO}_2$
    potassium depletion

Administration of alkali
inappropriate treatment of acidotic states
chronic alkali ingestion

Fig. 3.10 Causes of non-respiratory alkalosis.

anions. If there is a relative deficit of chloride as, for example, with loss of gastric juice and treatment with some diuretics, electrochemical neutrality during sodium reabsorption must be maintained by increased bicarbonate reabsorption and by hydrogen and potassium ion excretion. In states of mineralocortoid excess, alkalosis is perpetuated by the increased hydrogen ion excretion in the urine, which occurs secondarily to the increased sodium reabsorption.

The correction of a non-respiratory alkalosis requires reversal both of the primary cause and of the mechanism responsible for its perpetuation. The expected compensatory change would be an increase in $P\text{CO}_2$, which would increase the ratio $P\text{CO}_2/[\text{HCO}_3^-]$ and thus $[H^+]$ (see Equation 3.5). A low arterial $[H^+]$ inhibits the respiratory centre, causing hypoventilation, and thus an increase in $P\text{CO}_2$. However, since an increase in $P\text{CO}_2$ is itself a powerful stimulus to respiration, this compensation, particularly in acute non-respiratory alkalosis, may be self-limiting. In more chronic disorders, significant compensation may occur, presumably because the respiratory centre becomes less sensitive to carbon dioxide. Should hypoventilation lead to significant hypoxaemia, however, this will provide a powerful stimulus to respiration and prevent further compensation.

A non-respiratory alkalosis due to loss of gastric acid may also occur in patients undergoing nasogastric aspiration. It is not usually a feature of vomiting if the pylorus is patent, since the additional loss of alkaline secretions from the upper small intestine counteracts the effect of the retention of bicarbonate ions generated by gastric parietal cells. Vomiting with pyloric stenosis is an unusual cause of non-respiratory alkalosis but the disturbance can be severe; other causes rarely result in such a severe disturbance.

Management

The management of a non-respiratory alkalosis depends upon the severity of the condition and upon the cause. When hypovolaemia and hypochloraemia are present, they can be simultaneously corrected by an infusion of isotonic sodium chloride solution ('normal saline'), which will also improve renal perfusion and allow excretion of the bicarbonate load. In such cases, it is common practice to provide potassium supplements, although often this is not necessary. It is very rarely necessary to attempt rapid correction of non-respiratory alkalosis, for example by administration of ammonium chloride.

The mild alkalosis commonly associated with potassium depletion, which may, for example, be diuretic induced, rarely requires treatment *per se* although the hypokalaemia may require correction. The management of a state of mineralocorticoid excess is considered in *Chapter 8*.

The biochemical features of non-respiratory alkalosis can be summarized as follows:

Non-respiratory alkalosis	
$[H^+]$	↓
pH	↑
$P\text{CO}_2$	↑
$[\text{HCO}_3^-]$	↑↑

Respiratory alkalosis

The main causes of respiratory alkalosis are shown in *Fig. 3.11*. The common feature and cause of the alkalosis is a fall in $P\text{CO}_2$, which reduces the ratio of $P\text{CO}_2$ to bicarbonate concentration (see Equation 3.5). In acute respiratory alkalosis, the $[H^+]$ falls by approximately 5.5 nmol/L for each 1.0 kPa (7.5 mmHg) fall in $P\text{CO}_2$.

Case history 3.4

A 45-year-old man was admitted to hospital with a history of persistent vomiting. He had a long history of dyspepsia but had never sought advice for this, preferring to treat himself with proprietary remedies. On examination he was obviously dehydrated and his respiration was shallow.

Investigations

arterial blood:

	hydrogen ion	28 nmol/L (pH 7.56)
	P_{CO_2}	7.2 kPa (54 mmHg)
	bicarbonate (derived)	45 mmol/L
serum:	sodium	146 mmol/L
	potassium	2.8 mmol/L
	urea	34.2 mmol/L

A barium meal, performed after this metabolic imbalance had been corrected, showed pyloric stenosis, thought to be due to scarring caused by peptic ulceration.

Comment

The patient is alkalotic and, since the P_{CO_2} is high, this must be non-respiratory in origin. The increase in P_{CO_2} is a result of compensatory hypoventilation leading to carbon dioxide retention. In chronic non-respiratory alkalosis, as in this case, each increment of 1 mmol/L in bicarbonate concentration typically gives rise to an increase in P_{CO_2} of approximately 0.1 kPa (0.75 mmHg).

The alkalosis is a result of loss of unbuffered hydrogen ions in gastric juice with concomitant retention of bicarbonate. The raised urea is consistent with the clinical signs of dehydration resulting from fluid loss. (It may be noted that when dehydration is caused by conditions other than gastric fluid loss, a raised plasma urea concentration is more likely to be accompanied by a low plasma bicarbonate concentration and high plasma potassium concentration, as a consequence of impaired renal perfusion.) Fluid loss stimulates renal sodium reabsorption, but sodium can only be reabsorbed either with chloride or in exchange for hydrogen and potassium ions. Gastric juice has a high concentration of chloride and patients losing gastric secretions become hypochloraemic. This means that less sodium than usual can be reabsorbed with chloride. However, it appears that the defence of ECF volume takes precedence over acid–base homoeostasis and further sodium reabsorption occurs in exchange for hydrogen ions (perpetuating the alkalosis) and potassium ions (leading to potassium depletion). This explains the apparently paradoxical finding of acidic urine in patients with severe non-respiratory alkalosis. Potassium is also lost in the gastric juice, and thus patients frequently become potassium-depleted and yet are losing potassium in the urine.

The fall in P_{CO_2} causes a small decrease in bicarbonate concentration. Compensation occurs through a reduction in renal hydrogen ion excretion, which further decreases plasma bicarbonate concentration. Renal compensation in a respiratory alkalosis develops slowly, as it does in a respiratory acidosis. If a steady P_{CO_2} is maintained, maximal compensation with a new steady state develops within 36–72 h.

Management

As with other disturbances of acid–base homoeostasis, the management of patients with respiratory alkalosis should be directed towards the underlying cause, although this is frequently not possible. Fortunately, a chronic compensated respiratory alkalosis is not, in itself, dangerous. Increasing the inspired P_{CO_2} by

Causes of respiratory alkalosis

Hypoxia
high altitude
severe anaemia
pulmonary disease

Increased respiratory drive
respiratory stimulants, e.g. salicylates
cerebral disturbances, e.g. trauma, infection and
   tumours
hepatic failure
Gram-negative septicaemia
primary hyperventilation syndrome
voluntary hyperventilation

Pulmonary disease
pulmonary oedema
pulmonary embolism

Mechanical overventilation

Fig. 3.11 Major causes of respiratory alkalosis.

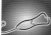 **Case history 3.5**

As part of a class experiment in physiology, a medical student volunteered to have a sample of arterial blood taken. The demonstrator took some time to explain the procedure to the class, during which time the student became increasingly anxious. As the blood was being drawn she complained of tingling in her fingers and toes.

Investigations
arterial blood:

hydrogen ion	30 nmol/L (pH 7.52)
P_{CO_2}	3.5 kPa (26.3 mmHg)
bicarbonate (derived)	21 mmol/L

Comment
The student is alkalotic with a low P_{CO_2}, thus the disturbance is respiratory in origin. The extent of the decrease in [H$^+$] indicates that there is neither compensation nor an additional acid–base disturbance. The low P_{CO_2} is a result of anxiety-induced hyperventilation and no compensation would be expected to have occurred in this short time. The symptoms are a result of a decrease in the concentration of ionized calcium, an effect of alkalosis.

making the patient re-breathe into a paper bag may abort the clinical features of acute hypocapnia in acute hyperventilation, but is only a temporary measure, and carries a risk of causing hypoxia.

The biochemical features of respiratory alkalosis can be summarized as follows:

Respiratory alkalosis

	acute	chronic
[H$^+$]	↓	slight ↓ or low–normal
pH	↑	slight ↑ or high–normal
P_{CO_2}	↓	↓
[HCO$_3^-$]	slight ↓	↓

INTERPRETATION OF ACID–BASE DATA

A thorough understanding of the pathophysiology of acid–base homoeostasis is essential for the correct interpretation of laboratory data, but these data should always be considered in the clinical context.

The starting point in any evaluation should be the hydrogen ion concentration or pH. This will indicate whether the predominant disturbance is an acidosis or an alkalosis. However, a normal value does not exclude an acid–base disorder. There may be either a fully compensated disturbance or two primary disturbances whose effects on hydrogen ion concentration cancel each other out.

If the P_{CO_2} is abnormal, there must be a respiratory component to the disturbance. If the P_{CO_2} is raised in an acidosis, the acidosis is respiratory and comparison of the hydrogen ion concentration with that predicted for an acute change in P_{CO_2} will indicate whether there is an additional metabolic component; this may be compensatory. If the P_{CO_2} is low in an acidosis, the acidosis is non-respiratory and there is an additional respiratory component, which will often reflect compensation. A similar rationale applies to alkalotic

Case history 3.6

A young woman was admitted to hospital unconscious, following a head injury. A skull fracture was demonstrated on radiography and a computerized tomography (CT) scan revealed extensive cerebral contusions. The respiratory rate was increased, at 38/min. Three days after admission, the patient's condition was unchanged.

Investigations

arterial blood:

hydrogen ion	36 nmol/L (pH 7.44)
P_{CO_2}	3.6 kPa (29.3 mmHg)
bicarbonate (derived)	19 mmol/L

Comment

This is a compensated respiratory alkalosis. The P_{CO_2} is reduced as a result of hyperventilation. The [H+] is at the lower limit of normal. Abnormalities of respiration (hypo- and hyperventilation) are common in patients with head injuries. Hyperventilation can occur with injuries involving the brain stem and as a result of raised intracranial pressure. Even though a low P_{CO_2} is also characteristic of the respiratory compensation in non-respiratory acidosis, the history and normal [H+] preclude this diagnosis. Also, a much lower bicarbonate concentration would be expected in a non-respiratory acidosis.

Case history 3.7

A young woman was admitted to hospital 8 h after she had taken an overdose of aspirin.

Investigations

arterial blood:

hydrogen ion	30 nmol/L (pH 7.53)
P_{CO_2}	2.0 kPa (15 mmHg)

Comment

The patient is alkalotic and the low P_{CO_2} indicates a respiratory cause. However, the [H+] is not as low as would have been expected as a result of an acute fall in P_{CO_2}. The data would be appropriate for a chronic, compensated respiratory alkalosis, but such a low P_{CO_2} would be exceptional and this interpretation is not compatible with the history. The alternative is that there is an acute respiratory alkalosis with a coexistent non-respiratory acidosis. This combination is characteristic of salicylate poisoning, where initial respiratory stimulation causes a respiratory alkalosis but later the metabolic effects of salicylate tend to predominate, producing an acidosis.

This case history illustrates the importance of considering the clinical setting when analyzing acid–base data. Calculation of the anion gap might have been helpful here. It would have been increased by the presence of organic anions, indicating a coexisting non-respiratory acidosis, but is normal in compensated respiratory alkalosis.

states. An algorithm for the analysis of acid–base data is given in *Fig. 3.12*.

Since the derived bicarbonate is calculated from the P_{CO_2} and [H+], it does not provide any more information than these two measurements alone. However, knowing the bicarbonate concentration may simplify the interpretation of acid–base data. Its concentration is always decreased in non-respiratory acidosis and increased in non-respiratory alkalosis, regardless of whether or not there is compensation.

Mixed acid–base disturbances occur frequently and appear complex. Correct diagnosis requires a logical approach and a clear understanding both of the relevant pathophysiology and of the quantitative relationships

between [H+] and P_{CO_2}. The biochemical changes that are characteristic of the various acid–base disturbances are shown in *Fig. 3.13*. With this physiological approach, calculated parameters such as 'standard bicarbonate' and 'base excess' are obsolete.

The standard bicarbonate is a calculated estimate of the bicarbonate concentration that would be present if the P_{CO_2} were normal and thus reflects only the non-respiratory influences on bicarbonate. The base excess is a calculated estimate of the non-respiratory influences on total buffering capacity. These parameters were introduced with a view to distinguishing between the

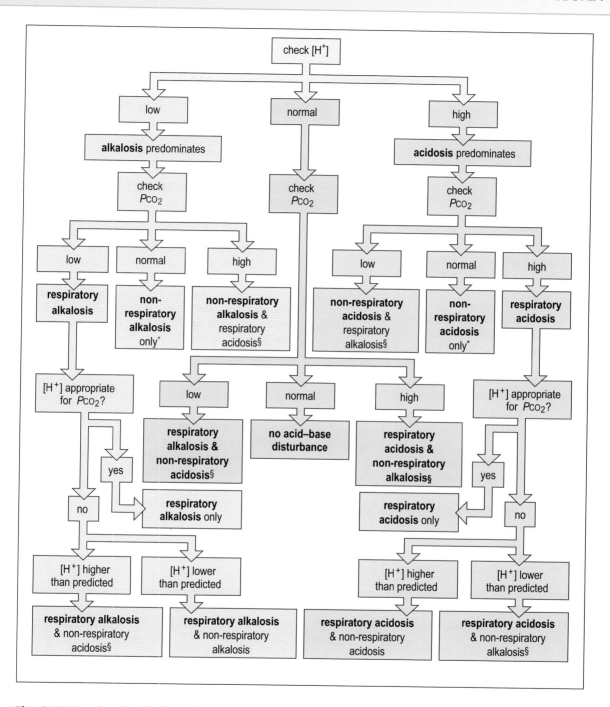

Fig. 3.12 An algorithm for the analysis of acid–base data. Where two disturbances are shown, the predominant one is in bold type.

§ indicates a disturbance that would be expected to develop as a result of physiological compensation, but could be a coexisting pathological process.

*Because compensation for non-respiratory disorders develops so rapidly, 'pure' (i.e. uncompensated) non-respiratory disorders do not occur unless the normal respiratory response is prevented (e.g. in a ventilated patient). Acutely, compensation for non-respiratory alkalosis is less efficient than for acidosis.

Case history 3.8

An elderly man was admitted to hospital in a confused state. He was dyspnoeic and had a cough productive of sputum. He was unable to give a coherent history but one of the casualty officers knew him to be an insulin-dependent diabetic patient with a long history of chronic bronchitis.

Investigations

arterial blood:

hydrogen ion	66 nmol/L (pH 7.18)
$P\text{CO}_2$	7.4 kPa (55.5 mmHg)

Comment

The patient is acidotic and the raised $P\text{CO}_2$ indicates a respiratory component. However, the $[H^+]$ is higher than would be expected in an acute respiratory acidosis with a $P\text{CO}_2$ at this level. Therefore, there must in addition be a non-respiratory component to the acidosis.

On the basis of these data alone, it is not possible to determine whether the respiratory disturbance is acute or chronic. These results could, for example, represent the results of the concurrent development of an acute respiratory and a non-respiratory acidosis. On the other hand, they are also compatible with the presence of non-respiratory acidosis in a patient with chronic carbon dioxide retention. Given that the patient is known to suffer from chronic bronchitis, the second interpretation is more likely.

respiratory and non-respiratory components in acid–base disorders, but they take no account of normal physiological responses. An abnormal standard bicarbonate or base excess indicates the presence of a non-respiratory acidosis or alkalosis. It does not, however, indicate whether this is either part of a mixed disturbance of acid–base homoeostasis or related to normal physiological compensation.

OXYGEN TRANSPORT AND ITS DISORDERS

In patients with respiratory disorders, a disturbance of the partial pressure of oxygen ($P\text{O}_2$) may be of greater clinical significance than either an abnormal $P\text{CO}_2$ or abnormal $[H^+]$. Although both oxygen and carbon dioxide are transported between the alveoli and the bloodstream, albeit in opposite directions, their respective partial pressures do not necessarily change in a reciprocal fashion. There are two reasons for this: first, carbon dioxide is generally more diffusible than oxygen, with the result that, in pulmonary oedema and interstitial lung disease, hypoxaemia develops but the $P\text{CO}_2$ may not increase; second, very little oxygen is carried in physical solution in the blood, and haemoglobin is normally nearly fully saturated with oxygen. As a result, hyperventilation cannot increase the arterial $P\text{O}_2$ significantly, but can reduce the $P\text{CO}_2$. A raised $P\text{O}_2$ is only seen in patients given supplementary oxygen, which results in an increased inspired $P\text{O}_2$.

The oxyhaemoglobin dissociation curve, which relates $P\text{O}_2$ to the percentage of the maximum saturation of haemoglobin with oxygen, is sigmoid (*Fig. 3.14*). As a

	Acidosis			Alkalosis		
	Non-respiratory	**Respiratory** acute	chronic	**Non-respiratory**	**Respiratory** acute	chronic
$[H^+]$	↑	↑	slight ↑ or high–normal	↓	↓	slight ↓ or low–normal
pH	↓	↓	slight ↓ or low–normal	↑	↑	slight ↑ or high–normal
$P\text{CO}_2$	↓	↑	↑	↑	↓	↓
$[HCO_3^-]$	↓↓	slight ↑	↑	↑↑	slight ↓	↓

Fig. 3.13 Biochemical changes characteristic of disturbances of acid–base homoeostasis.

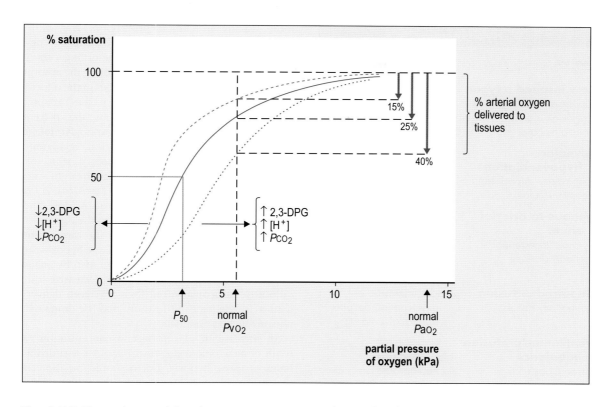

Fig. 3.14 The oxyhaemoglobin dissociation curve. Normal arterial and venous P_{O_2} are shown. The effect of a right or left shift in the amount of oxygen delivered to tissues is indicated. A right shift causes an increase, a left shift a decrease. P_{50} is the P_{O_2} at which haemoglobin is 50% saturated with oxygen. 2,3-DPG = 2,3-diphosphoglycerate.

consequence, a considerable drop in P_{O_2} can occur without a significant effect on the amount of oxygen carried in the blood. Saturation only falls below 90% when P_{O_2} falls below about 8 kPa, but if P_{O_2} decreases further, saturation declines rapidly.

There are many causes of hypoxaemia (*Fig. 3.15*). The reasons for the hypoxaemia associated with hypoventilation, venous-to-arterial shunting and impaired diffusion are self-evident. However, in many respiratory diseases, such as lung collapse and pneumonia, there is an imbalance between ventilation and perfusion of the alveoli. Blood leaving poorly ventilated, well-perfused alveoli will have a low P_{O_2} and a raised P_{CO_2}. The effect on P_{CO_2} can be compensated in normally perfused and ventilated alveoli by hyperventilation. This removes additional carbon dioxide, but cannot compensate for the low P_{O_2} in blood from poorly ventilated alveoli since the haemoglobin in blood from well-perfused

alveoli will be fully saturated and thus the amount of oxygen carried cannot be increased. The poorly perfused alveoli are effectively dead space. With moderate degrees of ventilation/perfusion imbalance, the P_{O_2} is reduced and the P_{CO_2} is either normal or even reduced. With severe imbalance, hyperventilation cannot compensate through increased removal of carbon dioxide from normally ventilated and perfused alveoli and the P_{CO_2} becomes elevated.

Although an adequate arterial P_{O_2} is essential for normal tissue oxygenation, it is not the only factor involved. The amount of oxygen delivered to tissues depends upon arterial oxygen *content* and their blood supply.

Oxygen content depends on haemoglobin concentration and on its saturation, which is a function of the affinity of haemoglobin for oxygen and the P_{O_2}. Haemoglobin saturation can be measured *in vitro* or,

Hypoxaemia	
Cause	**Mechanism**
Low inspired oxygen low barometic pressure low % oxygen in inspired air	low alveolar P_{O_2}
Alveolar hypoventilation respiratory depression neuromuscular disease	low alveolar P_{O_2}
Venous-to-arterial shunt cyanotic congenital heart disease	admixture of arterial blood (high P_{O_2}) with venous blood (low P_{O_2})
Impaired diffusion pulmonary fibrosis	inadequate arterial oxygenation despite normal alveolar P_{O_2}
Ventilation/perfusion imbalance chronic obstructive airways disease	blood perfuses non-aerated parts of lung and is not oxygenated

Fig. 3.15 Causes and mechanisms of hypoxaemia.

more usually in clinical practice, *in vivo*, with an oximeter. Pulse oximeters are lightweight devices designed to be clipped to an ear lobe or finger tip. They measure oxygen saturation by monitoring the absorption of light by oxy- and deoxyhaemoglobin in the underlying tissue. Various factors can affect the affinity of haemoglobin for oxygen, and thus the percentage saturation at a given P_{O_2}. 2,3-Diphosphoglycerate (2,3-DPG) is an important physiological regulator. An increase in red cell 2,3-DPG causes a shift in the oxyhaemoglobin dissociation curve to the right and this facilitates oxygen uptake by tissues (*Fig. 3.14*). 2,3-DPG levels are increased in chronic hypoxia. Acidosis and an increase in P_{CO_2} also shift the curve to the right.

Tissue blood supply depends on the cardiac output and local vascular resistance. Thus tissue hypoxia can be caused not only by hypoxaemia, but also by anaemia, impaired haemoglobin function, decreased cardiac output or vasoconstriction. Even if oxygen delivery to tissues is adequate, utilization may be impaired by poisons such as cyanide.

An increase in plasma lactate concentration (as a result of anaerobic metabolism) is often regarded as an index of tissue hypoxia, but it should be appreciated that it is a relatively late sign. By the time an increase is detectable, irreversible tissue damage may have occurred.

SUMMARY

- **Hydrogen ion homoeostasis** depends on buffering in the tissues and bloodstream, acid excretion by the kidneys and excretion of carbon dioxide (hydration of which forms carbonic acid) through the lungs.

- Blood **hydrogen ion concentration is directly proportional to the partial pressure of carbon dioxide (P_{CO_2}), and inversely proportional to the concentration of bicarbonate**, the principal extracellular buffer.

- **Acidosis** (increased [H^+]) can be caused by retention of carbon dioxide (**respiratory acidosis**), or ingestion/increased production/decreased excretion of acid or loss of bicarbonate (non-respiratory or **metabolic acidosis**). **Alkalosis** can be caused by hyperventilation (**respiratory alkalosis**), leading to a fall in P_{CO_2}, or increased excretion of acid (non-respiratory or **metabolic alkalosis**).

SUMMARY (cont'd)

- Physiological **compensatory mechanisms** operate to oppose the change in $[H^+]$: compensation in effect causes the generation of an opposing disturbance; for example, in respiratory acidosis, compensation is through increased renal acid excretion.

- Ultimate **correction** of an acidosis or alkalosis usually requires correction of the underlying cause.

- **Mixed disturbances**, with respiratory and non-respiratory components, occur frequently. Even in these cases, a diagnosis can be made based on clinical assessment and logical consideration of the arterial hydrogen ion concentration and partial pressure of carbon dioxide.

- **Maintenance of a normal arterial Po_2 requires** an adequate oxygen content in inspired gas and normal alveolar ventilation and perfusion. The **oxygen content of blood** depends on Po_2, red cell haemoglobin content and normal haemoglobin function; **oxygen delivery to tissues** additionally depends on the adequacy of tissue perfusion.

4 The kidneys

INTRODUCTION

The kidneys have three major functions: (i) excretion of waste, (ii) maintenance of extracellular fluid (ECF) volume and composition and (iii) hormone synthesis. Each kidney consists of approximately one million functional units, the nephrons.

The kidneys have a rich blood supply and normally receive about 25% of the cardiac output. Most of this is distributed initially to the capillary tufts of the glomeruli, which act as high pressure filters. Blood is separated from the lumen of the nephron by three layers: the capillary endothelial cells, the basement membrane and the epithelial cells of the nephron (*Fig. 4.1*). The endothelial and epithelial cells are in intimate contact with the basement membrane; the endothelial cells are fenestrated and contact between the epithelial cells and the membrane is discontinuous so that the membrane is exposed to blood on one side and to the lumen of the nephron on the other.

The glomerular filtrate is an ultrafiltrate of plasma; that is, it has a similar composition to plasma except that it is almost free of proteins. This is because the endothelium provides a barrier to red and white blood cells, and the basement membrane, although permeable to water and low molecular weight substances, is largely impermeable to macromolecules. This impermeability is related to both molecular size and electrical charge. Proteins with molecular weights lower than that of albumin (68 kDa) are filterable; negatively charged molecules are less easily filtered than those bearing a positive charge. Almost all the protein in the glomerular filtrate is reabsorbed and catabolized by proximal convoluted tubular cells, with the result that normal urinary protein excretion is less than 150 mg/24 h.

Filtration is a passive process. The total filtration rate of the kidneys is mainly determined by the difference between the blood pressure in the glomerular capillaries and the hydrostatic pressure in the lumen of the nephron, the nature of the glomerular basement membrane and the number of glomeruli. The normal glomerular filtration rate (GFR) is approximately 120 mL/min, equivalent to a volume of about 170 L/24 h.

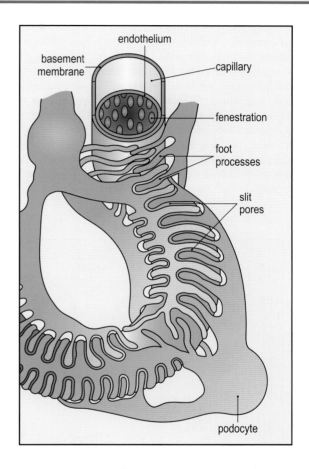

Fig. 4.1 Diagram of a glomerular capillary, showing fenestrations in endothelial cells, basement membrane and epithelial cells (podocytes) with slit pores between interdigitating foot processes.

However, urine production is only 1–2 L/24 h, depending on fluid intake; the bulk of the filtrate is reabsorbed further along the nephron.

The glomerular filtrate passes into the proximal convoluted tubule where much of it is reabsorbed. Under normal circumstances, all the glucose, amino acids, potassium and bicarbonate, and about 75% of the sodium, is reabsorbed isotonically here by energy-dependent mechanisms.

Medullary hyperosmolality, which is vital for the further reabsorption of water, is generated by the counter-current system, summarized in *Fig. 4.2*. Chloride ions, accompanied by sodium, are pumped out of the ascending limb of the loop of Henle into the surrounding interstitial fluid, and thence diffuse into the descending limb. Since the ascending limb of the loop of Henle is impermeable to water, the net effect is an exchange of sodium and chloride ions between the ascending and descending limbs. This alters the osmolality of both the fluid within the nephron and the surrounding interstitial fluid. A gradient of osmolality is set up between the isotonic cortico-medullary junction and the extremely hypertonic (approximately 1200 mmol/L) deep medulla. Diffusion of urea from the collecting duct into the interstitium and thence into the loop of Henle also makes an important contribution to medullary hypertonicity. It is noteworthy that urinary concentrating ability is impaired in malnourished children but can be restored by increasing their dietary protein intake or even adding urea to their diets.

The tubular fluid becomes increasingly dilute as it passes up the ascending limb of the loop of Henle, as a result of the continued removal of chloride and sodium ions. Fluid entering the distal convoluted tubule is hypotonic (approximately 150 mmol/L) with respect to the glomerular filtrate. Further dilution takes place in the early part of the distal convoluted tubule.

Approximately 90% of the filtered sodium and 80% of the filtered water has been reabsorbed from the glomerular filtrate by the time it reaches the beginning of the distal convoluted tubule. In the distal tubule, further sodium reabsorption takes place, in part controlled by aldosterone; this generates an electrochemical gradient that engenders the secretion of potassium and hydrogen ions. Ammonia is also secreted in the distal tubule and

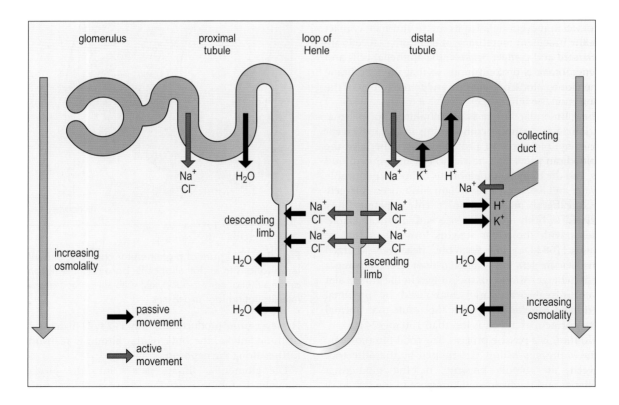

Fig. 4.2 Movements of major ions, passive movement of water and changes in osmolality in the nephron. In the ascending loop of Henle, chloride ions are actively transported and sodium ions accompany them to maintain electrochemical neutrality.

buffers hydrogen ions, being excreted as ammonium ions (*see p. 43*).

Whereas the proximal tubule is responsible for bulk reabsorption of the glomerular filtrate, the distal tubule exerts fine control over the composition of the tubular fluid, depending upon the requirements of the body.

Tubular fluid then passes into the collecting ducts, which extend through the hypertonic renal medulla and discharge urine into the renal pelvis. The cells lining the collecting ducts are normally impermeable to water. Vasopressin (antidiuretic hormone, ADH) renders them permeable by stimulating the incorporation of aqua-porins (water channels) into the cell membranes and allows water to be reabsorbed passively in response to the osmotic gradient between the duct lumen and the interstitial fluid. Thus, in the absence of vasopressin, a dilute urine is produced; in its presence, the urine is concentrated. Some reabsorption of sodium also occurs in the collecting ducts under the stimulus of aldosterone.

Since the normal GFR is approximately 120 mL/min, a volume of fluid equivalent to the entire ECF is filtered every two hours. Disease processes affecting the kidney therefore have a considerable potential for affecting water, salt and hydrogen ion homoeostasis and the excretion of waste products.

The kidneys are also important endocrine organs, pro-ducing renin, erythropoietin and calcitriol. The secretion of these hormones may be altered in renal disease. In addition, several other hormones are either inactivated or excreted by the kidneys and hence their concentrations in the blood can also be affected by renal disease.

BIOCHEMICAL TESTS OF RENAL FUNCTION

Diseases affecting the kidneys can selectively damage glomerular or tubular function, but isolated disorders of tubular function are relatively uncommon. In acute and chronic renal failure, there is effectively a loss of function of whole nephrons and, since the process of filtration is essential to the formation of urine, tests of glomerular function are almost invariably required in the investigation and management of any patient with renal disease. The principal function of the glomeruli is to filter water and low molecular weight components of the blood while retaining cells and high molecular weight components. The most frequently used tests are those that assess either the GFR or the integrity of the glomerular filtration barrier.

It should be noted that the GFR declines with age (to a greater extent in males than in females) and this must be taken into account when interpreting results.

Measurement of glomerular filtration rate

Clearance

An estimate of the GFR can be made by measuring the urinary excretion of a substance that is completely filtered from the blood by the glomeruli and is not secreted, reabsorbed or metabolized by the renal tubules. Experimentally, inulin (a plant polysaccharide) has been found to meet these requirements. The volume of blood from which inulin is cleared or completely removed in one minute is known as the inulin clearance and is equal to the GFR.

Measurement of inulin clearance requires the infusion of inulin into the blood and is not suitable for routine clinical use. The most frequently used clearance test is based on the measurement of creatinine. This endogenous substance is derived mainly from the turnover of creatine in muscle and daily production is relatively constant, being a function of total muscle mass. A small amount of creatinine is derived from meat in the diet. Creatinine clearance is calculated from the formula:

$$(4.1) \qquad \text{Clearance} = \frac{U \times \dot{V}}{P} \ \text{mL/min}$$

U = urinary creatinine concentration (μmol/L)
$\dot{V}$ = urine flow rate [mL/min or (L/24 h)/1.44]
P = plasma creatinine concentration (μmol/L)

Creatinine clearance in adults is normally of the order of 120 mL/min, corrected to a standard body surface area of 1.73m^2. It should be noted that the clearance formula is only valid for a steady state, i.e. when renal function is not changing rapidly.

The accurate measurement of creatinine clearance is difficult, especially in outpatients, since it is necessary to obtain a complete and accurately timed sample of urine. The usual collection time is 24 h, but patients may forget the time or forget to include some urine in the collection. Incontinent patients may find it impossible to make a urine collection. Patients have been known to add water or some other person's urine to their own collection, hoping to gain the doctor's approval for having been so prolific.

It may be more convenient and reliable to base the collection period on a patient's normal habits (e.g. overnight). The time at which the bladder is emptied before retiring to bed is noted; any urine passed during the night is collected as is the urine voided when the patient rises. The time is noted and a blood sample is taken that morning for the measurement of plasma creatinine. As long as the time over which the urine collection is made is known, and the collection is complete, any suitable time period can be used.

Creatinine is actively secreted by the renal tubules and, as a result, the creatinine clearance is higher than the true GFR. The difference is of little significance when the GFR is normal but when the GFR is low (<10 mL/min), tubular secretion makes a major contribution to creatinine excretion and creatinine clearance significantly over-estimates the GFR. The effect of creatinine breakdown in the gut also becomes significant when the GFR is very low. Lastly, in the calculation of creatinine clearance, two measurements of creatinine concentration and one of urine volume are required. Each of these has an inherent imprecision that can affect the accuracy of the overall result. Even in well-motivated subjects, studied under ideal conditions, the coefficient of variation of measure-ments of creatinine clearance can be as high as 10%, and it can be two or three times greater than this in ordinary patients.

Thus, although measurements of creatinine clearance are made frequently in clinical chemistry laboratories, they are potentially unreliable and should not be carried out unless there is a definite indication. In fact, accurate measurement of the GFR is required infrequently. Indications for its measurement include assessment of potential kidney donors, investigation of patients with minor abnormalities of renal function, and calculation of the initial doses of potentially toxic drugs that are eliminated from the body by renal excretion. An alter-native to a formal measurement of creatinine clearance is to calculate an estimate of the clearance from the serum creatinine concentration, using the Cockroft–Gault formula. This takes into account the effect of age, body weight and sex and obviates the imprecision arising from the need for an accurately timed and measured urine collection and the measurement of urine creatinine concentration, which are required for measurement of clearance. The formula is:

$$\text{Estimated clearance (mL/min)} = \frac{(140 - \text{age in years})(\text{weight in kg})}{\text{Serum [creatinine] in } \mu\text{mol/L} \times 0.81} \times \text{(for females) } 0.85$$

In practice, the majority of patients with established renal disease do not require repeated measurements of creatinine clearance: their renal function can be more reliably monitored by serial measurements of the plasma creatinine concentration (see below).

In hospitals with facilities for handling radioactive isotopes and measuring radioactivity, the technique of choice for measuring GFR is based on the injection of ^{51}Cr-labelled EDTA (ethylenediaminetetra-acetic acid) or ^{125}I-iothalamate. These substances are completely filtered by the glomeruli and are neither secreted nor reabsorbed by the tubules. Either serial blood samples are taken after injection of the isotope and the GFR is calculated from the rate of fall of plasma radioactivity as the isotope is cleared, or blood and urine are collected and the standard clearance formula used.

Plasma creatinine

Plasma creatinine concentration is the most reliable simple biochemical test of glomerular function. Ingestion of stewed meat can increase plasma creatinine concentration by as much as 30% seven hours after a meal and ideally blood samples should be collected after an overnight fast. Strenuous exercise also causes a transient, slight increase in plasma creatinine concen-tration. Plasma creatinine concentration is related to muscle bulk and therefore a concentration of 120 μmol/L could be normal for an athletic young man but would suggest renal impairment, though not necessarily of clinical significance, in a thin, 70-year-old woman. Although muscle bulk tends to decline with age, so too does the GFR and hence plasma creatinine concentra-tions remain fairly constant.

The reference range for plasma creatinine in the adult population is 60–120 μmol/L, but the day-to-day variation in an individual is much less than this range. Equation 4.1 indicates that plasma creatinine concen-tration is inversely related to the GFR. GFR can decrease by 50% before plasma creatinine concentration rises beyond the normal range; plasma creatinine concen-tration doubles for each further 50% fall in GFR. Consequently, a normal plasma creatinine does not necessarily imply normal renal function, although a raised creatinine does usually indicate impaired renal function (Fig. 4.3). Furthermore, a change in creatinine concentration, provided that it is outside the limits of normal biological and analytical variation, does suggest a change in GFR, even if both values are within the population reference range (see Case History 1.2).

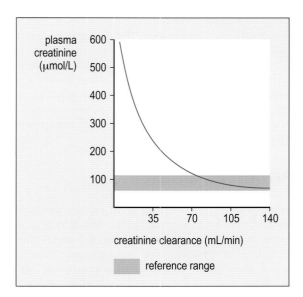

Fig. 4.3 Relationship between creatinine clearance and plasma creatinine concentration.

Causes of abnormal plasma urea to creatinine ratio	
Increased	**Decreased**
high protein intake	low protein intake
gastrointestinal bleeding	dialysis
hypercatabolic state	severe liver disease
dehydration	
urinary stasis	
muscle wasting*	
amputation*	

Fig. 4.4 Causes of an abnormal plasma urea to creatinine ratio. Causes of decreased creatinine synthesis; other conditions primarily affect urea concentration.

Changes in plasma creatinine concentration can occur, independently of renal function, due to changes in muscle mass. Thus a decrease can occur as a result of starvation and in wasting diseases, immediately after surgery and in patients treated with corticosteroids; an increase can occur during re-feeding. However, changes in creatinine concentration for these reasons rarely lead to diagnostic confusion.

In pregnancy the GFR increases. This usually more than balances the effect of increased creatinine synthesis during pregnancy and results in a decrease in plasma creatinine concentration.

Plasma urea

Urea is synthesized in the liver, primarily as a by-product of the deamination of amino acids. Its elimination in the urine represents the major route for nitrogen excretion. It is filtered from the blood at the glomerulus but significant tubular reabsorption occurs through passive diffusion.

Although plasma urea concentration is often used as an index of renal glomerular function, measurement of plasma creatinine provides a more accurate assessment. Urea production is increased by a high protein intake, in catabolic states, and by the absorption of amino acids and peptides after gastrointestinal haemorrhage. Conversely, production is decreased in patients with a low protein

intake and sometimes in patients with liver disease. Tubular reabsorption increases at low rates of urine flow (e.g. in fluid depletion) and this can cause increased plasma urea concentration even when renal function is normal.

Factors affecting the ratio of plasma urea to creatinine are summarized in *Fig. 4.4*. Changes in plasma urea concentration are a feature of renal impairment but it is important to consider possible extrarenal influences on urea concentrations before ascribing any changes to an alteration in renal function.

Urea diffuses readily across dialysis membranes and during renal dialysis a fall in plasma urea concentration is a poor guide to the efficacy of the process in removing other toxic substances from the blood.

Cystatin C

This low molecular weight peptide (13 kDa) is produced by all nucleated cells at a rate that is unaffected by inflammation and other pathological processes. It is cleared from the plasma by glomerular filtration and its plasma concentration reflects the GFR. It appears to provide a more sensitive indicator of decreased glomerular function than measurement of either plasma creatinine concentration or creatinine clearance, but at present it has been insufficiently evaluated to be adopted into routine practice in place of these measurements.

Assessment of glomerular integrity

Impairment of glomerular integrity results in the filtration of large molecules that are normally retained and is manifest as proteinuria. Proteinuria can, however, occur for other reasons (*see p. 78*).

With severe glomerular damage, red blood cells are detectable in the urine (haematuria). Whilst haematuria can occur as a result of lesions anywhere in the urinary tract, the red cells often have an abnormal morphology in glomerular disease. The presence of red cell casts (cells embedded in a proteinaceous matrix) in urinary sediment is strongly suggestive of glomerular dysfunction.

Tests of renal tubular function

Formal tests of renal tubular function are performed less frequently than tests of glomerular function. The presence of glycosuria in a subject with a normal blood glucose concentration implies proximal tubular malfunction which may be either isolated (renal glycosuria) or part of a generalized tubular defect (Fanconi syndrome). Amino aciduria can occur with tubular defects and can be investigated by amino acid chromatography. Tests of proximal tubular bicarbonate reabsorption may be required in the assessment of proximal renal tubular acidosis.

The only tests of distal tubular function in widespread use are the water deprivation test, to assess renal concentrating ability (*see p. 137*) and tests of urinary acidification, to diagnose distal renal tubular acidosis (*see p. 82*). The small amount of (principally low molecular weight) protein that is filtered by the glomeruli is normally absorbed by and catabolized in renal tubular cells. The presence of low molecular weight proteins in urine can indicate renal tubular damage. β_2-Microglobulin has been used for this purpose but is unstable in acidic urine. The measurement of α_2-microglobulin is more reliable but, in practice, specific evidence of tubular damage is rarely required clinically.

IMAGING AND RENAL BIOPSY

It is important to appreciate that biochemical tests of renal function are only one part of the repertoire of investigations available to the renal physician. Other techniques include: ultrasound (including Doppler studies to assess blood flow) and plain and contrast radiography (e.g. intravenous urography, arteriography), computerized tomography (CT) and magnetic resonance imaging (MRI), to provide anatomical information; static and dynamic isotope scanning, to provide functional information, and percutaneous renal biopsy, to provide a histopathological diagnosis. The detection of specific antibodies in serum (e.g. antiglomerular basement membrane antibodies, positive in Goodpasture's disease, a type of glomerulonephritis, and antineutrophil cytoplasmic antibodies, positive in systemic vasculitis) and other proteins (e.g. complement components, often low in systemic lupus erythematosus) can also provide valuable diagnostic information.

RENAL DISORDERS

Failure of renal function may occur rapidly, producing the syndrome of acute renal failure. This is potentially reversible since, if the patient survives the acute illness, normal renal function can be regained. However, chronic renal failure (CRF) develops insidiously, often over many years, and is irreversible, leading eventually to end-stage renal failure. Patients with end-stage renal failure require either long-term renal replacement treatment (i.e. dialysis) or a successful renal transplant in order to survive. Biochemical tests are essential to the management of renal failure, but seldom provide information of help in determining its cause.

The term 'glomerulonephritis' encompasses a group of renal diseases that are characterized by pathological changes in the glomeruli with an immunological basis, such as immune complex deposition. Glomerulonephritis may present in many ways: for example, as an acute nephritic syndrome with haematuria, hypertension and oedema, as acute or chronic renal failure, or as proteinuria leading to the nephrotic syndrome (proteinuria, hypoproteinaemia and oedema).

Many disorders primarily affect renal tubular function, but most are rare. Their metabolic and clinical consequences range from being trivial (as in isolated renal glycosuria), to being serious (as in cystinuria, *see p. 305*).

Acute renal failure

Acute renal failure (ARF) is characterized by a rapid loss of renal function, with retention of urea, creatinine, hydrogen ions and other metabolic products and, usually but not always, oliguria (<400 mL urine/24 h). Although potentially reversible, the consequences to homoeostatic mechanisms are so profound that this condition continues to be associated with a high mortality. Furthermore, ARF often develops in patients who are already severely ill.

Case history 4.1

A young man sustained multiple injuries in a motorcycle accident. He received blood transfusions and underwent surgery; 24 h after admission he had only passed 500 mL of urine. He was clinically dehydrated and his blood pressure was 90/50 mmHg.

Investigations

serum:	potassium	5.6 mmol/L
	urea	21.0 mmol/L
	creatinine	140 μmol/L
urine:	sodium	5 mmol/L
	urea	480 mmol/L

Comment

The diagnosis is prerenal uraemia. The urine contains little sodium and the urea has been concentrated by a factor of 22. These are normal physiological responses, implying that intrinsic renal function is intact and that the ability of the kidneys to function normally is constrained only by hypoperfusion. Osmolality was not measured, but in prerenal uraemia the urine to plasma osmolality ratio is characteristically greater than 1.5:1.

The distinguishing features of prerenal as opposed to intrinsic renal failure are listed in *Fig. 4.5*. These figures are not absolutely reliable. They are all invalidated if the patient has been given diuretics, and osmolalities are invalidated by the use of X-ray contrast media. In practice, it is often not possible to distinguish between prerenal and intrinsic renal failure using biochemical tests; furthermore, if untreated, prerenal failure progresses to intrinsic renal failure. A concentrated, sodium-poor urine is a more reliable indicator of prerenal uraemia than a dilute sodium-containing urine is of intrinsic renal failure, since the latter is appropriate for a well-hydrated healthy person. However, oliguria, although usually present, is not a constant feature of acute renal failure.

The increase in serum urea concentration in this patient is greater than the increase in creatinine. This is due in part both to passive reabsorption of urea and to increased synthesis from amino acids released as a result of tissue damage. The patient was given extra fluid intravenously and this resulted in a diuresis. The elicitation of this response is the only certain way of distinguishing prerenal from intrinsic renal failure. His serum urea and creatinine were normal 48 h later.

	Prerenal failure	Intrinsic failure
Urine sodium concentration	<20 mmol/L	>40 mmol/L
Urine:plasma urea concentration	>20:1	<10:1
Urine:plasma osmolality	>1.5:1	<1.1:1

Fig. 4.5 Biochemical values in oliguria due to prerenal and intrinsic renal failure. Intermediate values occur in incipient intrinsic renal failure.

ARF is conventionally divided into three categories, according to whether renal functional impairment is related to a decrease in renal blood flow (prerenal), to intrinsic damage to the kidneys (intrinsic), or to urinary tract obstruction (postrenal). Should any of these occur in a patient whose renal function is already impaired, the consequences are likely to be more serious. Some clues to the presence of chronic disease in a patient with ARF ('acute on chronic' renal failure) are discussed in *Case History 4.3*.

The term 'uraemia' (meaning 'urine in the blood') is often used as a synonym for renal failure (both acute and chronic). 'Azotaemia' is used in similar context and refers to an increase in the blood concentration of nitrogenous compounds.

Prerenal acute renal failure

This is caused by circulatory insufficiency, as may occur with severe haemorrhage, burns, fluid loss, cardiac failure or hypotension that leads to renal hypoperfusion and a decrease in GFR. Renal hypoperfusion induces intense renal vasoconstriction, which initially results in a decrease in GFR with relative preservation of tubular function. However, if adequate perfusion is not rapidly restored, prerenal uraemia may progress to intrinsic failure (acute tubular necrosis). It may be possible to prevent this if renal perfusion can be restored before structural damage has occurred.

Prerenal uraemia is essentially the result of a normal physiological response to hypovolaemia or a fall in blood pressure. Stimulation of the renin–angiotensin–aldosterone system and vasopressin secretion results in the production of a small volume of highly concentrated urine with a low sodium concentration. Renal tubular function is normal, but the decreased GFR results in the retention of substances normally excreted by filtration, such as urea and creatinine. Decreased excretion of hydrogen ions results in a tendency to metabolic acidosis, and of potassium to hyperkalaemia (often exacerbated by tissue damage and acidosis).

Intrinsic acute renal failure

A wide variety of conditions can cause intrinsic ARF (*Fig. 4.6*). Many cases are due to nephrotoxic drugs (e.g. aminoglycosides and non-steroidal anti-inflammatory drugs) or renal ischaemia secondary to hypoperfusion, leading to acute tubular necrosis. Causes include sepsis, severe haemorrhage, burns and cardiac failure. Specific renal diseases and systemic diseases affecting the kidneys are also important. The pathogenesis of this condition is complex: in any individual case several factors may be involved.

Although glomerular damage is uncommon in acute tubular necrosis, the GFR falls owing to glomerular hypoperfusion, itself a result of afferent arteriolar vaso-constriction. Failure of the GFR to recover after correction of the circulatory deficit is common. Contributory factors include intrarenal release of vasoactive substances, obstruction of the tubular lumen by debris and casts, or by interstitial oedema, and back-leak of glomerular filtrate through damaged tubular epithelium.

The characteristic biochemical changes in the plasma in ARF are summarized in *Fig. 4.7*. Hyponatraemia is common. It is due primarily to an excess of water relative to sodium: contributory factors may include

Intrinsic acute renal failure	
Causes	**Examples**
specific renal diseases and systemic disease affecting kidneys	rapidly progressive glomerulonephritis systemic lupus erythematosus
nephrotoxins	non-steroidal anti-inflammatory drugs (NSAIDs) aminoglycosides cephalosporins cis-platinum many other drugs and toxins
renal hypoperfusion	hypotension haemorrhage septicaemia low cardiac output burns crush injuries
intrarenal obstruction	Bence Jones protein

Fig. 4.6 Causes of acute renal failure.

Biochemical changes in plasma in acute renal failure	
Increased	**Decreased**
potassium urea creatinine phosphate magnesium hydrogen ion urate	sodium bicarbonate calcium

Fig. 4.7 Biochemical changes in plasma in acute renal failure.

increased water formation from oxidative metabolism, decreased excretion, continued intake of water or injudicious fluid administration. Hyperkalaemia occurs as a result of decreased excretion of potassium together with both a loss of intracellular potassium to the ECF (due to tissue breakdown) and intracellular buffering of retained hydrogen ions. In severe cases, plasma potassium concentration can increase by 1–2 mmol/L in a few hours, although the rise is usually less rapid. Decreased hydrogen ion excretion causes a non-respiratory acidosis.

Retention of phosphate and leakage of intracellular phosphate into the interstitial fluid leads to hyper-phosphataemia, which inhibits the 1α-hydroxylation of 25-hydroxycholecalciferol to calcitriol (*see p. 222*). The resulting decreased plasma concentration of calcitriol causes skeletal resistance to the actions of parathyroid hormone, causing hypocalcaemia. Hypercalcaemia in the oliguric phase of ARF suggests a diagnosis of malignancy (*see p. 224*). Hypermagnesaemia is also often present as a result of decreased magnesium excretion. In established ARF, what urine is produced has a similar osmolality and ionic composition to plasma. Proteinuria is always present and the urine is often dark, owing to the presence of haem pigments from the blood.

There are typically three phases to the course of acute tubular necrosis: the initial oliguric phase, a diuretic phase and a recovery phase. The oliguric phase typically lasts for 8–10 days but sometimes is much shorter or persists for several weeks. In an apparently increasing number of patients, there is no oliguric phase. Non-oliguric renal failure is particularly associated with aminoglycoside nephrotoxicity and burns. In general, it has a better prognosis than oliguric renal failure. When it occurs, the oliguric phase is followed by a diuretic phase, with increasing urine volume. This is due to an increase in GFR and initially there is often little improvement in tubular function. The composition of the urine is similar to that of protein-free plasma. During this phase, urine volume may exceed 5 L per day and, because of its high ionic concentration, there is a considerable risk of both dehydration and depletion of sodium and potassium.

Although the onset of the diuretic phase often heralds clinical improvement, plasma concentrations of urea and creatinine do not fall immediately since the GFR is still much lower than normal and insufficient to allow excretion of the surplus. The persisting high urea concentration in the blood, and hence in the glomerular filtrate, contributes to the diuresis by an osmotic effect. The acidosis also persists until tubular function is restored. Plasma calcium concentration may rise during this phase, particularly after crush injuries, owing to the release of calcium from damaged muscle. Temporary persistence of any elevation in the plasma concentration

Case history 4.2

A young man was admitted to hospital with severe abdominal injuries after being knocked down by a car. On examination, he was severely shocked with a swollen, tender abdomen. He was given intravenous fluids and blood, and was taken to the operating theatre. At laparotomy, his spleen was found to be ruptured: splenectomy was performed. There was also mesenteric damage and a tear in the duodenum: the damaged gut was resected.

Three days later he became hypotensive and pyrexial and was taken back to theatre. Free fluid was present in the peritoneal cavity and a leak was found in a segment of gangrenous small intestine. Appropriate surgical procedures were performed. Following this, the patient became oliguric despite adequate hydration.

Investigations

serum:		
	sodium	128 mmol/L
	potassium	5.9 mmol/L
	bicarbonate	16 mmol/L
	urea	22.0 mmol/L
	creatinine	225 μmol/L
	calcium	1.72 mmol/L
	phosphate	2.96 mmol/L
	albumin	28 g/L
urine:	urea	50 mmol/L
	sodium	80 mmol/L

Comment

These findings are typical of ARF in a septic, catabolic patient (*see Fig. 4.7*). He was treated with regular haemodialysis and parenteral nutrition; antibiotics were continued and his pyrexia settled. Eight days after the accident, the patient's urine output began to increase as shown in *Fig. 4.8*. The biochemical changes that occurred before and after the diuretic phase, until recovery of normal renal function, are also shown in *Fig. 4.8*.

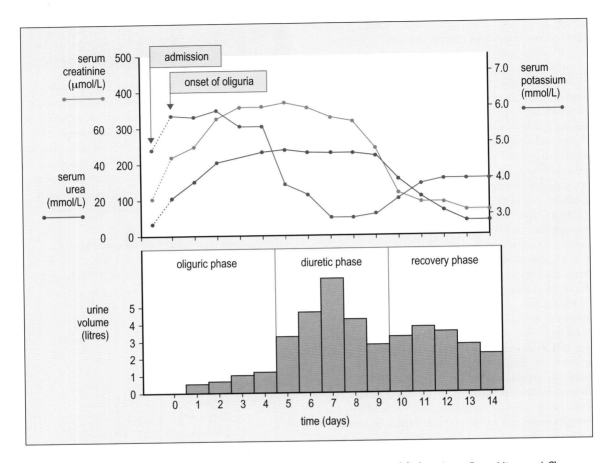

Fig. 4.8 Serum urea, creatinine and potassium in a case of acute renal failure (*see Case History 4.2*).

of parathyroid hormone will stimulate calcitriol synthesis and this may also contribute to hypercalcaemia.

Gradually, in the recovery phase, as the tubular cells regenerate and tubular function is restored, the diuresis subsides and the various abnormalities of renal function resolve. Patients who survive the acute illness usually recover completely. Some residual impairment of renal function is often demonstrable but it is not usually of clinical significance and may not be apparent from simple tests.

In very severe cases of ARF, particularly when pregnancy-related (e.g. due to antepartum haemorrhage), the ischaemic insult to the kidneys may exceed their regenerative capacity: there is renal cortical necrosis and no recovery of renal function. A type of renal failure occurring in patients with chronic liver disease is discussed in *Chapter 5*.

Postrenal renal failure

Obstruction to the flow of urine leads to an increase in hydrostatic pressure, which opposes glomerular filtration and, if prolonged, leads to secondary renal tubular damage. Causes of obstruction include renal calculi, prostatic enlargement (hypertrophic or neoplastic), other neoplasms of the urinary tract and retroperitoneal fibrosis. Obstruction that occurs above the level of the vesicourethral junction must be bilateral to have a major effect on urine flow. Complete anuria is rare with ARF from other causes and so is strongly indicative of the presence of obstruction. More often, however, obstruction is either intermittent or incomplete and urine production may even be normal in obstruction with overflow. The degree of reversibility of renal damage in obstructive renal failure depends to some extent on how longstanding it has been. It is more likely to be reversible if the obstruction is acute.

Management of ARF

Obstruction should always be excluded in a patient with renal failure, for example by ultrasound examination. If present, obstruction should either be relieved or, if this is not immediately possible, urinary drainage should be established by an appropriate procedure.

Many cases of intrinsic renal failure are preventable and, if a patient is judged to be in the prerenal phase, it is important to attempt to halt the progression to acute tubular necrosis by measures to improve renal perfusion (e.g. expansion of ECF volume). Volume repletion should be monitored by measurements of central venous pressure. Hypoxaemia, if present, must be corrected. Additional measures that can be employed include the judicious use of furosemide (frusemide), a loop diuretic, and/or low-dose dopamine, although there is only limited evidence of benefit from either.

If oliguria persists and acute tubular necrosis is diagnosed, it becomes necessary to minimize the severe adverse consequences of renal failure. The general principles of treatment include: strict control of sodium and water intake, to maintain normovolaemia; nutritional support, with some limitation of protein but adequate carbohydrate to minimize endogenous protein break-down; prevention of metabolic complications, such as hyperkalaemia and acidosis, and prevention of infection. Care should be taken to avoid the use of potentially nephrotoxic drugs.

When renal failure is short-lived and in non-oliguric acute renal failure, conservative measures alone may suffice. However, the majority of patients will require renal replacement treatment (e.g. haemofiltration or haemodialysis). The decision to start such treatment is usually primarily clinical, although laboratory data are also informative. In general, renal replacement should be started sooner rather than later. Factors that will prompt the decision include any of: evidence of uraemic encephalopathy; severe fluid overload; severe hyperkalaemia (e.g. plasma potassium >6.5 mmol/L); severe acidosis (e.g. $[HCO_3^-]$ <12 mmol/L, $[H^+]$ >80 nmol/L) or high (or rapidly rising) concentrations of urea (e.g. >730 mmol/L) or creatinine (e.g. >500 µmol/L).

Dialysis or haemofiltration may have to be continued into the early part of the diuretic phase until the GFR has recovered sufficiently for the plasma concentration of creatinine to start falling. The main problem during the diuretic phase is to supply sufficient water and electrolytes to compensate for the excessive losses. Fluid replacement should not automatically be isovolaemic since the diuresis is partly due to mobilization and excretion of excess ECF. From the onset of ARF until its resolution, it is essential to monitor the patient's plasma creatinine, sodium, potassium, bicarbonate, calcium and phosphate concentrations, urinary volume and sodium and potassium excretion.

The general principles of management are similar whatever the cause of ARF. In addition, specific measures may be indicated for certain diseases, for example the control of infection or hypertension and the use of immunosuppressive drugs in immunologically mediated renal disease.

Chronic renal failure

Many disease processes can lead to progressive, irreversible impairment of renal function. Glomerulonephritis, diabetes mellitus, hypertension, pyelonephritis and polycystic kidneys account for the majority of cases where a cause can be determined. In effect, all these conditions lead to a decrease in the number of functioning nephrons. Patients may remain asymptomatic until the GFR falls below 15 mL/min or lower. The natural history is of progression to end-stage renal failure, the state when conservative measures are no longer sufficient and dialysis or transplantation becomes necessary to save the patient's life. The time between presentation and end-stage renal failure is very variable: it may be a matter of weeks or as long as several years. In most patients, a graph of the reciprocal of serum creatinine concentration plotted against time approximates to a straight line. Such plots allow the physician to predict when renal replacement treatment is likely to become necessary. An increase in the slope (indicating an increase in the rate of deterioration of renal function) should alert the physician to a potentially treatable cause (e.g. hypovolaemia or infection).

Consequences

The major pathological and clinical features are similar in all patients with CRF, whatever the cause. The metabolic features are summarized in *Fig. 4.9*. Although there is impairment of urinary concentration, polyuria is never gross (not more than 4 L per day) because the GFR is so low. The urine tends to be of constant osmolality. The lack of urinary concentration is

End-stage renal disease		
Metabolic features	**Biochemical changes in plasma**	
impairment of urinary concentration and dilution	**Increased**	**Decreased**
impairment of electrolyte and hydrogen ion homoeostasis	potassium	sodium
retention of waste products of metabolism	urea	bicarbonate
decreased calcitriol synthesis	creatinine	calcium
decreased erythropoietin synthesis	hydrogen ion	
	phosphate	
	magnesium	

Fig 4.9 Metabolic and biochemical consequences of end-stage renal disease.

particularly noticed by the patient at night and nocturia is a common complaint. The ability to dilute the urine may be lost late in the course of renal failure and patients become very sensitive to the effects of either fluid loss or overload.

Sodium balance is usually maintained until the GFR falls below 20 mL/min. The majority of patients tend to retain sodium but severe renal sodium wasting is occasionally seen. This syndrome of 'salt-losing nephritis' occurs most often in patients whose renal disease particularly affects the tubules, for example analgesic nephropathy, polycystic disease and chronic pyelonephritis.

Hyperkalaemia is a late feature of CRF; it may be precipitated by a sudden deterioration in renal function or by the injudicious use of potassium-sparing diuretics.

Patients with CRF tend to be acidotic. The urinary buffering capacity is impaired as a result of decreased phosphate excretion and ammonia synthesis. The ability of individual nephrons to reabsorb filtered bicarbonate is often impaired, probably, in part, as an effect of the raised plasma concentration of parathyroid hormone (*see p. 222*). However, although plasma hydrogen ion concentration increases and bicarbonate decreases, these changes progress only slowly, owing to buffering of excess hydrogen ions in bone.

Most patients with CRF become hypocalcaemic and, in time, many develop renal osteodystrophy. This comprises secondary hyperparathyroidism or osteomalacia or both ('mixed renal osteodystrophy'). A fourth type, adynamic bone disease, characterized by reduced trabecular bone formation and resorption, is increasingly being recognized, particularly in patients given calcitriol or other 1α-hydroxylated derivatives of vitamin D.

The pathogenesis of renal osteodystrophy is complex (*Fig. 4.10*). Retention of phosphate causes a tendency to hyperphosphataemia, inhibiting calcitriol synthesis and leading to hypocalcaemia through a reduction in intestinal calcium absorption. Hypocalcaemia stimulates parathyroid hormone (PTH) secretion (secondary hyperparathyroidism). Other factors are also implicated in the increased secretion of PTH: reduced concentrations of calcitriol increase PTH synthesis through a direct effect on gene expression, and in advanced renal failure, the binding of calcitriol to its receptors in the parathyroid glands is inhibited. Decreased concentrations of calcitriol may also contribute to the resistance to the action of PTH on bone that occurs in advanced renal failure. High concentrations of PTH decrease the reabsorption of phosphate from each nephron, but eventually the falling GFR becomes the limiting factor in phosphate excretion and persistent hyperphosphataemia ensues. If the concentration of phosphate becomes so high that the solubility product of calcium and phosphate ($[Ca^{2+}] \times [Pi]$) is exceeded, metastatic calcification may occur. This is seen particularly in blood vessels and may in part contribute to the sclerotic deposits that can occur in bone. With advanced renal failure, the decrease in functioning renal tissue may also contribute to the decrease in calcitriol production. Another factor of importance is buffering of hydrogen ions by bone, which leads to demineralization.

Aluminium can cause osteomalacia. In the past, the presence of aluminium in softened water used to prepare dialysis fluid has caused problems, as has the absorption of aluminium from orally administered salts given to bind phosphate in the gut and prevent hyperphosphataemia.

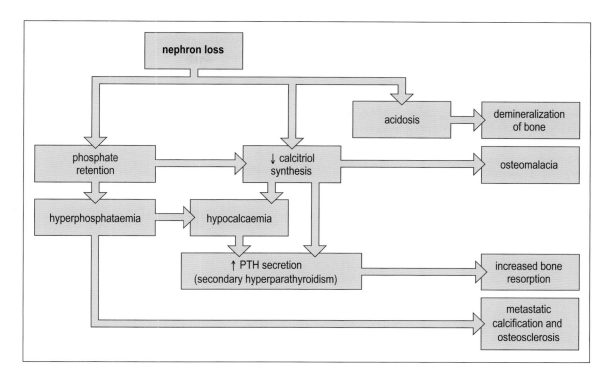

Fig. 4.10 Pathogenesis of renal osteodystrophy.

In addition to the effect on calcitriol synthesis, other endocrine consequences of chronic renal failure include decreased testosterone and oestrogen synthesis, abnormalities of thyroid function tests (seldom, however, associated with clinical thyroid disease), and abnormal glucose tolerance with hyperinsulinaemia due to insulin resistance. However, insulin-dependent diabetic patients who develop renal disease often have decreased insulin requirements since insulin is metabolized in the kidney.

A normochromic normocytic anaemia is usual in end-stage renal failure, owing to depression of bone marrow function by retained toxins and a decrease in the renal production of erythropoietin. A bleeding tendency may also be present and bleeding may exacerbate the anaemia.

Management of chronic renal failure

If the cause of CRF can be determined, appropriate treatment may reduce the rate of further loss of renal function, but seldom prevents it. Patients usually progress inexorably to end-stage renal failure but, before dialysis or transplantation becomes necessary, considerable amelioration of symptoms and biochemical abnormalities can be obtained by conservative measures.

Since the kidneys become unable to control water and sodium balance, it is essential that intake is matched to obligatory losses. Diuretics are often used to promote sodium excretion, since adequate dietary salt restriction may be unacceptable to the patient. At the same time, volume depletion must be avoided: it decreases renal blood flow and thus the GFR.

Hypertension is a frequent complication of CRF and also exacerbates it. Angiotensin-converting enzyme (ACE) inhibitors have been shown to reduce the rate of progression of renal impairment in patients with diabetic nephropathy independently of their effect on blood pressure and may be beneficial in renal failure from other causes. However, in patients with renal artery stenosis or advanced renal failure, ACE inhibitors can cause deterioration in function and hyperkalaemia. Patients' plasma creatinine and potassium concentrations

Case history 4.3

A 56-year-old man presented to his family doctor with weight loss, generalized weakness and lethargy of six months' duration. During this time, he had been passing more urine than usual, particularly at night. He had become impotent. On examination, the patient was found to be slightly anaemic and had a blood pressure of 180/110 mmHg. His urine contained protein but no glucose. A blood sample was taken for analysis.

Investigations

serum:		
	sodium	130 mmol/L
	potassium	5.2 mmol/L
	bicarbonate	16 mmol/L
	urea	43.0 mmol/L
	creatinine	640 µmol/L
	glucose (random)	6.4 mmol/L
	calcium	1.92 mmol/L
	phosphate	2.42 mmol/L
	alkaline phosphatase	205 U/L
	haemoglobin	9.1 g/dL

Comment

The doctor's first thought was that this patient had diabetes mellitus, but the absence of glycosuria militated against this and the results are typical of chronic renal failure. The history suggests slowly progressive, rather than acute, renal failure. The presence of anaemia and the raised alkaline phosphatase (due to renal osteodystrophy) are consistent with this diagnosis, although they are not specific findings.

The kidneys are small in most cases of chronic renal failure (unless due to amyloid or polycystic disease) and the demonstration of small kidneys by radiography or ultrasonography in a patient with renal disease is another indicator of chronicity. So, too, is the presence of hypertension.

Many other clinical features may be present in patients with end-stage renal disease (*Fig. 4.11*). The causes of many of these features are unknown, but they are presumably related to the retention of toxins which cannot be excreted. These 'uraemic toxins' include phenolic acids, polypeptides, polyamines and many other substances.

Clinical features of chronic renal failure

Neurological
lethargy
peripheral neuropathy

Musculoskeletal
growth failure
bone pain
myopathy

Gastrointestinal
anorexia
hiccough
nausea and vomiting
gastrointestinal bleeding

Cardiovascular
anaemia
hypertension
pericarditis

Dermal
pruritus
pallor
purpura

Genitourinary
nocturia
impotence

Fig. 4.11 Clinical features of chronic renal failure.

should be measured 1–2 weeks after starting treatment or increasing the dose.

Bicarbonate can be given orally to control acidosis. Hyperkalaemia is usually of less significance in CRF than in ARF, because it develops more slowly. It can usually be controlled with oral ion-exchange resins given in their calcium or sodium forms. Hyperphosphataemia can be controlled by giving oral calcium carbonate (which also helps correct acidosis). Osteodystrophy can be prevented, or treated if it does develop, by giving calcitriol or other 1α-hydroxylated derivatives of vitamin D, but care is necessary to avoid provoking hypercalcaemia.

Some limitation of dietary protein is beneficial to reduce the formation of nitrogenous waste products, but the limitation should not usually be so severe as to cause negative nitrogen balance. In patients who are not candidates for maintenance dialysis or transplantation, however, a very low protein intake can cause considerable symptomatic improvement in the terminal stage of renal failure, and may even slow the rate of decline in renal function. It is important to maintain an adequate intake of essential amino acids and carbohydrate.

Treatment of anaemia with recombinant erythropoietin has considerably improved the quality of life for patients on dialysis; it may also be used pre-dialysis, but with caution, as it can exacerbate hypertension.

The major cause of death in patients with CRF is cardiovascular disease. In addition to treating hypertension, other cardiovascular risk factors should be managed appropriately. Dyslipidaemia is common in patients with CRF; treatment may both reduce the risk of cardiovascular disease and help to preserve renal function.

Renal replacement treatment

Renal replacement treatment may be required for patients with ARF (*see p. 73*) and for patients with end-stage renal failure. Techniques include dialysis, haemofiltration and combinations of the two and, in patients with end-stage renal failure, transplantation. Dialysis-related techniques do not replace the endocrine functions of the kidney: patients on long-term dialysis require treatment with erythropoietin and vitamin D derivatives, and must follow a special diet. Patients who successfully undergo renal transplantation are free of these restrictions, but must take immunosuppressive drugs to prevent rejection.

The principle of dialysis is that blood is exposed to dialysis fluid from which it is separated by a semipermeable membrane. In haemodialysis, an extracorporeal circuit and artificial membrane are used and substances move from the plasma to the dialysate by diffusion. A controlled pressure gradient can be used to remove fluid. In peritoneal dialysis, dialysate is instilled into the peritoneal cavity, and the peritoneum acts as the semipermeable membrane. Haemodialysis is usually performed intermittently; peritoneal dialysis can be intermittent but is often performed continuously.

In haemofiltration, a membrane capable of a high rate of fluid transfer is used but there is no dialysis fluid. A pressure gradient, which can be generated in various ways, drives fluid and solutes across the membrane by a process called convection. Fluid and electrolyte balance is maintained by infusion of a suitable fluid into the extracorporeal circuit. Haemofiltration is usually performed continuously. The technique of haemodiafiltration removes fluid and solutes by a combination of diffusion and convection.

The factors governing the choice of renal replacement technique are complex. In ARF, the preferred technique is usually semicontinuous haemofiltration or haemodiafiltration; most patients with end-stage renal failure requiring chronic renal replacement are treated by intermittent haemodialysis (typically three times weekly) or peritoneal dialysis. Peritoneal dialysis is usually performed continuously (continuous ambulatory peritoneal dialysis, CAPD) and involves exchanges of 2 L of fluid three to four times daily. CAPD is a relatively simple technique and can be performed without specialized equipment. In CAPD, the dialysate is made hypertonic with glucose to facilitate removal of fluid, but diffusion of this glucose into the patient can lead to diabetes and hypertriglyceridaemia. Peritoneal dialysis can also lead to loss of protein. All renal replacement techniques can lead to loss of amino acids, trace minerals and vitamins.

Clearance rates by diffusion fall off rapidly with increasing molecular weight, but convection, which more nearly reflects normal glomerular function, allows fairly uniform clearance of all substances that can pass through the semipermeable membrane, typically decreasing significantly only with molecular weights exceeding 10 kDa. However, since the 'uraemic toxins' are primarily low molecular weight substances, dialysis is an effective technique for renal replacement.

The efficacy of dialysis in end-stage renal failure can be measured by calculating the function Kt/V, where K is the urea clearance of the dialyser, t is the dialysis time and V is the volume of distribution of urea (equal to the total body water). Kt/V correlates with outcome: effective symptom control requires a value of Kt/V of 1 or more, that is the urea clearance per session should be equal to total body water. Current targets in the UK are a value of Kt/V of >1.2 in patients on thrice weekly haemodialysis, and >1.7 in patients on CAPD.

Patients who have undergone transplantation require careful clinical and biochemical monitoring to assess graft function and to provide warning of incipient graft rejection. Features of graft rejection include oliguria and pyrexia but these may not be present and a rise in plasma creatinine concentration may be the first sign. However, an increase in creatinine can also occur with nephrotoxicity due to ciclosporin, a frequently used immunosuppressive drug. Indicators of tubular damage, for example the urinary activity of the tubular enzyme N-acetyl-glucosaminidase, have been studied as possible indicators of early rejection, but none is specific to the process and they are not widely used.

Proteinuria and the nephrotic syndrome

The glomeruli normally filter 7–10 g of protein per 24 h, but almost all is reabsorbed by endocytosis and subsequently catabolized in the proximal tubules. Normal urinary protein excretion is less than about 150 mg/24 h. Approximately half of this is Tamm–Horsfall protein, a glycoprotein secreted by tubular cells; less than 30 mg is albumin.

The presence or absence of proteinuria is usually assessed using a reagent-impregnated strip (dip-stick), which is dipped into the urine. This reliably detects albumin at concentrations greater than 200 mg/L but is less sensitive to other proteins. False positive results are obtained with urine that is alkaline, contaminated by various antiseptics or contains X-ray contrast media. It should be appreciated that a particular concentration of protein will be more significant if a large volume of urine is being produced, since it will represent a greater total excretion than if urine volume is low.

The mechanisms of proteinuria are summarized in *Fig. 4.12*. Glomerular proteinuria may be sufficiently gross to cause hypoproteinaemia and oedema (the nephrotic syndrome).

Mechanisms of proteinuria

Overflow
due to presence in plasma of a high concentration of a low molecular weight protein, which is filtered in a quantity exceeding tubular reabsorptive capacity, e.g. Bence Jones protein

Glomerular
due to increased glomerular permeability, e.g. albumin

Tubular
due to impaired or saturated reabsorption of protein filtered by normal glomeruli, e.g. β_2-microglobulin

Secreted
due to secretion by kidneys or epithelium of urinary tract, e.g. Tamm–Horsfall protein

Fig. 4.12 Mechanisms of proteinuria.

Investigation of proteinuria

If a patient's urine gives a positive reaction for protein using a dip-stick, the presence of protein should be confirmed by an independent test in the laboratory. If Bence Jones proteinuria is suspected, a specific test must be used since this protein is not detectable by dip-stick. Before investigating renal function, incidental extrarenal causes of proteinuria, such as fever, strenuous exercise and burns, should be excluded: such proteinuria is usually not of long-term significance. Orthostatic proteinuria (*see below*) should also be excluded.

When the presence of proteinuria has been confirmed, urinary protein excretion should be measured and simple tests of renal function, measurement of complement (C3) and renal ultrasound performed. If the results are all normal and protein excretion is less than 500 mg/24 h, the patient need not be subjected to further investigation but should be followed up. With protein excretion in excess of this, or with abnormal test results, further investigation, usually including biopsy, is necessary to determine the cause. Proteinuria in excess of 2 g/24 h is virtually always pathological and usually signifies glomerular disease.

Orthostatic proteinuria is a benign condition in which proteinuria is present only when subjects are upright. It occurs in approximately 5% of young adults. The prevalence decreases with increasing age. Orthostatic proteinuria occurs as a result of an increase in the hydrostatic pressure in the renal veins, itself a result of pressure of the liver on the inferior vena cava. It is of no clinical significance and can confidently be diagnosed if a sample of urine collected immediately on rising in the morning is protein-free.

Electrophoresis of a concentrated specimen of urine may help to distinguish between the various types of proteinuria. In tubular proteinuria, for example, the predominant proteins are of low molecular weight, being filtered proteins that are incompletely reabsorbed. In glomerular proteinuria, higher molecular weight proteins are present. Electrophoresis of concentrated urine is the best technique for the detection of Bence Jones proteinuria.

In minimal change glomerulonephritis, the most frequent cause of nephrotic syndrome in children, the proteinuria is typically highly selective – that is, higher molecular weight proteins tend to be retained – while in most other causes of the condition both high and low molecular weight proteins are excreted (low selectivity).

Measurement of selectivity, by comparing the clearances of IgG and albumin or transferrin, used to be used to indicate whether nephrotic syndrome was caused by minimal change glomerulonephritis, and to avoid the need for biopsy to make the diagnosis. However, the relationship is not constant, and most renal physicians now routinely treat nephrotic syndrome in children with steroids in the first instance, and only biopsy non-responders. Minimal change disease is less common as a cause of nephrotic syndrome in adults, and biopsy is usually considered essential.

The nephrotic syndrome

Hypoproteinaemia with oedema may develop if large amounts of protein are excreted in the urine. For this to occur, proteinuria must usually exceed 5 g/24 h. Although the ability of the liver to synthesize protein is greater than this, much of the filtered protein is catabolized after endocytosis by renal tubular cells and is thus lost from the circulation, even though it is not excreted in the urine. Conditions in which the nephrotic syndrome may occur are shown in *Fig. 4.13*.

The amount of proteinuria is not necessarily a useful guide to the severity of renal disease; for example, in minimal change glomerulonephritis, which has a good prognosis, the proteinuria may exceed that seen in patients with more aggressive glomerular lesions.

The clinical and biochemical features of the nephrotic syndrome are summarized in *Fig. 4.13*. There are two aspects to management: treatment of the underlying disorder, where the disorder can be identified and treatment is possible, and treatment of the consequences of protein loss. Minimal change glomerulonephritis often responds to corticosteroids or immunosuppressive drugs, but other types of glomerulonephritis are generally much less responsive to treatment.

General measures to counteract the consequences of protein loss include a high protein, low salt diet, although decreased appetite and impaired absorption of nutrients owing to oedema of the gut may be limiting factors. A high protein intake must be introduced with caution when there is concurrent renal failure. It is important not to cause too rapid a diuresis since this can lead to hypovolaemia and thus impair renal function; potassium depletion must also be avoided. Spironolactone is the diuretic of first choice, but thiazides or furosemide (frusemide) may be necessary in addition. Prevention of infection is vital and antibiotics are often administered prophylactically. The risk of thrombosis, especially renal vein thrombosis, which may cause a rapid increase in proteinuria, may warrant the prophylactic use of anticoagulants.

The nephrotic syndrome		
Causes	**Clinical and biochemical features**	
	Feature	**Mechanism**
minimal change glomerulonephritis membranous glomerulonephritis: idiopathic	proteinuria	glomerular damage
	oedema	low plasma albumin secondary hyperaldosteronism
associated with carcinoma, drugs or infection, e.g. malaria, hepatitis B	increased susceptibility to infection	low plasma immunoglobulins and complement
systemic lupus erythematosus	thrombotic tendency	hyperfibrinogenaemia and low antithrombin III
diabetic nephropathy		
other forms of glomerulonephritis	hyperlipidaemia	increased apolipoprotein synthesis

Fig. 4.13 The nephrotic syndrome: causes and clinical and biochemical features.

Case history 4.4

An 8-year-old girl was admitted to hospital with generalized oedema. Her urine had become frothy and the family doctor had found proteinuria.

Investigations

serum:	sodium	130 mmol/L
	potassium	3.6 mmol/L
	bicarbonate	32 mmol/L
	urea	2.0 mmol/L
	creatinine	45 μmol/L
	calcium	1.70 mmol/L
	total protein	35 g/L
	albumin	15 g/L
	triglyceride	16 mmol/L
	cholesterol	12 mmol/L
24 h urine protein excretion		12 g

The serum was grossly lipaemic.

Comment

The presence of proteinuria, hypoproteinaemia and oedema constitutes the nephrotic syndrome. The oedema is, in part, a result of redistribution of ECF between the vascular and interstitial compartments; secondary aldosteronism, with evidence of potassium depletion, is often present as a consequence.

Loss of protein is not confined to albumin. Plasma concentrations of hormone-binding proteins, transferrin and antithrombin III are also reduced. On the other hand, there is usually an increase in the concentrations of high molecular weight proteins such as α_2-macroglobulin, coagulation factors (fibrinogen, factor VIII, etc.) and the apolipoproteins. The increase in apolipoproteins causes secondary hypercholesterolaemia and hypertriglyceridaemia and these may in turn cause spurious hyponatraemia. In adults with persistent nephrotic syndrome, accelerated atherosclerosis may develop. Changes in the concentrations of coagulation factors can predispose to venous thrombosis, particularly in the renal veins. The hypocalcaemia is related in part to decreased protein binding and in part to renal excretion of vitamin D metabolites bound to vitamin D-binding globulin. Loss of immunoglobulins and complement components renders patients with nephrotic syndrome very susceptible to infection.

The GFR may be low, normal or increased in patients with the nephrotic syndrome. In minimal change glomerulonephritis, it is often increased and the low urea and creatinine concentrations in this patient reflect this. The quantity of protein excreted must be judged in relation to the GFR. A decrease in excretion is usually due to a decrease in glomerular permeability but it may occur because of a decrease in GFR. This may be due to the underlying disease or to a fall in plasma volume.

Renal tubular disorders

Renal tubular disorders can be congenital or acquired; they can involve single or multiple aspects of tubular function. The congenital conditions are all rare: their clinical sequelae relate to the consequences of loss of substances that are normally completely or partially reabsorbed by the tubules.

The Fanconi syndrome

This is a generalized disorder of tubular function characterized by glycosuria, amino aciduria, phosphaturia and acidosis. It can occur secondarily to a variety of conditions (*Fig. 4.14*). One of these is cystinosis, or Lignac–Fanconi disease, a rare inherited disease (only 1 in 40,000 live births in the UK) in which there is a defect in the transport of cystine out of lysosomes. This leads to cystine accumulation and the deposition of cystine crystals in many body tissues, including the kidney. Affected infants fail to thrive, develop rickets and polyuria with dehydration and eventually progress to renal failure. There is no specific treatment. Cystinosis should not be confused with cystinuria, a disorder of tubular transport.

Primary Fanconi syndrome can also develop in young adults; it is inherited, but the nature of the defect is not known.

Renal tubular acidosis (RTA)

The lesion in proximal (type 2) RTA is impairment of bicarbonate reabsorption. Type 2 RTA is a component of the Fanconi syndrome but can also occur as an isolated phenomenon. A transient form can occur in infants. Bicarbonate can be completely reabsorbed if the plasma bicarbonate concentration is low, and thus patients may excrete normal amounts of acid but at the expense of systemic acidosis. Treatment consists of administering large amounts of bicarbonate, for example 10 mmol/kg body weight/24 h. Distal (type 1 or classical) RTA occurs more frequently. It can be either inherited or acquired, for example secondarily to hypercalcaemia or autoimmune diseases. There is a defect in hydrogen ion excretion and the urine cannot be acidified. Consequences include osteomalacia, hypercalciuria, nephrocalcinosis, renal calculi and often hypokalaemia. In general, hyperkalaemia is more usual in acidotic states, but in these types of RTA the impaired ability of the kidneys to excrete hydrogen ions necessitates increased potassium excretion when sodium is reabsorbed in the distal tubules, and this may cause potassium depletion and hypokalaemia. Treatment involves the administration of bicarbonate in sufficient quantities to buffer normal hydrogen ion production (1–3 mg/kg body weight/24 h) and potassium supplements.

The most frequently encountered type of RTA is type 4. It is associated with hypoaldosteronism, either secondary to adrenal disease, or to renal disease in which there is decreased renin secretion (hyporeninaemic hypoaldosteronism, e.g. in diabetic nephropathy) or resistance to aldosterone (e.g. in obstructive nephropathy). In contrast to the other types of RTA, there is hyperkalaemia. The urine can be maximally acidified, but only at the expense of a systemic acidosis. The clinical features are primarily those of the underlying cause. Management is directed at the underlying cause and correction of the hyperkalaemia.

The diagnosis of RTA requires a high index of suspicion. Typically, there is hyperchloraemia and a normal anion gap. Other causes of this combination (e.g. loss of alkaline fluid from the gut and treatment with carbonic anhydrase inhibitors) must be excluded. Measurement of urine pH and plasma potassium concentration will usually indicate the correct diagnosis. Confirmation of the diagnosis of type 1 RTA may require a formal urinary acidification test (*see Fig. 4.15*). Diagnosis of type 2 RTA may occasionally require determination of the renal threshold for bicarbonate.

Defects of urinary concentration

Impairment of urinary concentration is a feature of nephrogenic diabetes insipidus, a primary tubular disorder. It is also a feature of cranial diabetes insipidus and chronic renal failure and can occur with hypercalcaemia, hypokalaemia and certain drugs, notably lithium. In nephrogenic diabetes insipidus, vasopressin secretion is normal but there is a defect involving either its receptors or one of the post receptor-binding events required for its normal action. Hypercalcaemia and hypokalaemia also interfere with this cyclic AMP-mediated pathway.

Glycosuria

Benign renal glycosuria is discussed on *p. 208*. Renal glycosuria can also occur in association with other tubular

---

Causes of Fanconi syndrome

idiopathic inherited metabolic disease:
    cystinosis (Lignac–Fanconi disease)
    galactosaemia
    fructose intolerance
    glycogen storage diseases
    tyrosinaemia
    Wilson's disease
nephrotoxins:
    heavy metals
    drugs
paraproteinaemia
amyloid

Fig. 4.14 Causes of the Fanconi syndrome.

Urinary acidification test	
Procedure	**Results**
take blood for bicarbonate measurements after overnight fast	normal response: urine pH <5.2 in at least one sample if this pH is not obtained, serum bicarbonate should be measured. Test should be repeated if serum bicarbonate is not below the lower limit of normal
measure pH of freshly passed urine: if urine pH <5.5, RTA is excluded if urine pH >5.5 *and* plasma [HCO$_3^-$] <16 mmol/L RTA is diagnosed	
if urine pH >5.5 *and* plasma [HCO$_3^-$] >16 mmol/L give ammonium chloride (100 mg/kg body weight) orally	type 1 RTA: urine pH ≥6.5
measure pH of freshly passed urine hourly for 8 h	

Fig. 4.15 Urinary acidification test. This test should not be performed in patients with liver disease.

abnormalities, for example as part of the Fanconi syndrome.

Amino aciduria

Renal amino aciduria can occur in combination with normal plasma concentrations of amino acids as a result of defective tubular reabsorption, for example Hartnup disease and cystinuria. Overflow amino aciduria occurs secondarily to elevated plasma concentrations when the tubular transport mechanism is saturated, as in, for instance, phenylketonuria.

Cystinuria has an incidence of about 1 in 7000 live births. Defective tubular reabsorption of cystine, ornithine, arginine and lysine leads to their excretion in the urine. The loss of these amino acids would alone be of little consequence, but cystine is relatively insoluble and cystinuria predisposes the patient to renal calculus formation. The management of cystinuria is discussed on *p. 305*.

Hypophosphataemic rickets

This condition, also known as vitamin D-resistant rickets, has a dominant X-linked pattern of inheritance. A defect in tubular phosphate reabsorption leads to severe rickets. This does not respond to treatment with vitamin D alone, even if administered in massive doses, but can be treated effectively with a combination of oral phosphate supplements and vitamin D, usually given as a 1α-hydroxylated derivative.

Hypophosphataemic rickets should not be confused with inherited vitamin D-dependent rickets type I, an autosomal recessive condition. The defect is in the 1α-hydroxylation of 25-hydroxycholecalciferol. This condition can be treated with 1α-hydroxylated derivatives of vitamin D alone, and is discussed, together with vitamin D-dependent rickets type II, in *Chapter 15 (p. 280)*.

Urinary calculi

Pathogenesis

Stones or calculi can form in urine when it is super-saturated with the crystalloid components of the calculus. Factors predisposing to this, and the commoner types of calculus that occur clinically, are shown in *Fig. 4.16*.

Hypercalciuria is present in up to 25% of patients with calcium oxalate/phosphate stones. It may be associated with hypercalcaemia, for example, due to primary hyperparathyroidism. Frequently, however, hypercalciuria is idiopathic: patients are normocalcaemic and the primary abnormality is an increase in intestinal calcium absorption.

Hyperoxaluria predisposes to renal calculus formation. Primary hyperoxaluria is a rare inherited metabolic disorder. Two types have been described: increased hepatic oxalate synthesis is common to both. In type 1 there is increased urinary excretion of oxalic, glycoxylic and glycolic acids; renal failure develops in the majority of cases and calcium oxalate crystals develop in many

Urinary calculi

Factors predisposing to formation
dehydration
urinary tract infection
persistently alkaline urine
hypercalciuria
hyperuricosuria
hyperoxaluria
urinary stagnation (due to obstruction)
lack of urinary inhibitors of crystallization

Composition
calcium oxalate (± phosphate)
calcium phosphate
magnesium ammonium phosphate ('triple
  phosphate')
uric acid
cystine

Biochemical investigations
analysis of calculus (if available)
plasma:
  calcium
  bicarbonate
  phosphate
  urate
urine:
  pH
  qualitative test for cystine
  24 h volume
  24 h excretion of calcium, oxalate, urate and
    citrate*
  consider urinary acidification test for RTA

* citrate is an inhibitor of calculus formation; its excretion is
reduced in type 1 RTA.

Fig. 4.16 Renal calculi: composition, factors predisposing to their formation and biochemical investigations.

body issues. Type 2 is a more benign condition in which there is increased urinary excretion of oxalic and glyceric acids; renal failure does not occur. Secondary hyperoxaluria is usually caused by increased intestinal absorption of dietary oxalate, with or without increased oxalate ingestion. This may be seen in patients with a variety of gastrointestinal disorders, in particular with inflammatory bowel diseases and conditions associated with malabsorption. In these circumstances, non-absorbed free fatty acids bind to calcium. This limits the amount of calcium available to combine with oxalate to form calcium oxalate, which is insoluble and is normally excreted in the faeces. As a result, an increased amount of oxalate remains in solution and can be absorbed into the bloodstream.

Investigation

The history and examination may suggest an underlying cause for urinary calculi, such as inadequate fluid intake. Biochemical tests that should be performed on plasma and urine are shown in *Fig. 4.16*. If available, a calculus should be analysed, although identification of urate or cystine stones is more helpful for management than that of stones containing calcium. The urine must be examined for evidence of infection in all patients presenting with urinary calculi. The radiographic appearance of a retained stone may be characteristic; for example, 'staghorn' calculi contain mixed phosphates and are related to chronic infection; pure uric acid stones (not containing calcium) are radiolucent, as are pure cystine stones. An intravenous urogram may show a predisposing anatomical abnormality. Most calculi can be detected by ultrasound.

Management

Small calculi are often passed spontaneously. Larger calculi may require surgical removal or disintegration by ultrasound. Any urinary tract infection should be treated. The identification of the cause of urinary calculus formation should make it possible to design an effective regimen to prevent further stone formation. This is particularly important in patients who form stones recurrently.

The management of cystinuria is considered on *p. 305*. Hyperuricaemia should be treated with allopurinol (*see p. 288*). Alkalinization of the urine increases the solubility of both cystine and uric acid but may be difficult to achieve. A high fluid intake is appropriate in all patients with a tendency to form urinary calculi.

If patients who form calcium stones are hypercalcaemic, the underlying cause should be treated. In the normocalcaemic majority, dietary manipulation to correct excessive intake of calcium or oxalate is appropriate. However, calcium restriction below maintenance levels is inadvisable since oxalate absorption may be increased and there may be adverse effects on the skeleton. In patients who do not respond to such measures, thiazide diuretics (which decrease urinary calcium excretion) are often very effective at preventing recurrence.

SUMMARY

- The kidneys have four major functions: the control of extracellular fluid volume and composition, hydrogen ion homoeostasis, excretion of waste products of metabolism and hormone production.

- The best simple test of overall renal *function* is the plasma creatinine concentration; the presence of proteinuria is a sensitive, although not specific, indicator of *damage* to the kidneys.

- **Acute renal failure** (ARF) is a life-threatening condition in which there is a potentially reversible deterioration in renal function. Causes include renal hypoperfusion, specific renal diseases and nephrotoxic drugs. When hypoperfusion is responsible, it may be possible to prevent the development of intrinsic renal damage by restoration of normal perfusion. Biochemical features of ARF include increases in plasma urea and creatinine concentrations, hyperkalaemia, hyperphosphataemia, acidosis and fluid retention. Patients are often oliguric and require dialysis or haemofiltration until renal function recovers.

- In **chronic renal failure** (CRF), renal function is irreversibly lost; patients eventually require transplantation or long-term dialysis. Causes include diabetes, vascular diseases, glomerulonephritis and pyelonephritis. CRF usually develops slowly and, because the kidneys have considerable functional reserves, patients tend to present late in the course of the illness. Retention of urea, creatinine and other waste products and disturbance of sodium and water homoeostasis are characteristic; severe acidosis and hyperkalaemia are only late features of the condition. Bone disease, with hypocalcaemia and hyperphosphataemia, and anaemia result from impairment of renal endocrine function.

- The **nephrotic syndrome** comprises proteinuria, hypoproteinaemia and oedema and can be a result of a variety of diseases affecting the glomeruli. The clinical and biochemical features stem from the loss of protein from the body. In addition to albumin, the loss of which is responsible for the oedema, the loss of other proteins leads to increased susceptibility to infection and hypercoagulability. Uraemia may or may not be present, depending on the nature of the underlying glomerular damage.

- The formation of **urinary calculi** is essentially the result of supersaturation of the urine. Factors predisposing to calculus formation include the excretion of high solute loads, for example of calcium, oxalate or urate, inadequate water intake and infection.

- **Disorders of renal tubular function** can lead to decreased excretion of substances that are excreted by the tubules (e.g. hydrogen ions) or to increased excretion of substances that are normally reabsorbed (e.g. glucose). They can be inherited or acquired.

5 The liver

INTRODUCTION

The liver is of vital importance in intermediary metabolism and in the detoxification and elimination of toxic substances (*Fig. 5.1*). Damage to the organ may not obviously affect its activity since the liver has considerable functional reserve and, as a consequence, simple tests of liver function (e.g. plasma bilirubin and albumin concentrations) are insensitive indicators of liver disease. Tests reflecting liver cell damage (particularly the measurement of the activities of hepatic enzymes in plasma) are often superior in this respect. The categorization of such tests as 'liver function tests' is clearly a misnomer, but seems likely to endure. Various tests have been devised to provide a quantitative assessment of functional hepatic cell activity (*see p. 90*) but they are as yet infrequently used in routine clinical practice.

The results of the standard biochemical liver function tests rarely provide a precise diagnosis on their own since they reflect the basic pathological processes common to many conditions. However, biochemical tests are cheap, non-invasive and widely available, and are of value in directing the use of other diagnostic tests, notably imaging and liver biopsy. They are also useful in detecting the presence of liver disease and in following its progress.

The liver has a dual blood supply: approximately two-thirds from the portal vein, which drains much of the gut and through which most of the nutrients absorbed from the gut reach the liver, and the remainder from the hepatic artery, which supplies most of the liver's oxygen. Blood leaves the liver through hepatic veins, which drain into the inferior vena cava.

The metabolic activity of the liver takes place within the parenchymal cells, which constitute 80% of the organ mass; the liver also contains Kupffer cells of the reticuloendothelial system. Parenchymal cells are contiguous with the venous sinusoids, which carry blood from the portal vein and hepatic artery, and with the biliary canaliculi, the smallest ramifications of the biliary system (*Fig. 5.2*). Substances destined for excretion in the bile are secreted from hepatocytes into

Major functions of the liver
Carbohydrate metabolism   gluconeogenesis   glycogen synthesis and breakdown
Fat metabolism   fatty acid synthesis   cholesterol synthesis and excretion   lipoprotein synthesis   ketogenesis   bile acid synthesis   25-hydroxylation of vitamin D
Protein metabolism   synthesis of plasma proteins (including some   coagulation factors but not immunoglobulins)   urea synthesis
Hormone metabolism   metabolism and excretion of steroid hormones   metabolism of polypeptide hormones
Drugs and foreign compounds   metabolism and excretion
Storage   glycogen   vitamin A   vitamin B_{12} iron
Metabolism and excretion of bilirubin

Fig. 5.1 Major functions of the liver.

the canaliculi, pass through the intrahepatic ducts and reach the duodenum via the common bile duct.

The most common disease processes affecting the liver are:

- hepatitis, with damage to liver cells
- cirrhosis, in which increased fibrous tissue formation leads to shrinkage of the liver, decreased hepatocellular function and obstruction of bile flow

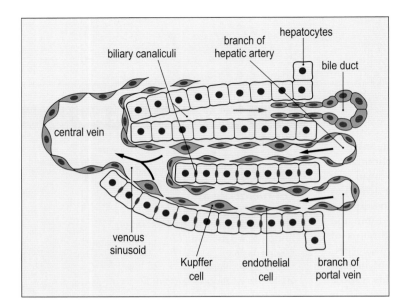

Fig. 5.2 Microstructure of the liver. The liver consists of acini in which sheets of hepatocytes, one cell thick, are permeated by sinusoids carrying blood (black arrow) from the portal venules and hepatic arterioles to the central vein. Bile (red arrow) is secreted from the hepatocytes into canaliculi, which drain into the bile ducts.

- tumours, most frequently secondary; for example, metastases from cancers of the large bowel, stomach and bronchus.

Patients with liver disease often present with characteristic symptoms and signs, but the clinical features may be non-specific and, in some patients, liver disease is discovered incidentally. Because of the intimate relationship between the liver and biliary system, extrahepatic biliary disease may present with clinical features suggestive of liver disease or may have secondary effects on the liver; for instance, obstruction to the common bile duct may cause jaundice and, if prolonged, a form of cirrhosis.

BILIRUBIN METABOLISM

Bilirubin is derived mainly from the haem moiety of haemoglobin molecules and is liberated when senescent red cells are removed from the circulation by the reticuloendothelial system (*Fig. 5.3*); the iron in haem is reutilized but the tetrapyrrole ring is degraded to bilirubin. Other sources of bilirubin include myoglobin and the cytochromes.

Unconjugated bilirubin is not water-soluble; it is transported in the bloodstream bound to albumin. In the liver, it is taken up by hepatocytes in a process involving specific carrier proteins. Bilirubin is then transported to the smooth endoplasmic reticulum, where it undergoes conjugation, principally with glucuronic acid, to form a diglucuronide; this process is catalyzed by the enzyme bilirubin-uridyl diphosphate (UDP) glucuronyl transferase. Conjugated bilirubin is water-soluble and is secreted into the biliary canaliculi, eventually reaching the small intestine via the ducts of the biliary system. Secretion into the biliary canaliculi is the rate-limiting step in bilirubin metabolism. In the gut, bilirubin is converted by bacterial action into urobilinogen, a colourless compound. Some urobilinogen is absorbed from the gut into the portal blood; hepatic uptake of this is incomplete; a small quantity reaches the systemic circulation and is excreted in the urine. Most of the urobilinogen in the gut is oxidized in the colon to a brown pigment, stercobilin, which is excreted in the stool.

Some 300 mg of bilirubin is produced daily but the healthy liver can metabolize and excrete ten times this amount. The measurement of plasma bilirubin concentration is thus an insensitive test of liver function.

The bilirubin normally present in the plasma is mainly (approximately 95%) unconjugated; since it is protein bound, it is not filtered by the renal glomeruli and, in health, bilirubin is not detectable in the urine. Bilirubinuria reflects an increase in the plasma concentration of conjugated bilirubin, and is always pathological.

Jaundice, the yellow discoloration of tissues due to bilirubin deposition, is a frequent feature of liver disease. Clinical jaundice may not be discernible unless

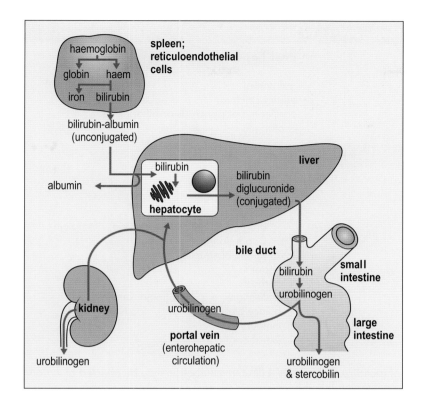

Fig. 5.3 Excretion of bilirubin by the liver. Bilirubin, which is bound to albumin in the plasma, is taken up into hepatocytes, conjugated in the smooth endoplasmic reticulum and excreted via the bile ducts into the gut, where it is converted to urobilinogen. Most of the urobilinogen is oxidized to stercobilin in the colon and excreted in the stool. Some urobilinogen is absorbed from the small intestine and enters the enterohepatic circulation. While most is excreted in the bile, some reaches the systemic circulation and is excreted in the urine.

the plasma bilirubin concentration is more than two and half times the upper limit of normal, i.e. more than 50 μmol/L. Hyperbilirubinaemia can be caused by increased production of bilirubin, impaired metabolism, decreased excretion or a combination of these. Causes of jaundice are listed in *Fig. 5.4*.

BIOCHEMICAL ASSESSMENT OF LIVER FUNCTION

Bilirubin

Hyperbilirubinaemia is not always present in patients with liver disease, nor is it exclusively associated with liver disease. For example, it is not usually present in patients with well-compensated cirrhosis but it is a common feature of advanced pancreatic carcinoma.

Unconjugated hyperbilirubinaemia

When an excess of bilirubin is unconjugated, the concentration in adults rarely exceeds 100 μmol/L. In the absence of liver disease, unconjugated hyper-bilirubinaemia is most often due either to haemolysis or to Gilbert's syndrome, an inherited abnormality of bilirubin metabolism.

In haemolysis, hyperbilirubinaemia is due to increased production of bilirubin, which exceeds the capacity of the liver to remove and conjugate the pigment. Nevertheless, more bilirubin is excreted in the bile, the amount of urobilinogen entering the enterohepatic circulation is increased and urinary urobilinogen is increased. Laboratory findings in haemolytic (pre-hepatic) jaundice are summarized in *Fig. 5.5*.

Activity of the hepatic conjugating enzymes is usually low at birth but increases rapidly thereafter; the transient 'physiological' jaundice of the newborn reflects this. With excessive haemolysis, as in Rhesus incompatibility, or a lack of enzyme activity, as occurs in prematurity and in the Crigler–Najjar syndrome, there may be a massive rise in the plasma concentration of unconjugated bilirubin. If bilirubin concentration exceeds approximately 340 μmol/L, its uptake into the brain may cause severe brain damage (kernicterus).

Major causes of jaundice	
Pre-hepatic	**Post-hepatic**
haemolysis ineffective erythropoiesis	gallstones biliary stricture carcinoma of pancreas or biliary tree cholangitis
Hepatic	

pre-microsomal:
    drugs, e.g. rifampicin, which interfere
      with bilirubin uptake
microsomal:
    prematurity
    hepatitis, e.g. viral or drug-induced
    Gilbert's syndrome
    Crigler–Najjar syndrome
	post-microsomal:
	    impaired excretion:
	      hepatitis
	      drugs, e.g. methyltestosterone, rifampicin
	      Dubin–Johnson syndrome
	    intrahepatic obstruction:
	      hepatitis
	      cirrhosis
	      infiltrations, e.g. lymphoma, amyloid
	      biliary atresia
	      tumours
	      extrahepatic sepsis

Fig. 5.4 Classification and major causes of jaundice. In hepatitis, bilirubin metabolism may be affected at various steps. The jaundice is usually due mainly to conjugated bilirubin.

Conjugated hyperbilirubinaemia

This condition is due to leakage of bilirubin from either hepatocytes or the biliary system into the bloodstream when its normal route of excretion is blocked. The water-soluble conjugated bilirubin entering the systemic circulation is excreted in the urine, giving it a deep orange–brown colour. In complete biliary obstruction, no bilirubin reaches the gut, no stercobilin is formed and the stools are pale in colour. The differential diagnosis of jaundice due to conjugated bilirubin is considered on pp. 96–97.

Hyperbilirubinaemia can be due to an excess of either or both conjugated and unconjugated bilirubin. The separate measurement of conjugated and unconjugated bilirubin concentration is useful in the diagnosis of neonatal jaundice, where there may be some doubt as to the relative contribution of defective conjugation and other causes; it is less often required in adults. If the plasma bilirubin concentration is less than 100 µmol/L and other tests of liver function are normal, it can be inferred that the raised levels are due to the unconjugated form of the pigment. The urine can be tested to confirm this since, with unconjugated hyperbilirubinaemia, there is no bilirubin in the urine.

A third fraction of bilirubin, consisting of conjugated bilirubin bound covalently to albumin, is found in the plasma of patients with longstanding conjugated hyperbilirubinaemia. This substance has a half-life similar to that of albumin. Its persistence in the plasma during the resolution of liver disease or after the relief of obstruction explains the persistence of jaundice in the absence of bilirubinuria that can occur in these circumstances.

Plasma enzymes

Enzymes used in the assessment of hepatic function include aspartate and alanine aminotransferases (formerly called transaminases and still abbreviated AST and ALT, respectively), alkaline phosphatase (ALP) and γ-glutamyl transferase (GGT). In general, these enzymes are not specific indicators of liver dysfunction. The hepatic isoenzyme of ALP is an exception, and ALT is more specific to the liver than AST.

Laboratory findings that may be present in haemolytic jaundice	
plasma bilirubin	unconjugated rarely >100 μmol/L except in neonates
plasma enzymes	aspartate aminotransferase and hydroxybutyrate dehydrogenase slightly increased
plasma haptoglobins	decreased
urine urobilinogen	increased
peripheral blood	increased reticulocytes decreased haemoglobin abnormal red cell morphology on blood film positive Coombs' (direct antiglobulin) test

Fig. 5.5 Laboratory findings that may be present in haemolytic jaundice.

Increased aminotransferase activities reflect cell damage; plasma levels may be 20 times the upper limit of normal (ULN) in patients with hepatitis. In cholestasis, plasma ALP activity is increased. This is due mainly to increased enzyme synthesis, stimulated by cholestasis. In severe obstructive jaundice, the plasma ALP activity may be up to ten times the ULN.

In practice, however, increases in the plasma activities of aminotransferases and ALP are often present in patients with liver disease, although one may predominate. In primarily cholestatic disease there may be secondary hepatocellular damage and increased plasma aminotransferase activities, while cholestasis frequently occurs in hepatocellular disease. Increased GGT activity is found in both cholestasis and hepatocellular damage: this enzyme is a very sensitive indicator of liver disease but is non-specific. Thus, although certain patterns of plasma enzyme activities are frequently observed in various types of liver disease, they are not reliably diagnostic.

Plasma enzyme activities are very useful in following the progress of liver disease once the diagnosis has been made. Falling aminotransferase activity suggests a decrease in hepatocellular damage and falling ALP activity suggests a resolution of cholestasis. However, in severe acute hepatic failure, a decrease in aminotransferase activity may misleadingly suggest an improvement when it is actually due to almost complete destruction of parenchymal cells.

Other causes of increased plasma activities of the aminotransferases, GGT and ALP are discussed in *Chapter 13*.

Plasma proteins

Albumin is synthesized in the liver and its concentration in the plasma is in part a reflection of the functional capacity of the organ. Plasma albumin concentration tends to decrease in chronic liver disease, but is usually normal in the early stages of acute hepatitis owing to its long half-life (approximately 20 days). There are many other causes of hypoalbuminaemia, as discussed on *p. 238*, but a normal plasma albumin concentration in a patient with chronic liver disease implies adequate synthetic function; a fall implies a significant deterioration.

The prothrombin time, usually expressed as a ratio (the international normalized ratio, INR) to a control value, is a test of plasma clotting activity and reflects the activity of vitamin K-dependent clotting factors synthesized by the liver, of which factor VII has the shortest half-life (4–6 h). An increase in the prothrombin time is often an early feature of acute liver disease, but a prolonged prothrombin time may also reflect vitamin K deficiency. The cause can be determined by administering the vitamin parenterally: in vitamin K deficiency, the prothrombin time should return to normal within 18 h.

A polyclonal increase in immunoglobulins is a frequent finding in patients with chronic liver disease (particularly of autoimmune origin) and may cause an increase in plasma total protein concentration even when albumin concentration is decreased. Plasma IgA is often increased in alcoholic liver disease, IgG in autoimmune hepatitis and IgM in primary biliary cirrhosis, but these changes are non-specific. More useful diagnostic information may be obtained from measuring individual autoantibodies: antimitochondrial antibody is increased in almost all patients with primary biliary cirrhosis, and antismooth muscle and antinuclear antibodies in many patients with autoimmune hepatitis. Viral infection can be detected by measurement of viral antigens and antibodies.

Diagnostically useful changes in the concentrations of other plasma proteins are shown in *Fig. 5.6*.

Plasma proteins of diagnostic value in liver disease		
Protein	**Condition**	**Change in concentration**
albumin	chronic liver disease	↓
γ-globulins	cirrhosis, especially autoimmune	↑
α_1-antitrypsin	cirrhosis due to α_1-antitrypsin deficiency	↓
caeruloplasmin	Wilson's disease	↓
α-fetoprotein	primary hepatocellular carcinoma	greatly ↑
transferrin	haemochromatosis	normal but 100% saturated with iron
ferritin	haemochromatosis	greatly ↑

Fig. 5.6 Plasma proteins of diagnostic value in liver disease.

Other tests of liver function

Given the imperfections of the simple tests of liver function that have been discussed above, it is not surprising that many tests have been devised with a view to providing greater diagnostic sensitivity and specificity. Various dynamic tests, which give an indication of functional hepatic cell mass, are available, but are infrequently used. They may be considered as analogous to the use of clearance measurements for renal function, in that by utilizing marker substances that are excreted or metabolized by the liver, they measure either the rate of their removal from the blood or the rate of formation of a metabolite. Such tests include the ^{14}C-aminopyrine breath test, a test of cytochrome P450-dependent demethylation, and the galactose elimination capacity, a measure of galactose phosphorylation. These tests are more sensitive than conventional tests but are more time-consuming; their use is likely to be limited to special situations (e.g. the monitoring of novel treatments, assessment of prognosis, etc.). The simplest of the newer quantitative tests of liver function (requiring only a single blood sample) is measurement of the formation of monoethylglycinexylidide (MEGX) after administration of a bolus of lidocaine (lignocaine). Unfortunately, the reference range is wide, and serial, rather than isolated, measurements are likely to prove more useful.

Plasma bile acid concentrations are increased in liver disease but, while this is a highly specific finding, bile acid measurements are in general no more sensitive than conventional tests. They do, however, have a special role in liver disease developing during pregnancy (*see p. 101*). Measurements of bilirubin conjugates in plasma show considerable promise as sensitive tests of hepatic function but are technically demanding. So too is measurement of plasma glutathione-S-transferase α-isoenzyme activity, which appears to be a more sensitive and organ-specific indicator of liver damage than the aminotransferases.

Non-biochemical investigation of hepatobiliary disease

Many other types of investigation can provide valuable information in patients suspected of having liver disease. Ultrasound examination can reveal gallstones, dilatation of the biliary system and the characteristic hyper-reflectivity of hepatic fatty infiltration. Cholangiography – examination of the biliary system with X-ray contrast media, given either intravenously or retrogradely, through an endoscope (endoscopic retrograde cholangiopancreatography, ERCP) – can reveal structural abnormalities of the biliary system. Arteriography can reveal the typical pathological circulation in hepatic tumours. CT and MRI can demonstrate space-occupying lesions, both solid and cystic. The 'gold standard' of diagnosis, particularly in chronic liver disease and cancer, is histology, usually of tissue obtained by percutaneous biopsy.

LIVER DISEASE

Acute hepatitis

Acute hepatitis is usually caused by viral infection (particularly with hepatitis viruses A, B, C, D and E but also Epstein–Barr virus and cytomegalovirus) or toxins (e.g. alcohol, paracetamol, carbon tetrachloride and various fungal toxins). There is considerable variation in the severity and time course of the disease but the pattern of changes in the standard liver function tests reflects the common underlying pathological process and is similar whatever the cause.

Patients may present with jaundice but there is often a pre-icteric stage with relatively non-specific symptoms such as anorexia and malaise.

Early in the course of acute hepatitis, bilirubin and urobilinogen are usually readily detectable in the urine by a simple dip-stick technique. For as long as the plasma bilirubin is raised, bilirubin continues to be excreted in the urine. Urobilinogen may disappear from the urine at the height of the jaundice, when there may be complete cholestasis because no bilirubin reaches the gut, but it reappears as the hepatitis resolves and biliary excretion returns to normal. These changes (*Fig. 5.7*) are of no practical value in the management of hepatitis, but the detection of bilirubin in the urine is a simple and valuable diagnostic pointer to hepatitis in the pre-icteric stage of the illness.

Many cases of viral hepatitis resolve completely. In severe cases, hepatic failure may develop, but most patients who survive the acute illness eventually recover

Typical biochemical changes during acute hepatitis		
	Pre-icteric	Icteric
plasma bilirubin	N/↑	↑↑
plasma aminotransferases	↑↑↑	↑
plasma alkaline phosphatase	N	N/↑
urinary bilirubin	↑	↑
urinary urobilinogen	↑	absent

Fig. 5.7 Typical biochemical changes during acute hepatitis. N = normal.

Case history 5.1

A 20-year-old student developed a flu-like illness with loss of appetite, nausea and pain in the right hypochondrium. On examination, the liver was just palpable and was tender. Two days later he developed jaundice, his urine became darker in colour and his stools became pale.

Investigations

	on presentation	one week later
serum:		
bilirubin	38 μmol/L	230 μmol/L
albumin	40 g/L	38 g/L
AST	450 U/L	365 U/L
ALP	70 U/L	150 U/L
GGT	60 U/L	135 U/L
urine:		
bilirubin	positive	positive
urobilinogen	positive	negative

Comment

The first set of results is characteristic of early hepatitis, with a raised aminotransferase reflecting cell damage. This usually precedes the rise in bilirubin and the development of jaundice. Impairment of the hepatic secretion of conjugated bilirubin and of urobilinogen uptake from the portal blood causes both these substances to be excreted in the urine.

The second set of results shows the expected high serum bilirubin but with a fall in AST as the phase of maximum cellular damage has passed. An increase in ALP, usually of not more than three times the ULN, is common at this stage. In hepatitis, the bilirubin in plasma is both conjugated and unconjugated, with the former predominating. Conjugated bilirubin is excreted in the urine and the pale stool reflects the decreased biliary excretion. The serum albumin has remained normal in this acute illness.

completely, aminotransferase activities falling to normal in 10–12 weeks. In some cases of infection with hepatitis B and C viruses, aminotransferase activities remain elevated; antigenaemia persists and chronic liver disease ensues. Infection with hepatitis A never leads to chronic disease.

Chronic hepatitis

Chronic hepatitis is defined as hepatic inflammation persisting for more than six months. There are many causes. Autoimmune hepatitis, chronic infection with hepatitis B or C, and alcohol are particularly important.

Autoimmune hepatitis (formerly called chronic active hepatitis) typically occurs in young women although it can occur in either sex at any age. It can also present acutely. The aetiology is unknown. There is a strong association with other autoimmune diseases. Auto-antibodies (antinuclear and antismooth muscle) are frequently present in the serum in high titre. Antiliver–kidney microsomal antibodies are characteristic of a type of autoimmune hepatitis that more frequently presents in childhood and is more often acute in onset with a more aggressive course.

Plasma aminotransferase activities are usually elevated in chronic hepatitis, but other liver function tests are often normal unless cirrhosis develops. Although the natural history of autoimmune hepatitis is of progression to cirrhosis, this is often preventable if immunosuppressive treatment (usually with azathioprine and corticosteroids) is started early in the course of the condition.

Acute liver failure

This term encompasses a range of clinical syndromes of severe liver dysfunction and encephalopathy developing within six months of the first clinical evidence of disease. It is now preferred to the term 'fulminant hepatic failure'.

Acute liver failure can be hyperacute (encephalopathy developing within seven days of the onset of jaundice), acute (8–28 days) or sub-acute (jaundice preceding encephalopathy by 4–12 weeks). It is a rare condition: toxins (e.g. paracetamol) and hepatitis are the most frequent causes. The underlying hepatic lesion is usually potentially reversible since the liver has a considerable capacity for regeneration, but the metabolic disturbance is profound and the prognosis poor; acute hepatic failure is often accompanied by renal failure.

Metabolic features of acute hepatic failure include severe hyponatraemia, hypocalcaemia and hypoglycaemia. Hydrogen ion homoeostasis is frequently disturbed. Lactic acidosis may develop as a result of the failure of hepatic gluconeogenesis from lactate, but may be masked by a respiratory alkalosis caused by toxic stimulation of the respiratory centre. Generalized depression of the brain stem may lead to respiratory arrest. In some cases (although not usually with paracetamol poisoning) a metabolic alkalosis predominates: this is in part related to excessive urinary potassium loss, due to intracellular potassium depletion and secondary aldosteronism, and in part to the accumulation of basic substances, such as ammonia, in the blood.

Despite the fact that renal failure may also be present, the plasma urea concentration is often low, reflecting decreased hepatic synthesis. The plasma creatinine concentration is theoretically a more reliable guide both to renal function and to whether the patient should be haemodialyzed, but some methods of measuring creatinine are subject to interference by bilirubin and produce invalid results in patients with jaundice. The prothrombin time is greatly prolonged as a result of impaired hepatic synthesis of clotting factors, and bleeding is an almost universal clinical problem.

Management

Management involves support of vital functions and correction of the metabolic imbalances. Respiratory failure may necessitate artificial ventilation and haemodialysis may be necessary if renal failure occurs. Close cooperation between the laboratory and clinical staff is vital in the management of acute hepatic failure. Artificial hepatic support has little to offer at present (although early trials of 'artificial livers' based on cultivated human liver cells show promise in providing temporary support, while the patient's own liver undergoes regeneration), and hepatic transplantation should be considered in the most severely ill.

As with cirrhosis, the advent of liver transplantation as treatment for acute hepatic failure has highlighted a need for good prognostic tests. Various multifactorial scoring systems have been described based, for example, on the prothrombin time (which is prolonged), severity of acidosis, factor V concentration (reduced) or factor V:VIII ratio (also reduced).

Cirrhosis

Causes of cirrhosis include chronic excessive alcohol intake, autoimmune disease (e.g. autoimmune hepatitis), primary biliary cirrhosis, persistence of hepatitis B or C virus and various inherited metabolic diseases, such as Wilson's disease, haemochromatosis and α_1-antitrypsin deficiency.

Due to the great functional capacity of the liver, metabolic and clinical abnormalities may not become apparent until late in the course of the disease; until this time, the cirrhosis is said to be 'compensated'. There are no reliable, simple biochemical tests to diagnose subclinical disease; dynamic tests of hepatic function (*see p. 90*) have the potential to do this but are time-consuming and are not in routine clinical use.

Procollagen type III peptide (PIIINP) is a peptide produced during collagen synthesis; its concentration in plasma reflects the rate of development of fibrosis, one of the features of cirrhosis, although it can also be increased by inflammation and necrosis. It has a role in the monitoring of patients being treated with methotrexate, a cytotoxic drug (*see p. 341*). Methotrexate can cause hepatic fibrosis. It was recommended that patients being treated with methotrexate should undergo regular liver biopsy, but the need for this can be reduced by monitoring patients' plasma PIIINP concentrations.

Encephalopathy, characterized by a decrease in consciousness and impairment of higher functions, is often present in decompensated cirrhosis and may also be a feature of severe acute hepatitis. Substances implicated in encephalopathy include ammonia, which accumulates when urea synthesis is impaired, and false neurotransmitters, such as octopamine and β-phenylethanolamine. These false neurotransmitters are derived from the amino acids tyrosine and phenylalanine, respectively, by bacterial decarboxylation in the gut, and are normally detoxified in the liver.

Treatment of hepatic encephalopathy involves appropriate management of any precipitating factors such as gastrointestinal haemorrhage, restriction of dietary protein intake, and the provision of enemas or laxatives (e.g. lactulose) to empty the bowels of nitrogen-containing material. Neomycin, a non-absorbable antibiotic, can be used to sterilize the gut in order to reduce the production of toxins by bacteria. An adequate energy intake is essential and fluid and electrolyte balance must be maintained. If ascites is present, sodium restriction is essential.

 Case history 5.2

A middle-aged female publican was admitted to hospital following a haematemesis. Endoscopy revealed the presence of oesophageal varices. The only biochemical abnormality was an elevated GGT (245 IU/L). Her varices were treated by sclerotherapy and no further bleeding occurred. The patient was told to abstain from alcohol. She was readmitted one year later, jaundiced, drowsy and with clinical signs of chronic liver disease.

Investigations

serum:		
	albumin	25 g/L
	bilirubin	260 µmol/L
	ALP	315 U/L
	AST	134 U/L
	GGT	360 U/L

Comment

The patient had continued to drink and the resulting liver damage eventually affected hepatic function. The decreased serum albumin, elevated serum bilirubin and enzyme changes are consistent with cirrhosis and active liver cell damage; the prothrombin time was also prolonged.

Hepatic decompensation may be precipitated in chronic liver disease by sepsis, bleeding into the gut, for example from varices, erosions and ulcers, and by various drugs, including diuretics. Diuretics may be given to treat ascites, a common feature of chronic liver disease, but must be used with caution. The pathogenesis of ascites is complex. Portal hypertension due to hepatic venous obstruction causes splanchnic arterial vasodilatation. This leads to underfilling of the arterial circulation and stimulation of renal sodium and water retention. Hypoalbuminaemia may also contribute.

Case history 5.3

A 40-year-old woman presented with jaundice. There was no history of contact with hepatitis, recent foreign travel, injections or transfusions. She did not drink alcohol. She had been well in the past but had suffered from increasingly intense pruritus during the previous 18 months.

Investigations

serum:	total protein	85 g/L
	albumin	28 g/L
	bilirubin	340 μmol/L
	ALP	522 U/L
	AST	98 U/L
	GGT	242 U/L

Comment

The very high alkaline phosphatase indicates a cholestatic jaundice; the low albumin is consistent with chronic liver disease. The clue to the diagnosis is the high total protein, implying a serum globulin level of 57 g/L. This is often seen in autoimmune liver disease. Further investigations revealed a high titre of antimitochondrial antibodies, characteristic of primary biliary cirrhosis. This diagnosis was confirmed by histological examination of tissue obtained by percutaneous liver biopsy.

Pruritus in chronic liver disease is due to the accumulation of bile salts. Measurement of plasma bile salts has been suggested as a sensitive test of hepatocellular function but has not been adopted routinely, except in pregnancy (*see p. 90*).

Renal failure is a recognized complication of chronic liver disease, particularly end-stage alcoholic cirrhosis. It may take the form of acute tubular necrosis, due, for example, to haemorrhage or infection, but more frequently is functional in nature, that is, the kidneys are histologically normal and tubular function is intact, the urine being concentrated and having a low sodium concentration. There is, however, no sustained benefit from extracellular fluid volume expansion. This 'hepatorenal syndrome' may arise spontaneously or be precipitated by fluid loss (diarrhoea, inappropriate use of diuretics). Response to treatment is generally poor and there is progressive azotaemia, fluid retention and severe hypotension, although death is usually from liver rather than renal failure. The pathogenesis is incompletely understood: intense renal vasoconstriction, probably secondary to systemic arterial underfilling, is an important factor.

Disturbance of endocrine function is common in patients with chronic liver disease. The most obvious is the feminization of males, with gynaecomastia, impotence, decreased body hair, testicular atrophy, etc. Altered metabolism of both androgens and oestrogens, and an increase in the plasma concentration of sex hormone binding globulin (*see p. 178*) may be responsible.

Once established, hepatic cirrhosis is irreversible. If possible, any underlying cause should be treated appropriately. Specific complications, including ascites, bleeding (e.g. from oesophageal varices resulting from portal hypertension) and malabsorption, may also be amenable to treatment. Causes of death include hepatic encephalopathy, uncontrollable bleeding and septicaemia.

The development of liver transplantation as treatment for cirrhosis has brought about a need for accurate prognostic tests. Several prognostic indices have been developed based upon a combination of clinical features and the results of biochemical tests such as the prothrombin time and plasma albumin and bilirubin concentrations. Surgery should not be undertaken while the short-term prognosis for the patient is still good, nor delayed until he or she is moribund.

Alcohol and the liver

Alcohol is a common cause of liver disease. There are three main categories. Fat accumulation in the liver (hepatic steatosis) occurs frequently in people who abuse alcohol; it may give rise to asymptomatic hepatomegaly with modest increases in plasma aminotransferases, a more marked increase in GGT activity, but a normal bilirubin concentration. Frank alcoholic hepatitis often develops after a bout of heavy drinking in patients with a history of excessive alcohol ingestion. Third, chronic alcohol ingestion is a common cause of cirrhosis. This risk is greater for women than for men but cirrhosis is not inevitable even in heavy drinkers: only 10–20% of chronic alcoholics develop cirrhosis. The most important aspect of management, apart from general supportive measures and treatment of any complications, is to persuade the patient to abstain totally from alcohol. If this can be achieved, the prognosis in alcoholic cirrhosis is better than in cirrhosis due to other causes. Other aspects of alcohol toxicity are considered in *Chapter 20*.

Non-alcoholic fatty liver disease

In addition to excessive alcohol ingestion, hepatic steatosis has many other causes, numerically the most important being obesity and diabetes. Other causes include parenteral feeding (particularly with an excess of energy substrates, *see p. 359*), starvation, some inherited metabolic disorders (e.g. glycogen storage disease type 1) and drugs, particularly amiodarone, an antiarrythmic agent.

Patients may complain of discomfort in the right upper quadrant of the abdomen, but are usually asymptomatic; plasma bilirubin and albumin concentrations are normal but aminotransferase activities can be up to two to three times the upper reference limit, with the ratio of aspartate to alanine aminotransferase (AST/ALT) activities typically being one or less; γ-glutamyl transferase activity is usually elevated, to an extent that reflects the amount of fat deposition.

Liver biopsy shows fatty infiltration, but, as with the patient in *Case History 5.4*, the diagnosis is usually made on the basis of the clinical features and the elimination of other causes. In the majority of patients, the prognosis is good, and the condition resolves if the underlying cause can be treated effectively. In some, however, there is progression through steatohepatitis to fibrosis, impaired liver function and, eventually, cirrhosis. The cause of this progression is unknown, but may be related to increased oxidative stress. In some patients who have progressed to end-stage liver disease and undergone transplantation, the condition has recurred.

Tumours and infiltrations

The liver is a common site for tumour metastasis. Primary liver tumours are rare in the western world but occur frequently in other geographical areas. Primary tumours are associated with cirrhosis, persistence of serological markers for hepatitis B and C, and various carcinogens, including aflatoxins. Plasma α-fetoprotein is elevated at diagnosis in approximately 70% of

Case history 5.4

A 54-year old woman with newly diagnosed diabetes was referred to a diabetic clinic for initial investigation and treatment. Physical examination was unremarkable except for a body mass index of 36 kg/m^2 (ideal 20–25).

Investigations

serum:	creatinine	92 μmol/L
	bilirubin	16 μmol/L
	AST	72 U/L
	ALP	142 U/L
	GGT	98 U/L
	albumin	43 g/L
	cholesterol	5.2 mmol/L
	triglyceride (fasting)	7.4 mmol/L
blood:	HbA$_{1c}$	9.2%

Comment

Because of the abnormal results of liver function tests, she was more extensively investigated. Serological tests for hepatitis viruses and autoantibodies were negative and there was no evidence of haemochromatosis; ultrasound examination of the liver showed hyper-reflectivity, typical of fatty infiltration. The patient strongly denied excessive alcohol intake, maintaining that she drank only an occasional glass of wine 'to be sociable, when we go out'. A presumptive diagnosis of non-alcoholic fatty liver disease was made; she was given dietary advice and prescribed metformin. Six months later, her body mass index had fallen to 31 and HbA$_{1c}$ was 7%, indicating satisfactory glycaemic control. Repeat liver function tests were normal, and fasting triglyceride concentration was 3.2 mmol/L.

patients with primary hepatocellular carcinomas and is a valuable marker for this tumour, although it can also be increased, usually to a lesser extent, in acute and chronic hepatitis and in cirrhosis. Infiltrative conditions that can affect the liver include lymphomas and amyloidosis. Patients with such conditions, and with intrahepatic tumours, are often not jaundiced. The only

Case history 5.5

An elderly woman consulted her general practitioner because of weight loss and constipation. She had lost approximately 8 kg in weight in two months and had lost her appetite. She had previously opened her bowels daily but had recently had intervals of several days between movements and had passed only small amounts of stool on each occasion. On examination she was anaemic and had obviously lost weight. The liver was enlarged and had an irregular edge; a mass was palpable in the right iliac fossa.

Investigations

serum: albumin	30 g/L
ALP	314 U/L
bilirubin, AST and GGT	normal
stool occult blood	positive

A barium enema revealed a carcinoma of the caecum; an isotopic liver scan showed multiple filling defects characteristic of tumour deposits.

Comment

An increase in serum ALP in a patient with carcinoma could be due to metastases in bone or liver. When the source of the enzyme is not obvious clinically, it can usually be inferred from isoenzyme studies. With hepatic metastases there is often no increase in plasma bilirubin concentration unless lymph nodes at the porta hepatis are involved and obstruct the major bile ducts. Although tumour deposits within the liver can cause obstruction of small bile ducts, which is reflected by the increase in ALP, bilirubin leaking into the bloodstream can be taken up and excreted by parts of the liver not affected by tumour.

Hypoalbuminaemia is common in malignant disease and is usually multifactorial. Poor nutrition, increased catabolism (cancer cachexia) and replacement of normal hepatic tissue by tumour are all possible contributory causes in this case.

Carcinoma of the caecum is often clinically silent and may not present until extensive secondary spread has occurred.

biochemical abnormality may be an increase in plasma ALP activity.

The investigation of jaundice

In adults, jaundice due to unconjugated hyperbilirubinaemia is usually mild. Gilbert's syndrome, haemolysis and interference with hepatic bilirubin uptake by drugs are the major causes. Other liver function tests are normal and bilirubin is absent from the urine. Gilbert's syndrome (*see below*) is usually diagnosed by exclusion of other causes; features of haemolytic jaundice are summarized in *Fig. 5.5*.

In liver disease of whatever type, although there may be decreased uptake and conjugation of bilirubin, impaired excretion is the major cause of hyperbilirubinaemia and the retained bilirubin is conjugated. The differential diagnosis of jaundice due to conjugated hyperbilirubinaemia thus includes hepatitis and causes of intra- and extrahepatic cholestasis, that is obstruction of the flow of bile from the liver into the gut (*see Fig. 5.4*). Valuable diagnostic information may be provided by the history and examination. Biochemical tests can also give valuable information; for example, a high plasma aminotransferase activity suggests the presence of hepatocellular damage while a very high ALP activity suggests cholestasis. Serology, for detection of autoantibodies or evidence of viral infection, is essential.

It is rarely possible to distinguish reliably between intra- and extrahepatic cholestasis from the results of biochemical tests alone. Once hepatitis has been excluded, the next step is usually ultrasound examination, followed by appropriate further investigations depending on whether this provides evidence of biliary obstruction (*see Fig. 5.8* and *p. 90*).

The investigation of jaundice that develops following surgery is discussed in *Case History 5.7*. Cholestasis, sometimes leading to jaundice, is a recognized complication of parenteral nutrition. It is discussed in detail in *Chapter 20*.

Inherited abnormalities of bilirubin metabolism

There are four conditions in which jaundice is caused by an inherited abnormality of bilirubin metabolism: Gilbert's, Crigler–Najjar, Dubin–Johnson and Rotor syndromes. Their characteristics are summarized in

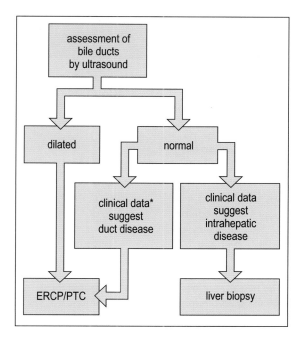

Fig. 5.8 Procedures for the investigation of cholestatic jaundice. ERCP = endoscopic retrograde cholangiopancreatography; PTC = percutaneous transhepatic cholangiography (second choice procedure). *For example, biliary pain.

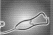 **Case history 5.6**

A retired publican presented to his family practitioner with a three-month history of epigastric pain radiating into the back and not related to meals. He was given antacids but returned one month later with more severe pain and weight loss. Over the past week his urine had become dark in colour and his stools pale. He had also become jaundiced. On examination, apart from the jaundice and signs of recent weight loss, no abnormality was found.

Investigations

serum:		
	total protein	72 g/L
	albumin	40 g/L
	bilirubin	380 µmol/L
	ALP	510 U/L
	AST	80 U/L
	GGT	115 U/L

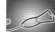 **Case history 5.6 (cont'd)**

Ultrasound examination demonstrated the presence of dilated bile ducts.

A barium meal and follow-through revealed indentation of the second part of the duodenum by an extrinsic mass, thought to be a carcinoma of the head of the pancreas.

A computerized tomogram of the abdomen also suggested the presence of tumour within the pancreas and this was confirmed at laparotomy.

Comment

The results of the biochemical tests suggest that the jaundice is due to biliary obstruction and militate against, although do not exclude, the presence of liver disease. The clinical features are very suggestive of a carcinoma of the head of the pancreas obstructing the common bile duct as it enters the duodenum. However, the biochemical results, although compatible with this diagnosis, could also be caused by a calculus obstructing the common bile duct, a metastatic tumour involving lymph nodes at the hilum of the liver or intrahepatic cholestasis.

Pancreatic carcinoma often presents with pain and cholestatic jaundice. The plasma concentration of the tumour marker CA19-9 is often elevated (*see* p. 332), but by the time the condition is diagnosed, it is usually too advanced for treatment to be curative.

Fig. 5.9. Gilbert's syndrome affects 2–3% of the population but the others are rare.

The jaundice of Gilbert's syndrome is typically mild and present only intermittently. It is often noticed after an infection or a period of decreased food intake, possibly because fasting increases plasma concentrations of free fatty acids, which compete with bilirubin for transport by albumin and uptake into liver cells. There may be mild malaise and hepatic tenderness but there are no other abnormal physical signs. The liver is histologically normal and there are no sequelae.

Gilbert's syndrome is usually diagnosed on the basis of the clinical features and the exclusion of haemolysis.

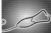 **Case history 5.7**

An elderly man was admitted to hospital with acute abdominal pain. Clinically, he had generalized peritonitis and radiography suggested a perforated viscus. At laparotomy, he was found to have a ruptured diverticulum of the sigmoid colon. Peritoneal lavage was carried out and a defunctioning colostomy was constructed. Seventy-two hours later he was still very ill; he was hypotensive despite adequate fluid replacement and treatment with inotropic drugs; faeculent material was leaking from his wound, and he was slightly jaundiced.

Investigations

serum: bilirubin   84 µmol/L
        AST   124 U/L
        ALP   152 U/L

Comment

Postoperative jaundice is a common clinical problem. Causes include:

- increased bilirubin formation, e.g. due to haemolysis of transfused stored blood or resorption of haematomas
- hepatocellular damage, e.g. due to drugs, shock, transfusion-transmitted or coincidental hepatitis
- intrahepatic cholestasis, e.g. due to sepsis, hypotension, drugs or parenteral nutrition
- extrahepatic obstruction, e.g. due to calculi or perioperative damage to the bile ducts.

Postoperative jaundice is often multifactorial, as in this patient who was both hypotensive and septic. The elevated ALP is consistent with cholestasis but the elevated aminotransferase could be due to damage to other tissues besides the liver. The cause of cholestasis in septic patients is uncertain: impaired hepatic secretory capacity, obstruction due to swelling of Kupffer cells and changes in the composition of bile may all play a part.

 Case history 5.8

A medical student recovering from an attack of influenza was noticed to be slightly jaundiced. Worried that he might have hepatitis, the student had some blood taken for biochemical tests.

Investigations

serum: bilirubin   60 µmol/l
        ALP   74 U/L
        AST   35 U/L
        haemoglobin   16 g/dL
        reticulocytes 1%
urine: bilirubin   negative

Comment

The negative urine bilirubin indicates that the excess bilirubin in the serum is unconjugated. There is no evidence of hepatocellular damage and the normal haemoglobin and reticulocyte count indicate that haemolysis cannot be the cause of the raised bilirubin. By elimination, the diagnosis is Gilbert's syndrome.

The hyperbilirubinaemia is due to a defect in the regulatory part of the gene coding for bilirubin UDP-glucuronyl transferase; in some cases there is also decreased hepatic uptake of bilirubin. In cases where there is a family history, the pattern of inheritance is characteristic of an autosomal dominant, single gene defect.

If there is any doubt, provocative tests may be helpful. An increase in plasma bilirubin concentration of 20 µmol/L in response to either a 400 kcal food intake over 48 hours or an infusion of nicotinic acid (50 mg intravenously over 30 seconds, with blood samples taken every half hour for two hours, then hourly for three hours) is characteristic.

Isolated abnormalities of 'liver enzymes'

With the widespread use of biochemical profiling, abnormalities of liver enzymes are often discovered incidentally, that is in the absence of clinical evidence of

Inherited disorders of bilirubin metabolism		
Syndrome	**Defect**	**Clinical features**
Gilbert's	decreased conjugation of bilirubin and decreased uptake in some cases (autosomal dominant)	mild, fluctuant unconjugated hyperbilirubinaemia which increases on fasting normal biopsy normal lifespan
Crigler–Najjar	Type 1 (autosomal recessive) absence of conjugating enzyme	severe unconjugated hyperbilirubinaemia early death due to kernicterus partial response to phototherapy, none to phenobarbital
	Type 2 (?autosomal recessive) partial defect of conjugating enzyme	severe unconjugated hyperbilirubinaemia, but good response to phenobarbital and phototherapy often survive to adulthood
Dubin–Johnson	decreased hepatic excretion of bilirubin (autosomal recessive)	mild, fluctuant conjugated hyperbilirubinaemia hepatic pigment disposition (melanin) increased coproporphyrin I/III ratio in urine bilirubinuria normal lifespan
Rotor	unknown (autosomal recessive)	similar to Dubin–Johnson but no hepatic pigmentation

Fig. 5.9 Inherited disorders of bilirubin metabolism. The precise nature of the metabolic defect in Dubin–Johnson syndrome is not known.

hepatobiliary disease. An isolated increase in ALP is usually due to bone disease: hepatic causes usually result in an increase in GGT and the combination should prompt further investigation. An isolated increase in GGT is usually due to enzyme induction (e.g. by alcohol or drugs) and not to liver damage. Isolated increases in aminotransferases are common. They can indicate clinically silent hepatitis; non-alcoholic steatohepatitis (NASH, *see* p. 95) is a more frequent cause. The possibility that drugs (whether prescribed, over-the-counter, recreational or contained in herbal remedies) are responsible should always be considered. Abnormalities of liver function tests are seen frequently in acutely ill patients: causes include intrahepatic cholestasis secondary to sepsis and hepatic congestion secondary to heart failure.

Uncommon liver diseases

Wilson's disease is an inherited abnormality (autosomal recessive) of copper metabolism, characterized by decreased biliary excretion of copper and decreased incorporation of copper into caeruloplasmin, a plasma protein. Copper is deposited in the liver, the basal ganglia of the brain and the cornea of the eye. Patients with Wilson's disease may present either in childhood with a fulminating hepatitis, accompanied in many cases by haemolysis and a renal tubular defect, or in young adults with cirrhosis or manifestations of disease of the basal ganglia (e.g. dysarthria, tremor and choreiform movements).

The biochemical features of Wilson's disease are a reduced plasma caeruloplasmin concentration, low–normal or low plasma copper (with increased binding to albumin) and increased urinary copper excretion. The decrease in caeruloplasmin is not unique to Wilson's disease, but is also seen in chronic hepatitis and malnutrition. The definitive diagnostic test is the demonstration of a high copper content in liver tissue obtained by biopsy; increased hepatic copper deposition is also seen to a lesser extent in primary biliary cirrhosis and in neonatal biliary atresia but these conditions have other distinguishing features.

Wilson's disease is treated with penicillamine, which chelates copper and increases its urinary excretion; in chronic cases this often halts the progress of the disease. When patients present with fulminant hepatitis the prognosis is poor, but some cases have been treated successfully by liver transplantion; since the genetic defect is expressed in the liver, transplantation effectively cures the disease.

Haemochromatosis (*see p. 317*), an inherited disorder characterized by excessive iron uptake from the gut and iron deposition in the tissues, can affect many organs, including the liver.

α_1-Antitrypsin deficiency (*see p. 240*), an inherited condition characterized either by the absence of this protein from the plasma or by the presence of an abnormal form of the protein, is another rare cause of cirrhosis.

Liver transplantation

Liver transplantation is now increasingly used for the treatment of irreversible, severe liver disease. Donor organs are scarce and careful patient selection is vital. Following surgery, the major complications include haemorrhage, renal failure, immediate non-function of the graft, infection and rejection. The results of measurements of plasma aminotransferases and other liver function tests may suggest the development of complications, but diagnosis usually rests on imaging techniques or biopsy. The monitoring of immuno-suppressive treatment with ciclosporin and tacrolimus is discussed in *Chapter 19*.

Gallstones and biliary tract disease

Gallstones are composed primarily of cholesterol with varying amounts of bilirubin and calcium salts. Cholesterol is maintained in solution in bile by virtue of the surface-active properties of bile salts and lecithin, but while a change in the proportion of these components may predispose to stone formation, other factors are also involved. Stones consisting primarily of bilirubin diglucuronide may develop in patients with chronic haemolytic anaemias.

Gallstones may be clinically silent. They can, however, cause biliary colic and obstruction and predispose to cholecystitis, cholangitis and pancreatitis. Biochemical tests may be of value in the management of these conditions, but the analysis of biliary calculi is of no importance in the routine diagnosis or surgical management of patients with gallstones.

Primary sclerosing cholangitis (PSC) is a cholestatic liver disease characterized by inflammation and progressive fibrosis of the biliary system, leading to cirrhosis and liver failure. Though it can occur at any age, most patients are young men, and some two-thirds have inflammatory bowel disease (usually ulcerative colitis). The cause is unknown, but an immunological basis seems likely. The majority of patients are positive for perinuclear antineutrophil cytoplasmic antibodies (ANCA), but these are by no means specific to this condition, occurring, for example, in up to 50% of patients with autoimmune hepatitis. Between 10 and 30% of patients with primary sclerosing cholangitis develop cholangiocarcinoma, an aggressive tumour of bile ducts. Measurement of tumour markers may be of value in monitoring PSC. Plasma CA 19-9 concentrations are elevated in PSC and reflect disease activity; CA 19-9 concentrations rise to very high levels in cholangiocarcinoma. Plasma CEA (carcinembryonic antigen, *see p. 330*) concentrations are usually normal in uncomplicated PSC and rise more modestly in cholangiocarcinoma. An increase in a weighted index of the concentration of both markers is predictive of the onset of cholangiocarcinoma in a majority of cases.

Liver disease in children

Jaundice is common in neonates and is frequently physiological (*see Chapter 21*). Such jaundice is due to unconjugated bilirubin and does not persist beyond two weeks after birth. Separate measurement of conjugated bilirubin ('split bilirubin') can be helpful. If more than 25% of plasma bilirubin is conjugated, hepatobiliary disease should be considered. Clinical features that suggest liver disease include pale stools and dark urine, bruising or bleeding, hepatomegaly, failure to thrive and (rarely) dysmorphic features. The causes of conjugated hyperbilirubinaemia in the neonate include neonatal hepatitis (due to intrauterine infection, e.g. with cytomegalovirus, rubella or toxoplasmosis, or perinatal infection, e.g. with herpes simplex), biliary abnormalities (biliary atresia, choledochal cysts) and metabolic disorders (α_1-antitrypsin deficiency, tyrosinaemia type 1, galactosaemia, cystic fibrosis, etc.).

Beyond the neonatal period, the causes of liver disease include viral hepatitis, autoimmune disease and metabolic disorders. In contrast to babies presenting in the neonatal period, older children with liver disease may not be jaundiced.

Liver disease in pregnancy

Pregnancy can reveal previously undiagnosed liver disease or exacerbate known pre-existing disease, particularly primary biliary cirrhosis. Some liver diseases, however, occur only during pregnancy. Two conditions typically cause cholestasis: hyperemesis gravidarum and intrahepatic cholestasis of pregnancy.

In hyperemesis gravidarum, severe vomiting, usually in the first trimester, can cause dehydration and undernutrition. There may be mild jaundice and plasma liver enzyme activities may be increased up to four times normal. Fat accumulation in the liver has been demonstrated on biopsy and is probably related to under-nutrition, as the abnormalities can be reversed by improving nutrient intake. Intrahepatic cholestasis of pregnancy typically occurs in the last trimester. The major clinical feature is pruritus, later accompanied by mild jaundice. Plasma bilirubin concentration rarely exceeds 100 μmol/L; plasma alkaline phosphatase activity can be increased up to ten times normal, but bile acid concentrations may be increased up to a hundredfold and this may be the only biochemical abnormality. The condition resolves rapidly after delivery but is associated with an increased risk of premature labour and stillbirth. The cause is unknown but there is evidence that it has a genetic basis.

There are also hepatitic syndromes specific to pregnancy. Acute fatty liver of pregnancy is a severe, uncommon condition, which typically presents late in pregnancy, with malaise, anorexia, vomiting and abdominal pain, followed by jaundice and a substantial risk of progression to acute liver failure and biochemical findings typical of that condition. Hyperuricaemia is an early biochemical abnormality. Untreated, mortality is up to 20%, but rapid resolution usually follows delivery. A greater than expected number of cases are associated with a genetic defect of long-chain fatty acid oxidation.

Pregnancy-induced hypertension (pre-eclampsia, see p. 188) is characterized by the development of hypertension, proteinuria and oedema, typically in the third trimester or late in the second. A small number of patients progress to eclampsia, with severe hypertension, seizures and coma. Treatment of hypertension may be required but delivery is usually curative. In the HELLP syndrome [haemolysis, elevated liver enzymes (aminotransferases up to ten times normal) and low platelet count ($<100 \times 10^{12}$/L)], pre-eclampsia is associated with nausea, vomiting, abdominal pain and disseminated intravascular coagulopathy (DIC). There is moderate, and mainly unconjugated, hyperbilirubinaemia, but (in contrast to acute fatty live of pregnancy) encephalopathy does not occur. The pathogenesis of pregnancy-induced hypertension is uncertain, but there is increasing evidence that implicates disordered prostaglandin metabolism.

Drugs and the liver

The liver plays a central role in the metabolism of many drugs, converting them to polar, water-soluble metabolites, which can be excreted in bile and urine. The enzymes involved are located in the smooth endoplasmic reticulum of the hepatocytes. Metabolism usually involves two types of reaction: phase 1 metabolism, for example oxidation or demethylation by cytochrome P450-linked enzymes; and phase 2 metabolism in which phase 1 metabolites are conjugated with polar molecules, for example glucuronic acid or glutathione.

Drug-induced liver damage may be predictable, arising when a toxic metabolite is produced by a phase 1 reaction at a rate which exceeds the detoxicating capacity of the phase 2 reaction, as occurs, for example, in a paracetamol overdose. However, many drugs may have toxic effects when used in therapeutic doses (*Fig. 5.10*); this response (idiosyncratic hepatotoxicity) is unpredictable and is independent of the dose of the drug administered. Some idiosyncratic reactions to drugs,

Some drugs causing liver disease

Dose-dependent hepatotoxicity
paracetamol (in overdose)
salicylates (high doses only)
tetracyclines (high doses only)
azathioprine
methotrexate

Idiosyncratic hepatotoxicity
isoniazid*
halothane
methyldopa*
rifampicin
dantrolene*

Dose-dependent cholestasis
methyltestosterone

Idiosyncratic cholestatic hepatitis
chlorpromazine
erythromycin estolate
chlorpropamide
tolbutamide
nitrofurantoin*

Fig. 5.10 Some drugs causing liver disease.
Rifampicin also impairs bilirubin uptake and excretion,
and induces hepatic enzymes involved in drug
metabolism. * Signifies that chronic hepatitis can occur.

such as halothane-induced liver damage, have an immunological basis: the binding of a metabolite to a liver cell protein alters its antigenicity and provokes an immune response.

Some drugs are associated with the development of cholestasis: this may be an idiosyncratic response, as is the case with chlorpromazine, and additionally there is often evidence of liver cell damage. Other drugs, for instance 17α-alkyl-substituted steroids, including some anabolic steroids, predictably cause cholestasis without hepatocellular damage when administered in high doses.

Minor degrees of hepatic dysfunction occur relatively frequently as results of idiosyncratic responses, but overt hepatotoxicity is fortunately rare. The simple tests of liver function and damage are important for the detection of hepatotoxicity during trials of new drugs.

Other adverse effects of drugs on the liver include hepatic fibrosis or cirrhosis (particularly with methotrexate), granuloma formation, vascular disease and the development of tumours.

Test / Condition	Acute hepatitis	Chronic hepatitis	Cirrhosis	Cholestasis	Malignancy and infiltrations
Bilirubin	N to ↑↑	N to ↑	N to ↑	↑ to ↑↑↑	N
Aminotransferases	↑↑↑	↑	N to ↑	N to ↑	N to ↑
Alkaline phosphatase	N to ↑	N§	N to ↑↑	↑↑↑	↑↑
Albumin	N	N to ↓	N to ↓	N	N to ↓
γ-Globulins	N	↑	↑	N	N
Prothrombin time	N to ↑*	N to ↑	N to ↑*	N to ↑†	N

Fig. 5.11 Typical patterns of abnormalities of simple liver function tests in various liver diseases. The severity of the abnormalities is dependent on the degree of liver damage and its effect on liver function.
N = Normal.
* Not corrected by parenteral vitamin K.
§ May be increased if cirrhosis is present.
† Corrected by parenteral vitamin K.

SUMMARY

- The liver has a central role in intermediary metabolism and is also responsible for the detoxification of many foreign compounds, deamination of amino acids and synthesis of urea, synthesis and excretion of bile, metabolism of some hormones, synthesis of plasma proteins and storage of certain vitamins.

- Because of its considerable functional reserve, **biochemical tests tend to be insensitive indicators of hepatic function, although they can be highly sensitive indicators of damage to the liver**. The results of biochemical tests often indicate the nature of a liver disease (*Fig. 5.11*), but less often indicate a specific diagnosis. They are, however, invaluable in monitoring the course of liver disease and the response of patients to treatment. **Imaging techniques and biopsy are more often diagnostic**.

- The most frequently performed biochemical tests are the measurement of plasma **bilirubin** and **albumin** concentrations and the measurement of the activities of the **aminotransferases**, **alkaline phosphatase** (ALP) and **γ-glutamyl transferase** (GGT) in the plasma.

- A raised plasma bilirubin concentration is a frequent but not invariable finding in patients with liver disease. However, **conjugated hyperbilirubinaemia can result from extrahepatic biliary obstruction** and a mild, **unconjugated hyperbilirubinaemia is often a result of haemolysis**.

- Greatly increased plasma aminotransferase activities are characteristic of hepatocellular damage; greatly increased ALP activity is characteristic of biliary obstruction. However, the aminotransferases may be increased irrespective of either the nature or cause of hepatocellular damage and ALP may be increased with both intra- and extrahepatic obstruction. In many patients with liver disease, moderate increases in both enzymes are observed. Furthermore, changes in neither of these enzymes are specific to liver disease.

- Plasma **GGT activity** is frequently increased in liver disease but an isolated increase may indicate excessive alcohol consumption; the finding of an increase in GGT in a patient with an increased plasma ALP activity implies a hepatic origin for the latter.

- **Albumin** is synthesized by the liver but, because of its long plasma half-life, plasma albumin concentration tends to be decreased only in chronic liver disease. Many other factors can also affect albumin concentration. Blood clotting factors are synthesized in the liver and the **prothrombin time** provides a sensitive and rapidly responsive index of hepatic synthetic capacity.

- **Serological** tests for specific **autoantibodies** are valuable in the differential diagnosis of chronic liver disease. Serology for evidence of **viral infection** is valuable in both acute and chronic liver disease. Other tests which may be useful in specific liver diseases include the measurement of α-fetoprotein (liver cancer), α_1-antitrypsin (α_1-antitrypsin deficiency) and copper and caeruloplasmin (Wilson's disease).

6 The gastrointestinal tract

INTRODUCTION

The digestion and absorption of food is a complex process, which depends upon the integrated activity of the organs of the alimentary tract. Food is mixed with the various digestive fluids, which contain enzymes and cofactors, and is broken down into small molecules which are absorbed by the intestinal epithelium. Complex carbohydrates such as starch are converted to mono- and disaccharides, the latter undergoing further hydrolysis by intestinal brush border disaccharidases (e.g. lactase) to allow absorption of the constituent monosaccharides. Proteins are broken down by proteases (secreted as inactive precursors) and peptidases to oligopeptides and amino acids. The absorption of fat is a complex process. Mechanical mixing and the action of bile salts create an emulsion of triglycerides (strictly, triacylglycerols, *see Chapter 14*), which is a substrate for pancreatic lipase. This enzyme converts triglycerides to free fatty acids and monoglycerides. These are then incorporated with bile salts into mixed micelles and are absorbed from these into intestinal epithelial cells where they are re-esterified.

All these processes require the intimate mixing of enzymes, cofactors and substrates, and the maintenance of the optimum pH for enzyme activity. Disorders of the stomach, pancreas, liver and small intestine can result in the malabsorption of nutrients.

In addition to its importance in the absorption of water and nutrients, the mucosal lining of the gastrointestinal tract has an important barrier function, providing protection against the action of hydrogen ions and enzymes, and preventing invasion of its wall by its normal bacterial flora. The small intestine also contributes to this protective function through its immune function. In gastrointestinal disease, this barrier function may be compromised and bacteria may gain access to the circulation and cause a septicaemia.

The gut also secretes numerous hormones, most of which act on the gut itself or on related organs.

Gastrin	
Functions	**Control of secretion**

stimulation of:
  gastric acid
    secretion
  pepsin secretion
  gastric motility
  growth of gastric
    mucosa
	stimulated by:
	  increased vagal
	    discharge
	  gastric distension
	  food, particularly
	    amino acids and
	    peptides, in
	    stomach
	  calcium in blood

	inhibited by:
	  gastric acidity
	  gastrointestinal
	    hormones,
	    e.g. secretin

Fig. 6.1 Gastrin: functions and control of secretion.

THE STOMACH

In the stomach, food mixes with acidic gastric juice, which contains the proenzyme of pepsin, and intrinsic factor, essential for the absorption of vitamin B_{12}. Secretion of gastric juice is under the combined control of the vagus nerve and the hormone gastrin.

Gastrin is secreted by G-cells in the antrum of the stomach itself and has several physiological functions (*Fig. 6.1*). It is a polypeptide hormone, present in the bloodstream mainly in two forms, G-17 and G-34, containing 17 and 34 amino acids respectively. Other gastrin molecules have been identified in the blood, but the physiological significance of this heterogeneity is not known. All the variants have an identical C-terminal amino acid sequence.

Disorders and investigation of gastric function

Biochemical tests are of limited use in the diagnosis of gastric disorders: the stomach can be directly inspected by endoscopy, and contrast radiography can also provide valuable information. Biochemical tests can be used to investigate conditions in which it is suspected that gastric acid secretion may be abnormal, particularly in atypical or recurrent peptic ulceration.

Most peptic ulceration is associated with colonization of the stomach with *Helicobacter pylori*. This organism decreases the resistance of gastric mucosa to acid, and stimulates gastrin, and hence acid, secretion. Increased acid secretion is important in the pathogenesis of duodenal ulcers. Eradication of this organism is curative. The diagnosis is by serology. *Helicobacter* can split urea to form ammonia and carbon dioxide, and this is the basis for a breath test, formerly used for diagnosis but now occasionally to confirm eradication or to indicate persisting infection after treatment. The sensitivity of this test is 96% and specificity virtually 100%. Isotopically labelled (^{13}C- or ^{14}C-) urea is given orally and the isotope is measured in the expired breath. Excretion is increased if infection is present. H_2-receptor antagonists (which block H_2-histamine receptors), inhibitors of H^+,K^+-ATPase (proton pump inhibitors) and sucraflate, which protects the mucosa, are all effective in relieving symptoms and promoting healing. H_2-receptor antagonists can be given chronically to prevent recurrence in patients who do not have *H. pylori* or in whom attempts at eradication fail. Surgery is now rarely required in peptic ulcer disease.

In a small number of patients, peptic ulceration is atypical: for example, duodenal ulcers are resistant to medical treatment or recur, or there are multiple or jejunal ulcers. Atypical peptic ulceration is a feature of Zollinger–Ellison syndrome, a rare condition in which hypergastrinaemia is caused by a gastrinoma of the pancreas, duodenum or, less frequently, the G-cells of the stomach. Approximately 60% of gastrinomas are malignant and in approximately 30% of cases they occur as part of a syndrome of multiple endocrine neoplasia (MEN). Plasma gastrin concentrations typically exceed 200 ng/L (normal <50). In addition to having recurrent or atypical peptic ulceration, patients sometimes have steatorrhoea, owing to inhibition of pancreatic lipase by the excessive gastric acid.

The first-line biochemical test in such patients is the measurement of fasting plasma gastrin concentration. This is frequently elevated, but some patients with gastrinomas have normal or only slightly elevated plasma gastrin concentrations and there are other causes of hypergastrinaemia (*see Fig. 6.2*), including achlorhydria. This is a condition most frequently seen in patients with atrophic gastritis but is also present in pernicious anaemia; it can occur in association with gastric carcinoma, and may be present even in patients with peptic ulceration. If the cause of hypergastrinaemia is in doubt and in patients with atypical peptic ulceration but whose gastrin concentrations are not clearly elevated, it may be helpful to measure plasma gastrin concentration following the administration of secretin. This hormone increases gastrin secretion from gastrinomas, but reduces it or has no effect in hypergastrinaemia from other causes. Measurement of gastric acid secretion may also help to distinguish between the causes of hyper-gastrinaemia. It is typically >15 mmol/h in patients with gastrinomas but low and resistant to stimulation in patients with achlorhydria. Maximal gastric acid secretion can be measured by the pentagastrin test. Protocols for the test vary but in essence it involves measurement of acid in fluid aspirated through a nasogastric tube in the resting state and after the administration of pentagastrin, a synthetic analogue of gastrin. Basal acid secretion is normally <10 mmol/h in males (<6 mmol/h

Causes of hypergastrinaemia		
Disorder	**Gastric acid secretion**	**Gastrin response to secretin**
Zollinger–Ellison syndrome	greatly ↑	↑
hypersecretion of gastrin by antral G-cells	greatly ↑	none or ↓
pernicious anaemia	↓	↓
post vagotomy	↓	↓
chronic renal failure	variable	↓

Fig. 6.2 Some causes of hypergastrinaemia.

in females); stimulated secretion is normally <45 mmol/h in males and <35 mmol/h in females.

Zollinger–Ellison syndrome is treated by surgical removal of the tumour, where possible. Vagotomy and long-term treatment with inhibitors of gastric acid secretion may also be necessary and may be the only possible treatment if the tumour cannot be resected.

It should be noted that inhibitors of gastric acid secretion can themselves cause increased gastrin secretion: H_2-inhibitors should be stopped three days, and proton pump inhibitors two weeks, before taking blood for gastrin measurement. As the hormone is very labile, the blood must be mixed with aprotinin, a protease inhibitor, immediately after venesection, to prevent degradation.

THE PANCREAS

The pancreas is an essential endocrine organ producing insulin, glucagon, pancreatic polypeptide and other hormones; its endocrine functions are discussed in *Chapter 11*. The exocrine secretion of the pancreas is an alkaline, bicarbonate-rich juice containing various enzymes essential for normal digestion: the proenzyme forms of the proteases, trypsin, chymotrypsin and carboxypeptidase, and the lipolytic enzyme lipase, co-lipase and amylase.

The secretion of pancreatic juice is primarily under the control of two hormones secreted by the small intestine: secretin, a 27 amino acid polypeptide, which stimulates the secretion of an alkaline fluid, and cholecystokinin (CCK), which stimulates the secretion of pancreatic enzymes and contraction of the gallbladder. Like gastrin, CCK is a heterogeneous hormone: the predominant form in the gut is a 33 amino acid polypeptide, but an eight amino acid form is present in some parts of the central nervous system and appears to function as a neuro-transmitter. Both secretin and CCK are secreted in response to the presence of acid, amino acids and partly digested proteins in the duodenum.

Pancreatic disorders and their investigation

The major disorders of the exocrine pancreas are acute pancreatitis, chronic pancreatitis, pancreatic cancer and cystic fibrosis. Biochemical investigations are essential in the diagnosis and management of the first of these, of limited use in the second, and of little use in the third. Cystic fibrosis, an inherited metabolic disease causing progressive loss of pancreatic function, is discussed in *Chapter 16*. Clinical evidence of impaired exocrine function is usually only seen in advanced pancreatic disease. Endocrine function is usually well preserved, although glucose intolerance or frank diabetes can develop in severe or advanced disease. Endocrine disease of the pancreas is discussed in *Chapter 11*.

Acute pancreatitis

This condition presents as an acute abdomen with severe pain and a variable degree of shock. The most frequent known causes are excessive alcohol ingestion and gallstones; many cases are idiopathic. Less common causes include infection (usually viral), hypertrigly-ceridaemia and hypercalcaemia. The pancreas becomes acutely inflamed and, in severe cases, haemorrhagic.

The initial lesion involves intracellular activation of enzyme precursors, leading to the generation of oxygen free radicals and an acute inflammatory response. This may extend beyond the pancreas and lead to adult respiratory distress syndrome (ARDS), circulatory and renal failure. Sepsis, probably as a result of bacterial translocation from the gut, is a life-threatening com-plication. Some degree of organ failure occurs in approximately 25% of patients and the mortality is 5–10%.

The clinical diagnosis is supported by finding a high serum amylase activity. This enzyme is secreted by salivary glands and the exocrine pancreas. Its activity in serum is usually (though not invariably) raised in acute pancreatitis, levels >10 × ULN (upper limit of normal) being virtually diagnostic. However, the increase may not be so great, and elevated levels may be seen in other conditions presenting with acute abdominal pain, particularly perforated duodenal ulcer (*see Fig. 6.3*). Amylase is a relatively small molecule, and is rapidly excreted by the kidneys (hence the increase in activity in renal failure); in mild pancreatitis, rapid clearance may be reflected by a normal serum level but increased urinary amylase. Extra-abdominal causes of a raised plasma amylase activity rarely cause increases of more than 5 × ULN. Macroamylasaemia is an example of a high plasma enzyme activity being due to reduced clearance. In this condition, amylase becomes complexed with

Case history 6.1

A 53-year-old man, who admitted to a heavy alcohol intake over many years, developed severe abdominal pain, which radiated through to the back. The pain had started quite suddenly, 18 hours before admission to hospital. He had no previous history of gastrointestinal disease. On examination, the patient was mildly shocked and his abdomen was tender in the epigastric region with slight guarding. There was no evidence of either intestinal obstruction or perforation of a viscus on radiographic examination. Blood was taken for urgent biochemical investigation.

Investigations

serum:		
urea	10 mmol/L	
creatinine	90 µmol/L	
calcium	2.10 mmol/L	
albumin	30 g/L	
glucose	12 mmol/L	
amylase	5000 U/L	

Comment

The diagnosis of acute pancreatitis is based on the clinical history, evidence of inflammation (usually by CT scanning) and the finding of a high serum (or sometimes urinary) amylase activity. It is effectively a diagnosis of exclusion: the finding of a very high serum amylase activity is very suggestive but is not on its own diagnostic, as many other conditions can cause elevated activity. It is necessary to consider all the available evidence, and to exclude other causes of an acute abdomen. In this case, the history is suggestive of pancreatitis and the clinical findings, although non-specific, are consistent with this diagnosis. The radiological findings militate against, but do not exclude, intestinal obstruction and perforation, two important differential diagnoses.

The slightly raised urea, with normal creatinine, can be explained by renal hypoperfusion due to shock. Loss of protein-rich exudate into the peritoneal cavity frequently causes a fall in plasma albumin concentration and contributes to the hypocalcaemia that is often present, especially in severe cases of acute pancreatitis. The formation of insoluble calcium salts of fatty acids, released within and around the inflamed pancreas by pancreatic lipase, also contributes to the hypocalcaemia. Hyperglycaemia may occur, but is usually transient.

another protein (in some cases an immunoglobulin) to form an entity of much greater apparent molecular weight; renal clearance is reduced as a result. This has no direct clinical sequelae but can misleadingly suggest the presence of pancreatic damage.

Measurement of the pancreas-specific isoenzyme of amylase can improve the diagnostic specificity of plasma amylase determinations. Measurement of serum lipase activity has been reported to be a more specific test for acute pancreatitis but the test is little used in the UK. A combination of lipase and amylase measurement has been reported to have specificity and sensitivity of approximately 90%.

In severe pancreatitis, methaemalbumin may be detectable in the plasma, but this finding is not sufficiently consistent to be of diagnostic value. The plasma of patients with pancreatitis may be lipaemic (due to hypertriglyceridaemia) and there may be a mild increase in bilirubin concentration and alkaline phosphatase activity. An early elevation in plasma aspartate transaminase activity is characteristic of pancreatitis caused by gallstones.

Several prognostic scoring systems that include biochemical data have been developed for acute pancreatitis to identify patients at greatest risk who should be managed in an intensive care facility. Three or more

Causes of an increased plasma amylase
>10 × ULN
acute pancreatitis
>5 × ULN
perforated duodenal ulcer
intestinal obstruction
other acute abdominal disorders
acute oliguric renal failure
diabetic ketoacidosis
ruptured Fallopian tube
usually <5 × ULN
salivary gland disorders, e.g. calculi and
inflammation (including mumps)
chronic renal failure
macroamylasaemia
morphine administration (spasm of sphincter of
Oddi)

Fig. 6.3 Causes of an increased plasma amylase activity. The values shown are typical, but higher or lower activities can occur in individual cases.

Ranson's criteria
On admission:
age >55 years*
white blood count >16 × 10^9/L*
blood glucose >11 mmol/L*
serum lactate dehydrogenase (LDH)
>350 U/L*
serum aspartate aminotransferase (AST)
>250 U/L*
During initial 48 h:
packed cell volume decrease >10%
serum urea increase >1.8 mmol/L*
serum calcium <2.00 mmol/L
$P\text{O}_2$ <8 kPa
base deficit >4 mmol/L*
fluid sequestration >6 L

Fig. 6.4 Ranson's criteria of severity in acute pancreatitis.
*These figures are for pancreatitis not due to gallstones; slightly different figures apply to gallstone-induced pancreatitis. Data taken from Ranson JH, *et al.* *Surg. Gynecol. Obstet.* 1974; 39: 69–81.

Ranson's signs (*see Fig. 6.4*) constitute severe pancreatitis: mortality is <1% if only one or two signs are present, but >40% with five or more. The APACHE-II scoring system (applicable to many acute conditions) is more complicated but more powerful: it is based on the measurement of twelve physiological measurements, the patient's age and evidence of chronic illness on admission.

The management of acute pancreatitis is essentially conservative. Patients should be given nothing by mouth. Fluid and electrolyte balance should be maintained by intravenous infusion and adequate analgesia provided. Enteral (nasojejunal) or parenteral feeding may be required. Prophylactic antibiotics are recommended in severe cases. Progress can be monitored by serial measurements of amylase and C-reactive protein, and by imaging (ultrasound and CT scanning).

Chronic pancreatitis

Chronic pancreatitis is an uncommon condition, which usually presents with abdominal pain or malabsorption and occasionally with impaired glucose tolerance. The malabsorption is due to impaired digestion of food, but there is considerable functional reserve and pancreatic lipase output must be reduced to only 10% of normal before steatorrhoea is produced. Such a reduction only occurs in extensive disease or if the main pancreatic duct is obstructed. Alcohol is an important aetiological factor and there may be a history of recurrent acute pancreatitis.

Tests of exocrine function (*see below*) are unhelpful in the investigation of pain thought to be of pancreatic origin, but are used to establish that pancreatic insufficiency is present in patients who present with malabsorption. Measurements of plasma amylase and lipase activities are of no value: they are normal or low in patients with chronic pancreatitis, except in acute exacerbations. Measurements of faecal enzymes are discussed on *p. 110*. Pancreatic calcification is frequently visible on plain abdominal X-ray of patients with advanced chronic pancreatitis. Ultrasound imaging will exclude gallstones or a dilated biliary system, and show the morphology of the pancreas. If abnormal, it should be followed by CT scanning. Endoscopic retrograde cholangiopancreatography (ERCP) is capable of revealing the characteristic anatomical changes of chronic pancreatitis long before the results of functional tests become abnormal. Percutaneous pancreatic biopsy (CT or ultrasound guided) is feasible but requires considerable skill.

The damage to the organ in chronic pancreatitis is irreversible. Management involves treatment of the underlying cause, if known, pain relief and avoidance of alcohol. Pancreatic extracts are indicated when features of malabsorption are present. Diabetes is treated with insulin. Surgery may be required when there is intractable pain.

Tests of pancreatic function

These fall into two groups: direct tests, involving analysis of fluid aspirated from the duodenum, and indirect tests, in which intubation of the patient is not required. The former are now rarely performed. Examples include the measurement of bicarbonate concentration and amylase or trypsin activity in duodenal fluid either following a test meal (Lundh test) or the administration of secretin and CCK. Bicarbonate concentration and enzyme activities are decreased in chronic pancreatic insufficiency.

Examples of the more widely used indirect tests include the fluorescein dilaurate and p-aminobenzoic acid (PABA) tests. Both utilize the same principle, measuring the excretion of an orally administered substance in a form dependent on pancreatic enzyme activity for its absorption. In the fluorescein dilaurate test (see Fig. 6.5), the substance is fluorescein dilaurate.

This is hydrolyzed in the gut by pancreatic esterase to yield fluorescein, which is absorbed from the gut, conjugated in the liver to fluorescein glucuronide and excreted in the urine, where it can be measured. The urinary excretion is compared with that following an equivalent amount of free fluorescein, thereby eliminating any influence of intestinal, hepatic or renal function on the result. However, since pancreatic esterase is dependent on bile salts for its activity, the test effectively assesses combined pancreatico-biliary function: results may wrongly suggest pancreatic deficiency if bile salt secretion is defective.

In the PABA test, benzoyltyrosyl-PABA (BT-PABA) is given orally together with a tracer quantity of isotopically labelled PABA. PABA is absorbed and excreted in the urine but pancreatic chymotrypsin is required to release PABA from BT-PABA. The amounts of radioactivity and excreted PABA are measured and compared with the doses administered to provide a ratio that reflects pancreatic exocrine function.

Pancreatic elastase and chymotrypsin activities in faeces are reduced in chronic pancreatic insufficiency. Measurements of both enzymes are used as tests for this condition: both show high sensitivity and specificity for the condition, with elastase being slightly superior in both respects.

Carcinoma of the pancreas

Pancreatic carcinoma may be difficult to diagnose (see Case History 5.6). Presentation often occurs as a result of metastases rather than as a direct effect of the primary tumour. Other presentations include obstructive

Fluorescein dilaurate test	
Procedure	**Results**

day 1 (test):
    give 0.5 mmol fluorescein dilaurate orally
    ensure adequate fluid intake
    collect urine for 10 h
    measure amount of fluorescein excreted
	$\dfrac{\text{fluorescein excreted on day 1}}{\text{fluorescein excreted on day 2}} \times 100 = \dfrac{\text{test}}{\text{control}}\ \text{index}$
	
	 normal pancreatic function: $\dfrac{\text{test}}{\text{control}}$ index >30%

day 2 (control):
    give 0.5 mmol fluorescein orally
    follow same procedure as day 1
	pancreatic insufficiency: $\dfrac{\text{test}}{\text{control}}$ index <20%

Fig. 6.5 Fluorescein dilaurate test.

jaundice, when a tumour in the head of the pancreas obstructs the common bile duct, and malabsorption. Biochemical tests of pancreatic function are rarely of any use in diagnosis, and other techniques, particularly imaging, are far more powerful diagnostic tools. The plasma concentration of the tumour markers carcinoembryonic antigen (CEA) and CA 19-9 are elevated in up to 80% of patients with pancreatic malignancy, but can be elevated with other (particularly colorectal) cancers and sometimes in non-malignant disease. Unfortunately, pancreatic cancer often presents late; by the time it is diagnosed, metastases are often present, and only palliative surgical procedures are feasible.

THE SMALL INTESTINE

The small intestine is the site of absorption of all nutrients; most of this absorption takes place in the duodenum and jejunum, but vitamin B_{12} and bile salts are absorbed in the terminal ileum. Approximately 8 L of fluid enter the gut every 24 h. This is derived from ingested food and water and from the digestive juices, including those secreted by the small intestine itself. Most of this fluid, and the salts it contains, is reabsorbed in the jejunum, ileum and large intestine.

The small intestine can be affected by many disease processes, but the major effects on function relate to the consequences of impaired absorption of nutrients and fluid, and to disruption of its barrier function.

Investigation of intestinal function

Tests of carbohydrate absorption

A variety of tests involving the ingestion of carbohydrates and the measurement of their plasma concentrations or urinary excretion have been developed for the investigation of small intestinal function. The best known is the xylose absorption test, which involves the administration of a test dose of D-xylose, a plant sugar. This is absorbed from the jejunum without prior digestion. It is only partly metabolized in the body, mainly being excreted unchanged in the urine, where it can be measured. Accurately timed urine collection is essential. Misleadingly low results are obtained if the glomerular filtration rate is decreased,

as occurs in renal failure and many normal elderly people. Other factors that can produce misleading results include delayed gastric emptying, oedema and obesity. An alternative approach is to measure serum xylose concentration 60 minutes after administering xylose.

This test is cheap and simple to perform. Although abnormal results are almost always found in severe coeliac disease and disorders of the proximal small intestine causing malabsorption, xylose absorption may be normal in milder disease. It cannot therefore be used to screen for malabsorption but may be helpful in the differential diagnosis of steatorrhoea. Xylose absorption is usually normal in patients with pancreatic disease and small intestinal disease affecting only the terminal ileum. It may be decreased in patients with bacterial overgrowth of the small intestine, due to bacterial fermentation. This provides the basis of a test for bacterial overgrowth (see p. 114). The diagnostic performance of the xylose test is improved by giving the xylose (5.0 g) together with 3-O-methyl-D-glucose (2.5 g) and comparing the absorption of the two sugars by measurement of their plasma concentrations. The normal molar [xylose]/[3-O-methyl-D-glucose] ratio is 1:3; it is reliably decreased in mucosal disease and a normal result effectively excludes untreated coeliac disease. In practice, however, the ease with which the proximal small intestine can now be biopsied has greatly reduced the need for and use of such investigations.

Some small intestinal conditions, including inflammatory bowel diseases (IBD), give rise to increased gut permeability; this can be assessed together with absorptive capacity by giving an oral mixture of D-xylose and 3-O-methyl-D-glucose together with L-rhamnose (1.0 g) and lactulose (5.0 g) and measuring their urinary excretions. The percentage dose excreted is calculated; the normal lactulose/rhamnose excretion ratio is <0.06; it is increased in untreated coeliac disease and in active small intestinal Crohn's disease, in which gut permeability to lactulose is increased but the absorption of rhamnose is decreased. However, this test is not widely used, in part because the analyses required are technically demanding.

Intestinal permeability can more easily be assessed by measuring the faecal concentration of the neutrophil protein, calprotectin. This is increased in almost all patients with IBD, correlates well with disease activity and is predictive of relapse in patients in remission. Of great practical importance is the fact that faecal calprotectin is usually normal in patients with irritable bowel syndrome (IBS), so that the demonstration of a normal value obviates the need of more extensive investigation of patients in whom a diagnosis of IBD or IBS is being considered.

Suspected intestinal disaccharidase deficiency can be investigated by administering the appropriate disaccharide (50 g) orally and measuring the blood glucose response. If the result is abnormal, specificity can be improved by comparing the result with that obtained following administration of the equivalent quantities (25 g each) of the constituent monosaccharides. Administration of the disaccharide usually provokes symptoms in patients with the corresponding enzyme deficiency: the faeces become acidic (pH <6.0) because fermentation produces organic acids, and faecal osmolality is increased (>350 mmol/kg) owing to the presence of the non-absorbed disaccharide. A more reliable test is to measure breath hydrogen after giving the disaccharide (*Fig. 6.6*): because it is not absorbed, the disaccharide reaches the colon where another of the products of bacterial fermentation is hydrogen. The definitive test for disaccharidase deficiencies is measurement of the appropriate enzyme in a biopsy sample.

The most common disaccharidase deficiency affects lactase. It may be congenital or acquired; it often occurs transiently when there is damage to gut mucosa, such as after gastroenteritis. Less common are sucrase–isomaltase and maltase deficiencies.

Tests of amino acid absorption

Tests of amino acid absorption from the gut are only used as research procedures. Generalized malabsorption of amino acids occurs only with extensive small bowel disease. Malabsorption of specific amino acids occurs in certain inherited metabolic disorders; for example, deficiency of tryptophan can occur in Hartnup disease, an inherited disorder of the transport of neutral amino acids. In cystinuria, there is impaired transport of the dibasic amino acids lysine, cystine, ornithine and arginine, but this condition is not associated with a deficiency syndrome.

Loss of protein from the gut in a protein-losing enteropathy can be assessed by measuring faecal radioactivity after parenteral administration of isotopically labelled proteins (e.g. ^{51}Cr-albumin, or polyvinyl-pyrrolidine). Such investigations are not commonly performed, however, since the cause of any hypoproteinaemia is usually obvious in such conditions.

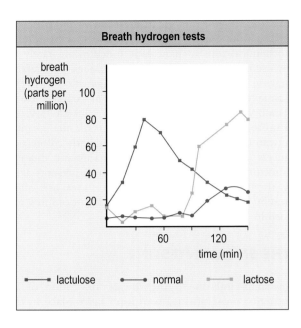

Fig. 6.6 Breath hydrogen tests. Hydrogen is not produced by mammalian cells; its presence in expired air is due to bacterial fermentation of unabsorbed carbohydrate. Typical results are shown from the test performed in a patient with bacterial colonization of the small intestine when challenged with oral lactulose (10 g), where the lactulose acts as a substrate for bacterial metabolism, and in a patient with intestinal lactase deficiency when challenged with oral lactose (50 g) compared with a normal individual given lactose. Hydrogen is generated by the fermentation of unabsorbed lactose in the colon, with the result that the increase in breath hydrogen occurs later than with small intestinal bacterial overgrowth.

Tests of fat absorption

Because the absorption of fat is a complex process, the effects of fat malabsorption are often a prominent feature of generalized malabsorption. For this reason, and because fat malabsorption can occur with gastric, pancreatic, hepatic and intestinal disease, tests of fat absorption can be used to diagnose generalized malabsorption (*see p. 115*). However, the presence of generalized malabsorption can often be reliably inferred from clinical findings (particularly steatorrhoea) and the results of simple tests (*see p. 115*). Further tests will then be required to determine the *cause* of malabsorption, but formal tests to confirm its *presence* are now required only infrequently.

Faecal fat test

Fat absorption has traditionally been assessed by measuring the excretion of fat in faeces. After digestion, dietary fat is normally absorbed completely in the small intestine; a small quantity of fat (<18 mmol/24 h) is excreted in faeces but this is derived from enterocytes.

With malabsorption of fat, its excretion in the faeces is increased. However, a major problem with its measurement is the need to obtain an accurately timed faecal collection. Collections should preferably be made for five consecutive days, although, for practical reasons, three-day collections are often used. Accuracy of timing can be improved by using a non-absorbable coloured marker such as carmine. This is administered orally and faecal collection is started when the marker appears in the stool; a second marker is given 120 (or 72) hours after the first, and collection is terminated when this appears.

This test is unpleasant for all concerned and is only of value if performed correctly. Dietetic guidance should be sought to ensure that the patient consumes 90–100 g fat per day for 48 hours before and during the period of collection: if less fat is ingested, minor degrees of malabsorption may be missed.

Triolein breath test

Due to the unpleasantness of the faecal fat test and its impracticality as an outpatient procedure, there has been considerable enthusiasm for the development of alternative tests. The triolein breath test is probably the most reliable alternative (*Fig. 6.7*). This test takes only a few hours and can be performed on a day ward. The principle of the test is that when isotopically labelled triolein is given orally, digested and absorbed, some of the label appears in the breath as isotopically labelled carbon dioxide, which can be measured using appropriate equipment. The triolein is labelled with either ^{13}C, a stable isotope, or ^{14}C, which is radioactive. Since it is the specific activity of the expired carbon dioxide that is measured, a constant rate of production of carbon dioxide from all other sources must be assumed; patients must be fasting and must rest throughout the test.

The triolein breath test is not reliable in patients with diabetes, obesity, thyroid disease or chronic respiratory insufficiency and is not suitable for use in pregnancy.

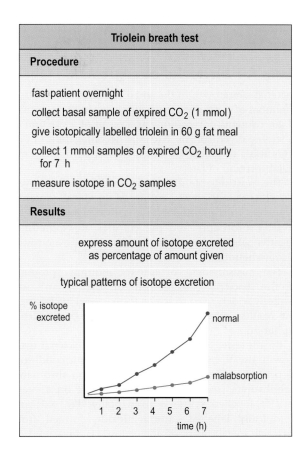

Fig. 6.7 Triolein breath test. CO_2 samples are collected by bubbling expired air into vials containing 1 mmol hyamine, which reacts with the CO_2. An indicator is used which changes colour when the reaction is complete. Individual laboratories should determine their own lower limit of normal for isotope excretion.

Properly performed, however, it is a sensitive test for fat malabsorption and results correlate well with those of faecal fat excretion. However, neither test differentiates between the different causes of fat malabsorption.

Modifications of the triolein test have been described in which the respective absorptions of labelled triglyceride and labelled free fatty acids are compared, with the intention of distinguishing between pancreatic and intestinal causes of malabsorption. In practice, the triolein breath test is best used to diagnose fat malabsorption in doubtful cases. Specific tests (e.g. of pancreatic function) should be used to diagnose the cause.

Tests for bacterial overgrowth

Bacterial overgrowth in the small intestine can occur in a number of conditions, particularly when there is stasis of gut contents, for example as a result of a stricture or in jejunal diverticulosis. Bacterial deconjugation of bile acids leads to failure of mixed micelle formation and malabsorption of fat.

The most reliable diagnostic test for bacterial overgrowth is aspiration and culture of duodenal contents. However, this method has disadvantages: it is an invasive procedure and the cultures are sometimes negative when other evidence of bacterial overgrowth is overwhelming.

The measurement of urinary indicans (products of the bacterial metabolism of tryptophan) was formerly widely used to screen for bacterial overgrowth, but results correlate poorly with those of duodenal aspiration.

Breath tests can be used to diagnose bacterial overgrowth. Breath hydrogen is increased in this condition, particularly after administration of a non-absorbable carbohydrate (see Fig. 6.6). In the xylose breath test, $^{13}C/^{14}C$-labelled xylose is given orally (Fig. 6.8) and isotopically labelled carbon dioxide, formed from bacterial metabolism of the xylose, is measured in expired breath. This procedure is similar to that for the triolein test. This test appears to be more specific and sensitive than the $^{13}C/^{14}C$-glycocholic acid test, the principle of which is that bacteria deconjugate the glycocholic acid (a bile acid), releasing isotopically labelled glycine, which is absorbed in the proximal small gut and metabolized, producing labelled carbon dioxide. Intact bile acids are absorbed in the terminal ileum.

Tests of terminal ileal function

Terminal ileal function can be investigated using the Schilling test of vitamin B_{12} absorption as this vitamin is absorbed in the terminal ileum. The test involves giving vitamin B_{12} with and without intrinsic factor (necessary for its absorption) and measuring the subsequent urinary excretion. The test involves the use of radioactive isotopes and is now rarely used. Malabsorption of vitamin B_{12} occurs in pernicious anaemia, an autoimmune disease, and suspected pernicious anaemia is now usually investigated by

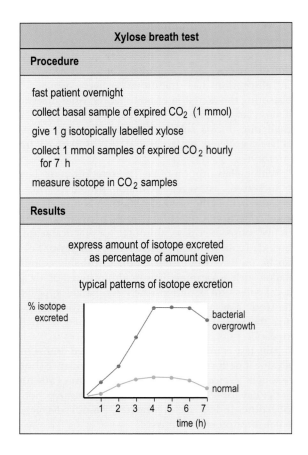

Xylose breath test
Procedure
fast patient overnight
collect basal sample of expired CO_2 (1 mmol)
give 1 g isotopically labelled xylose
collect 1 mmol samples of expired CO_2 hourly for 7 h
measure isotope in CO_2 samples
Results

express amount of isotope excreted as percentage of amount given

typical patterns of isotope excretion

Fig. 6.8 Xylose breath test for the diagnosis of intestinal bacterial overgrowth. CO_2 is collected as in the triolein test.

measuring serum vitamin B_{12} concentration and anti-parietal cell and anti-intrinsic factor antibodies.

Non-biochemical tests of intestinal function

The mucosa of the small intestine can be biopsied endoscopically under direct vision. This procedure has almost entirely replaced the use of peroral suction biopsy using a Crosbie capsule. Small intestinal biopsy is the definitive procedure for the diagnosis of coeliac disease (gluten-induced enteropathy, see Case History 6.2). The diagnosis of disaccharidase deficiencies can also be confirmed by measuring the enzyme in an intestinal biopsy.

Characteristic radiographical appearances are seen in patients with certain intestinal diseases, for example Crohn's disease (*see Case History 6.4*). Biochemical tests, however, continue to be used for diagnosis of the malabsorption syndrome.

DISORDERS OF INTESTINAL FUNCTION

Malabsorption

The term malabsorption strictly refers to impaired absorption of the products of digestion, whilst maldigestion is failure of digestion, which may be responsible for non-absorption of nutrients, for example in pancreatic insufficiency. In practice, since the resultant clinical syndromes are basically the same, the term malabsorption is commonly used to encompass both disorders.

The clinical features of malabsorption are varied and stem from either deficiency of nutrients or retention of nutrients within the bowel lumen. The clinical features and common causes of malabsorption are shown in Fig. 6.9.

More than one mechanism can be responsible for malabsorption in individual cases. After gastric surgery, for example, impaired mixing of food with digestive juices, decreased stimuli to their secretion, rapid transit and bacterial colonization of a blind afferent loop may all contribute to malabsorption.

Investigations are required for two purposes: to diagnose malabsorption and to determine its cause. If the diagnosis is obvious clinically (e.g. if steatorrhoea is present), only tests to determine the cause are required. If the diagnosis is uncertain, simple tests (*see Fig. 6.10*) should be performed first; if the results of these are normal, malabsorption is unlikely and further expensive or invasive tests can often be avoided.

Coeliac disease

This condition, also known as gluten-sensitive enteropathy, is the commonest cause of malabsorption

Simple tests for the diagnosis of malabsorption

serum albumin, calcium, phosphate, alkaline phosphatase
full blood count
red cell indices [mean red cell volume (MCV), mean corpuscular haemoglobin (MCH)]
serum iron, ferritin
vitamin B_{12}, folate
prothrombin time

Fig. 6.10 Simple tests for the diagnosis of malabsorption.

Malabsorption

Clinical features	Causes
Retention of non-absorbed nutrients diarrhoea,* steatorrhoea abdominal discomfort and distension* flatulence* **Decreased absorption of nutrients** anaemia* (iron, folate and vitamin B_{12} deficiency) glossitis, angular stomatitis* (iron deficiency) osteomalacia and rickets (vitamin D deficiency) oedema (hypoalbuminaemia) bleeding tendency (vitamin K deficiency) weight loss,* growth failure in children*	pancreatic enzyme deficiency, e.g. chronic pancreatitis and cystic fibrosis bile salt deficiency, e.g. biliary obstruction and hepatic disease intestinal, e.g. coeliac disease, tropical sprue, Crohn's disease and partial resection bacterial overgrowth, e.g. gastric surgery, internal fistulae, strictures and jejunal diverticulosis

Fig. 6.9 Malabsorption: clinical features and common causes. There may be several reasons for the development of malabsorption in individual cases. *Indicates the most common features.

Case history 6.2

A 3-year-old boy was referred for the investigation of failure to thrive: he was below the third centile for height and the tenth for weight, although both parents were tall. The boy had frequent diarrhoea and did not appear to enjoy his food. On examination, he was anaemic and had abdominal distension; there was obvious wasting of the muscles of the limbs, buttocks and shoulder girdle.

Investigations

Serum:	albumin	30 g/L
	tissue transglutaminase	
	antibody	strongly positive
haemoglobin		9.7 g/dL

A blood film showed hypochromic, microcytic red cells. A duodenal biopsy showed total villous atrophy.

Comment

There are many causes of growth failure. In this case, the history and findings on examination suggest a gastrointestinal disorder. Hypoproteinaemia and a hypochromic, microcytic anaemia, characteristic of iron deficiency, are common in patients with malabsorption. The positive serology for tissue transglutaminse antibody suggests coeliac disease, and this diagnosis is supported by the biopsy appearance.

A gluten-free diet was started and the boy's symptoms regressed. Three months later, the intestinal villi appeared almost normal on biopsy. The diagnosis was confirmed when symptoms returned after a gluten challenge and a further biopsy was again abnormal.

 Case history 6.3

A middle-aged publican presented with flatulence and abdominal distension. On questioning, he admitted to weight loss and to passing frequent, bulky, foul-smelling bowel motions which were difficult to flush away.

Investigations

serum:	calcium	2.10 mmol/L
	phosphate	0.70 mmol/L
	glucose (fasting)	12 mmol/L
	alkaline phosphatase	264 U/L
	albumin	40 g/L

A plain abdominal radiograph revealed pancreatic calcification.

Comment

The clinical features are characteristic of malabsorption (*Fig. 6.9*). The patient is hypocalcaemic and hypophosphataemic with a raised alkaline phosphatase due to vitamin D deficiency with secondary hyperparathyroidism. With gross steatorrhoea, further investigations to establish that the patient has malabsorption are not necessary, but the cause must be determined.

The presence of pancreatic calcification is very suggestive of alcohol-induced chronic pancreatitis. The raised fasting concentration of glucose, indicating glucose intolerance, is compatible with chronic pancreatitis and no further investigations of pancreatic function were performed. The patient was advised to abstain from alcohol. He was given pancreatic extract to add to his food and the symptoms regressed. This therapeutic response provides further confirmation of the diagnosis of pancreatic insufficiency.

in the UK. Malabsorption is caused by villous atrophy, affecting particularly the mucosa of the proximal small intestine. Coeliac disease is a result of sensitivity to gliadin, a component of gluten, a protein present in wheat and other cereal flours. It varies considerably in severity. It may present in infancy (typically on weaning) with severe failure to thrive, apathy, muscle wasting and steatorrhoea, in later childhood (with growth failure, anaemia or bone disease) or in adults (typically with diarrhoea and often a long history of being unwell). Complete withdrawal of gluten from the diet leads to regrowth of villi and eventual resolution of symptoms.

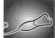 **Case history 6.4**

A 35-year-old woman was referred for the investigation of diarrhoea and abdominal pain. She had lost weight and was clinically anaemic. She had had two previous episodes of the same symptoms, lasting for several weeks on each occasion in the preceding two years, but had not sought medical advice.

Investigations

serum:	albumin	28 g/L
	haemoglobin	8.5 g/dL
	red cell volume	110 fL

A ^{14}C-triolein breath test was performed; the excretion of ^{14}C-carbon dioxide was very low and for a few hours after having had a fat meal the woman experienced abdominal discomfort and distension. A barium meal and follow-through revealed narrowing and ulceration of the terminal ileum, with an ileo-ileal fistula.

Comment

Weight loss is a common feature of gastrointestinal disease, even without malabsorption, and the breath test was used to screen for possible malabsorption.

The patient did not have steatorrhoea; this was ascribed to her habitual low-fat diet, prescribed for familial hypercholesterolaemia some years before. The development of symptoms when she was challenged with fat suggests that her symptoms might have been more florid if she had had a normal fat intake. There was nothing in the history specifically to suggest a biliary or pancreatic disorder and the diagnosis was made radiologically.

The radiographical appearances are typical of Crohn's disease, an inflammatory disease of the gut in which ulceration and fibrosis occur and may lead to the formation of strictures and fistulae. Although the condition can affect any part of the gut, the ileum is most often involved. The course is often one of remission and exacerbations.

In the acute illness, mesalazine, steroids or azathioprine may be used and nutritional support may be necessary. Surgery may be required for intestinal obstruction or fistulae, or if medical treatment fails. Malabsorption in Crohn's disease may be due to either damage to the ileum or bacterial overgrowth of a stagnant loop, a possible consequence of internal fistula formation.

Diagnosis is by intestinal biopsy. The characteristic villous atrophy resolves on exclusion of gluten from the diet and recurs following a gluten challenge. Various antibodies (e.g. against gliadin, reticulin, endomysium and tissue transglutaminase) are present in the plasma in active disease. The antigen in endomysium is tissue transglutaminase and the detection of tissue trans-glutaminase antibody provides the most sensitive (approximately 85%) and specific (approximately 97%) serological screening test for coeliac disease. Serum total IgA concentration should also be measured: most laboratories measure the IgA antibody and false negative tests occur in IgA deficiency (seen in 10% of patients).

Intestinal failure

Intestinal failure is a condition in which the ability of the intestine to absorb fluids and nutrients threatens a person's nutritional status and hence health. Unless very short-lived, it is an indication for nutritional support. Acute, reversible intestinal failure can be a complication of surgery (e.g. as a result of sepsis or fistula formation), chemotherapy or irradiation. Chronic intestinal failure is most frequently a consequence of the short bowel syndrome, when a large segment of small intestine has been resected because, for example, of ischaemia following vascular occlusion. Other causes of chronic intestinal failure include Crohn's disease, radiation enteritis, systemic sclerosis and amyloid.

The gut has considerable reserve capacity, and the severity of dysfunction in short gut syndrome is related to the site of resection, the length of the segment resected and the extent to which adaptation (an increase in the absorptive capacity of the remaining gut) occurs. Adaptation can occur to a greater extent in the ileum than in the jejunum. The volume of fluid lost through an ileostomy decreases with time: little or no reduction occurs with a jejunostomy. Less dysfunction follows resection of mid-jejunum than of proximal small intestine (essential for the absorption of most nutrients) or of ileum (essential for bile acid and vitamin B_{12} absorption). Preservation of the ileocaecal valve reduces colonization of the small intestine by colonic bacteria and increases transit time. In practice, patients with less than 75 cm of residual small intestine following bowel resection almost invariably require long-term parenteral nutrition. Patients with up to 200 cm usually require oral or enteral supplementation. Most patients will require parenteral nutrition initially but the early introduction of at least some enteral nutrition promotes adaptation and helps protect the barrier function of the gut. Provided that it does not cause a significant increase in fluid loss, enteral provision can be gradually increased and parenteral support decreased, care being taken to ensure that the patient's nutritional requirements are fully met. The provision of nutritional support is discussed in *Chapter 20*.

The major problem in the first few days following gut resection is fluid and mineral loss; accurate measurement and replacement of the losses is essential. This loss may decrease as adaptation occurs, or be controllable with drugs.

Long-term complications of the short bowel syndrome include persistent diarrhoea, nutrient deficiencies, gallstones (due to bile salt wasting) and renal calculi (due to hyperoxaluria, *see p. 83*). Deficiencies of some nutrients are commoner than of others. Vitamin B_{12} deficiency can complicate ileal resection; zinc and

Gastrointestinal hormones		
Hormone	**Location**	**Function**
gastrin	gastric antrum	stimulates gastric acid secretion and growth of gastric and intestinal mucosa
cholecystokinin	duodenum, jejunum	stimulates pancreatic enzyme secretion and gallbladder contraction
secretin	duodenum, jejunum	stimulates pancreatic bicarbonate secretion
pancreatic polypeptide (PP)	pancreas	inhibits exocrine pancreatic secretion
gastric inhibitory polypeptide (GIP)	duodenum, jejunum	releases insulin in response to glucose (hence also known as glucose-dependent insulinotrophic polypeptide); inhibits gastric acid secretion
vasoactive intestinal polypeptide (VIP)	entire GI tract	neurotransmitter; regulates GI motility and secretion
motilin	duodenum, jejunum	stimulates GI motility

Fig. 6.11 Some gastrointestinal (GI) hormones: locations and their principal functions.

magnesium deficiency are common with persistent diarrhoea, and malabsorption of vitamin D and calcium, together with resistance to the action of vitamin D, the basis of which is poorly understood, can cause metabolic bone disease. Persisting lactase deficiency may limit milk intake, further compromising calcium status.

The metabolism of dietary carbohydrate as a result of abnormal microbial colonization of the gut can cause metabolic acidosis due to the production of lactic acid. The cause of the acidosis may go unrecognized as the lactate produced is the D(−)-isomer rather than the L(+)-isomer, which is formed during glycolysis. The D(−)-isomer is not measured in most assays for lactate.

Other intestinal disorders

Given the amount of fluid that enters the gut each day, there is considerable potential for fluid and electrolyte depletion in situations of impaired reabsorption. Dehydration can complicate prolonged vomiting and diarrhoea, and enterocutaneous fistulae. Magnesium and potassium depletion are also frequently associated with excessive loss of fluid from the gastrointestinal tract.

In some cases there is increased secretion of fluid into the gut; for example, in cholera, massive fluid loss can occur very rapidly. Secretory diarrhoea also occurs with villous adenomata of the rectum, tumours that secrete large volumes of potassium-rich mucus, and with tumours secreting vasoactive intestinal polypeptide (VIP) which cause profuse, watery diarrhoea, the Werner–Morrison syndrome.

GASTROINTESTINAL HORMONES

The principal functions of gastrin, secretin, CCK, insulin and glucagon have been well understood for some time. In recent years, a number of other gastro-intestinal polypeptide hormones have been discovered (*Fig. 6.11*). Although many of their properties are known, their exact physiological functions are incompletely understood.

At present, assays for these hormones are available only in specialized laboratories and the indication for measuring them for diagnostic purposes is largely con-fined to cases of suspected hormone-secreting tumours, for example, in the Werner–Morrison syndrome.

SUMMARY

- **The gastrointestinal tract is responsible for the digestion and absorption** of food. This process also depends upon **normal hepatic and pancreatic function** and is controlled by both neural and humoral mechanisms.

- Formal assessment of gastric acid secretion is now seldom required, but measurement of the hormone **gastrin**, which stimulates gastric acid secretion, is valuable in patients with atypical peptic ulceration, since this may be due to a gastrin-secreting tumour.

- Many **other gut hormones** have been described. The measurement of some of them may similarly be useful in the investigation of patients suspected of having a hormone-secreting tumour.

- The **malabsorption syndrome** can be a result of intestinal, pancreatic or hepatic dysfunction. Significant malabsorption can readily be excluded by simple tests on blood or serum. If malabsorption is obvious clinically, for instance because of weight loss and gross steatorrhoea, tests for malabsorption add nothing to the diagnosis. Such tests, for example the triolein breath test, should be used only in doubtful cases. Once a diagnosis of malabsorption has been made, investigations are required to determine the cause if this is not obvious clinically. Biochemical, histological and radiological data may all be useful in this context.

SUMMARY (cont'd)

- **Intestinal failure** most frequently complicates resection of the small intestine or Crohn's disease. Excessive fluid loss is a common problem, and nutritional support is required, sometimes in the long term.

- **Acute pancreatitis** typically presents as an acute abdomen. Increased serum amylase activity is characteristic of, though not specific to, this condition. In acute pancreatitis, shock, renal failure, hypocalcaemia and hyperglycaemia may be complicating factors. The major predisposing factors are gallstones and alcohol. When severe, acute pancreatitis has a poor prognosis.

- **Chronic pancreatitis** usually presents with pain and/or malabsorption. Alcohol is the commonest cause. The pancreatic damage is irreversible; treatment is aimed at relieving symptoms.

- Approximately 8 L of fluid are secreted into the gut each day, the great majority of which is reabsorbed. **The loss of fluid and salts from the gut** because of vomiting, diarrhoea or a fistula can lead to severe salt and water depletion.

The hypothalamus and the pituitary gland

INTRODUCTION

The pituitary gland consists of two parts, the anterior pituitary, or adenohypophysis, and the posterior pituitary, or neurohypophysis. Though very closely related anatomically, they are embryologically and functionally quite distinct. The anterior pituitary comprises primarily glandular tissue, while the posterior pituitary is of neural origin. The pituitary gland is situated at the base of the brain, in close relation to the hypothalamus (*Fig. 7.1*), which has an essential role in the regulation of pituitary function.

ANTERIOR PITUITARY HORMONES

The anterior pituitary secretes several hormones, some of which are trophic, that is they stimulate the activity of other endocrine glands (*Fig. 7.2*). The secretion of

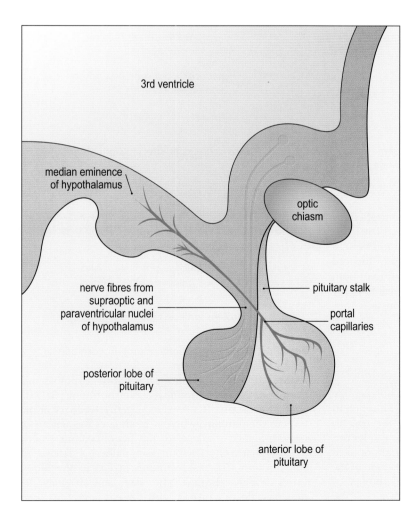

Fig. 7.1 Diagrammatic, sagittal section through part of the brain to show the anatomical relationship of the pituitary gland and hypothalamus. The portal blood vessels, through which hypothalamic hormones reach the anterior pituitary, and nerve fibres, which transport hypothalamic hormones to the posterior pituitary, are shown.

Anterior pituitary hormones		
Hormone	**Target organ**	**Action**
growth hormone (GH)	liver	somatomedin synthesis, hence growth stimulation
	others	metabolic regulation
prolactin	breast	lactation
thyroid-stimulating hormone (TSH)	thyroid	thyroid hormone synthesis and release
follicle-stimulating hormone (FSH)	ovary	oestrogen synthesis
		oogenesis
	testis	spermatogenesis
luteinizing hormone (LH)	ovary	ovulation
		corpus luteum, hence progesterone production
	testis	testosterone synthesis
adrenocorticotrophic hormone (ACTH)	adrenal cortex	glucocorticoid synthesis and release
	skin	pigmentation
β-lipotrophin		precursor of endorphins

Fig. 7.2 Anterior pituitary hormones and their actions. All the actions shown are stimulatory; trophic hormones stimulate both synthesis and release of hormones by their target organs.

hormones by the anterior pituitary is controlled by hormones secreted by the hypothalamus, which reach the pituitary through a system of portal blood vessels. The secretion of hypothalamic hormones is influenced by higher centres in the brain, and the secretion of both hypothalamic and pituitary hormones is regulated by feedback from the hormones whose production they stimulate in target organs.

Growth hormone

Growth hormone (GH) is a 191 amino acid polypeptide hormone. It is essential for normal growth, although in the main it acts indirectly by stimulating the liver to produce insulin-like growth factor-1 (IGF-1), also known as somatomedin-C. IGF-1 has considerable amino acid sequence homology with insulin and shares some of the actions of this hormone. GH also has a number of metabolic effects, which are summarized in *Fig. 7.3*. The

Metabolic actions of growth hormone
increases lipolysis (hence ketogenic)
increases hepatic glucose production and decreases tissue glucose uptake (hence diabetogenic)
increases protein synthesis (hence anabolic)

Fig. 7.3 Metabolic actions of growth hormone.

release of GH is controlled by two hypothalamic hormones, growth hormone-releasing hormone (GHRH) and somatostatin. IGF-1 exerts negative feedback at the level of the pituitary, where it modulates the actions of GHRH, and at the level of the hypothalamus where, together with GH itself, it stimulates the release of somatostatin. The concentration of GH in the blood varies widely through the day and it may be undetectable (<1 mU/L) with present assays for long periods. Physiological secretion occurs in sporadic bursts, lasting for one to two hours, mainly during sleep. Peak concentrations may be as high as 40 mU/L. Secretion can be stimulated by stress, exercise, a fall in blood glucose concentration, fasting and ingestion of certain amino acids. Such stimuli can be used in provocative tests for diagnosing GH deficiency, particularly in children. GH secretion is inhibited by a rise in blood glucose and this effect provides the rationale for the use of the oral glucose tolerance test in the diagnosis of excessive GH secretion. Excessive secretion (due usually to a pituitary tumour) causes gigantism in children and acromegaly in adults; deficiency causes growth retardation in children and can cause fatigue, loss of muscle strength, impaired psychological wellbeing and an adverse cardiovascular risk profile (elevated plasma total and LDL-cholesterol concentrations and hyperfibrinogenaemia) in adults.

Somatostatin, the 14 amino acid hypothalamic peptide that inhibits GH secretion, has many other actions both within the hypothalamo–pituitary axis and elsewhere. For example, it inhibits the release of thyroid-stimulating hormone (TSH) in response to thyrotrophin-releasing hormone (TRH) and it is present in the gut and pancreatic islets, where it inhibits the secretion of many gastrointestinal hormones including gastrin, insulin and glucagon. The physiological significance of these actions is poorly understood. Rare somatostatin-secreting tumours of the pancreas have been described and somatostatin secretion can also occur from medullary carcinomas of thyroid and small cell carcinomas of the lung. Somatostatin analogues are used therapeutically to stop bleeding from the upper gastrointestinal tract, to inhibit hormone secretion by tumours and to treat acromegaly.

Prolactin

Prolactin is a 198 amino acid polypeptide hormone; its principal physiological action is to initiate and sustain lactation. Prolactin secretion is controlled by the hypothalamus through the release of dopamine, which inhibits the process. There is no known hypothalamic prolactin-releasing hormone. Although both TRH and vasoactive intestinal polypeptide (VIP) stimulate prolactin secretion, it is not thought that this is physiologically important. Increased prolactin secretion occurs with prolactin-secreting tumours and is also frequently seen with other pituitary tumours if they obstruct blood flow from the hypothalamus and thus the dopamine-dependent inhibition of prolactin secretion. In the absence of dopamine, prolactin secretion is autonomous.

The secretion of prolactin is pulsatile, increases during sleep and stress, and in women is dependent upon oestrogen status, making it difficult to define a precise upper limit for plasma prolactin concentration in normal men and women, although 500 mU/L is often regarded as the upper reference value in non-pregnant women and 300 mU/L in men. There is no useful lower reference value for plasma prolactin concentration. Its secretion increases during pregnancy but concentrations fall to normal within approximately seven days after birth if a woman does not breast feed. With breast feeding, concentrations start to decline after about three months, even if breast feeding is continued beyond this time. The consequences of hyperprolactinaemia are discussed on p. 134. Prolactin deficiency is uncommon but does occur, for example with pituitary infarction: its principal manifestation is failure of lactation.

Thyroid-stimulating hormone

Thyroid-stimulating hormone (TSH) is a glycoprotein (molecular weight 28 kDa) composed of an α- and a β-subunit; the α-subunit is common to TSH and the gonadotrophins and is almost identical to that of human chorionic gonadotrophin (hCG), but the β-subunit is unique to TSH.

The normal plasma concentration of TSH in health is approximately 0.3–5.0 mU/L, but the lower value in particular is dependent on the assay used. TSH binds to specific receptors on thyroid cells and in doing so stimulates the synthesis and secretion of thyroid hormones. Secretion of TSH is stimulated by the hypothalamic tripeptide TRH and this effect, and probably the release of TRH itself, is inhibited by high circulating concentrations of thyroid hormones.

Thus thyroid hormone synthesis is regulated by a negative feedback system: if plasma concentrations of thyroid hormones decrease, TSH secretion increases, stimulating thyroid hormone synthesis; if they increase, TSH secretion is suppressed. In primary hypothyroidism, TSH secretion is increased; in hyperthyroidism it is decreased. TSH deficiency can cause hypothyroidism but hyperthyroidism due to TSH-secreting tumours is very rare.

Gonadotrophins

Follicle-stimulating hormone (FSH) and luteinizing hormone (LH) are both glycoproteins of molecular weight approximately 30 kDa consisting of two subunits: the β-subunits are unique to each hormone but the α-subunit is the same in each, is present also in TSH and is similar to that in hCG.

The synthesis and release of both hormones are stimulated by the hypothalamic decapeptide, gonadotrophin-releasing hormone (GnRH), these effects being modulated by circulating gonadal steroids. GnRH is secreted episodically, resulting in pulsatile secretion of gonadotrophins with peaks in plasma concentration occurring at approximately 90-minute intervals. In males, LH stimulates testosterone secretion by Leydig cells: both testosterone and oestradiol, derived from the Leydig cells themselves and from the metabolism of testosterone, feed back to block the action of GnRH on LH secretion. FSH, in concert with high intratesticular testosterone concentrations, stimulates spermatogenesis; its secretion is inhibited by inhibin (*Fig. 7.4*), a hormone produced during spermatogenesis.

In the female, the relationships are more complex. Oestrogen (mainly oestradiol) secretion by the ovary is stimulated primarily by FSH in the first part of the menstrual cycle; both hormones are necessary for the development of Graafian follicles. As oestrogen concentrations in the blood rise, FSH secretion declines until oestrogens trigger a positive feedback mechanism, causing an explosive release of LH and, to a lesser extent, FSH. The increase in LH stimulates ovulation and development of the corpus luteum, but rising concentrations of oestrogens and progesterone then inhibit FSH and LH secretion; inhibin from the ovaries also appears to inhibit FSH secretion. If conception does not occur, declining concentrations of oestrogens and progesterone from the regressing corpus luteum trigger menstruation and LH and FSH release, initiating the maturation of further follicles in a new cycle (*Fig. 7.5*). Before puberty, plasma concentrations of LH and FSH are very low and unresponsive to exogenous GnRH. With the approach of puberty, FSH secretion increases before that of LH.

Increased concentrations of gonadotrophins are seen in ovarian failure in women, whether pathological or after the natural menopause. High concentrations of

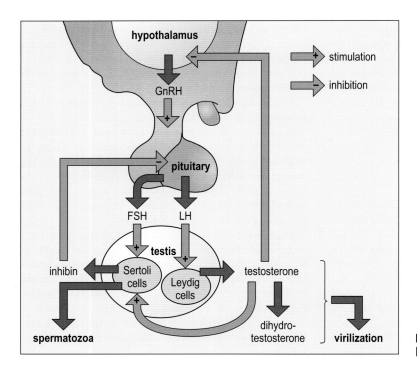

Fig. 7.4 Control of testicular function by pituitary gonadotrophins.

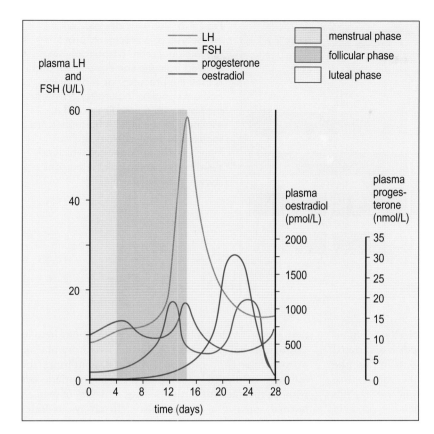

plasma LH and FSH (U/L)

LH
FSH
progesterone
oestradiol

menstrual phase
follicular phase
luteal phase

plasma oestradiol (pmol/L)

plasma proges-terone (nmol/L)

time (days)

Fig. 7.5 Changes in the plasma concentration of pituitary gonadotrophins during the menstrual cycle. The resultant changes in oestrogens (17β-oestradiol) and progesterone concentration are also shown.

FSH are seen in azoospermic men and LH is increased if testosterone secretion is decreased.

Gonadotrophin-secreting tumours (secreting either LH or FSH) of the pituitary are uncommon. Decreased gonadotrophin secretion, leading to secondary gonadal failure, is more common. It can either be an isolated phenomenon, due to hypothalamic dysfunction, or occur with generalized pituitary failure. A case of hypogonadotrophic hypogonadism is described in *Case History 10.1.*

Adrenocorticotrophic hormone

Adrenocorticotrophic hormone (ACTH) is a polypeptide (molecular weight 4500 Da), comprising a single chain of 39 amino acids. Its biological function, which is to stimulate adrenal glucocorticoid (but not mineralo-corticoid) secretion, is dependent upon the N-terminal 24 amino acids. ACTH is a fragment of a much larger precursor, pro-opiomelanocortin (molecular weight 31 kDa) (*Fig. 7.6*), which is the precursor not only of ACTH but also of β-lipotrophin, itself the precursor of endogenous opioid peptides (endorphins). The control of the release of β-lipotrophin and the endorphins has not been fully elucidated, but ACTH release is controlled by a hypothalamic peptide, corticotrophin-releasing hormone (CRH). ACTH secretion is pulsatile and also shows diurnal variation, the plasma concentration being highest at approximately 0800 h and lowest at midnight. Secretion is greatly increased by stress and is inhibited by cortisol. Thus cortisol secretion by the adrenal cortex is controlled by negative feedback, but this and the circadian variation can be overcome by the effects of stress. The normal range for plasma ACTH at concentration at 0900 h is <50 ng/L.

Increased secretion of ACTH by the pituitary is seen with pituitary tumours (Cushing's disease) and in primary adrenal failure (Addison's disease). The

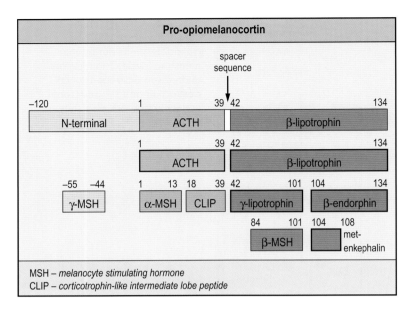

Fig. 7.6 ACTH is derived by proteolysis of a precursor, pro-opiomelanocortin. β-Lipotrophin is derived from the same precursor and is itself the precursor of endorphins and enkephalins (naturally occurring peptides with opioid-like activity). Melanocyte-stimulating hormones are secreted in some species, but not humans. (Those hormones which are secreted physiologically in humans are shown in heavier outlines.)

hormone may also be secreted ectopically by non-pituitary tumours. Excessive ACTH synthesis is associated with increased pigmentation. This is due to the melanocyte-stimulating action of ACTH. Although a separate melanocyte-stimulating hormone (MSH) has been described in other animals, it does not occur in humans. Decreased secretion of ACTH may be an isolated phenomenon but is more commonly associated with generalized pituitary failure.

MEASUREMENT OF ANTERIOR PITUITARY HORMONES

The investigation of suspected pituitary hypofunction should begin with measurement of pituitary and target organ hormones in a blood sample taken at 0900 h. TSH deficiency will be apparent from a low total or free thyroxine concentration without the elevation of TSH characteristic of primary hypothyroidism. Plasma TSH concentration may be normal or low in hypopituitarism: it is rarely undetectable.

In males, a normal plasma testosterone concentration indicates normal LH secretion. In hypopituitarism, plasma testosterone concentration is low and LH and FSH concentrations are normal or low. In pre-menopausal females, amenorrhoea with a low plasma oestradiol concentration and normal or low gonadotrophins suggests hypothalamic or pituitary

dysfunction. A clomiphene test (*see p. 180*) may help to distinguish between these. A normal ovulatory plasma progesterone concentration (*see p. 187*) indicates the integrity of the hypothalamo–pituitary–ovarian axis without the need for further testing; a history of regular, normal menstrual cycles also effectively excludes gonadotrophin deficiency. In normal post-menopausal women, plasma gonadotrophin concentrations are grossly elevated; in hypopituitarism, they are normal or low.

Tests involving the administration of TRH and GnRH followed by measurement of TSH and gonadotrophins have traditionally been used in the investigation of pituitary disease, often combined with the insulin hypoglycaemia test (IHT, see below). However, the use of these tests has been criticized on the grounds that the responses to these releasing hormones only reflect the readily releasable pituitary pools of the hormones concerned and do not assess the physiological integrity of the pituitary. Normal responses can occur in spite of other evidence of pituitary hypofunction. The response to the releasing hormones is often delayed in patients with hypothalamic, as opposed to pituitary, dysfunction, but such delayed responses can also occur in pituitary disease. In practice, the releasing hormone tests often add little to what can be deduced from clinical observation and the results of basal hormone measurements.

Because GH is secreted sporadically, it may be undetectable in the plasma of normal individuals. Thus while a concentration of >20 mU/L in a single sample excludes significant deficiency, a low concentration is not necessarily indicative of deficiency. Growth hormone secretion can be assessed using the IHT: a peak plasma concentration <20 mU/L after adequate hypoglycaemia (blood glucose concentration <2.2 mmol/L) is reliable evidence of GH deficiency. Because the IHT is potentially hazardous, various other tests of GH secretion have been devised, involving the administration of, for example, GHRH, glucagon, arginine, yeast extract or L-dopa, although the relevance of these pharmacological stimuli to the physiological secretion of GH is questionable. GH concentrations >20 mU/L are usually regarded as excluding GH deficiency but lesser responses are not conclusive evidence of deficiency. Vigorous exercise also stimulates GH secretion, but even with standardized protocols an apparently sub-normal response may not indicate GH deficiency. More reliable information may be provided by the measurement of GH secretion during sleep, by means of frequent blood sampling through an indwelling cannula, but there are obvious practical drawbacks to this procedure.

Measurements of IGF-1 are increasingly being used together with GH stimulation tests in the investigation of suspected GH deficiency. A low plasma concentration of IGF-1, together with an impaired or absent GH response to stimulation, confirms GH deficiency. Some patients, who appear clinically to have GH deficiency, have normal or elevated plasma GH concentrations but because of a receptor or intracellular signalling defect are resistant to its action. This syndrome is known as Laron dwarfism: patients have low plasma IGF-1 concentrations. It should be noted that, while plasma IGF-1 concentrations are much more stable than those of GH, they do vary with age and nutritional status: measured values should always be assessed with reference to age- and sex-matched reference values.

The integrity of the hypothalamo–pituitary adrenal axis can also be tested using the IHT. A rise in plasma cortisol concentration to at least 550 nmol/L after adequate hypoglycaemia indicates a normal axis. It has been shown that if the basal plasma cortisol concentration is <100 nmol/L, the cortisol response to hypoglycaemia is never normal, whereas it invariably is normal if the basal concentration is >400 nmol/L. A formal IHT may therefore not be necessary in patients whose basal plasma cortisol concentrations are outside the range 100–400 nmol/L. The protocol for the IHT is given in *Fig. 7.7*. The short ACTH stimulation test (Synacthen test, *see p. 148*), used primarily in the investigation of adrenal failure, has also been advocated as a test for ACTH deficiency. This may seem illogical, but the rationale is that ACTH deficiency causes adrenal atrophy and thus decreases adrenal responsiveness to ACTH. A good correlation between the results of the IHT and short ACTH stimulation tests has been demonstrated: a plasma cortisol concentration >550 nmol/L 30 minutes after the administration of synthetic ACTH (250 µg, i.v.) excludes ACTH deficiency. Experience with the low dose (1 µg) Synacthen test in this context is presently limited, but it may be less sensitive in identifying partial failure of ACTH secretion.

Prolactin secretion is increased by stress but in practice the measurement of prolactin in an IHT adds nothing to the information provided by a single basal measurement.

Insulin hypoglycaemia test

In this test, the stress of insulin-induced hypoglycaemia is used to assess the secretion of GH and ACTH by the pituitary (in practice, cortisol is usually measured for the reasons explained above and because the assay of ACTH is technically more demanding). The test is potentially hazardous because of the possible sequelae of hypoglycaemia. A doctor should always be present when the test is performed. It is contraindicated in patients with a history of fits or ischaemic heart disease and it should not be performed in patients whose 0900 h serum cortisol concentration is low. In children, it should only be performed in specialized units. Concentrated dextrose solution must be available for immediate administration should severe hypoglycaemia develop. Giving glucose because of severe symptomatic hypoglycaemia does not invalidate the results of the test. The stress need only be very brief to be effective. It is important that documented hypoglycaemia is obtained, since if it does not occur a lack of response might be due to the inadequacy of the stimulus rather than to pituitary failure. If hypoglycaemia does not develop, a further dose of insulin must be given. The protocol for this test and the normal responses are shown in *Fig. 7.7*. It can be combined with releasing hormone tests although, as discussed, the results of these tests often provide little additional useful information.

It may be preferable to give the insulin by continuous intravenous infusion. The rate can be adjusted until hypoglycaemia develops, whereupon the infusion is stopped. This is a more certain and safer way of

Combined test of anterior pituitary function					

Procedure

1. fast patient overnight and weigh

2. insert and heparinize i.v. cannula

3. draw and discard 1 mL of blood before collecting each sample and heparinize cannula after each sample is drawn

4. after 30 min take basal blood sample and analyze for glucose, cortisol (or ACTH), FSH, LH, TSH, free thyroxine, GH and testosterone/oestradiol

5. give 200 µg TRH, 100 µg GnRH and 0.15 U/kg body weight soluble insulin

6. take blood samples for analysis as follows:

time (min)	assay				
	glucose	cortisol	FSH, LH	TSH	GH
0	*	*	*	*	*
15	*				
20			*	*	
30	*	*			*
45	*				
60	*	*	*	*	*
90	*	*			*
120	*	*			*

7. repeat insulin dose at 45 min if patient has not become clinically (sweating) or biochemically (blood glucose < 2.2 mmol/L) hypoglycaemic and extend sampling accordingly

Normal response

cortisol	increment peak	>200 nmol/L >550 nmol/L (the same criteria apply if glucagon is used)
GH	peak	>20 mU/L (after glucagon: 15 mU/L in males, 20 mU/L in females)
FSH	peak	>1.5 times basal level
LH	peak	>5 times basal level
TSH	increment	≥ 2 mU/L (elderly) ≥ 5 mU/L (young adults)

Fig. 7.7 Combined test (triple bolus test) of anterior pituitary function. In patients thought to be very likely to be hypopituitary, the insulin dose should be 0.1 U/kg body weight; in patients with Cushing's disease or acromegaly, a dose of 0.30 U/kg may be used. When glucagon (1 mg intramuscularly) is used instead of insulin, blood samples for cortisol and GH should be taken at 30 min intervals from 90 to 240 min after the injection (GH and cortisol responses occur later than when insulin is used).

producing hypoglycaemia than giving a single bolus of insulin. When the induction of hypoglycaemia is contraindicated, glucagon can be used to stimulate cortisol and GH secretion instead of insulin.

DISORDERS OF ANTERIOR PITUITARY FUNCTION

Hypopituitarism

Hypopituitarism can result from hypothalamic or pituitary disease (*see Fig. 7.8*). Tumours of the pituitary are the most common cause. When these are functional, clinical features of hormone excess may also be present. Partial hypopituitarism is seen more frequently than complete loss of pituitary function. The presenting features depend on several factors, including the extent and severity of the hormone deficiencies; age is particularly important. Decreased GH secretion is an early feature of pituitary failure, but whilst its effects can be dramatic in children, they are less obvious in adults. In general, GH and gonadotrophin secretion (LH before FSH) are affected before that of ACTH. It is very uncommon for hypothyroidism to be the presenting feature of pituitary failure. Isolated deficiency of some of the anterior pituitary hormones can occur but this is usually congenital. In most such cases it is due to failure of secretion of the relevant hypothalamic hormone. Haemorrhage into a pituitary tumour can cause 'pituitary apoplexy'. The onset is sudden, usually with headache, signs of meningism, visual deterioration and loss of consciousness. Immediate treatment with intravenous fluids and hydrocortisone is required, often followed by surgery. Some of the many causes and clinical features of hypopituitarism are indicated in *Fig. 7.8*.

Suspected anterior pituitary hypofunction is investigated using the tests described on *p. 126*. It may be accompanied by hypofunction of the posterior pituitary (causing diabetes insipidus); the investigation of this condition is discussed on *pp 136–140*. Diabetes insipidus is uncommon, except with large pituitary tumours, but can develop, often transiently, after surgery. Even in patients with impaired vasopressin (antidiuretic hormone, ADH) secretion, diabetes insipidus may not be apparent if ACTH secretion is also impaired, since cortisol, the secretion of which is dependent on ACTH, is necessary for normal water excretion.

Anorexia nervosa

Anorexia nervosa, a disorder characterized by self-imposed starvation and a preoccupation with body size, may clinically resemble hypopituitarism. Amenorrhoea, due to decreased gonadotrophin secretion, is common to both conditions. However, pubic and axillary hair, which may be lost in hypopituitarism, is normal in anorexia nervosa and there may even be additional (lanugo) hair on the body. The weight loss of anorexia nervosa is usually severe in comparison with that which can occur in hypopituitarism. Plasma cortisol and GH concentrations tend to be elevated in anorexia nervosa.

Growth hormone deficiency

GH deficiency is an uncommon but important cause of growth retardation. Other causes are summarized in *Chapter 21*. GH may be undetectable in plasma in normal children, which means that, while a random concentration of greater than 20 mU/L excludes significant deficiency, a low concentration in a random blood sample is not diagnostic.

Growth hormone deficiency is treated with regular injections of biologically synthesized human growth hormone. Since most cases of isolated GH deficiency are now known to be caused by GHRH deficiency, GHRH may have a therapeutic role in the future. In adults with GH deficiency, treatment with GH improves body composition. Improvements in bone mineral density, cardiovascular risk profile and psychological wellbeing have been shown in some studies but not in others. Treatment of adults with GH is recommended only in severe deficiency, and should be discontinued if it is of no demonstrable benefit. The effects of treatment are monitored clinically and by measuring plasma IGF-1 concentration, the aim being to avoid values exceeding the upper limit of the age-adjusted reference range. The use of GH to promote anabolism in severely catabolic patients is under investigation. Its use to increase muscle mass in the absence of evidence of deficiency (e.g. in weightlifters) is inadvisable since harmful side-effects can result.

Pituitary tumours

Pituitary tumours may be purely destructive but are often functional, producing excessive quantities of a hormone. Even tumours which appear to be non-functional may secrete small (clinically insignificant)

Hypopituitarism

Causes

Tumours
pituitary tumours:
  adenoma
  craniopharyngioma
cerebral tumours:
  primary
  secondary

Miscellaneous
sarcoidosis
histiocytosis X
haemochromatosis

Hypothalamic disorders
tumours
functional disturbances, e.g. anorexia
  nervosa and starvation, causing reversible
  hypogonadotrophic hypogonadism
isolated GH and gonadotrophin secretion due
  to impaired secretion of hypothalamic-
  releasing hormones

Vascular disease
post-partum necrosis (Sheehan's syndrome)
infarction, especially of tumours
severe hypotension
cranial arteritis

Trauma

Infection
meningitis, especially tuberculous
syphilis

Iatrogenic
surgery
therapeutic skull irradiation (in malignancy)
prolonged treatment with glucocorticoids or
  thyroid hormones causing isolated ACTH
  and TSH suppression, respectively

Clinical features

Hormone	Features of deficiency
growth hormone	children: growth retardation adults: decreased muscle bulk and strength impaired psychological wellbeing osteopenia atherogenic lipid profile any tendency to hypoglycaemia may be accentuated
prolactin	failure of lactation
gonadotrophins	children: delayed puberty females: oligomenorrhoea, infertility, atrophy of breasts and genitalia males: impotence, azoospermia, testicular atrophy both sexes: decreased libido, loss of body hair, fine wrinkling of skin
ACTH	weight loss, weakness, hypotension, hypoglycaemia and other features of glucocorticoid deficiency, usually of insidious onset unless stressed; decreased skin pigmentation; loss of pubic and axillary hair in women
TSH	weight gain, cold intolerance, fatigue, etc.
vasopressin	thirst, polyuria

Fig. 7.8 Main causes and clinical features of hypopituitarism.

Case history 7.1

A 50-year-old man tripped and fell as he was running for a bus. He hit his head against the kerb and was knocked out for a few seconds. An ambulance was called and he was taken to the local hospital.

There was no sign of physical injury on examination but a skull radiograph showed enlargement of the pituitary fossa. The casualty officer questioned the patient further. Over the preceding 12 months he had lost his libido and found it necessary to shave less frequently than before; he had also noticed some loss of axillary and pubic hair. He frequently felt dizzy when getting out of bed in the morning and despite spending a lot of time in the sun had not acquired his usual summer tan.

Investigations

serum: cortisol (0900 h)   300 nmol/L
        GH   <2 mU/L
        free thyroxine   12 pmol/L
        TSH   2 mU/L
        testosterone   4 nmol/L
        LH   <1.5 U/L
        FSH   <1.0 U/L
        prolactin   <50 mU/L

combined glucagon, TRH and GnRH stimulation test:

serum: cortisol (maximum)   350 nmol/L at 180 min
        LH, FSH   no increment over basal values
        GH   no increment over basal value
        TSH   5 mU/L at 20 min; 3 mU/L at 60 min

Comment

The clinical features are typical of hypopituitarism (*Fig. 7.8*) and the test results confirm this diagnosis. GH, gonadotrophin and prolactin concentrations are all low; the cortisol concentration is in the lower part of the normal range. These hormones show little or no response to appropriate stimuli. The low testosterone is secondary to the lack of gonadotrophins. In view of the overwhelming evidence for the diagnosis, it was not considered necessary to perform a Synacthen test. The serum free thyroxine is near the lower end of the normal range; if this were related to incipient thyroid failure, a higher TSH concentration would be expected. There is a TSH response to TRH, but even this is towards the lower limit of normal.

Cortisol replacement therapy was started immediately and testosterone and thyroxine were also given. Within a few hours, the patient became polyuric and signs of water depletion developed. His serum sodium concentration, which was low on admission (128 mmol/L), rose to 149 mmol/L. Diabetes insipidus, due to impaired release of vasopressin, can be masked by simultaneous cortisol deficiency and revealed when replacement therapy is started, as in this case.

The patient was given synthetic vasopressin, which controlled his polyuria. He subsequently underwent surgery and a chromophobe adenoma was successfully removed. On follow-up, there was no evidence of recovery of pituitary function and he remained on replacement therapy.

Case history 7.2

A ten-year-old boy was referred to hospital for investigation of short stature. He had always been small, but his parents became worried when his seven-year-old brother overtook him in height. He had been measured two years before and had only grown 3 cm since then. On examination, there was no abnormality apart from his short stature. The history and appropriate tests excluded many of the recognized causes of growth retardation (*see p. 372*).

Investigations

serum GH: 4 mU/L (after vigorous exercise)
4 mU/L (during documented hypoglycaemia induced by insulin)

Comment

The diagnosis of GH deficiency depends upon the demonstration of subnormal growth velocity and subnormal plasma GH concentrations. Both features are present in this case. If plasma GH concentration is normal (>20 mU/L), either after exercise or in a sample obtained while the child is asleep, this obviates the need to perform the more invasive and hazardous insulin hypoglycaemia test. Exercise should be according to a standard protocol to ensure that it provides a sufficient stimulus to GH secretion. In this case, the response was subnormal and to confirm GH deficiency the insulin hypoglycaemia test was performed: the response was again subnormal.

A fall in blood glucose concentration is sufficient to stimulate GH secretion in normal people, but it is advisable to achieve documented hypoglycaemia (blood glucose <2.2 mmol/L) to ensure an adequate stimulus. Sex steroids are important in determining the magnitude of the response. Equivocal responses in children with pubertal delay require that the test is repeated after priming with sex steroids.

There was no other evidence of pituitary hypofunction in this boy and no evidence of a destructive pituitary lesion. A diagnosis of idiopathic GH deficiency was made. He began treatment with GH and grew at a normal rate thereafter, although he was always shorter than his peers. Typically, the lost height is not completely restored when GH deficiency is treated.

quantities of the glycoprotein pituitary hormones or just the α-subunit. Non-functional tumours usually present over the age of 60 years. The order of frequency with which hormone secretion occurs in patients with pituitary tumours is prolactin (relatively common) > GH > ACTH > gonadotrophins > TSH (very rare). Any pituitary tumour may give rise to clinical features due to the destruction of normal pituitary tissue, that is hypopituitarism, and of intracranial space-occupying lesions such as headache, vomiting and papilloedema. Visual field defects may develop when an upward growing tumour impinges on the optic chiasm and occasionally a patient's sight may be threatened.

Biochemical measurements are important to assess pituitary function in patients with pituitary tumours. Demonstration of the tumour itself and its anatomical extent requires imaging. Plain skull X-ray may demonstrate erosion of bone; magnetic resonance imaging (MRI) is usually preferred to computerized tomography (CT) for the demonstration of tumours. Formal assessment of visual fields is essential.

Growth hormone excess: acromegaly and gigantism

Acromegaly and gigantism are usually (95% of cases) the result of excessive GH secretion by a pituitary tumour. Acromegaly is an occasional feature of multiple endocrine neoplasia (MEN type 1). Approximately 5% of cases are the result of ectopic secretion of GHRH (e.g. by a bronchial carcinoid tumour). Excessive GH secretion causes increased growth of soft tissues and bone. If this occurs before the epiphyses have fused, growth of long bones occurs, leading to gigantism. More commonly, GH-secreting tumours occur in adults, producing acromegaly, with increased growth of soft tissues, hands, feet, jaw and internal organs. The GH concentration in a random serum sample is usually raised, but because GH secretion is normally episodic, the clinical diagnosis should be confirmed biochemically by demonstrating a failure of GH suppression in response to an oral glucose tolerance test. In normal subjects, plasma GH concentration falls to less than 2 mU/L during this procedure. In acromegaly and gigantism, GH fails to suppress normally and there may even be an increase in concentration. The glucose response may indicate impaired glucose tolerance (approximately 25% of patients) or, less frequently (10%), diabetes mellitus.

In many patients with acromegaly, TRH causes an increase in GH secretion; the reason for, or relevance of, this observation is unclear. Plasma IGF-1 concentrations are elevated in patients with acromegaly: measurements of IGF-1 are helpful in the assessment of otherwise borderline cases, and are used to follow the response of patients to treatment; there is less fluctuation in its concentration than in that of growth hormone.

The clinical features of excessive GH secretion are related to both the somatic and the metabolic effects of the hormone (*Fig. 7.9*). In addition, features due directly to the presence of the pituitary tumour are often present. Hyperprolactinaemia, due either to interference with the normal inhibition of prolactin secretion or (less frequently) to its secretion by the tumour itself, occurs in 30% of patients with acromegaly but there may be impaired secretion of other pituitary hormones.

Treatment of acromegaly and gigantism is aimed at reducing excessive GH secretion, preventing or treating deficiencies of other pituitary hormones and preventing damage to surrounding structures, particularly the optic nerves, by the tumour. In practice, it is often difficult to achieve all these goals. The main modes of treatment are surgery, external irradiation and medical therapy. Trans-sphenoidal resection of the pituitary tumour is the treatment of choice in the majority of cases. Occasionally, with large tumours with suprasellar extension, transfrontal craniotomy is necessary. If there is continuing evidence of excessive GH secretion, external irradiation or, more frequently, medical therapy, can be used. The most effective drugs are octreotide and lanreotide, long-acting analogues of somatostatin. Dopamine agonists (e.g, bromocriptine, cabergoline), which stimulate GH secretion in normal subjects but inhibit it in many patients with acromegaly, are also used. A GH receptor antagonist (pegvisomant) has been introduced recently.

When there is accompanying hypopituitarism, replacement treatment is with cortisol, gonadal steroids

Clinical features of excessive growth hormone secretion		
Somatic	**Metabolic**	**Local effects of tumour**
increased growth of: skin, subcutaneous tissues skull and jaw hands, feet long bones, if before fusion of epiphyses	elevated, non-suppressible plasma GH concentration	headache
	glucose intolerance	visual field defects
	clinical diabetes mellitus	hypopituitarism
nerve compression (particularly carpal tunnel syndrome) excessive sweating, greasy skin, acne goitre cardiomegaly, hypertension increased risk of colonic cancer	hypercalcaemia, hyperphosphataemia	diabetes insipidus

Fig. 7.9 Clinical features of excessive GH secretion. Features of hyperprolactinaemia (due to co-secretion of the hormone or a decrease in dopaminergic inhibition of prolactin secretion) may also be present.

Case history 7.3

A 40-year-old man consulted his GP because he had become impotent. He had also been embarrassed by excessive sweating in the absence of exertion. His wife thought that his facial features had become coarser, and he had recently had to buy a larger pair of shoes than normal because his old ones had become uncomfortable. The GP found mild hypertension and a trace of glycosuria and referred him to an endocrine clinic with a presumptive diagnosis of acromegaly.

Investigations

oral glucose tolerance test:

blood glucose	(initial)	8.5 mmol/L
	(2 h)	11.5 mmol/L
serum GH	(initial)	22 mU/L
	(minimum)	20 mU/L

0900 h serum:		
prolactin		800 mU/L
testosterone		11 nmol/L
LH		2.0 U/L
FSH		1.5 U/L
free T4		16 pmol/L
TSH		0.8 mU/L
cortisol		400 nmol/L
cortisol (30 min after Synacthen)		700 nmol/L

visual fields: partial bitemporal hemianopia

skull radiograph: enlarged pituitary fossa with erosion of anterior clinoid processes

pituitary CT scan: pituitary tumour with suprasellar extension

Comment

The clinical diagnosis is confirmed by the high basal GH concentration, which is not suppressed by glucose. The glucose tolerance test is diagnostic of diabetes: abnormal glucose tolerance is seen in about 35% of cases of acromegaly.

The basal prolactin concentration is elevated; testosterone concentration is low–normal secondary to low gonadotrophin secretion (gonadotrophins would be increased in primary testicular failure). The pituitary–thyroid and pituitary–adrenal axes appear normal.

The presence of a tumour is confirmed by the radiographic appearances; the optic chiasm lies immediately above the pituitary and compression of it can cause either visual field defects, characteristically a bitemporal hemi- or quadrantanopia, or threaten complete visual failure.

(or gonadotrophins), thyroxine and vasopressin, either alone or in combination, are given as required. All patients with acromegaly and gigantism must be followed up and reassessed regularly for evidence of either recurrence or further loss of normal pituitary function.

Hyperprolactinaemia

Hyperprolactinaemia is a common endocrine abnormality. It is an important cause of infertility in both males and females, impotence in males and menstrual irregularity in females. These effects are thought to be

Hyperprolactinaemia

Causes

Physiological
stress, sleep, pregnancy, suckling

Drugs
dopaminergic receptor blockers,
   e.g. phenothiazines, haloperidol
dopamine-depleting agents,
   e.g. methyldopa, reserpine
others, e.g. oestrogens, TRH

Pituitary disorders
prolactin-secreting tumour (prolactinoma)
tumours blocking dopaminergic inhibition
   of prolactin secretion
pituitary stalk section and surgery

Others
hypothyroidism
ectopic secretion
chronic renal failure

Clinical features

Females
oligomenorrhoea, amenorrhoea
infertility
galactorrhoea

Males
impotence
infertility
gynaecomastia

Fig. 7.10 Causes and clinical features of hyperprolactinaemia.

mediated through inhibition of the pulsatility of GnRH by prolactin. The causes and clinical features of hyperprolactinaemia are summarized in *Fig. 7.10*. There may also be features related to the cause of the hyperprolactinaemia. The causes include various drugs, which either block pituitary dopaminergic receptors or deplete the brain of dopamine, in addition to pituitary tumours (prolactinoma) and destructive pituitary lesions that interfere with the normal inhibition of prolactin secretion. Prolactinomas are usually small (microadenomas, <10 mm diameter) but larger tumours (macroadenomas) can occur that erode the

pituitary fossa and extend outside its confines. Overall, prolactinomas occur more frequently in women but affected men are more likely to have a macroadenoma.

Prolactin is secreted in response to both stress and TRH, and plasma concentrations also depend on oestrogen status. It is therefore difficult to define an upper limit of normal for plasma prolactin concentration. Slightly elevated concentrations of prolactin are less likely to be of significance in well-oestrogenized women. Plasma prolactin concentrations in patients with microadenomas are usually less than 5000 mU/L. Prolactin-secreting tumours >10 mm diameter are usually associated with plasma prolactin concentrations >5000 mU/L. Lower concentrations in patients with large pituitary tumours are usually a result of disruption of the delivery of dopamine to the pituitary. Because prolactin-secreting tumours often respond rapidly to medical treatment, urgent measurement of prolactin may be required in a patient with a large pituitary tumour associated with visual failure.

Drugs, hypothyroidism and, in amenorrhoeic women, pregnancy, must be excluded as causes of hyperprolactinaemia. Apparently high concentrations of the hormone (up to 5000 mU/L) can sometimes be due to macroprolactin – a complex of prolactin with an immunoglobulin that is detected by immunoassays, but does not cause the clinical features of hyperprolactinaemia.

Numerous dynamic tests have been proposed to aid in the diagnosis of suspected prolactin-secreting tumours. The most widely used is the measurement of the prolactin response to TRH, which is diminished in most patients with prolactinomas. However, this is not a consistent, or a specific, finding and neither the TRH nor any other dynamic test is of established value in the diagnosis of prolactinomas. If a tumour is diagnosed, patients must be tested for deficient secretion of other anterior pituitary hormones. With small tumours, other pituitary functions are usually normal. Formal assessment of visual fields is mandatory in patients with macroprolactinomas.

The majority of patients with small prolactin-secreting tumours respond to treatment with a dopamine agonist (e.g. cabergoline or bromocriptine). Prolactin concentration usually falls to normal and many women regain fertility. Long-term treatment is usually necessary although, in some patients, hyperprolactinaemia does not recur on withdrawal of the drug. Patients who do not respond to or are intolerant of medical treatment are treated by trans-sphenoidal surgery. Medical treatment reduces prolactin secretion and causes tumour shrinkage in the majority of patients with larger tumours. Surgery is sometimes required but tends to be less successful than with small tumours. External irradiation may be helpful in some cases.

Cushing's disease

Cushing's disease, in which increased secretion of cortisol by the adrenal cortex is secondary to increased secretion of ACTH by the anterior pituitary, is discussed in *Chapter 8*. Patients who have been treated for Cushing's disease by adrenalectomy alone may later develop hyperpigmentation and the clinical features of a large pituitary tumour (Nelson's syndrome). The pigmentation is due to the melanocyte-stimulating activity of ACTH and its precursors. Nelson's syndrome is uncommon in patients in whom treatment for Cushing's disease has included pituitary surgery or irradiation in addition to adrenalectomy.

Other conditions related to pituitary tumours

Tumours that secrete TSH or gonadotrophins are rare. Occasionally, TSH-secreting tumours develop in patients with long-standing untreated hypothyroidism but these regress when replacement treatment is given. Approximately 30% of pituitary tumours, usually chromophobe adenomas, are non-functioning. They can present with features of hypopituitarism or because of the physical presence of the tumour and are occasionally diagnosed incidentally from a skull radiograph taken for some other purpose.

Even apparently non-functioning tumours may secrete small but clinically insignificant quantities of hormones. Some secrete only the α-subunit of the glycoprotein hormones and measurement of plasma α-subunit concentration may be useful in assessing the success of treatment in such cases.

POSTERIOR PITUITARY HORMONES

The posterior pituitary secretes two hormones: vasopressin (ADH) and oxytocin. These hormones are synthesized in the hypothalamus and pass down nerve axons into the posterior pituitary, from where they are released into the circulation. Oxytocin is involved in the control of uterine contractility and of milk release from the lactating breast. Disorders of its secretion are probably uncommon and are not clinically important. In contrast, vasopressin is essential to life and disorders of its secretion are well recognized.

Vasopressin

Vasopressin has a vital role in the control of the tonicity of the extracellular fluid, and hence indirectly of the intracellular fluid, and of water balance. Excessive secretion results in dilutional hyponatraemia, with a risk of water intoxication; decreased secretion results in diabetes insipidus, a condition in which there is uncontrolled excretion of water with a tendency to severe dehydration. The syndromes of excessive secretion of vasopressin are discussed on *p. 26*; they are frequently seen in conditions that do not affect the pituitary directly. Diabetes insipidus, on the other hand, is usually due to pituitary or hypothalamic disease (cranial diabetes insipidus, CDI) (*Fig. 7.11*), although it

Causes of diabetes insipidus
Cranial
tumours:
craniopharyngioma
secondary tumours
pituitary tumours with suprasellar extension
granulomatous disease
meningitis and encephalitis
vascular disorders
trauma (may be transient)
surgery (often transient)
idiopathic
familial
Nephrogenic
familial
metabolic:
hypokalaemia
hypercalcaemia
drugs:
lithium
demeclocycline
post-obstructive uropathy
chronic renal disease:
pyelonephritis
polycystic disease
amyloid
sickle cell disease

Fig. 7.11 Causes of diabetes insipidus.

Fluid deprivation test

Procedure

allow fluids overnight before test and give light breakfast with no fluid; no smoking permitted

weigh patient

allow no fluid for 8 h; patient must be under constant supervision during this time

every 2h:
  weigh patient (stop test if weight falls by >5% initial body weight*)
  patient empties bladder: measure urine volume and osmolality
  measure plasma osmolality (stop test if osmolality >300 mmol/kg*)

after 8 h allow patient to drink (no more than twice urine volume of period of fluid deprivation, to avoid acute hyponatraemia) and give 2 µg desmopressin i.m.

measure urine osmolality every 4 h for a further 16 h

*end-point diagnostic of diabetes insipidus; allow access to fluid and assess response to desmopressin

Interpretation of results: see Fig. 7.15

Fig. 7.12 Fluid deprivation test. The first eight hours test for the ability to concentrate the urine and hence differentiate between diabetes insipidus and primary polydipsia. The period after the administration of desmopressin tests for the kidneys' ability to respond to vasopressin and therefore differentiates between cranial and nephrogenic diabetes insipidus. The results of this test may be equivocal, necessitating further investigation.

can also be due to a failure of the kidneys to respond to the hormone (nephrogenic diabetes insipidus, NDI), either because of a defect in the vasopressin receptor or in signal transduction, or because of inadequate medullary hypertonicity.

In diabetes insipidus, the lack of vasopressin (or resistance to its actions) results in polyuria (typically >3 L urine/24 h) and thirst. Unless the hypothalamic thirst centre is also damaged, thirst leads to increased fluid intake (polydipsia). The differential diagnosis includes

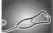 ### Case history 7.4

A middle-aged woman, who had undergone mastectomy and local radiotherapy for carcinoma of the breast two years previously, attended for her regular outpatient appointment. There was no sign of recurrence but she complained of increasing thirst over the previous months and that she was passing copious amounts of urine. The thirst became intolerable if she went without water for more than a few hours and her sleep was disturbed by the frequent need to pass urine and have a drink. There was no glycosuria; serum creatinine, potassium and calcium concentrations were all normal. She was admitted for investigation.

Investigations

random plasma: osmolality   295 mmol/kg
                sodium   144 mmol/L
urine osmolality   90 mmol/kg

Fluid deprivation test: after six hours' water deprivation her weight had fallen from 60 kg to 57 kg; the test was therefore stopped.

at end of test: plasma osmolality   307 mmol/kg
                 urine osmolality   220 mmol/kg

She was then allowed to drink and was given a dose of desmopressin. Following this, her urine osmolality rose to 810 mmol/kg.

Comment

The history of intolerable thirst with a slightly raised plasma osmolality yet dilute urine is very suggestive of diabetes insipidus and this diagnosis is confirmed by the failure to conserve water and concentrate the urine during water deprivation. She responded to desmopressin, indicating that vasopressin deficiency, rather than renal insensitivity to the hormone, was the cause of her symptoms.

She was treated successfully with regular administration of desmopressin and her symptoms resolved. A skull radiograph was normal but CT scanning revealed a small lesion in the region of the hypothalamus. The patient died one year later, with extensive cerebral metastatic deposits from her breast carcinoma.

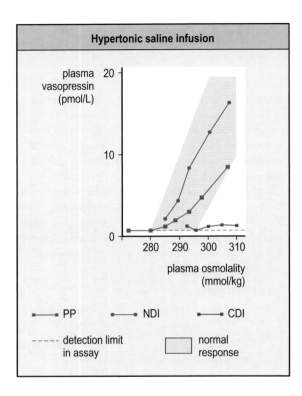

Fig. 7.13 Hypertonic saline infusion. Typical responses to the intravenous infusion of 5% saline are shown for patients with nephrogenic diabetes insipidus (NDI), cranial diabetes insipidus (CDI) and primary polydipsia (PP).

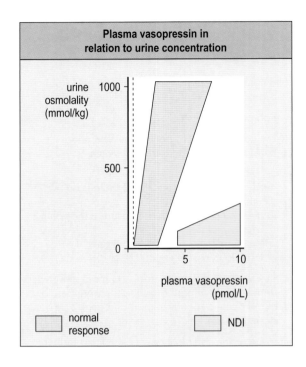

Fig. 7.14 Plasma vasopressin in relation to urine concentration during fluid deprivation. In nephrogenic diabetes insipidus (NDI), vasopressin concentrations are inappropriately high in relation to urine osmolality.

other conditions causing polyuria and polydipsia, for example diabetes mellitus, chronic renal failure, hypercalcaemia and hypokalaemia. Simple tests will eliminate these possibilities. Children with diabetes insipidus may present with enuresis.

A compulsive desire to drink (psychogenic or primary polydipsia) also causes polyuria. However, in this case polyuria is secondary to increased fluid intake, while in diabetes insipidus the opposite applies, polydipsia being a response to polyuria. In both conditions, the urine is dilute. If a random urine osmolality is greater than 750 mmol/kg, diabetes insipidus is excluded. Plasma sodium concentration and osmolality are usually normal in both conditions although they may be high–normal in diabetes insipidus (and frankly elevated if patients are denied water) and low–normal in primary polydipsia.

If there is doubt about the diagnosis, a fluid deprivation test should be performed (*Fig. 7.12*). This is effectively a biological assay for vasopressin. Patients with diabetes insipidus may become dangerously dehydrated if denied access to fluid; they may also exercise considerable ingenuity to obtain fluid. Close supervision is therefore essential; the test should be performed during the day, and fluid deprivation not be required overnight.

In a normal subject, the urine becomes concentrated in response to fluid deprivation and plasma osmolality does not exceed 295 mmol/kg. In diabetes insipidus, the urine does not become concentrated and plasma osmolality rises. In patients who are water overloaded before the test is started, the urine may not become concentrated; plasma osmolality is usually low and may remain so since vasopressin secretion is only stimulated if it rises above 285 mmol/kg. Thus the urine becomes concentrated only if the plasma osmolality exceeds this level.

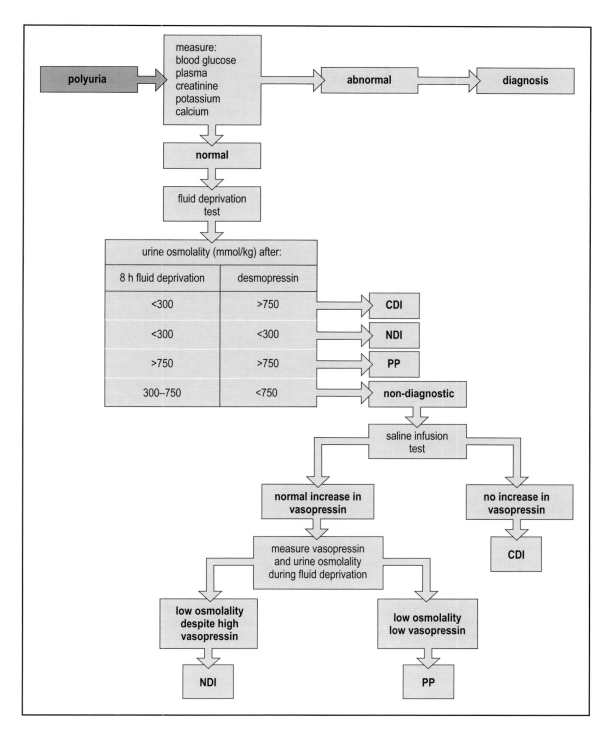

Fig. 7.15 An algorithm for the investigation of polyuria. CDI = cranial diabetes insipidus, NDI = nephrogenic diabetes insipidus, PP = primary polydipsia.

At the end of the eight-hour period, the patient is allowed to drink water and is given 1-desamino-D-arginine-vasopressin (desmopressin), a synthetic analogue of vasopressin. In CDI, the urine should become concentrated; in patients with NDI, it remains dilute. If the water deprivation test is to be carried out on a patient with anterior pituitary disease, adequate cortisol replacement must be provided.

If the results of a fluid deprivation test are equivocal, the plasma vasopressin response to hypertonic saline infusion should be assessed. The response is normal in patients with NDI or primary polydipsia, but decreased in patients with CDI (*Fig. 7.13*). The former two conditions can be distinguished by comparing plasma vasopressin concentration with urine osmolality after a period of fluid deprivation (*Fig. 7.14*). In NDI, plasma vasopressin is much higher than normal. Alternatively, since vasopressin measurements are not widely available, a closely supervised therapeutic trial of desmopressin treatment can be used. This causes an improvement in CDI, has no effect in NDI and causes increasing hyponatraemia in primary polydipsia. An algorithm for the investigation of polyuria is given in *Fig. 7.15*.

About 5% of cases of CDI are familial, with autosomal dominant inheritance. There are two inherited forms of NDI. In the X-linked recessive condition, the vasopressin receptor is functionally abnormal. In the other (very rare) autosomal recessive condition, there is defective synthesis of aquaporin-2 (a water channel protein).

Management of diabetes insipidus

Patients must always have access to adequate fluid and, whenever possible, the underlying disease should be treated. Cranial diabetes insipidus is usually treated with desmopressin, given orally or as a nasal spray. If polyuria is only mild (i.e. urine volume <4 L/24 h) specific treatment may not be necessary. Patients must learn to monitor their fluid output and input in order to avoid water intoxication. This may be a particular problem if the sensation of thirst is blunted.

Patients with NDI, because they do not respond to vasopressin, must maintain an adequate water intake to avoid dehydration. Hydronephrosis and hydroureter secondary to bladder distension may occur and lead to renal impairment. Thiazide diuretics, which induce a state of sodium depletion, stimulating renal sodium and water retention, may reduce the polyuria. Potassium supplements or the concomitant use of a potassium-sparing diuretic may be necessary to prevent hypokalaemia.

SUMMARY

- The **anterior pituitary gland** secretes **growth hormone** (GH) and **prolactin**, and trophic hormones that control the activity of the gonads (LH and FSH: **luteinizing hormone** and **follicle-stimulating hormone**), thyroid (TSH: **thyroid-stimulating hormone**) and the adrenal cortex (ACTH: **adrenocorticotrophic hormone**). The secretion of all these hormones is regulated by **hypothalamic hormones**, which reach the pituitary through a portal system of blood vessels. The trophic hormones are in addition controlled by feedback mechanisms involving the hormones produced by the respective target organs.

- **Anterior pituitary hypofunction** (hypopituitarism) can result in the inadequate production of one or more hormones; the clinical manifestations depend upon the particular pattern of deficiency. Hypopituitarism may either be the result of disease affecting the pituitary itself or be secondary to hypothalamic disease, with failure of production of hypothalamic hormones. Hypopituitarism is investigated by measuring basal and stimulated concentrations of pituitary hormones.

SUMMARY (cont'd)

- **Pituitary tumours** can cause hypopituitarism by destroying normal pituitary tissue, but may be functional and produce syndromes related to excessive hormone secretion. Pituitary tumours producing prolactin, GH and ACTH are well recognized, but secretion of gonadotrophins or TSH is rare. In addition to their endocrine effects, both functional and non-functional tumours can give rise to clinical features characteristic of intracranial space-occupying lesions.

- The **posterior pituitary gland** secretes **oxytocin** and **vasopressin**. Both are synthesized in the hypothalamus and reach the posterior pituitary through nerve axons. Because of this, damage to the posterior pituitary may only cause temporary failure of hormone secretion. Oxytocin stimulates uterine contraction during labour but does not appear to be an essential hormone.

- **Vasopressin** is essential as it controls water excretion by altering the permeability of the renal collecting tubules to water in response to changes in extracellular fluid osmolality. **Excessive vasopressin secretion produces water retention** with a dilutional hyponatraemia. **Defective vasopressin secretion results in diabetes insipidus**, with uncontrolled renal water loss. Diabetes insipidus can also be due to renal insensitivity to vasopressin; the two types can be distinguished from each other, and from psychogenic polydipsia, by assessing the response to a fluid deprivation test or the infusion of hypertonic saline.

8 The adrenal glands

INTRODUCTION

The adrenal glands have two functionally distinct parts: the cortex and the medulla. The adrenal cortex is essential to life; it produces three classes of steroid hormone: glucocorticoids, mineralocorticoids and androgens. The medulla, which is functionally part of the sympathetic nervous system, is not essential to life and its pathological importance is related mainly to the occurrence of rare catecholamine-secreting tumours.

Glucocorticoids, of which the most important is cortisol, are secreted in response to adrenocorticotrophic hormone (ACTH), which is itself secreted by the pituitary in response to hypothalamic corticotrophin releasing hormone (CRH). Cortisol exerts negative feedback control on ACTH release. Glucocorticoids have many physiological functions (*Fig. 8.1*) and are particularly important in mediating the body's response to stress.

The most important mineralocorticoid is aldosterone. This is secreted in response to angiotensin II, produced as a result of the activation of the renin–angiotensin system by a decrease in renal blood flow and other indicators of decreased extracellular fluid (ECF) volume (*Fig. 8.2*). Secretion of aldosterone is also directly stimulated by hyperkalaemia. The main action of aldosterone is to stimulate sodium reabsorption in the distal convoluted tubules in the kidneys in exchange for potassium and hydrogen ions; it thus has a central role in the determination of the ECF volume. ACTH does not have a major physiological role in aldosterone secretion. A single injection of ACTH increases plasma aldosterone concentration, but ACTH infusion does not cause a sustained increase. Curiously, the secretion of aldosterone by adrenal tumours is affected by ACTH (*see p. 157*).

The adrenal cortex is also a source of androgens, including dehydroepiandrosterone (DHEA), DHEA sulphate (DHEAS) and androstenedione. The clinical effects of excessive adrenal androgens can be a prominent feature of adrenal disorders in females.

ADRENAL STEROID HORMONE BIOSYNTHESIS

The hormones secreted by the adrenal cortex are synthesized from cholesterol by a sequence of enzyme-catalyzed reactions (*Fig. 8.3*). An awareness of these pathways is important for the understanding of congenital adrenal hyperplasia, a group of conditions each caused by a lack of one of these enzymes.

MEASUREMENT OF ADRENAL STEROID HORMONES

Adrenal steroid hormones are measured by specific immunoassays: chemical measurements of 17-oxosteroids and 17-oxogenic steroids (adrenal androgens and cortisol-like substances, respectively) are obsolete. The plasma concentrations of these hormones can fluctuate for various reasons and the results of single estimations must be interpreted with caution.

The measurement of urinary cortisol excretion is valuable in investigations of Cushing's syndrome. Urinary

---

Functions of glucocorticoids

increase protein catabolism

increase hepatic glycogen synthesis

increase hepatic gluconeogenesis

inhibit ACTH secretion (negative feedback mechanism)

sensitize arterioles to action of noradrenaline, hence involved in maintenance of blood pressure

permissive effect on water excretion; required for initiation of diuresis in response to water loading

Fig. 8.1 Principal physiological functions of glucocorticoids.

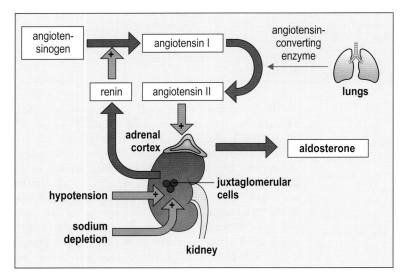

Fig. 8.2 Stimulation of aldosterone secretion through activation of the renin–angiotensin system. Renin, released into the plasma from the juxtaglomerular cells of the kidney in response to various stimuli, catalyzes the formation of angiotensin I from angiotensinogen, an α_2-globulin. Angiotensin I is metabolized to an octapeptide, angiotensin II, by angiotensin-converting enzyme during its passage through the lungs. Angiotensin II stimulates the release of aldosterone from the adrenal cortex; it is a powerful pressor agent and also stimulates thirst and the secretion of vasopressin.

'steroid profiling', in which steroids are separated and quantitated by gas–liquid chromatography, is particularly valuable in the investigation of suspected congenital adrenal hyperplasia; it may also be helpful in the investigation of suspected adrenal carcinoma.

Cortisol

Ninety-five per cent of cortisol in the blood is bound to protein, principally to the cortisol-binding globulin, transcortin. Free cortisol concentration, and thus the amount of cortisol that can be excreted unchanged in the urine, is very small. Transcortin is almost fully saturated at normal cortisol concentrations. Because of this, if cortisol production increases, the concentration present in the plasma in the free form, and thus the amount that is excreted, increases to a disproportionately greater extent than the total. For this reason, measurement of the 24-hour urinary excretion of cortisol, provided that an accurate urine collection can be made, is a sensitive way of detecting increased, but not decreased, secretion of the hormone.

Plasma cortisol concentrations show a diurnal variation, being highest in the morning and lowest at night (*Fig. 8.4*). Blood for cortisol measurement should usually be drawn between 0800 h and 0900 h; however, samples are taken at 2300 h to detect loss of the diurnal variation, an early feature of adrenal hyperfunction (Cushing's syndrome). Random measurements are rarely of any value in the diagnosis of adrenal disease,

except that a high concentration in a sick patient may reasonably be taken to exclude adrenal failure.

Cortisol is secreted in response to stress, mediated through ACTH, and thus stress must be kept to a minimum if results are to be interpreted correctly. Investigations of adrenal hypo- or hyperfunction often involve measurement of cortisol after attempting to stimulate or suppress its secretion.

When interpreting plasma cortisol results, it should be remembered that the synthetic glucocorticoid prednisolone may cross-react with cortisol in immunoassays for the hormone. Cross-reaction does not occur with dexamethasone, nor with spironolactone, an aldosterone antagonist used as a diuretic.

Aldosterone

Aldosterone secretion is stimulated through the action of renin; therefore, it is often helpful to measure the plasma renin activity at the same time as the concentration of aldosterone, to establish whether aldosterone secretion is autonomous or under normal control. Calculation of the plasma aldosterone:renin ratio in a random blood sample is a useful screening test for excessive aldosterone secretion: it is excluded by a low value (*see p. 156*). Plasma aldosterone concentration varies with posture: the use of samples taken from patients while they are inert or supine is discussed further in connection with the investigation of excessive secretion of aldosterone (*see p. 156*).

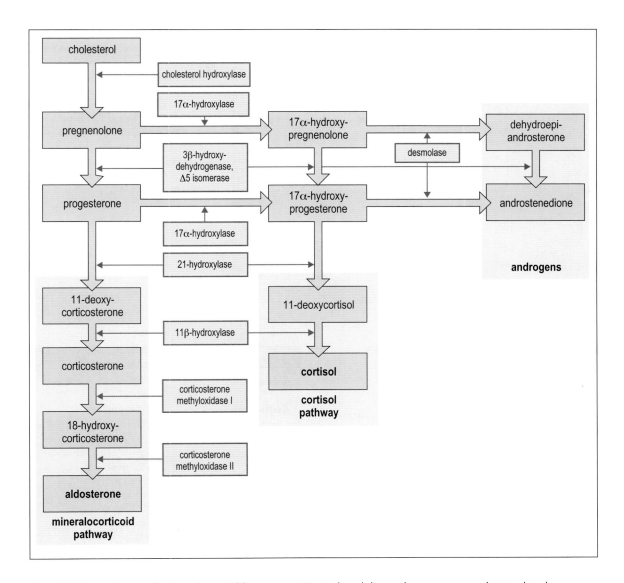

Fig. 8.3 Biosynthesis of adrenal steroid hormones. Cortisol and the androgens are synthesized in the zona reticularis and zona fasciculata of the adrenal glands. Corticosterone methyloxidase II, required for the synthesis of aldosterone, is present only in the zona glomerulosa. Androstenedione can be converted to testosterone in peripheral tissues but, in adult males, adrenal androgens, and the testosterone derived from them, make only a minor contribution to total androgenic activity.

Androgens

Measurements of adrenal androgens are of value in the diagnosis and management of congenital adrenal hyperplasia (*see p. 157*) and in the investigation of virilization in women (*see Chapter 10*).

DISORDERS OF THE ADRENAL CORTEX

Patients with adrenal disorders can present with clinical features related to either hypo- or hyperfunction. In congenital adrenal hyperplasia, a combination of features may be present.

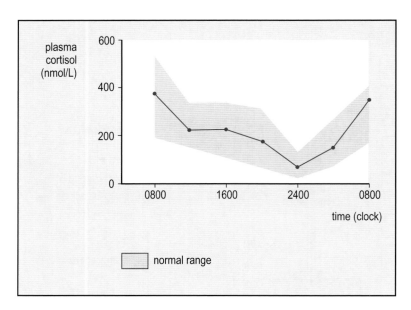

Fig. 8.4 Diurnal variation in plasma cortisol concentration. Plasma cortisol levels are at their highest shortly after waking and then decline throughout the day to reach a nadir in the late evening. Because of this variation, it is important that blood samples are taken at times that coincide either with the peak or the trough, random samples being of little value. The graph shows mean values and the range in a sample of healthy people.

Adrenal hypofunction (Addison's disease)

The common causes and clinical features of this uncommon but life-threatening condition are listed in *Fig. 8.5*. The cases originally described by Addison were caused by tuberculosis, but autoimmune disease is now the major cause in the UK. In such cases, adrenal autoantibodies are usually present and there may be associated organ-specific autoimmune disease (e.g. pernicious anaemia).

The commonest cause of adrenal hypofunction is suppression of the pituitary–adrenal axis by glucocorticoids used therapeutically. Although, during treatment, patients may develop features of Cushing's syndrome, a sudden withdrawal of steroids or failure to increase the dose during stress (e.g. surgery) may precipitate acute adrenal failure. Normal pituitary–adrenal function is regained only slowly when steroids are withdrawn and it is essential that the dosage is reduced gradually when steroid treatment is to be discontinued.

The majority of the clinical features of adrenal failure are due to the lack of glucocorticoids and mineralocorticoids. Increased pigmentation is a result of the high concentrations of ACTH, which occur because of the loss of negative feedback by cortisol: ACTH has some melanocyte-stimulating activity.

Adrenal hypofunction	
Causes	**Clinical features**

Common
glucocorticoid treatment
autoimmune adrenalitis
tuberculosis
	Common
	tiredness, generalized
	  weakness, lethargy
	anorexia, nausea,
	  vomiting
	weight loss
	dizziness and postural
	  hypotension
	pigmentation
	loss of body hair
	  (women)

Less common adrenalectomy secondary tumour deposits amyloidosis haemochromatosis histoplasmosis adrenal haemorrhage	**Less common** hypoglycaemia depression

Fig. 8.5 Causes and clinical features of primary adrenal hypofunction.

Case history 8.1

A 17-year-old girl presented with a two-month history of tiredness and lethargy. She had noticed that she became dizzy when she stood up. On examination, she had pigmentation of the buccal mucosa and palmar creases and in an old appendicectomy scar. Her blood pressure was 120/80 mmHg lying down, but fell to 90/50 mmHg when she stood up.

Investigations

serum:	sodium	128 mmol/L
	potassium	5.4 mmol/L
	urea	8.5 mmol/L
blood glucose (fasting)		2.5 mmol/L

short ACTH stimulation test:
plasma cortisol:

0900 h	150 nmol/L
30 min after ACTH	160 nmol/L
60 min after ACTH	160 nmol/L
plasma ACTH (0900 h)	500 ng/L
(normal <50 ng/L)	

anti-adrenal antibodies were detectable at high concentration

Comment

On the basis of these results, a diagnosis of primary adrenal failure was made. Her symptoms resolved rapidly after starting glucocorticoid and mineralocorticoid replacement and she remained well thereafter. Postural hypotension is a common finding in adrenal failure: it is due to a decrease in ECF volume caused by a lack of aldosterone leading to sodium loss. This decrease in ECF volume may also cause a degree of prerenal uraemia, as demonstrated in this case. Hyponatraemia is not always present in adrenal failure, particularly in the early stages. Sodium is lost isotonically from the kidneys, but the lack of cortisol may cause water retention and with severe hypovolaemia, vasopressin (antidiuretic hormone, ADH) secretion is stimulated. Deficiency of aldosterone is also responsible for potassium retention and thus hyperkalaemia.

The fasting blood glucose is at the low end of the reference range in this patient: the unopposed action of insulin may cause symptomatic hypoglycaemia.

The 0900 h cortisol is at the lower limit of the reference range and there is virtually no response to ACTH. Except in very severe cases, cortisol is measurable in the plasma, even though the concentration is low–normal or frankly low. However, this represents the adrenal glands' maximal output since they are already stimulated by the high concentration of endogenous ACTH.

Ten years later, her periods ceased. Her premature menopause was due to autoimmune ovarian failure. There is a recognized association between autoimmune adrenal failure and other organ-specific autoimmune diseases.

Adrenal failure usually has an insidious onset, with non-specific symptoms, but can develop acutely. Adrenal crisis is a medical emergency. The clinical features include severe hypovolaemia, shock and hypoglycaemia. It may be precipitated by stress (e.g. due to infection, trauma or surgery) in patients with incipient adrenal failure. Patients being treated with glucocorticoids, whether in physiological doses (replacement therapy) or pharma-

ACTH stimulation tests*	
Short test	**Long test**
Procedure	**Procedure**
take blood sample at 0900 h for measurement of cortisol	day 1: inject 1 mg depot ACTH i.m.
inject 250 µg ACTH i.m. or i.v.	days 2 and 3: repeat
take further blood samples after 30 and 60 min for cortisol measurement	day 4: perform short ACTH test
Normal results	**Results**
plasma cortisol after ACTH increment of 200 nmol/L with peak of >550 nmol/L	primary adrenal insufficiency: plasma cortisol at 0900 h on day 4 <200 nmol/L (usually <100 nmol/L) with no increment following ACTH
	secondary adrenal insufficiency (hypothalamic or hypopituitarism): increment in plasma cortisol of at least 200 nmol/L above baseline

Fig. 8.6 ACTH stimulation tests for the diagnosis of adrenal failure. It is important to note that blood should be taken for ACTH assay before giving ACTH. It is not necessary to withhold any treatment until after the tests are completed, provided that the drug being used does not cross-react with cortisol, since exogenous steroids do not affect the response of the adrenal gland to ACTH in the short term. *Also known as Synacthen tests: Synacthen is synthetic ACTH.

cological doses (e.g. in severe inflammatory conditions) are also susceptible to adrenal failure in these circumstances if the dosage is not increased. Haemorrhage into the adrenal glands may occur as a complication of anticoagulant treatment and in meningococcal septicaemia, and can result in acute adrenal failure.

Adrenal failure can occur secondarily to pituitary failure as a result of decreased stimulation by ACTH. Other features of hypopituitarism may be present (*see p. 129*); in contrast to patients with primary adrenal failure, abnormal pigmentation does not occur.

In secondary adrenal failure, hypotension can occur because the sensitivity of arteriolar smooth muscle to catecholamines is reduced by a lack of cortisol. Hyponatraemia may sometimes be present, since the lack of cortisol reduces the ability of the kidneys to excrete a water load, but there is no renal salt wasting since aldosterone secretion is not dependent upon ACTH.

Unless a patient is being treated with synthetic corticosteroids, a plasma cortisol concentration of <50 nmol/L in a blood sample drawn at 0900 h is effectively diagnostic of adrenal failure, while a concentration >550 nmol/L excludes the diagnosis. However, in the majority of patients with adrenal failure, whether primary or secondary, the plasma cortisol concentration lies between these extremes, and an ACTH stimulation test must be performed to establish the diagnosis. The normal response to a single dose of soluble ACTH (Synacthen) ('short Synacthen test') is shown in *Fig. 8.6*. If the response is in any way abnormal the patient should be assumed to have adrenal failure. In both primary and secondary adrenal failure, the response in the short ACTH stimulation test is absent or blunted (*see Case History 8.1*). This should be regarded as a screening test for adrenal failure; unless the clinical features leave no doubt that primary adrenal disease is responsible, a long ACTH stimulation test can be performed (*Fig. 8.6*). In this test, depot ACTH, which has a longer duration of action, is given daily for three days, and a short ACTH stimulation test is performed on day 4. Plasma cortisol concentration increases in response to ACTH in secondary, but not primary, adrenal failure. Alternatively, a single dose of depot ACTH can be given, with plasma cortisol estimations made at various times up to 24 hours, but this is likely to be less sensitive if secondary adrenal failure is long-standing.

The best differentiation between primary and secondary adrenal failure is provided by measurement of plasma ACTH. In primary adrenal failure, pituitary ACTH production is greatly increased because of the lack of negative feedback by cortisol, whereas in secondary adrenal failure the plasma concentration of ACTH is low.

Although, ideally, these tests should be done before starting treatment, when a severely ill patient is judged clinically to have adrenal failure, treatment should not be delayed. A blood sample can be taken immediately for later cortisol measurement. Treatment can then be commenced with a synthetic glucocorticoid that does not cross-react with cortisol in the laboratory assay (e.g. dexamethasone) and an ACTH stimulation test performed as soon as is convenient. The results will not be vitiated by the treatment if only a short time elapses before the test is done. Patients presenting acutely with adrenal failure require intravenous hydrocortisone and fluid replacement with 0.9% sodium chloride. Plasma potassium and glucose concentrations should be monitored and intravenous glucose provided if necessary.

All patients with adrenal failure require life-long replacement therapy, usually with both hydrocortisone and 9α-fludrocortisone, a synthetic mineralocorticoid. Hydrocortisone replacement is usually given in three unequal doses (e.g. 10 mg in the morning and 5 mg at midday and in the early evening). The adequacy of replacement can be assessed clinically and by measuring plasma cortisol concentration at intervals throughout the day (cortisol 'day curve'): this allows detection of a concentration that is too high shortly after a dose or too low shortly before the next dose is due. Mineralocorticoid treatment can be assessed by measuring plasma renin activity: elevated activity implies inadequate replacement and complete suppression, excessive replacement. Hydrocortisone has some intrinsic mineralocorticoid activity, and occasionally patients may be free of symptoms on hydrocortisone alone, particularly if they maintain a high salt intake.

Long-term follow up is essential to ensure the continuing adequacy of replacement treatment and to

 Case history 8.2

A 40-year-old woman presented with a history of tiredness, constipation and general malaise. The clinical diagnosis of hypothyroidism was confirmed by a serum TSH of 60 mU/L and she was started on replacement therapy with thyroxine. Shortly afterwards, she developed abdominal pain, vomiting and diarrhoea after a meal including cold chicken. These symptoms persisted and were unusually severe, and her GP referred her to the emergency clinic at the local hospital. On examination she was severely dehydrated and hypotensive; blood was taken for investigations and intravenous saline infusion was started.

Investigations

serum:	sodium	120 mmol/L
	potassium	5.6 mmol/L
	urea	12 mmol/L
	glucose	2.5 mmol/L

The medical registrar wondered if she might have adrenal failure, and on more careful examination noticed that she had pigmentation over her knees and knuckles. He asked the laboratory to save the remaining serum for cortisol measurement and started intravenous hydrocortisone. Her condition improved rapidly; the laboratory later reported that the cortisol concentration was <50 nmol/L.

Comment

Adrenal failure often develops insidiously but adrenal crisis can be precipitated at any time by stress. Another factor of relevance in this case is the hypothyroidism. Organ-specific autoimmune diseases can occur in association, and treatment of hypothyroidism in a patient with coexistent incipient adrenal failure can cause this to become clinically overt.

check for the development of other autoimmune endocrine disease. The dose of hydrocortisone should be increased during intercurrent illness, trauma, surgery, etc.

Adrenal hyperfunction

In Cushing's syndrome there is over-production primarily of glucocorticoids, though mineralocorticoid and androgen production may also be excessive. In Conn's syndrome mineralocorticoids alone are produced in excess.

Cushing's syndrome

The causes and clinical features of Cushing's syndrome are listed in *Fig. 8.7*. Cushing's disease, that is adrenal hyperfunction secondary to a pituitary corticotroph adenoma, accounts for 60–70% of cases of spontaneously arising Cushing's syndrome (i.e. not caused by treatment with steroids). The clinical features are due primarily to the glucocorticoid effects of excessive cortisol but cortisol precursors and indeed cortisol itself have some mineralocorticoid activity. Thus sodium retention, leading to hypertension, and potassium wasting, causing a hypokalaemic alkalosis, are common findings except in iatrogenic disease (synthetic glucocorticoids have no mineralocorticoid activity). Increased production of adrenal androgens may also contribute to the clinical presentation.

Pseudo-Cushing's syndrome, in which patients appear cushingoid and may have some of the biochemical abnormalities of true Cushing's disease, can occur in severe depression and in alcoholics. Alcohol-related pseudo-Cushing's syndrome usually resolves rapidly on withdrawal of alcohol. Patients with severe obesity may also look cushingoid, but Cushing's syndrome is a very rare cause of obesity.

There are two diagnostic steps in the investigation of a patient with suspected Cushing's syndrome: the demonstration of increased cortisol secretion and the elucidation of the cause. It is common to see patients who look cushingoid but it is much less common that Cushing's syndrome is the cause. It is, therefore, often useful to carry out preliminary tests on an outpatient basis, aimed at excluding those patients who do not have adrenal disease and identifying those who may, and who thus merit further investigation. Tests used for

Cushing's syndrome
Causes
corticosteroid or ACTH treatment
pituitary hypersecretion of ACTH (Cushing's disease)
adrenal adenoma
adrenal carcinoma
ectopic ACTH secretion by tumours, e.g. carcinoma of bronchus and carcinoid tumours
Clinical features
truncal obesity ('moon face', buffalo hump, protruberant abdomen)
thinning of skin
purple striae
excessive bruising
hirsutism, especially in adrenal carcinoma
skin pigmentation (only if ACTH elevated)
hypertension
glucose intolerance
muscle weakness and wasting, especially of proximal muscles
menstrual irregularities, hirsutism
back pain (osteoporosis and vertebral collapse)
psychiatric disturbances: euphoria mania depression

Fig. 8.7 Causes and clinical features of Cushing's syndrome.

this purpose (*Fig. 8.8*) are the measurement of 24 h urinary cortisol excretion and the overnight or low-dose dexamethasone suppression test. Isolated measurements of plasma cortisol concentration are of no value. They are often normal during the day in patients with Cushing's syndrome.

Normal 24 h urinary cortisol excretion is <300 nmol. Increased excretion is characteristic of Cushing's syndrome (though it can also occur in pseudo-Cushing's and severe obesity), but care is required in the interpretation of results. If the urine collection is incomplete, the true excretion will be underestimated. This problem may be obviated by expressing the results as a fraction of the urinary creatinine excretion.

Screening tests for Cushing's syndrome	
Test	**Normal result**
24 h urinary cortisol excretion	<300 nmol/24 h
overnight/48 h low-dose dexamethasone suppression test	plasma cortisol <50 nmol/L at 0900 h

Fig. 8.8 Screening tests for Cushing's syndrome. The values for cortisol concentration used for diagnosis may vary slightly between laboratories. Cushing's syndrome is excluded by normal results in these tests.

Dexamethasone is a synthetic glucocorticoid that binds to cortisol receptors in the pituitary and suppresses ACTH release (and thus the secretion of cortisol by the adrenals) in normal individuals. In the overnight test, 1 mg is given at night and blood is drawn for measurement of cortisol at 0900 h the next morning. In normal individuals, this should be <50 nmol/L. A failure of suppression is characteristic of Cushing's syndrome but is not specific since it may also be seen in pseudo-Cushing's syndrome and as a result of stress. Fewer false positives occur if dexamethasone is given at a dose of 0.5 mg 6-hourly for 48 h, with cortisol being measured on the morning after the last dose. False negatives virtually never occur with either protocol. It is important that, if urinary cortisol excretion is to be measured, the period of collection does not include the time when dexamethasone is being given.

The insulin hypoglycaemia test, also used in the investigation of pituitary function (*see p. 128*), can be helpful in the diagnosis of Cushing's syndrome, since the normal increase in plasma cortisol concentration that occurs in response to hypoglycaemia is abolished even in mild Cushing's syndrome, while in patients with pseudo-Cushing's a normal response occurs.

Loss of diurnal variation of cortisol secretion is an early feature of Cushing's syndrome and the diagnosis is excluded if the plasma cortisol concentration at 2300 h or 2400 h is normal (<100 nmol/L). Since the patient must be resting and not stressed, plasma cortisol measurement at night is not a practical outpatient procedure. It necessitates hospital admission, itself a stressful event, with the result that false positive results are common. However, if care is taken to minimize stress (ideally blood is taken from the sleeping patient through a previously inserted cannula after two or three days in hospital), a raised value does indicate pathological over-production of cortisol.

Tests that are useful in elucidating the cause of Cushing's syndrome include the high-dose dexamethasone suppression test, the corticotrophin-releasing hormone (CRH) test and measurement of plasma ACTH. The former involves giving 2 mg dexamethasone 6-hourly for 48 h; plasma cortisol concentration is measured at 0900 h on the morning following the last dose. In Cushing's disease, the cortisol concentration characteristically decreases to less than 50% of the pre-treatment value. Failure of suppression suggests ectopic ACTH secretion or an adrenal tumour. Plasma ACTH concentrations are often very high with ectopic secretion and are low with adrenal tumours. Moderately elevated values are seen in Cushing's disease.

Exceptions to these results occur frequently. Many patients with ectopic ACTH have a characteristic clinical presentation, with weight loss, severe muscle weakness, pigmentation, hypertension, hypokalaemic alkalosis and diabetes, but without the classical somatic manifestations of Cushing's disease. In other cases, however (particularly when due to carcinoid tumours), ectopic ACTH secretion may produce a clinical syndrome that is clinically and biochemically identical to Cushing's disease. Imaging techniques, for example chest X-ray and pituitary and abdominal CT scanning, may reveal a tumour, while selective venous blood sampling for ACTH measurement, to locate the source of ACTH secretion, can also be helpful.

The CRH test can be useful to differentiate between Cushing's disease and ectopic ACTH secretion. In Cushing's disease, CRH (100 µg, i.v.) typically increases plasma ACTH concentration by 50% over baseline after 60 minutes, and cortisol concentration by 20%, whereas with ectopic ACTH secretion or an adrenal tumour there is typically no response.

The management of Cushing's syndrome depends upon the cause. Adrenal adenomas and, if possible, carcinomas, should be resected. The treatment of choice for Cushing's disease is trans-sphenoidal hypophysectomy. Bilateral adrenalectomy was formerly used and still may sometimes be required since the adrenals may become semi-autonomous. Bilateral adrenalectomy must always be followed by treatment to the pituitary (usually external irradiation) to prevent continued

Case history 8.3

A 35-year-old male window cleaner presented with muscle weakness. This mainly affected his thighs with the result that he sometimes had to use his hands to help himself up from a sitting position. He was also finding it difficult to climb ladders at work. He had no other complaints.

On examination, he had a cushingoid appearance with truncal obesity, proximal muscle wasting, violaceous abdominal striae and a plethoric, 'moon face'. His blood pressure was 180/110 mmHg. He admitted that he had noticed the changes in his appearance developing over the past nine months but had been too shy to seek medical advice. It was only when he became concerned that he might not be able to continue working that he consulted his doctor. He was admitted to hospital for further investigation.

Investigations

serum: sodium		136 mmol/L
potassium		3.2 mmol/L
bicarbonate		33 mmol/L
blood glucose (fasting)		7.5 mmol/L
serum cortisol:	(0900 h)	930 nmol/L
	(2400 h)	900 nmol/L
plasma ACTH	(0900 h)	130 ng/L
		(normal <50 ng/L)
urine cortisol excretion		840 nmol/24 h

dexamethasone suppression test:
0900 h serum cortisol after
0.5 mg dexamethasone four times
daily for two days (low dose)   880 nmol/L

0900 h serum cortisol after
2.0 mg dexamethasone four times
daily for two days (high dose)   320 nmol/L

Comment

The diagnosis is Cushing's disease. The clinical features are typical. The high 0900 h cortisol, lack of diurnal variation and high urinary cortisol excretion all suggest adrenal hyperfunction. An overnight dexamethasone suppression test was not performed because the presentation was so typical that an outpatient screening test was considered unnecessary. However, the formal two-stage test gave a result typical of Cushing's disease, with no change at the low dose and decreased cortisol secretion with the high dose.

In Cushing's disease, the pituitary usually remains susceptible to feedback by glucocorticoids, but is apparently less sensitive than normal (i.e. a higher concentration of cortisol is necessary to suppress ACTH; *Fig. 8.9b*). In Cushing's syndrome caused by adrenal tumours, whether adenomas or carcinomas, and also in ectopic ACTH secretion, there is usually no response to dexamethasone, even at the higher dose, since pituitary ACTH secretion is already suppressed by the high plasma cortisol concentrations (*Fig. 8.9c*). This patient's plasma ACTH is raised: with adrenal tumours, feedback of cortisol to the pituitary suppresses ACTH while with ectopic ACTH secretion, ACTH concentrations are very high (*Fig. 8.9d*). The results of biochemical tests in the various forms of Cushing's syndrome are summarized in *Fig. 8.10*.

Case history 8.3 (cont'd)

Measurements of plasma ACTH concentration are of great value in establishing the cause of Cushing's syndrome. However, the hormone is very labile and plasma must be separated rapidly, using a refrigerated centrifuge, and kept deep-frozen until the assay is performed if valid results are to be obtained.

This patient has a hypokalaemic alkalosis, a result of renal potassium wasting, and hypertension, a result of sodium retention. The fasting blood glucose is elevated: impaired glucose tolerance is common in Cushing's syndrome but clinical features of diabetes are uncommon, except in ectopic ACTH secretion. If the patient is coincidentally diabetic there may be a marked deterioration in control.

A skull radiograph in this patient showed a normal pituitary fossa: in Cushing's disease, the pituitary tumour secreting ACTH is usually very small, but may be revealed by MRI or CT scanning.

growth of the pituitary tumour. If this is not done, the tumour may increase in size and give rise to clinical symptoms and signs. The latter includes pigmentation, due to the secretion of excessive quantities of ACTH (Nelson's syndrome). Patients who have undergone hypophysectomy or bilateral adrenalectomy will require appropriate steroid replacement therapy for life. When surgery is not possible, and in all cases pending surgery, symptomatic relief may ensue from the use of drugs that block cortisol synthesis, such as metyrapone, which inhibits steroid-11-hydroxylase.

Conn's syndrome

This condition is characterized by excessive production of aldosterone. The principal causes and the clinical features are shown in *Fig. 8.11*. In about two-thirds of cases, the cause is an adrenal adenoma. Most other cases are a result of diffuse hypertrophy of the zona glomerulosa of the adrenal cortex. A rare cause is glucocorticoid-remediable aldosteronism, an inherited (autosomal dominant) condition in which aldosterone synthesis is under the control of ACTH. The clinical features of Conn's syndrome are mainly a result of the hypokalaemia, itself a consequence of increased renal potassium excretion. Many patients are asymptomatic, and are diagnosed when hypokalaemia is found during the investigation of hypertension. Hypertension is a consequence of aldosterone-induced sodium retention. Conn's syndrome is an uncommon cause of hypertension but is important because it is treatable. Its prevalence has been thought to be low (1–2% of patients with hypertension), but this is probably an underestimate, as a result of only patients with frank

hypokalaemia having been screened for the condition. The true prevalence is probably of the order of 5%.

Primary aldosteronism may be mimicked by treatment with carbenoxolone and by the ingestion of liquorice. Both these substances have metabolites that inhibit 11β-hydroxysteroid dehydrogenase. This enzyme converts cortisol to an inactive metabolite, cortisone, but does not affect aldosterone. Its inhibition in mineralocorticoid-sensitive tissues in effect potentiates the action of cortisol as a mineralocorticoid. For the same reason, an inherited defect in this enzyme (which mimics the effect of inhibition) is the cause of the syndrome of apparent mineralocorticoid excess, a rare cause of hypertension and hypokalaemic alkalosis. It, and related conditions, are discussed on *p. 274*.

High aldosterone concentrations are also seen in patients whose plasma renin activity is increased. This is secondary aldosteronism, since the adrenal glands are responding to their normal trophic stimulus, in contrast to the automonous secretion of aldosterone in Conn's syndrome, which is termed primary aldosteronism.

Secondary aldosteronism is far more common than the primary form and is associated with a variety of conditions (*Fig. 8.12*) in which renin secretion is increased. Patients may or may not be hypertensive, depending on the underlying condition.

When investigating a patient with hypokalaemia and hypertension, many possible causes of secondary aldosteronism can be eliminated either on clinical grounds or on the basis of simple tests. Plasma sodium concentration is usually high–normal or slightly elevated in primary aldosteronism; in secondary aldosteronism, the concentration is usually <138 mmol/L. If necessary, measurement of plasma renin activity under appropriate

Cushing's syndrome

a. Normal

production of cortisol by adrenal cortex
stimulated by ACTH

cortisol exerts a negative feedback effect on
release of ACTH by pituitary

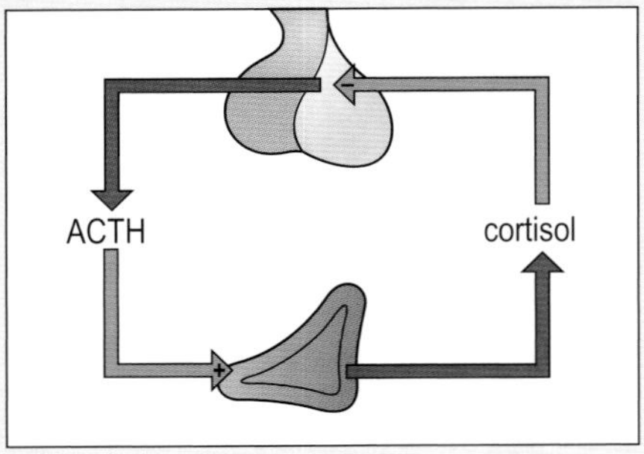

b. Cushing's disease

ACTH secretion increased

pituitary insensitive to feedback
by normal levels of cortisol

higher levels of cortisol required to produce
negative feedback effect on ACTH secretion

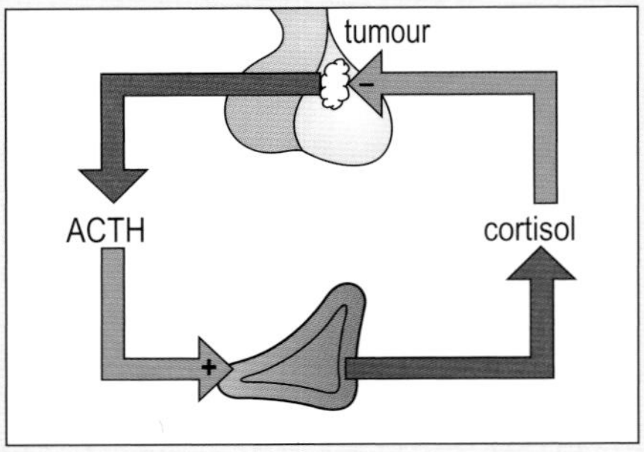

c. Adrenal tumours

autonomous cortisol production

high circulating cortisol inhibits ACTH secretion

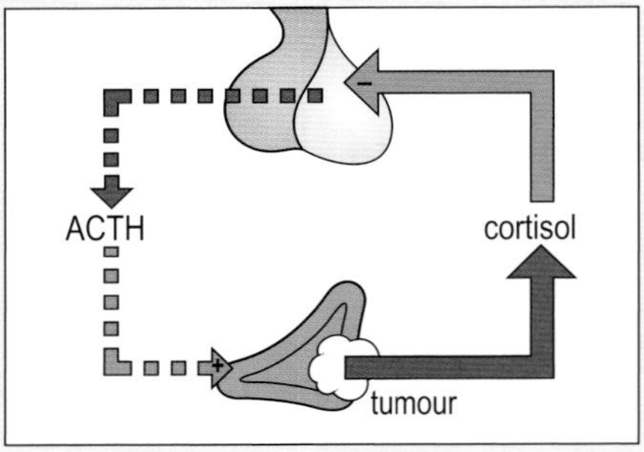

d. Ectopic ACTH secretion

high level of ACTH secreted by tumour
stimulates excessive cortisol production

inhibition of secretion of ACTH by pituitary

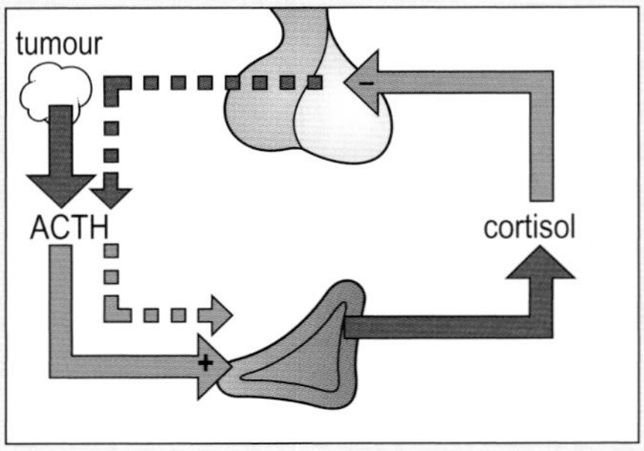

Fig. 8.9 Pituitary–adrenal relationships in Cushing's syndrome.

Typical results of adrenal function tests in Cushing's syndrome					
Condition	Basal cortisol (nmol/L)	Dexamethasone suppression test		CRH test	Plasma ACTH (ng/L)
		Low dose	High dose		
Cushing's disease	↑ (<1000)	no suppression	suppression	response	↑ (<200)
adrenal tumour	↑ (variable)	no suppression	no suppression	no response	↓
ectopic ACTH secretion	greatly ↑ (>1000)	no suppression	no suppression	no response	greatly ↑ (>200)

Fig. 8.10 Typical results of adrenal function tests in Cushing's syndrome. With ectopic ACTH secretion by carcinoid tumours, the results of these tests may be identical to those seen in Cushing's disease, as the tumour may have glucocorticoid receptors which will respond to dexamethasone.

Conn's syndrome
Causes
adrenal adenoma bilateral hypertrophy of zona glomerulosa cells glucocorticoid-remediable aldosteronism
Clinical features
hypertension muscle weakness (occasionally paralysis) latent tetany and paraesthesiae polydipsia and polyuria

Fig. 8.11 Causes and clinical features of Conn's syndrome. Most patients are hypertensive but asymptomatic.

Conditions associated with secondary aldosteronism
Common congestive cardiac failure cirrhosis of liver with ascites nephrotic syndrome
Less common renal artery stenosis sodium-losing nephritis Bartter's and Gitelman's syndromes* renin-secreting tumours

Fig. 8.12 Conditions associated with secondary aldosteronism. *Bartter's and Gitelman's syndromes are rare, inherited disorders of renal sodium reabsorption. Sodium loss stimulates aldosterone secretion and leads to hypokalaemia. In Gitelman's syndrome, there is also hypercalciuria and hypomagnesaemia.

conditions (*see below*) will distinguish between primary and secondary aldosteronism. It is low in the former condition, but elevated in the latter.

Primary aldosteronism should be suspected in any hypertensive patient who has a low plasma potassium concentration, but the commonest cause of this association is treatment with loop or thiazide diuretics. In these circumstances, plasma potassium concentration should be checked after withdrawal of the diuretic for a fortnight before proceeding to further investigations. Other causes of hypokalaemia should be excluded. The hypokalaemia of Conn's syndrome is a result of excessive renal potassium excretion. Hypokalaemia from other causes should lead to maximal renal potassium retention. Thus, in a hypokalaemic patient who is not on diuretics, renal potassium excretion of more than 30 mmol/24 h is very suggestive of primary aldosteronism. However, in early cases, or if patients have a low salt intake (as is often recommended in hypertension), plasma potassium concentration may be normal or only slightly low.

There should be three stages to the diagnosis of aldosteronism: screening, diagnosis and establishment of the cause. Screening involves measuring aldosterone and plasma renin activity in the same sample and does not require that hypotensive medication is stopped or

Screening for Conn's syndrome using the plasma aldosterone:renin activity ratio		
Ratio	**Interpretation**	**Action**
<800	diagnosis excluded	seek other causes
>1000, <2000	diagnosis possible	confirmatory tests
>2000	diagnosis very likely	establish cause

Fig. 8.13 Screening for Conn's syndrome using the plasma aldosterone:renin activity ratio. Aldosterone is measured in pmol/L, renin in pmol/mL/h.

that posture is standardized. The interpretation of results is indicated in *Fig. 8.13*. Unless the results are clearly normal or abnormal, confirmation or exclusion of the diagnosis is most simply made by performing a saline infusion test. This involves the infusion of 1.25 L of 0.9% saline over a period of two hours: if plasma aldosterone concentration remains >240 pmol/L, the diagnosis is confirmed. Sodium loading increases the amount of sodium reaching the distal renal tubules and should inhibit aldosterone secretion. Caution is required, particularly in the elderly, because of a small risk of provoking cardiac failure. A more elaborate procedure, regarded by some as the definitive investigation, involves a combination of sodium loading and the administration of fludrocortisone over a period of four days. There is a risk of provoking profound hypokalaemia and potassium replacement may be required. However, this test requires admission to hospital, whereas the saline infusion test can be done as an outpatient. Many antihypertensive drugs, e.g. β-blockers and angiotensin-converting enzyme inhibitors, can affect the secretion of aldosterone and it may be necessary to modify a patient's treatment before performing either of these investigations. α-Adrenergic antagonists can usually be given but the advice of the laboratory should be sought concerning this.

Plasma aldosterone concentration and renin activity are affected by posture. Standing increases renin secretion, and hence that of aldosterone, in normal subjects, because of the decrease in renal blood flow. The response of aldosterone to posture may help to distinguish between Conn's syndrome due to a tumour

 Case history 8.4

A 35-year-old woman was found to have a blood pressure of 190/110 mmHg by her GP at a routine health check. He prescribed a thiazide diuretic but a week later she returned to the surgery complaining of severe muscle weakness and constipation. The doctor arranged an urgent consultation at the local hospital where her serum potassium was found to be 2.6 mmol/L. The diuretic was stopped, her blood pressure was controlled with prazosin and she was given oral potassium supplements. After three weeks her serum potassium concentration was only 3.0 mmol/L. A 24-hour urine collection contained 70 mmol potassium. Conn's syndrome was thought so likely that she was admitted to hospital for further investigation.

Investigations

plasma aldosterone
    (0900 h, recumbent) 1320 pmol/L
                           (normal 100–450 pmol/L)
    (1300 h, ambulant)   510 pmol/L

plasma renin activity
    (0900 h)   <0.5 pmol/min/mL
                     (normal 1.1–2.7 pmol/mL/h)

Comment

A CT scan of the abdomen showed a small mass arising from the left adrenal gland. This was removed surgically. She made a rapid recovery after the operation and repeated checks showed her to be normokalaemic and normotensive.

Giving a diuretic may provoke symptomatic hypokalaemia in mild aldosteronism. The hypokalaemia in this condition is characteristically resistant to potassium supplementation. In primary aldosteronism, the plasma aldosterone:renin ratio is typically >1000, as in this patient.

The fall in aldosterone concentration after four hours is characteristic of Conn's syndrome due to an adrenal tumour.

or to adrenal hyperplasia. A blood sample is taken in the morning, the patient having stayed recumbent since waking. A further blood sample is taken after the patient has been ambulant for four hours. In the majority of patients with adenomas, plasma aldosterone concentration decreases by 50% in relation to the value in the sample drawn while the patient was recumbent; with bilateral hyperplasia there is often an increase. This differential response is due to adenomas being sensitive to ACTH (the concentration of which falls during the morning) while in adrenal hyperplasia, the adrenals are sensitive to angiotensin II (the concentration of which rises when the patient is ambulant). Plasma cortisol concentration must be measured at the same time. Only if it falls can it be certain that the predicted fall in ACTH has occurred. As in Cushing's syndrome, imaging techniques and selective blood sampling may be required to diagnose the cause of Conn's syndrome in equivocal cases. Glucocorticoid-remediable aldosteronism can be diagnosed using a genetic test.

If Conn's syndrome is shown to be due to a tumour, this should be removed surgically. In patients with bilateral adrenal hyperplasia, treatment with spironolactone, a diuretic that antagonizes the action of aldosterone, may be sufficient to control the blood pressure. Spironolactone is also used in patients with tumours while they await surgery. Glucocorticoid-suppressible hyperaldosteronism is treated with dexamethasone.

Congenital adrenal hyperplasia (CAH)

This term encompasses a group of inherited metabolic disorders of adrenal steroid hormone biosynthesis. Their clinical features depend upon the position of the defective enzyme in the synthetic pathway, which determines the pattern of hormones and precursors that is produced (*see Fig. 8.3*).

21-Hydroxylase deficiency, with an incidence of 1 in 12,000 of live births in the UK, accounts for around 95% of all cases of CAH. The majority of the remaining 5% are due to deficiency of 11β-hydroxylase. 21-Hydroxylase deficiency is often incomplete and adequate cortisol synthesis can be maintained by increased secretion of ACTH by the pituitary. It is this that causes hyperplasia of the glands. Because of the metabolic block, the substrate of the enzyme (17α-hydroxyprogesterone)

accumulates and there is increased formation of adrenal androgens (*see p. 145*).

Female infants affected by CAH may be born with ambiguous genitalia but when the enzyme deficiency is only partial the condition may not present until early adulthood with hirsutism, amenorrhoea or infertility (late onset CAH). Males may present with pseudo-precocious puberty in their second or third year of life but are not virilized at birth. In about one-third of neonates with 21-hydroxylase deficiency, the enzyme deficiency is complete; these present shortly after birth with a life-threatening salt-losing state, in which cortisol and aldosterone production are insufficient to maintain normal homoeostasis. The partial and complete forms of 21-hydroxylase deficiency appear to be two separate entities, the manifestations of the condition running true to type within affected families.

Diagnosis is made by demonstrating an elevated concentration of 17α-hydroxyprogesterone (17-OHP) in the plasma at least two days after birth (before this time, maternally derived 17-OHP may still be present in the infant's blood). Treatment involves replacement of cortisol, and mineralocorticoid if necessary, which should suppress the excessive ACTH production and hence the excessive androgen synthesis. Treatment is monitored by measurement of either plasma 17-OHP or androstenedione.

Partial 11β-hydroxylase deficiency is also more common than complete deficiency of the enzyme. Increased androgen production causes virilization, which tends to be more severe than in 21-hydroxylase deficiency (but again is not present in males at birth). Hypertension develops, owing to the accumulation of 11-deoxycorticosterone, a substrate of the defective enzyme that has salt-retaining properties. The diagnosis rests upon the demonstration of an increased plasma concentration of either 11-deoxycortisol or its urinary metabolite. Treatment is with cortisol alone: although aldosterone secretion is defective, 11-deoxycorticosterone provides adequate mineralocorticoid activity.

Other forms of CAH involving, for example, 17-hydroxylase, 18-hydroxylase (thus affecting aldosterone secretion only) and steroid 3β-hydroxydehydrogenase, Δ5 isomerase, are very rare. Some indication of their consequences, in terms of adrenal steroid metabolism, should be apparent from studying *Fig. 8.3*. They are also referred to in *Chapter 16 (see p. 300)*.

A case history of congenital adrenal hyperplasia is presented in *Chapter 10*.

Case history 8.5

A 75-year-old woman presented with anxiety, palpitation and sweating. Her pulse was 80/min, regular, and blood pressure 160/100 mmHg. She had previously been investigated for abdominal pain, for which no cause had been found. Tests of thyroid function were normal. A 24 h urine collection was made.

Results

urine hydroxy-methoxymandelic acid (HMMA)	99 µmol/24 h (ref range <35)
urine adrenaline	1.0 µmol/24 h (ref range <0.1)
urine noradrenaline	0.38 µmol/24 h (ref range <0.57)

A CT scan of the abdomen showed a mass arising from the left adrenal gland, and an isotopic scan of the adrenals, using meta-^{131}I-iodobenzyl-guanidine, showed a single left adrenal mass.

Comment

The clinical features suggested thyrotoxicosis but this was excluded by the results of thyroid function testing. The clinical features were also consistent with a phaeochromocytoma, but a high index of suspicion may be necessary to initiate the appropriate investigations. The screening test was positive, and the high adrenaline excretion suggested that the tumour would be of adrenal origin. The biochemical localization was confirmed by the imaging procedures, and at operation, carried out after three days' treatment with phenoxybenzamine and propranolol (respectively α- and β-adrenergic antagonists), a 5 cm left adrenal phaeochromocytoma was removed.

DISORDERS OF THE ADRENAL MEDULLA

The main interest in the adrenal medulla for clinical biochemistry relates to phaeochromocytomas. These are tumours that secrete catecholamines, the normal secretory product of the organ, and which are a rare (approximately 0.5% of all cases), but treatable, cause of hypertension. Approximately 10% of phaeochromocytomas are found in extramedullary tissue that shares the same embryological origin, that is chromaffin tissue derived from neuroectoderm. Catecholamines can also be produced by tumours of embryologically related tissue, for example the carotid bodies, and by neuroblastomas, rare tumours occurring only in infants and young children and usually presenting as a rapidly enlarging abdominal mass.

Patients with phaeochromocytomas typically present with symptoms such as headache, palpitation, sweating, pallor, tremor and abdominal discomfort. These often occur sporadically. Hypertension is common: although this may be episodic, it is usually sustained. Although phaeochromocytomas are rare, hypertension is a common condition, and therefore it is important to have available a screening test that identifies those patients likely to have a phaeochromocytoma and who should be subjected to more definitive investigation, and eliminates those in whom this probability is very low.

The metabolism of catecholamines is outlined in *Fig. 8.14*. Adrenaline (epinephrine) and noradrenaline (norepinephrine) are metabolized by catechol-O-methyltransferase (COMT) to metadrenaline and normetadrenaline, respectively. They are also converted by the consecutive action of monoamine oxidase and COMT to 4-hydroxy-3-methoxymandelic acid (HMMA), also known as vanillylmandelic acid (VMA).

Approaches to screening and diagnosis vary between laboratories, and the laboratory staff should be contacted to ensure that appropriate samples are collected. Screening tests include the measurement of urinary HMMA or metanephrines (i.e. metadrenaline and normetadrenaline). Diagnosis is based on measurements of urinary or plasma catecholamines. All these tests have good specificity but measurement of catecholamines, although technically difficult, has the highest sensitivity. Measurement of metanephrines is more sensitive than measurement of HMMA. Constituents of a number of common foods, including bananas, vanilla, tea and coffee, may react in some methods used for measuring HMMA.

Following diagnosis, the site of the tumour is identified by an imaging technique, guided by the fact that extra-adrenal phaeochromocytomas tend to secrete nor-adrenaline in excess of adrenaline, the reverse being true of tumours of the adrenal medulla itself (*see Case History 8.5*).

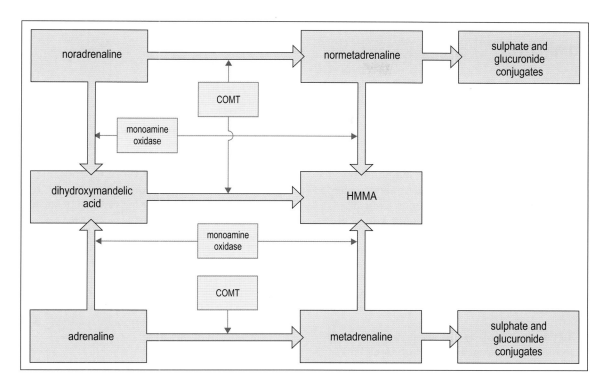

Fig. 8.14 Metabolism of catecholamines. COMT = catechol-O-methyltransferase; HMMA = 4-hydroxy-3-methoxymandelic acid.

Additional investigations are rarely necessary for diagnosis, but when the results of catecholamine measurements are equivocal, the pentolinium test may be helpful. Pentolinium is a sympathetic ganglion-blocking drug that reduces catecholamine secretion in normal subjects but not in patients with phaeochromocytomas; in such patients, secretion is autonomous. Blood is taken for catecholamine measurement before and 15 minutes after giving 2.5 mg pentolinium by intravenous injection.

Although phaeochromocytomas are benign in 90% of cases, all tumours should be removed surgically. However, this is a potentially hazardous operation since large quantities of catecholamines may be released into the circulation during the procedure. It should be noted that 10% of patients with phaeochromocytomas have multiple tumours. The tumours may be a component of multiple endocrine neoplasia (MEN) types 2A and B (*see p. 326*) and thus evidence of other relevant endocrine disorders should be sought in affected patients.

SUMMARY

- The **adrenal cortex** secretes three classes of steroid hormones: glucocorticoids, androgens and mineralocorticoids.

- The secretion of **cortisol** is controlled by adrenocorticotrophic hormone (ACTH); ACTH secretion is subject to feedback inhibition by cortisol. Control is also exerted from the higher centres through the hypothalamus. Cortisol secretion shows a diurnal variation, with peak plasma concentrations in the morning and a trough in the late evening. Cortisol is essential to life: it is involved in the response to stress and with other hormones regulates many pathways of intermediary metabolism. Its metabolic action is largely catabolic.

- ACTH also stimulates the production and secretion of **androgens**; these hormones have a role in determining secondary sexual characteristics in the female but do not appear to have a specific role in the male.

- **Aldosterone** is the most important mineralocorticoid; it stimulates sodium reabsorption in the distal tubules of the kidneys. It is an important determinant of the extracellular fluid volume. Its secretion is controlled by the renin–angiotensin system, in response to changes in blood pressure and blood volume.

- **Adrenal failure** is most frequently due to organ-specific autoimmune destruction of the glands, although there are many other causes. It can present acutely as a medical emergency with hypoglycaemia and circulatory collapse due to renal salt wasting. In more chronic cases, lassitude, weight loss and postural hypotension are frequent clinical features. Diagnosis depends upon demonstrating a failure of the adrenal to produce cortisol in response to ACTH (Synacthen test). Pituitary disease can cause secondary adrenal failure by reducing ACTH secretion.

- Over-production of adrenal cortical hormones can affect predominantly cortisol (producing **Cushing's syndrome**), or aldosterone (**Conn's syndrome**). Cushing's syndrome can also be secondary to excess ACTH production by a pituitary tumour or by a non-endocrine tumour (ectopic ACTH production), or be iatrogenic, due to treatment with corticosteroids or ACTH. Clinical features of Cushing's syndrome include characteristic somatic changes, muscle weakness, glucose intolerance, hypokalaemia and hypertension. Patients with Conn's syndrome develop hypertension and hypokalaemia. The diagnosis of both these conditions involves initial screening tests, the demonstration of high, non-suppressible concentrations of the hormones and then elucidation of the cause.

- The various forms of **congenital adrenal hyperplasia** are inherited metabolic disorders of adrenal steroid hormone biosynthesis. The clinical features derive from a mixture of under-production of either cortisol or aldosterone or both, and increased production of androgens. The most common type is steroid 21-hydroxylase deficiency.

- The **adrenal medulla** produces catecholamines but is not essential to life. There appear to be no clinical sequelae from decreased adrenal medullary activity, but tumours of the glands (neuroblastomas and phaeochromocytomas) can produce excessive quantities of catecholamines. These cause hypertension and other clinical features related to increased sympathetic activity.

9 The thyroid gland

INTRODUCTION

The thyroid gland secretes three hormones: thyroxine (T4) and triiodothyronine (T3), both of which are iodinated derivatives of tyrosine (*Fig. 9.1*), and calcitonin, a polypeptide hormone. T4 and T3 are produced by the follicular cells but calcitonin is secreted by the C cells, which are of separate embryological origin. Calcitonin is functionally unrelated to the other thyroid hormones. It has a minor role in calcium homoeostasis and disorders of its secretion are rare (*see Chapter 12*). Thyroid disorders in which there is either over- or under-secretion of T4 and T3 are, however, common.

Thyroxine synthesis and release are stimulated by the pituitary trophic hormone, thyroid-stimulating hormone (TSH). The secretion of TSH is controlled by negative feedback by the thyroid hormones (predominantly T4) (*see p. 123*), which modulate the response of the pituitary to the hypothalamic hormone, thyrotrophin-releasing hormone (TRH; *Fig. 9.2*). Glucocorticoids, dopamine and somatostatin inhibit TSH secretion. The physiological significance of this is not known but it may be relevant to the disturbances of thyroid hormones that can occur in non-thyroidal illness (*see p. 168*).

The major product of the thyroid gland is T4. Ten times less T3 is produced (the proportion may be greater

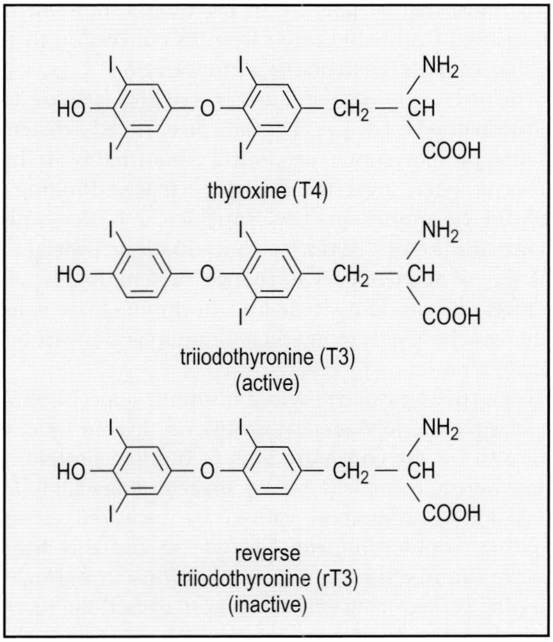

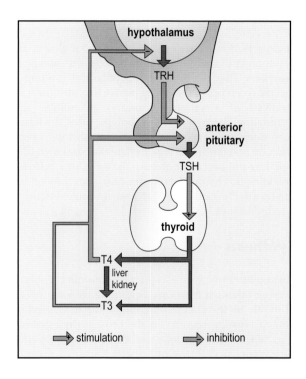

Fig. 9.2 Control of thyroid hormone secretion. TSH is released from the pituitary in response to the hypothalamic hormone, TRH, and stimulates the synthesis and release of thyroid hormones. TSH release is inhibited by thyroid hormones, which decrease the sensitivity of the pituitary to TRH. They may also inhibit TRH release by the hypothalamus.

Fig. 9.1 Chemical structure of the thyroid hormones, T4 and T3, and the inactive metabolite of T4, rT3.

in thyroid disease), most T3 (approximately 80%) being derived from T4 by deiodination in peripheral tissues, particularly the liver, kidneys and muscle. T3 is 3–4 times more potent than T4. Deiodination can also produce reverse triiodothyronine (rT3: *see Fig. 9.1*), which is physiologically inactive. It is produced instead of T3 in starvation and many non-thyroidal illnesses, and the formation of either the active or inactive metabolite of T4 appears to play an important part in the control of energy metabolism. The anterior pituitary is also active in converting T4 to T3. It is thought that the pituitary senses thyroid hormone status through a change in the concentration of T3 due to deiodination within anterior pituitary cells.

THYROID HORMONES

Functions

Thyroid hormones are essential for normal growth and development and have many effects on metabolic processes. They act by entering cells and binding to specific receptors in the nuclei, where they stimulate the synthesis of a variety of species of mRNA, thus stimulating the synthesis of polypeptides, including hormones and enzymes. Their most obvious overall effect on metabolism is to stimulate the basal metabolic rate, but the precise molecular basis of this action is not known. Thyroid hormones also increase the sensitivity of the cardiovascular and nervous systems to catecholamines.

Synthesis

Thyroid hormone synthesis involves a number of specific enzyme-catalyzed reactions, beginning with the uptake of iodide by the gland and culminating in the iodination of tyrosine residues in the protein thyroglobulin (*Fig. 9.3*); these reactions are all stimulated by TSH. Rare, congenital forms of hypothyroidism caused by inherited deficiencies of each of the various enzymes concerned have been described.

Thyroglobulin is stored within the thyroid gland in colloid follicles. These are accumulations of thyroglobulin-containing colloid surrounded by thyroid follicular cells. Release of thyroid hormones (stimulated by TSH) involves pinocytosis of colloid by follicular

cells, fusion with lysosomes to form phagocytic vacuoles, and proteolysis (*Fig. 9.4*). Thyroid hormones are thence released into the blood stream. Proteolysis also results in the liberation of mono- and diiodotyrosines (MIT and DIT); these are usually degraded within thyroid follicular cells and their iodine is retained and re-utilized. A small amount of thyroglobulin also reaches the bloodstream.

Thyroid hormones in blood

The normal plasma concentrations of T4 and T3 are 60–150 nmol/L and 1.0–2.9 nmol/L, respectively. Both hormones are extensively protein-bound: some 99.98% of T4 and 99.66% of T3 are bound, principally to a specific thyroxine-binding globulin (TBG) and, to a lesser extent, to prealbumin and albumin. TBG is approximately one-third saturated at normal concentrations of thyroid hormones (*Fig. 9.5*). It is generally accepted that only the free, non protein-bound, thyroid hormones are physiologically active. Although the total T4 concentration is normally 50 times that of T3, the different extents to which these hormones are bound to protein mean that the free T4 concentration is only 2–3 times that of free T3. In the tissues, most of the effects of T4 probably result from its conversion to T3, so that T4 itself is essentially a prohormone.

The precise physiological function of TBG is unknown; individuals who have a genetically determined deficiency of the protein show no clinical abnormality. It has, however, been suggested that the extensive binding of thyroid hormones to TBG provides a buffer which maintains the free hormone concentrations constant in the face of any tendency to change. Protein binding also reduces the amount of thyroid hormones that would otherwise be lost by glomerular filtration and subsequent renal excretion.

Total (free + bound) thyroid hormone concentrations in plasma are dependent not only on thyroid function but also on the concentrations of binding proteins. If these were to increase (*Fig. 9.6*), the temporary fall in free hormone concentration caused by increased protein binding would stimulate TSH release and this would restore the free hormone concentrations to normal: if binding protein concentrations were to fall, the reverse would occur. In either situation, there would be a change in the concentrations of total hormones, but the free hormone concentrations would remain normal.

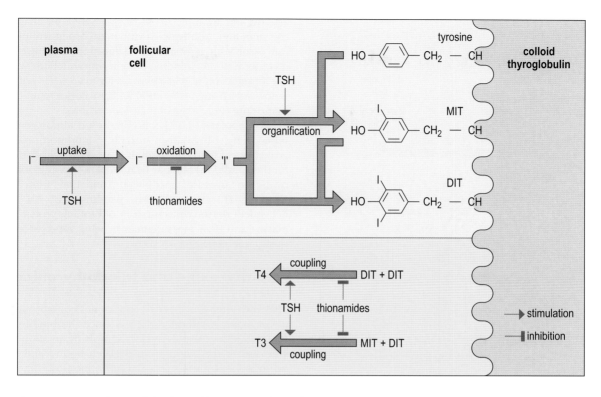

Fig. 9.3 Biosynthesis of the thyroid hormones. The iodination and condensation reactions involve tyrosine residues that are an integral part of the thyroglobulin polypeptide. The thyroid hormones remain protein-bound until they are released from the cell. The precise nature of the active iodine moiety ('I') is not known. Once formed, it is immediately incorporated into tyrosine residues to form monoiodotyrosine (MIT) and diiodotyrosine (DIT). Anti-thyroid thionamide drugs, such as carbimazole, act by inhibiting the formation of the active moiety or by preventing the coupling of DIT to form T4.

Thus measurement of total hormone concentrations can give misleading information.

This is a matter of considerable practical importance, since changes in the concentrations of the binding proteins occur in many circumstances (*Fig. 9.7*). Further, certain drugs, for example salicylates and phenytoin, displace thyroid hormones from their binding proteins, thus reducing total, but not free, hormone concentrations once a new steady state is attained. If an attempt is made to assess thyroid status in a patient who is not in a steady state, the results may be bizarre and misleading.

Only small amounts of T4 and T3 are excreted by the kidneys owing to the extensive protein binding. The major route of thyroid hormone degradation is by deiodination and metabolism in tissues, but they are also conjugated in the liver and excreted in bile.

TESTS OF THYROID FUNCTION

Laboratory tests of thyroid function are required to assist in the diagnosis and monitoring of thyroid disease. Most laboratories offer a standard 'profile' of thyroid function tests (usually TSH and free T4), and perform additional tests only if these results are equivocal or the clinical circumstances require it.

Total thyroxine and triiodothyronine

Measurement of plasma total T4 (tT4) concentration was formerly widely used as a test of thyroid function, but has the major disadvantage in that it is dependent on binding protein concentration as well as thyroid

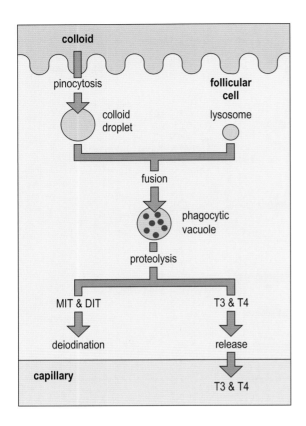

Fig. 9.4 Secretion of the thyroid hormones. Colloid is taken up into follicular cells by pinocytosis and undergoes lysosomal proteolysis, resulting in the release of thyroid hormones.

activity. For example, a slightly elevated plasma tT4 concentration, compatible with mild hyperthyroidism, can occur with normal thyroid function if there is an increase in plasma binding protein concentrations. With the introduction of reliable assays for free T4 (fT4), there is now little, if any, justification for laboratories continuing to measure tT4 as a test of thyroid function.

Plasma total T3 (tT3) concentration is almost always raised in hyperthyroidism (usually to a proportionately greater extent than tT4, hence it is the more sensitive test for this condition) but may be normal in hypothyroidism owing to increased peripheral formation from T4. However, tT3 concentrations, like those of tT4, are dependent on the concentration of binding proteins in plasma and their measurement is being superseded by measurements of free T3 (fT3).

Free thyroxine and triiodothyronine

The measurement of free hormone concentrations poses major technical problems since the binding of free hormones in an assay, for example by an antibody, will disturb the equilibrium between bound and free hormone and cause release of hormone from binding proteins. Various techniques have been developed that allow the estimation of free T4 and T3 concentrations in plasma. Such measurements, in theory, circumvent the problems associated with protein binding and have rendered obsolete techniques for the indirect assessment of free hormone concentrations, such as the resin uptake test, calculation of the free thyroxine index or measurement of the T4/TBG ratio. However, with gross abnormalities of binding protein concentrations, the results of measurements of free hormones may be misleading owing to technical limitations of the assays.

In pregnancy, TBG concentration increases, owing to increased synthesis stimulated by oestrogens, and leads to

	Plasma concentration		Extent of protein binding (%)	Half-life (days)
	total (nmol/L)	free (pmol/L)		
T4	60–150	9.0–26.0	99.98	6–7
T3	1.0–2.9	3.0–9.0	99.66	1–1.5

Fig. 9.5 Thyroid hormones in blood. Each laboratory should determine its own normal range for plasma concentrations.

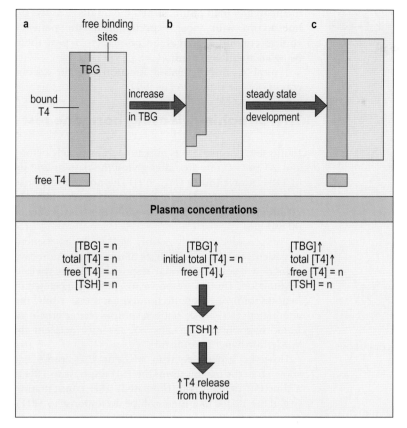

Fig. 9.6 Effect of an increase in TBG concentration on plasma T4 concentration. (a) In the initial steady state, TBG is one-third saturated with T4. (b) TBG concentration increases, causing more T4 to be bound, thus reducing the free T4 concentration. This stimulates TSH secretion which leads to an increase in the release of T4 from the thyroid. (c) T4 becomes redistributed between the bound and the free states, leading to a new steady state with the same free T4 concentration but an increased total T4.

an increase in tT4. Free T4 concentration may rise slightly in early pregnancy, possibly owing to the weak thyroid-stimulating properties of chorionic gonadotrophin, but returns to normal values by 20 weeks. In most women, fT4 remains within the non-pregnant reference range.

Just as tT3 concentration can be normal in hypo-thyroidism (especially in mild cases), so, too, can fT3 concentration, and its measurement is of no value in the diagnosis of this condition. Free T3 is, however, a sensitive test for hyperthyroidism. In hyperthyroid patients, both fT4 and fT3 are usually elevated (fT3 to a proportionately greater extent) but there are exceptions to this. In a small number of patients with hyperthyroidism, fT3 concentration is elevated but fT4 is not (though it is usually high–normal) – a condition called 'T3-toxicosis'. Occasionally fT4 is elevated but not fT3. This is usually due to concomitant non-thyroidal illness resulting in decreased conversion of T4 to T3, and fT3 concentration increases when this illness resolves.

Thyroid-stimulating hormone

Since the release of TSH from the pituitary is controlled through negative feedback by thyroid hormones, measurements of TSH can be used as an index of thyroid function.

If primary thyroid disease is suspected and the plasma TSH concentration is normal, it can be safely inferred that the patient is euthyroid. In overt primary hypothyroidism, TSH concentrations are greatly increased, often to ten or more times the upper limit of normal. Smaller increases are seen in borderline cases but TSH measurement is more sensitive than T4 under these circumstances. TSH can also increase transiently during recovery from non-thyroidal illness (*see below*). Plasma TSH concentrations are suppressed to very low values in hyperthyroidism, but low concentrations can also occur in individuals with sub-clinical disease and in euthyroid patients with non-thyroidal illness ('sick

Causes of abnormal plasma TBG concentrations
Increase
genetic
pregnancy
oestrogens, including oestrogen-containing oral contraceptives
Decrease
genetic
protein-losing states, e.g. nephrotic syndrome
malnutrition
malabsorption
acromegaly
Cushing's disease
corticosteroids (high dose)
severe illness
androgens

Fig. 9.7 Causes of abnormal plasma concentrations of TBG.

euthyroidism', *see below*). Indeed, in hospital patients, a low plasma TSH concentration is more often due to non-thyroidal illness than to hyperthyroidism, while a slightly elevated concentration is as frequently due to recovery from such illness as to mild or incipient hypothyroidism.

Clinical biochemistry laboratories undertake large numbers of tests of thyroid function. To simplify their procedures, many adopt the approach of measuring TSH as a first-line test of thyroid function, adding other tests as required, for example if the concentration of TSH is found to be outside the euthyroid reference range or if there is a strong suspicion that thyroid dysfunction is secondary to pituitary disease (though this is far less common than primary thyroid dysfunction). A combination of tests may also be required to assess patients being treated for thyroid disease, particularly in the early stages.

It should be noted that immunometric assays (such as is used for TSH) are subject to interference by naturally occurring heterophilic antibodies against the monoclonal antibodies used in the assay; such interference occurs only infrequently, but can give rise

to apparently high results. When the results of assays do not accord with those expected from the patient's clinical condition, it may be prudent to repeat them using an alternative method.

Typical results of thyroid function tests in various conditions are shown in *Fig. 9.8*.

Thyrotrophin-releasing hormone test

In this test, plasma TSH is measured immediately before, and 20 and 60 minutes after giving the patient 200 µg of TRH intravenously (*Fig. 9.9*). The normal response is an increase in TSH concentration of 2–20 mU/L in 20 minutes, with reversion towards the basal value at 60 minutes.

This test was formerly mainly used in the assessment of patients in whom other tests of thyroid function gave equivocal results. A normal response excludes thyroid dysfunction. The TSH response to TRH is exaggerated in hypothyroidism, even in borderline cases, while the attenuated (so-called 'flat') response characteristic of frank hyperthyroidism also occurs in incipient or borderline hyperthyroidism.

However, experience with modern TSH assays has shown that the magnitude of the TSH response to TRH is a function of basal (unstimulated) TSH concentration (e.g. if the TSH is low, there will be no response to TRH). Measuring the TSH response to TRH provides no additional information over that provided by a basal TSH measurement. The TRH test is now only used in the investigation of patients with pituitary or hypothalamic disease, to assess the capacity of the pituitary to secrete TSH. TSH secretion is rarely completely lost in pituitary disease, and thus the TSH response to TRH is more usually decreased than absent and may even be normal. In hypothalamic disease, the response is characteristically (though not invariably) delayed, plasma TSH concentration at 60 minutes exceeding that at 20 minutes.

Other tests of thyroid function

Other biochemical disturbances, not involving the thyroid hormones, occur in thyroid disease but are of no value diagnostically; examples are hypercalcaemia and hyperphosphataemia in some patients with thyrotoxicosis, and hypercholesterolaemia, hyponatraemia and elevated plasma creatine kinase activity in hypothyroidism.

		Plasma fT4		
		High	**Normal**	**Low**
Plasma TSH	**High**	TSH-secreting tumour (rare) (fT3 = ↑)	Borderline/ compensated hypothyroidism	Hypothyroidism (primary) Recovery from sick euthyroid state
	Normal	Euthyroid with T4 autoantibodies (uncommon)	Euthyroid	Sick euthyroid (fT3 = ↓) Hypopituitarism (other pituitary hormones = ↓)
	Low	Hyperthyroidism (fT3 = ↑)	T3 thyrotoxicosis (fT3 = ↑) Early in treatment of hyperthyroidism Sub-clinical hyper-thyroidism (fT3 = N/↑)	Hypopituitarism (other pituitary hormones = ↓) Sick euthyroid (severe) (fT3 = ↓)

Fig. 9.8 The results of thyroid function tests in various conditions.

Techniques involving the use of radioactive isotopes for the investigation of thyroid disease are of two types. Tests involving the quantification of radioactive iodine uptake were introduced before specific tests for thyroid hormones were available but they are now little used. Thyroid scintiscanning, however, is in common use. In this technique, a dose of an isotope, usually ^{99m}Tc-pertechnetate, is given, and its distribution within the thyroid is determined using a gamma camera. This technique allows the identification of 'hot' (active) or 'cold' (inactive and potentially malignant) nodules in patients with lumps in the thyroid. It can also distinguish between Graves' disease (uniformly increased uptake), multinodular goitre (patchy uptake) or an adenoma (single 'hot' spot) in patients with thyrotoxicosis, and detect aberrant or ectopic thyroid tissue.

Various autoantibodies to thyroid-related antigens may be detectable in the plasma of patients with thyroid disease. Graves' disease is caused by antibodies that bind to and stimulate the TSH receptor. Assays for these antibodies are not generally available, but their measurement may be valuable in the diagnosis of Graves' disease as a cause of thyrotoxicosis in the absence of the characteristic eye signs, and in the prediction of relapse of Graves' disease after a course of anti-thyroid drugs. Anti-peroxidase (formerly called anti-microsomal) and anti-thyroglobulin antibodies are present in the blood of almost all patients with autoimmune thyroiditis (particularly Hashimoto's disease and primary atrophic hypothyroidism) but are probably not pathogenic. They are also frequently present in Graves' disease. Autoantibodies to thyroid hormones may bind to T4 and T3 and can occasionally give rise to abnormal results in measurements of these hormones. The results are usually so bizarre that in practice they are rarely a cause of diagnostic confusion.

The measurement of thyroid autoantibodies may be helpful in patients in whom biochemical tests of thyroid function are equivocal, since their presence in high titre is consistent with thyroid disease. It is not, however, diagnostic. Most elderly individuals with thyroid autoantibodies are clinically and biochemically euthyroid.

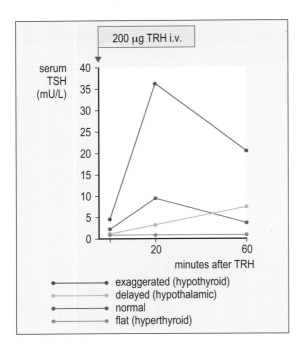

Fig. 9.9 TRH test: 200 µg is given intravenously and serum TSH is measured at 0, 20 and 60 minutes. Typical responses are shown.

Problems in the interpretation of thyroid function tests

As alluded to above, no biochemical test of thyroid function can be guaranteed to be reliable in patients with non-thyroidal illness. Abnormal results may occur in patients with infections, malignancy, myocardial infarction, following surgery, etc. who do not have thyroid disease. In general, thyroid function tests should not be performed on such patients unless there is a strong suspicion that they have thyroid disease.

Typically, during the acute phase of an illness, fT3 concentration and, less often, fT4 concentration is decreased. TSH is usually normal but may be undetectable in the severely ill. During recovery, TSH may rise transiently into the hypothyroid range as thyroid hormone concentrations return to normal. In chronic illness, for example chronic renal failure, free hormone concentrations are decreased (to an extent that may reflect the severity of the underlying disease); TSH is usually normal, but is occasionally decreased.

The occurrence of abnormalities of thyroid function tests in patients with non-thyroidal illness has been termed the 'sick euthyroid syndrome'. Causes include decreased peripheral conversion of T4 to T3; changes in the concentration of binding proteins (to an extent that may reveal technical limitations in the ability of free hormone assays to provide a true measurement of free hormone concentrations); increased plasma concentrations of free fatty acids, which displace thyroid hormones from their binding sites, and non-thyroidal influences on the hypothalamic–pituitary–thyroid axis, for example by cortisol, which can inhibit TSH secretion.

Furthermore, many drugs can influence the results of tests of thyroid function. Some examples are given in *Fig. 9.10*.

Case history 9.1

Knowing that thyroid disease is common in the elderly, a house physician requested thyroid function tests on an elderly woman admitted to hospital with severe cellulitis of the leg secondary to an infected ingrowing toenail.

Investigations

serum: TSH   0.1 mU/L
        fT4   8.0 pmol/L
        fT3   2.0 pmol/L

Comment

TSH, fT4 and fT3 are all low, results that at first glance might suggest thyroid failure secondary to hypopituitarism. However, a TSH this low would be unusual except in severe hypopituitarism: TSH secretion tends to be affected late in progressive pituitary disease. A random serum cortisol concentration was 950 nmol/L, indicating normal response of the hypothalamic–pituitary–adrenal axis to stress, and it was concluded that the thyroid function results were due to the 'sick euthyroid syndrome'. The infection was treated successfully and thyroid function tests were repeated prior to discharge: serum TSH concentration was 6 mU/L, fT4 was 12 pmol/L and fT3, 4.7 pmol/L.

Drugs and the thyroid	
Drug	**Effect**
corticosteroids dopaminergic drugs	inhibit TSH secretion
lithium, iodine, carbimazole, thiouracils	inhibit T3 and T4 secretion
oestrogens, phenothiazines	increase TBG
corticosteroids, androgens	decrease TBG
salicylates, phenytoin	compete with T4 for binding by TBG
β-blockers, amiodarone*	inhibit conversion of T4 to T3

Fig. 9.10 Drugs and the thyroid. *Amiodarone is an iodine-containing anti-arrhythmic drug. It can also both increase and decrease thyroid hormone synthesis and may occasionally cause clinical thyroid disease.

DISORDERS OF THE THYROID

The metabolic manifestations of thyroid disease relate to either excessive or inadequate production of thyroid hormones (hyperthyroidism and hypothyroidism, respectively). The clinical syndrome that results from hyperthyroidism is thyrotoxicosis. The term 'myxoedema' is often used to describe the entire clinical syndrome of hypothyroidism but strictly refers specifically to the dryness of the skin, coarsening of the features and subcutaneous swelling characteristic of severe hypothyroidism. Patients with thyroid disease may present with a thyroid swelling or goitre. Investigation may reveal hypo- or (more frequently) hyperthyroidism but there may be no functional abnormality. A goitre can be the presenting feature of thyroid cancer.

Hyperthyroidism

The major causes and clinical features of hyperthyroidism are shown in *Fig. 9.11*. Primary hyperthyroidism is far more common than secondary hyperthyroidism (TSH- or hCG-dependent). The commonest single cause is

Hyperthyroidism
Causes
*Graves' disease *toxic multinodular goitre *solitary toxic adenoma thyroiditis exogenous iodine and iodine-containing drugs, e.g. amiodarone excessive T4 or T3 ingestion ectopic thyroid tissue, e.g. struma ovarii functioning metastatic thyroid cancer hCG dependent: choriocarcinoma TSH dependent: pituitary tumour
* these account for >90% of cases
Clinical features
weight loss (but normal appetite) sweating, heat intolerance fatigue palpitation: sinus tachycardia or atrial fibrillation angina, heart failure (high output) agitation, tremor generalized muscle weakness, proximal myopathy diarrhoea oligomenorrhoea, infertility goitre eyelid retraction, lid lag

Fig. 9.11 Causes and clinical features of hyperthyroidism. Periorbital oedema, proptosis, diplopia, ophthalmoplegia, corneal ulceration, loss of visual acuity, pretibial myxoedema and thyroid acropachy are features of Graves' disease only.

Graves' disease, an autoimmune disease characterized by the presence of thyroid-stimulating antibodies in the blood. These autoantibodies bind to TSH receptors in the thyroid and stimulate them in the same way as TSH, through activation of adenylate cyclase and the formation of cyclic AMP.

The laboratory diagnosis of hyperthyroidism depends on the demonstration of a high plasma concentration of fT3 (and usually fT4) with a low TSH. These tests are

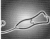

Case history 9.2

A 24-year-old physiotherapist consulted her GP because excessive moistness of her skin was causing embarrassment at work. She was also concerned that her eyes seemed to have become more prominent and that she had lost weight, although her appetite was unchanged. On examination, her doctor observed that her pulse was 92 per minute at rest and that she had a slightly enlarged thyroid gland.

Investigations

serum:
TSH	<0.1 mU/L
fT4	34 pmol/L
fT3	12 pmol/L

An isotopic scan of the thyroid showed an enlarged gland, with uniformly increased uptake. Autoantibodies to thyroid peroxidase and thyroglobulin were present in the serum in high titre.

Comment

The high fT3 and fT4 concentrations with low TSH are diagnostic of thyrotoxicosis, and the presence of autoantibodies and scan appearances are characteristic of Graves' disease. Although the clinical features are typical of thyrotoxicosis (see Fig. 9.11) they are often less so in milder cases and in the elderly. They may suggest an anxiety state (see Case History 9.3). Some clinical features are specific to Graves' disease and can have a course independent of the hyperthyroidism. Patients may present with the ocular manifestations of Graves' disease (ophthalmic Graves' disease) yet be clinically euthyroid. However, the TSH is usually suppressed even though fT3 may not be elevated, and such patients eventually become biochemically and clinically thyrotoxic. The combination of a low TSH with a normal (usually high–normal) fT3 ('sub-clinical' or 'borderline' hyperthyroidism) can occur early in the course of Graves' disease and other conditions causing thyrotoxicosis.

also used to monitor the response to treatment and for long-term follow-up. The concentrations of fT3 and fT4 fall as patients become euthyroid but some time may elapse before normal pituitary responsiveness to thyroid hormones is regained and there is an increase in TSH into the normal range. Thus while a normal TSH concentration indicates that a patient is euthyroid, a low value is not on its own indicative of persisting hyperthyroidism.

There are three options for the treatment of thyrotoxicosis: anti-thyroid drugs, radioactive iodine and surgery (sub-total thyroidectomy). Treatment with β-adrenergic blocking drugs may provide temporary symptomatic relief but has no effect on the underlying disease process. Very rarely, patients with thyrotoxicosis present with, or develop, thyroid storm or crisis, a medical emergency whose features include hyperpyrexia, dehydration and cardiac failure. The diagnosis of thyroid storm is made on clinical grounds and although thyroid function tests should be performed to confirm the diagnosis, treatment must not be delayed pending the results of the tests.

Unless they have a very large goitre, it is usual to treat younger patients with Graves' disease with anti-thyroid drugs. These suppress thyroid hormone synthesis, though not the release of preformed hormone, and thus there is usually a delay before any response is seen. Although one of the most frequently used drugs, carbimazole, is immunosuppressive, it probably does not have a significant effect on the underlying pathogenic process in Graves' disease.

Anti-thyroid drugs are given in high doses initially, but once the patient has become euthyroid, a decrease in dosage is often possible (titration regimen). An alternative approach is to continue with a high dose of the chosen drug and give thyroxine at a replacement dose, e.g. 150 μg/day (block and replacement regimen).

Untreated Graves' disease has a natural history of remission and relapse. Some patients (30–40%) have only a single episode of hyperthyroidism. It is usual to give anti-thyroid drugs for a period of 18 months to two years. Thyroid status is monitored during this time and thereafter. If the patient relapses, a further course of drug treatment or another mode of treatment is indicated.

Long-term follow-up of patients treated for Graves' disease is essential. Patients treated with anti-thyroid drugs may relapse, occasionally after many years; some, on the other hand, become hypothyroid. Recurrences of the disease also occur in patients treated surgically or with radioactive iodine. Up to 35% of patients treated surgically, and the majority of patients treated with radioactive iodine, will eventually become hypothyroid, sometimes as long as ten years or more after treatment. Hypothyroidism that develops within six months of either surgery or radioactive iodine treatment may be temporary, but abnormalities of thyroid function tests, in particular a slightly raised TSH, but normal plasma fT4 and fT3 concentrations, may persist though the patient remains clinically euthyroid. This is illustrated in *Fig. 9.12*.

The pathogenic thyroid-stimulating autoantibody in Graves' disease is an IgG immunoglobulin. In a pregnant woman with Graves' disease it can cross the placenta and may cause neonatal hyperthyroidism, even if the mother is euthyroid. Neonatal hyperthyroidism is a transient phenomenon since the maternal immunoglobulins are gradually cleared from the neonatal circulation, but treatment may be required in the short term.

Transient biochemical (but usually asymptomatic) hyperthyroidism occurs in up to 5% of women after pregnancy. The changes are usually maximal at 1–3 months after delivery and are often succeeded by symptomatic hypothyroidism (which sometimes persists) at 4–6 months.

Hypothyroidism

There are many causes of primary hypothyroidism (*Fig. 9.13*) but hypothyroidism can also occur secondarily to decreased trophic stimulation both in hypopituitarism and in hypothalamic disease. It is, however, very rare for patients with pituitary failure to present with clinical features of hypothyroidism alone. The commonest cause of hypothyroidism is atrophic myxoedema, the end result of autoimmune destruction of the gland. The clinical manifestations (*Fig. 9.13*) are variable and may result in the patient being referred to almost any specialist department in a hospital.

Clinical diagnosis is confirmed by the finding of a high plasma TSH concentration (unless the condition is secondary to hypopituitarism) and low fT4 concentration. Measurement of T3 is of no value in the diagnosis of hypothyroidism (*see p. 164*).

Hypothyroidism is treated by replacement of thyroid hormones, usually T4. It is usual to start with a small dose (e.g. 50 µg/day) and increase this at 4–6 week intervals on the basis of the results of thyroid function tests. In the elderly and patients with ischaemic heart disease, a lower starting dose (e.g. 25 µg) should be

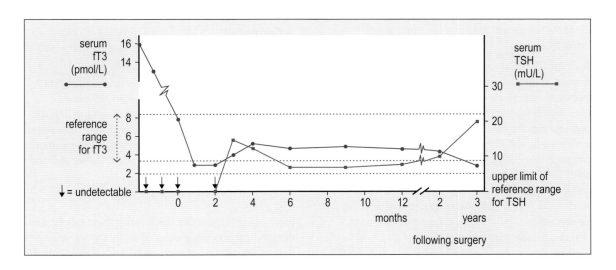

Fig. 9.12 Changes in serum fT3 and TSH concentrations following partial thyroidectomy for Graves' disease. The patient was rendered euthyroid prior to surgery with anti-thyroid drugs. Initially, TSH secretion remained suppressed but eventually rose in response to the low fT3. Normal thyroid hormone secretion by the remaining thyroid tissue was maintained by increased TSH stimulation, but eventually the patient became hypothyroid, as shown by the increased TSH. Hypothyroidism can also develop in patients treated with anti-thyroid drugs or radioiodine.

Case history 9.3

Shortly before her final examinations, a medical student experienced sleep disturbance, tachycardia with palpitation, and noticed that her hands were warm and sweaty. Her doctor was sure that her symptoms were due to anxiety, but was persuaded to take a blood sample for thyroid function tests.

Investigations

serum: TSH 1.3 mU/L
T4 165 nmol/L
T3 2.9 nmol/L
free T4 24 pmol/L

These results were considered to be equivocal and a TRH test was performed

serum TSH: 0 min 1.2 mU/L
20 min 5.4 mU/L
60 min 3.1 mU/L

Comment

This patient exemplifies the problems posed by the effect of changes in binding protein concentration on measurements of total thyroid hormone concentration.

The total T4 is elevated and T3 is at the upper limit of normal; free T4 is near the upper limit of normal; these results are consistent with mild or early thyrotoxicosis. However, the normal TSH suggests that the patient is euthyroid and this is confirmed by the normal TSH response to TRH (although this conclusion was predictable from the initial TSH). It transpired that the patient was taking an oestrogen-containing oral contraceptive pill and the resulting increase in plasma TBG concentration would explain the abnormal total hormone concentrations.

As discussed on *p. 166*, the TRH test rarely adds anything to the information provided by a single TSH measurement, except in suspected pituitary disease.

 Case history 9.4

A senior civil servant was persuaded to seek medical advice because of his increasingly bizarre behaviour. He had slowed up mentally, become indecisive and had given up his daily game of squash, claiming that he no longer had the energy to play. Whereas in the past he had annoyed his colleagues by opening windows even on cold days, he now no longer objected to them remaining closed. His appearance had changed, his skin appearing sallow and his hair coarse and lacking lustre.

His GP suspected hypothyroidism and elicited a history of recent constipation in addition to the other typical features. Bradycardia was present and when the peripheral reflexes were tested, slow quadriceps relaxation was noted. There was no goitre.

Investigations

serum: TSH >100 mU/L
fT4 3.9 pmol/L

Comment

The clinical diagnosis of hypothyroidism is confirmed by the very high serum TSH concentration, reflecting the lack of negative feedback from circulating thyroid hormones. Under such circumstances, measurement of fT4 is unnecessary for diagnosis, although, as discussed on *p. 163*, many laboratories routinely measure TSH and fT4 on all samples submitted for thyroid function tests.

used. There is a risk that the increase in metabolic rate and demand for oxygen prompted by hormone replacement may precipitate angina or myocardial infarction. Triiodothyronine has a more rapid onset of action and is preferable in the initial treatment of patients in myxoedema coma (*see below*).

In the laboratory, thyroid hormone replacement can be monitored by measuring plasma TSH and, if this is abnormal, fT4 concentrations (fT3 if the patient is being treated with T3). Ideally, the replacement dosage should be sufficient to maintain TSH within the reference

Hypothyroidism	
Causes	**Clinical features**
*atrophic hypothyroidism (this condition may represent the end-stage of Hashimoto's disease)	lethargy, tiredness
	cold intolerance
*autoimmune hypothyroidism (Hashimoto's thyroiditis)	dryness and coarsening of skin and hair
	hoarseness
*post-surgery, radioactive iodine, anti-thyroid drugs (e.g. carbimazole) and other agents (e.g. lithium)	weight gain
	slow relaxation of muscles and tendon reflexes
congenital	many others, including:
	anaemia, typically macrocytic, non-megaloblastic but pernicious in 10% of cases
dyshormonogenic	dementia, psychosis
	constipation
secondary (pituitary or hypothalamic disease)	bradycardia, angina, pericardial effusion
	muscle stiffness
iodine deficiency	carpal tunnel syndrome
	infertility, menorrhagia, galactorrhoea
*these account for >90% of cases	

Fig. 9.13 Causes and clinical features of hypothyroidism. Children with hypothyroidism may present with growth failure, delayed pubertal development or a deterioration in academic performance.

range. Too high a concentration indicates inadequate replacement; a suppressed TSH suggests excessive replacement and a risk of causing atrial fibrillation and, possibly, osteoporosis. In patients treated with T4, the plasma concentrations associated with a clinically euthyroid state are generally somewhat higher than the normal euthyroid range, because there is no contribution to endogenous hormone activity by secreted T3. If the dosage is changed, the results of thyroid function tests may not reach a new steady state for some time. The expected fall in TSH concentration lags behind the increase in that of fT4 when treatment is started, and, if the TSH has been suppressed because of over-replacement, months may elapse before normal thyrotrophic responsiveness to T4 is regained.

Compliance with and the adequacy of treatment should be checked annually by measurements of TSH and, if this is abnormal, fT4. Usually non-compliant patients who take their tablets regularly for a few days before a blood test will be revealed by their having a raised TSH but a normal or even elevated fT4.

Occasionally, patients with hypothyroidism present as an emergency with stupor and hypothermia. This 'myxoedema coma' has a high mortality. In addition to thyroid hormone replacement, usually with T3, possible coexistent adrenal insufficiency must be treated with hydrocortisone and appropriate measures taken to treat any infection, heart failure or electrolyte imbalance and to restore body temperature to normal.

Thyroiditis

Inflammation of the thyroid, or thyroiditis, may be due to infection (usually viral) or autoimmune disease. In viral thyroiditis, associated with coxsackie, mumps and adenovirus, the inflammation results in a release of preformed colloid and there is an increase in the concentration of thyroid hormones in the blood. Patients may become transiently, and usually only mildly, thyrotoxic. This phase persists for up to six weeks and is followed by a similar period in which thyroid hormone

Case history 9.5

A 55-year-old businesswoman underwent the medical screening programme provided by her company. Various tests were performed, including assessment of thyroid function.

Investigations

serum: TSH   8 mU/L
       fT4   12 pmol/L

Comment

Serum TSH concentration is slightly elevated, and fT4, though within the reference range, is near the lower end, compatible with early or borderline hypothyroidism. Thyroid failure can be an insidious condition and sufficient function of the failing thyroid may be maintained by increased secretion of TSH in the early stages. Measurement of fT4 concentration, though useful for subsequent comparison, may not be of practical help in management.

Patients with borderline hypothyroidism should be treated if they are symptomatic, but because not all patients will progress to frank hypothyroidism, the usual practice if they are asymptomatic is to review them at 4–6 monthly intervals and, if they remain aymptomatic, only treat them if plasma TSH concentration rises to more than 10 mU/L. Patients with borderline hypothyroidism should be tested for anti-thyroid autoantibodies. If present in high concentration, many physicians begin replacement treatment even in the absence of symptoms on the grounds that they indicate that progression to hypothyroidism is likely to occur. In the patient described in this case, thyroxine replacement was not given initially, but six months later, her serum TSH concentration had increased to 29 mU/L and fT4 was 9 pmol/L. After thyroxine replacement had been started, this patient commented that she now realized that she had been feeling 'run down' for some time beforehand. Because the clinical features of hypothyroidism can be so non-specific, patients may only appreciate, retrospectively, that they were present after replacement therapy has been started.

output may be decreased, although not sufficiently to cause symptoms. Thereafter, normal function is regained.

Hashimoto's thyroiditis, an autoimmune condition, has been mentioned as a cause of hypothyroidism. Autoantibodies are present in high titre, and the disease is associated with the presence of other organ-specific autoimmune diseases. Very occasionally, transient hyperthyroidism may occur early in the course of the disease due, as in viral thyroiditis, to increased release of preformed colloid.

Goitre and thyroid cancer

Goitre, or enlargement of the thyroid, can occur in patients with hyperthyroidism (e.g. in Graves' disease, toxic multinodular goitre or a thyroid adenoma), hypothyroidism (e.g. in Hashimoto's disease or iodine deficiency) and in euthyroid individuals with benign or malignant tumours of the gland. Physiological enlargement of the thyroid may occur during adolescence, unaccompanied by any change in function, but, otherwise, thyroid function tests should be performed even in apparently euthyroid patients presenting with a goitre since the results may provide a clue to the cause.

The biochemistry laboratory has no part to play in the diagnosis of thyroid cancer, with the exception of calcitonin-secreting medullary carcinoma. When patients with thyroid cancer are treated by ablative doses of radioactive iodine and put on replacement thyroxine, the efficacy of the treatment can be assessed by measuring plasma thyroglobulin concentrations. Since small amounts of thyroglobulin are normally released from the gland together with thyroid hormones, persistent thyroid activity can be inferred if thyroglobulin is present in the plasma.

SCREENING FOR THYROID DISEASE

Congenital hypothyroidism (usually due to thyroid agenesis or dysgenesis) is sufficiently serious and common (1 in 4000 live births in the UK but considerably higher in some other countries) for it to be worthwhile to screen for the condition. Untreated, affected children become cretins, with very low intelligence and impaired growth and motor function. Treatment by replacement of T4 is simple and effective but this must be started as soon after birth as a reliable diagnosis can be made. The screening method involves measurement of TSH in a capillary blood sample collected on to a Guthrie card (*see p. 302*) at 6–8 days of age. Screening for phenylketonuria is performed at the same time. Maternal thyroxine crosses the placenta and can affect the infant's pituitary–thyroid axis for a short period after birth.

Hypo- and hyperthyroidism are both common in the elderly (more so the former), with a combined prevalence of approximately 5%. Since both the conditions may present insidiously, and atypically, in the elderly, attempts have been made to screen for the conditions in this population. In practice, however, the influence of non-thyroidal illness on the results of thyroid function tests renders this a far from straightforward proposition. Furthermore, while there is evidence that the presence of a slightly raised plasma TSH together with the presence of thyroid autoantibodies indicates an increased risk of future clinical hypothyroidism, people with either one of these abnormalities alone may not be at significant risk.

SUMMARY

- The thyroid gland secretes two iodine-containing hormones, **thyroxine (T4)** and **triiodothyronine (T3)**. More T4 is secreted than T3. Some T4 is metabolized to T3 in peripheral tissues; T3 is the more active hormone. The synthesis and secretion of thyroid hormones is stimulated by the pituitary hormone thyroid-stimulating hormone (TSH). The release of TSH is in turn controlled by thyrotrophin-releasing hormone from the hypothalamus. T4 and T3 exert negative feedback inhibition on TSH release.

- Thyroid hormones are essential for **normal growth and development**, and also control **basal metabolic rate** and stimulate many metabolic processes.

- T4 and T3 are extensively **protein-bound in the blood** (T4 to an even greater extent than T3), to thyroxine-binding globulin, albumin and prealbumin, the free, physiologically active fractions being less than 1% of the total. Factors that affect the concentration of the binding proteins can alter total hormone concentrations without affecting the free fraction, and thus erroneously suggest the presence of an abnormality of thyroid function.

- Thyroid status is best assessed biochemically by **measurement of plasma TSH and fT4 concentrations**, with fT3 being measured in addition if hyperthyroidism is suspected. Typically, **in primary hypothyroidism, thyroid hormone concentrations (fT4 more so than fT3) are low and TSH is high; in hyperthyroidism, TSH is very low and fT3 and, usually, fT4 is high**. Drug treatment and non-thyroidal disease frequently cause the results of thyroid function tests to be abnormal in patients who do not have thyroid disease.

- Patients with thyroid disease may present as a result of overactivity of the gland (**hyperthyroidism**, causing thyrotoxicosis) or underactivity (**hypothyroidism**, causing myxoedema). Both conditions have **widespread systemic effects**. Patients in either category may have enlargement of the gland (goitre) but patients with goitres can be euthyroid. Both hyper- and hypothyroidism are commonly the result of autoimmune disease, although there are many other causes. The measurement of specific autoantibodies can provide useful diagnostic information in thyroid disease. Options for the treatment of hyperthyroidism include anti-thyroid drugs, radioactive iodine and surgery; patients with hypothyroidism require hormone replacement.

- The thyroid also secretes **calcitonin**, a polypeptide hormone with a minor role in calcium homoeostasis.

10 The gonads

INTRODUCTION

Androgens and testicular function

The testes are responsible for the synthesis of the male sex hormones (androgens) and the production of spermatozoa. The most important androgen, both in terms of potency and the amount secreted, is testosterone. Other testicular androgens include androstenedione and dehydroepiandrosterone (DHEA). These weaker androgens are also secreted by the adrenal glands but adrenal androgen secretion does not appear to be physiologically important in the male. In the female, however, it contributes to the development of certain secondary sexual characteristics, in particular the growth of pubic and axillary hair. The pathological consequences of increased adrenal androgen secretion are discussed in *Chapter 8* and on *p. 183*.

Testosterone is a powerful anabolic hormone. It is essential both to the development of secondary sexual characteristics in the male and for spermatogenesis. It is secreted by the Leydig cells of the testis under the influence of luteinizing hormone (LH). Spermatogenesis is also dependent on the function of the Sertoli cells of the testicular seminiferous tubules. These cells are follicle-stimulating hormone (FSH) dependent; they secrete inhibin, which inhibits FSH secretion, and androgen-binding protein, whose function is probably to ensure an adequate local testosterone concentration.

Testosterone concentrations in the plasma are very low before puberty but then rise rapidly to reach normal adult values. A slight decline in concentration may be seen in the elderly.

In the circulation, approximately 97% of testosterone is protein-bound, principally to sex hormone-binding globulin (SHBG) and to a lesser extent to albumin. The free fraction is readily available to tissues; albumin binds testosterone more loosely than SHBG and albumin-bound testosterone may be in part available. Free testosterone is considered a better indicator of effective androgen availability than total, but its measurement is technically difficult: in practice, the calculated ratio of testosterone:SHBG concentration is used as an index of free testosterone status. The biological activity of testosterone is mainly due to dihydrotestosterone (DHT). This is formed from testosterone in target tissues in a reaction catalyzed by the enzyme 5α-reductase. In a rare condition in which there is deficiency of this enzyme, DHT cannot be formed; male internal genitalia develop normally (Wolffian duct development in the fetus is testosterone dependent) but masculinization, which requires DHT, is incomplete. In states of androgen insensitivity, defects of the receptors for either testosterone or DHT, or both, can cause a spectrum of clinical abnormalities ranging from gynaecomastia to pseudohermaphroditism.

Testosterone is also present in females, at a much lower concentration, about one-third being derived from the ovaries and the remainder from the metabolism of adrenal androgens.

Specific assays are available for testosterone, DHT and other androgens, and SHBG. Measurement of urinary 17-oxosteroids – metabolites of androstenedione and testosterone – is now obsolete.

Oestrogens and ovarian function

The cyclical control of ovarian function during the reproductive years is discussed in *Chapter 7*. The principal ovarian hormone is 17β-oestradiol, but some oestrone is also produced by the ovaries. Oestrogens are also secreted by the corpus luteum and the placenta.

Oestrogens are responsible for the development of many female secondary sexual characteristics. They also stimulate the growth of ovarian follicles and the proliferation of uterine endometrium during the first part of the menstrual cycle. They have important effects on cervical mucus and vaginal epithelium, and on other functions associated with reproduction.

Plasma concentrations of oestrogens are low before puberty. During puberty, oestrogen synthesis increases and cyclical changes in concentration occur thereafter until the menopause, unless pregnancy occurs. After the menopause, the sole source of oestrogens is from the metabolism of adrenal androgens; plasma concentrations fall to very low values. In the plasma, oestrogens are transported bound to protein, 60% to albumin and the remainder to SHBG. Only 2–3% remains unbound. Oestrogens stimulate the synthesis of SHBG and also that of other transport proteins, notably thyroxine-binding globulin (TBG) and transcortin, and thus increase total thyroxine and total cortisol concentrations in the plasma.

Slowly rising or sustained high concentrations of oestrogens, together with progesterone, inhibit pituitary gonadotrophin secretion by negative feedback, but the rapid rise in oestrogen concentration that occurs prior to ovulation stimulates LH secretion (positive feedback).

Oestradiol is present in low concentrations in the plasma of normal men. Approximately one-third is secreted by the testis, the remainder being derived from the metabolism of testosterone in the liver and in adipose tissue.

Progesterone

Progesterone is an important intermediate in steroid hormone biosynthesis but is secreted in appreciable quantities only by the corpus luteum and the placenta. Its concentration in plasma rises during the second half of the menstrual cycle but then falls if conception does not take place. In the plasma, it is extensively bound to albumin and transcortin; only 1–2% is free. Progesterone has many important effects on the uterus, including preparation of the endometrium for implantation of the conceptus, and also on the cervix, vagina and breasts. It is pyrogenic and mediates the increase in basal body temperature that occurs with ovulation. Progesterone can be measured in plasma and this assay is used in the investigation of infertility in women (*see p. 187*).

Sex hormone-binding globulin

SHBG binds both testosterone and oestradiol in the plasma, though it has greater affinity for testosterone. The plasma concentration of SHBG in males is about half that in females. Factors that alter SHBG concentration (*Fig. 10.1*) alter the ratio of free testosterone to free oestradiol. If SHBG concentration decreases, the ratio of free testosterone to free oestradiol increases, though there is an absolute increase in the concentrations of both hormones. If SHBG concentration increases, the ratio decreases. Thus in either sex, the effect of an increase in SHBG is to increase oestrogen-dependent effects while a decrease in SHBG increases androgen-dependent effects (*Fig. 10.2*).

Factors affecting sex hormone-binding globulin concentration
Increase
oestrogens hyperthyroidism liver cirrhosis
Decrease
androgens hypothyroidism glucocorticoids malnutrition and malabsorption protein-losing states obesity, particularly in women

Fig. 10.1 Factors which cause an increase or a decrease in the plasma concentration of sex hormone-binding globulin (SHBG).

DISORDERS OF MALE GONADAL FUNCTION

Delayed puberty and hypogonadism in males

It is uncommon for a boy to enter puberty before the age of nine years. Precocious puberty is discussed in *Chapter 21*. Boys who have not entered puberty by the age of 14 years are considered to have delayed puberty. They often present earlier than this, more often with short stature (a result of the delayed pubertal growth spurt) rather than with concern about gonadal development. Delayed puberty can be constitutional (i.e. idiopathic, often associated with a family history), related to chronic illness (e.g. coeliac disease, cystic fibrosis) or a consequence of hypogonadism. Delayed puberty should be investigated to diagnose any pathological disorder: constitutional delayed puberty is essentially a diagnosis of exclusion.

The term hypogonadism implies defective spermatogenesis or testosterone production or both. It can be primary (that is, due to testicular disease) or occur secondarily to pituitary or hypothalamic disease. Primary hypogonadism is sometimes referred to as hypergonadotrophic hypogonadism (decreased feedback

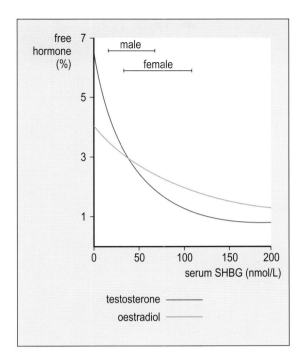

Fig. 10.2 Effect of a change in serum SHBG concentration on free oestradiol and testosterone concentrations. A decrease in SHBG increases free testosterone concentration more than free oestradiol and thus is androgenic; an increase in the concentration of SHBG is anti-androgenic. The normal ranges of SHBG in males and females are shown.

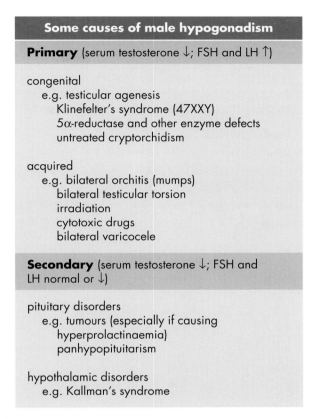

Fig. 10.3 Some causes of male hypogonadism.

causes increased gonadotrophin secretion) and secondary as hypogonadotrophic (the hypogonadism is a consequence of decreased gonadotrophin secretion because of either pituitary or hypothalamic disease). Some of the causes are indicated in *Fig. 10.3*. Primary hypogonadism can be due to only defective seminiferous tubule function or defective Leydig cell function or both. The former leads to infertility through decreased production of spermatozoa, but masculinization is usually normal. Defective Leydig cell function, on the other hand, results in a failure of testosterone-dependent functions including spermatogenesis. The effects of decreased testosterone secretion depend upon age at the time of onset of the disorder. Secondary sexual characteristics are in part preserved if secretion is lost after puberty.

The basic biochemical characteristics that distinguish between primary and secondary hypogonadism are not always clear-cut. This is partly because most currently available assays for gonadotrophins are insufficiently sensitive to distinguish between low and normal concentrations. The secretion of gonadotrophins and testosterone is pulsatile. Ideally, when basal concentrations or the effects of chronic stimulation are to be measured, analyses should be performed on several blood specimens drawn over the period of an hour.

The use of provocative tests of the hypothalamo–pituitary–gonadal axis in hypogonadism is discussed in *Case History 10.1*.

Although biochemical tests are important in establishing that a patient has primary, rather than secondary, gonadal failure, they are less useful in distinguishing between the various causes of primary hypogonadism. In general, seminiferous tubule defects are associated with a raised plasma FSH concentration; Leydig cell defects are associated with a raised plasma LH concentration. Human chorionic gonadotrophin (hCG), which has an action similar to LH, can be used to test Leydig cell

Case history 10.1

A 20-year-old man presented with impotence. On examination, he was eunuchoid; there was only sparse pubic and axillary hair, the genitalia were infantile, muscular development was poor and his span exceeded his height with a sole–pubic symphysis distance greater than symphysis to crown.

Investigations

serum: testosterone   3 nmol/L
      LH   <1.5 U/L
      FSH   <1.5 U/L

clomiphene test (3 mg/kg body weight clomiphene citrate daily for seven days):

serum: LH   <1.5 U/L
     FSH   <1.5 U/L

gonadotrophin-releasing hormone (GnRH) test (100 µg GnRH i.v.):

time (min)	FSH (U/L)	LH (U/L)
0	<1.5	<1.5
20	2.0	2.0
60	2.5	3.0

(after 100 µg GnRH subcutaneously daily for two weeks)

0	3.5	4.5
20	8.4	21.5
60	4.5	8.0

Comment

Boys with constitutional delayed puberty occasionally do not enter puberty until 16–18 years of age, but this patient is clearly hypogonadal. The low testosterone and gonadotrophins in this case suggest a lesion at the level of either the pituitary or hypothalamus. This is confirmed by the failure of response to clomiphene. This drug competes with gonadal steroids for hypothalamic receptors and in normal men results in an increase in gonadotrophin secretion and thus testosterone secretion. Patients with pituitary lesions may have clinical or biochemical evidence of other pituitary abnormalities (none was present in this case).

The GnRH test is sometimes used in an attempt to distinguish between pituitary and hypothalamic causes of hypogonadism but in practice is of limited value. In pituitary disease, it might be expected that the LH and FSH responses to GnRH would be diminished or absent, but they can be normal. In hypothalamic disease, the response can be delayed (greater at 60 min than 20 min, cf. TRH test, p. 166), normal, or decreased; in this case, it is both subnormal and delayed. The pituitary can become insensitive to exogenous GnRH in hypothalamic disease and repeated injections of the hormone may correct this. When the GnRH test was repeated after GnRH priming, this patient's response was normal, indicating a hypothalamic, rather than a pituitary, defect. He was later found to be anosmic (lacking a sense of smell). The association between anosmia and hypogonadotrophic hypogonadism is called Kallman's syndrome. The eunuchoid habitus is a direct consequence of testosterone deficiency; testosterone promotes epiphyseal fusion and when its secretion is inadequate, there is continued growth of long bones, which become disproportionate to the axial skeleton.

Had the FSH and LH concentrations been elevated in this patient, and with nothing in the history to suggest acquired testicular failure, the next investigation would have been karyotyping, to investigate for possible Klinefelter's syndrome.

Human chorionic gonadotrophin (hCG) test	
Procedure	**Results**
day 0: 0900 h; take blood for testosterone give 5000 U hCG i.m.	normal response: plasma testosterone level increases to above upper limit of reference range
day 4: 0900 h; take blood for testosterone	primary testicular failure: little or no response
	secondary testicular failure: response may be normal

Fig. 10.4 Human chorionic gonadotrophin test for primary testicular failure.

function (*Fig. 10.4*). Semen analysis will provide an indication of seminiferous tubule function and testicular biopsy is valuable in patients with low sperm counts if the cause is not obvious clinically. Careful clinical examination is essential in all cases of gonadal failure.

The treatment of hypogonadism in males should be directed towards the underlying cause wherever possible. Testosterone is given in testosterone deficiency syndromes, but if fertility is required, treatment must be with gonadotrophin replacement or, in hypothalamic disorders, pulsatile GnRH administration. Even in constitutional delayed puberty, a course of testosterone can be beneficial, giving a 'kick-start' to puberty, which often continues naturally thereafter.

Gynaecomastia

Breast development in males is usually related to a disturbance of the balance of oestrogens to androgens. It may occur physiologically in neonates as a result of exposure to maternal oestrogens. During puberty, approximately 50% of normal boys develop gynaecomastia due to temporarily increased secretion of oestrogens relative to androgens. In both instances the gynaecomastia resolves spontaneously. Mild gynaecomastia may also occur in the elderly, as a result of a decrease in testosterone secretion.

Gynaecomastia occurring at other times should be regarded as pathological. The principal causes are shown in *Fig. 10.5*. Drugs are responsible in 10–20% of patients. The cause may be obvious from either the history or clinical examination. Investigations that may help to establish the cause include measurement of plasma testosterone, oestradiol, gonadotrophins, hCG,

Some causes of gynaecomastia
Physiological
neonatal
pubertal
old age
Pathological
increased oestrogens
e.g. chronic liver disease*, end-stage renal failure, Cushing's syndrome, hyperthyroidism*, tumours
decreased androgens
e.g. Klinefelter's syndrome
androgen insensitivity
e.g. testicular feminization
refeeding after starvation
(LH secretion increased)
Pharmacological
oestrogens
digoxin (binds to oestrogen receptors)
cytotoxics (testicular damage)
anti-androgens (e.g. cyproterone; spironolactone has some anti-androgenic activity)
many others (phenothiazines, methyldopa, etc. mechanism uncertain)

Fig. 10.5 Some causes of gynaecomastia. *Increased SHBG may contribute in these conditions through reducing free testosterone concentrations.

SHBG and prolactin, and tests of renal, liver, thyroid, adrenal and pituitary function. Karyotyping is required to diagnose Klinefelter's syndrome, in which an additional X chromosome is present (47XXY); chest and skull imaging may also be helpful.

DISORDERS OF FEMALE GONADAL FUNCTION

Delayed puberty and hypogonadism in females

Few girls enter puberty before about eight years of age. Precocious puberty is discussed in *Chapter 21*. The great majority of girls will have entered puberty by about 13 years of age. Girls with delayed puberty usually present because of absence of breast development or amenorrhoea (*see below*). Girls with no breast development by the age of 13 or with primary amenorrhoea after the age of 15 should be further investigated. As in boys, constitutional delayed puberty is essentially a diagnosis of exclusion. The pathological causes (*see Fig. 10.6*) can be divided into hypogonadism (hypergonadotrophic, i.e. primary ovarian failure, and hypogonadotrophic, i.e. secondary to pituitary or hypothalamic disease) and chronic disease (e.g. coeliac disease, chronic renal failure).

The principles of treatment of female hypogonadism are similar to those in males: low doses of oral oestrogens are used initially to promote feminization, then

---

Some causes of female hypogonadism

Primary (serum oestradiol ↓; FSH and LH ↑)
congenital
 e.g. Turner's syndrome (45XO) and variants
  Noonan's syndrome (46XX)
acquired
 e.g. chemotherapy/radiotherapy

Secondary (serum oestradiol ↓; FSH and LH normal or ↓)
see causes of secondary male hypogonadism, *Fig. 10.3*

Fig. 10.6 Some causes of female hypogonadism.

---

sequential oestrogen and progestogen to induce menstruation. Treatment with gonadotrophins or GnRH is required to stimulate ovulation.

Amenorrhoea and oligomenorrhoea

Amenorrhoea can be primary (menstruation has never occurred) or secondary. Oligomenorrhoea is sparse or infrequent menstruation; it can be due to less severe forms of some of the causes of amenorrhoea. Primary amenorrhoea can occur as part of the syndrome of female hypogonadism but can also be present in normally feminized women.

The commonest cause of amenorrhoea in women of child-bearing age is pregnancy, and this possibility, however unlikely, must always be excluded. The finding of an apparently high plasma LH concentration may suggest pregnancy before a pregnancy test is performed: chorionic gonadotrophin cross-reacts in many assays for LH.

Pregnancy apart, amenorrhoea in normally feminized women is most frequently due to a hormonal disturbance that results in a failure of ovulation. Causes include disordered hypothalamo–pituitary function, related to weight loss (30–35% of cases in most series) or hyperprolactinaemia (10–12%), but idiopathic in some 10% of cases; ovarian dysfunction (e.g. autoimmune disease leading to premature menopause) (10–12%) and increased androgen production (particularly polycystic ovary syndrome and late-onset congenital adrenal hyperplasia) (30–35%). Weight loss can lead to decrease in the frequency of the pulsatility of GnRH secretion and thus decreased secretion of LH and FSH. Menstruation almost always ceases if weight loss falls below 75% of the ideal, and this can happen with smaller losses. Regular menstruation returns if weight is regained.

Severe stress and intensive exercise regimens, such as are adopted by long-distance runners, ballet dancers and gymnasts, can also lead to amenorrhoea, probably for complex neuroendocrinological reasons in addition to any effect of decrease in body weight.

Amenorrhoea due to excessive androgen secretion is often associated with hirsutism or even virilism. These conditions are discussed in the next section.

Uterine dysfunction is an uncommon cause of amenorrhoea. It can be excluded, if necessary, by the progestogen challenge test. If medroxyprogesterone acetate is given orally (10 mg daily for five days), the occurrence of vaginal bleeding 5–7 days later signifies that the uterus was adequately oestrogenized. If bleeding does not occur, the test is repeated, giving oestrogen (ethinyloestradiol, 50 mg daily for 21 days, with progestogen on the last five days). Absence of bleeding indicates uterine disease. If bleeding occurs, oestrogen deficiency is present.

The diagnosis of hormonal causes of amenorrhoea requires basal measurements of plasma FSH, LH and prolactin concentrations. A high FSH concentration is indicative of ovarian failure (and is more sensitive in this respect than LH). If LH, but not FSH, is elevated, and the patient is not pregnant, the most likely diagnosis is polycystic ovary syndrome, and pelvic ultrasonography should be performed. If LH and FSH concentrations are normal or low, a pituitary or hypothalamic disorder should be sought, by anatomical studies and dynamic testing of the hypothalamo–pituitary axis in a manner similar to that described for male hypogonadism. As in males, however, the results of such tests do not always distinguish between pituitary and hypothalamic disorders.

The management of amenorrhoea depends upon the cause, and whether fertility is required. In hyperprolactinaemia, the treatment is directed to the underlying cause wherever possible (e.g. withdrawal of drugs, treatment of hypothyroidism).

In ovarian, pituitary or hypothalamic disease, when fertility is not required, cyclical oestrogen and (if the patient has a uterus) progestogen replacement is given. In established ovarian failure, pregnancy is only possible using donated ova.

If fertility is required in pituitary failure, treatment is with human FSH and LH; hCG may be required to mimic the mid-cycle LH peak and stimulate ovulation. Careful monitoring of plasma oestradiol concentrations is necessary to detect hyperstimulation, which carries a risk of multiple pregnancy and the production of ovarian cysts.

Patients with hypothalamic disease may respond to clomiphene. This substance blocks oestradiol receptors in the hypothalamus and may stimulate GnRH (and thus LH and FSH) secretion. Non-responders are treated with pulsatile GnRH. Clomiphene is also useful in inducing ovulation in patients with polycystic ovary syndrome (PCOS). When it has not been possible to distinguish between hypothalamic and pituitary disease, a failure to respond to pulsatile GnRH suggests that amenorrhoea is due to pituitary dysfunction.

A simple protocol for the investigation of endocrine causes of amenorrhoea is given in *Fig. 10.7*.

The climacteric

During the climacteric, progressive ovarian failure causes a decline in ovarian oestrogen secretion and eventually menstruation ceases; the menopause is the last menstrual period. The only oestrogen produced after the menopause is the small amount derived from metabolism of adrenal androstenedione in adipose tissue. The plasma concentrations of pituitary gonadotrophins become greatly elevated, FSH tending to increase first; this change is a more reliable indication of ovarian failure than plasma oestrogen concentrations, which show considerable variability. Metabolic changes that occur after the menopause include increases in plasma low density lipoprotein concentration and plasma urate concentration. Oestrogen deficiency is a major factor contributing to the development of postmenopausal osteoporosis.

Many post-menopausal women are now given hormone replacement treatment (HRT). This can be effective in controlling the acute symptoms of the menopause and is of proven benefit in preventing postmenopausal osteoporosis, although long-term use carries an increased risk of certain malignancies. Oestrogen can be given alone in women who have had a hysterectomy, but cyclical progestogen must be given in addition to women who have not, to prevent endometrial hyperplasia and possible malignant transformation. Biochemical monitoring of HRT is not required routinely but, if symptoms of oestrogen deficiency persist in patients on HRT, it may be helpful to measure plasma oestradiol concentration.

Hirsutism and virilism

Hirsutism is an increase in body hair in an androgen-related distribution. In most instances, menstruation is normal, but hirsutism may be accompanied by menstrual irregularity and other features of virilism (e.g. clitoromegaly, male-pattern hair loss, etc.). There is considerable racial variation in the amount of body hair in women and what may be regarded as normal in some races may be thought excessive by others.

The cause is usually excessive exposure of tissues to androgens. This may be due either to increased androgen secretion or a low level of SHBG, which increases the free testosterone fraction. In some cases there appears to be an increased sensitivity to androgens. The causes of hirsutism and virilism are indicated in *Fig. 10.8*.

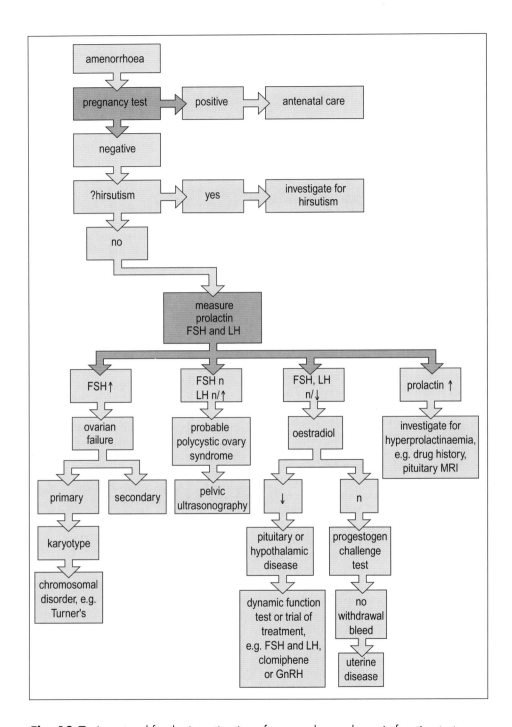

Fig. 10.7 A protocol for the investigation of amenorrhoea; dynamic function tests (GnRH, clomiphene) may distinguish between hypothalamic and pituitary causes although in practice this may only become clear when treatment aimed at restoring fertility is instituted.

Causes of hirsutism and virilization
Idiopathic
Ovarian polycystic ovary syndrome androgen-secreting tumours post-menopausal
Adrenal congenital adrenal hyperplasia Cushing's syndrome androgen-secreting tumours
Iatrogenic androgens progestogens

Fig.10.8 Causes of hirsutism and virilization. Idiopathic causes and the polycystic ovary syndrome account for the great majority of cases.

The commonest cause of hirsutism (probably more than 75% of cases) is polycystic ovary syndrome (PCOS), a condition of hyperandrogenization and chronic anovulation in the absence of specific underlying adrenal or pituitary disease. This is a functional definition although morphologically the ovaries do usually have multiple cysts. The condition shows considerable variation in its expression: many women previously classified as having 'idiopathic hirsutism' have a mild form of PCOS. It is familial, but the basis of its inheritance is uncertain. Its expression in men may be with premature balding.

The ovaries are the sources of the excess androgens in PCOS although the cause of the excessive secretion remains unclear. The diagnosis is based on clinical findings and ultrasonography. Plasma LH concentration is often elevated but, although this finding is relatively specific, it is insensitive, in that many patients who otherwise satisfy the diagnostic criteria for the condition have normal concentrations. Plasma testosterone concentration is moderately increased (*see below*). Plasma oestradiol concentrations are usually in the normal mid-follicular range.

Many patients with PCOS are overweight and the condition is associated with the 'metabolic syndrome' (*see p. 360*) of hyperinsulinaemia, insulin resistance and dyslipidaemia that is a recognized risk factor for the development of both type 2 diabetes mellitus and cardiovascular disease.

The management of PCOS depends on the severity of the condition and individual circumstances. Cosmetic treatment may be all that is required in mild cases in the absence of menstrual disturbance. The anti-androgen drug cyproterone can be used in more severe cases but not if fertility is required. Regularization of menstruation can often be achieved with a low-dose combined oral contraceptive. If fertility is required, treatment with clomiphene, an anti-oestrogen, will induce ovulation in more than 75% of cases; low-dose FSH may be helpful

 Case history 10.2

A young woman consulted her doctor because she was embarrassed by excessive hair on her upper lip, lower abdomen and thighs. She was moderately obese. Her periods had always been irregular.

Investigations

serum: testosterone 3.5 nmol/L
LH (early follicular) 14 U/L
FSH (early follicular) 3 U/L

ultrasound examination of the ovaries:
multiple cysts present, bilaterally

Comment

These findings are characteristic of the polycystic ovary syndrome; testosterone concentration is slightly elevated, and LH is high in relation to FSH. The clinical features of this condition include hirsutism, acne, menstrual disturbances and obesity, but there is considerable variation in their prevalence and severity. Neither are the typical hormonal changes always present. The pathogenesis of the condition is uncertain. The normal ovaries synthesize androgens (principally testosterone and androstenedione) but their secretion is increased in PCOS. Conversion of androgens to oestrogens in liver and adipose tissue inhibits secretion of FSH (preventing ovulation) and stimulates that of LH (further stimulating androgen secretion). Impaired glucose tolerance or frank type 2 diabetes is present in up to 30% of obese young women with PCOS.

in non-responders. Patients with an associated metabolic syndrome should be screened for diabetes, but all should be given dietary and lifestyle advice. There is some evidence that metformin, which reduces insulin resistance, may improve reproductive function as well as the metabolic profile in women with PCOS.

The appropriate investigation of hirsutism depends on the clinical context, although if menstruation is normal, no endocrine abnormality may be found. Measurement of LH, FSH, testosterone and, if available, SHBG, is desirable in all patients. Moderately elevated testosterone concentrations (2.5–5.0 nmol/L) occur in PCOS and late-onset congenital adrenal hyperplasia (CAH). Concentrations in excess of 5.0 nmol/L are strongly suggestive of an androgen-secreting tumour, which may be in an adrenal or an ovary.

The presence of other clinical features (e.g. of Cushing's syndrome) in a hirsute patient may suggest a specific diagnosis and thus appropriate further investigations. In patients with severe hirsutism or if menstrual disturbance or virilism is present, adrenal androgens and 17-hydroxyprogesterone (17-OHP) should be measured. A diagnosis of late-onset CAH is supported by the finding of an elevated concentration of 17-OHP, which increases to more than twice the upper limit of normal 60 minutes after an injection of synthetic ACTH (Synacthen, 250 µg i.m.). High concentrations of 17-OHP, dehydroepiandrosterone sulphate and androstene-dione are found in patients with adrenal tumours, but 17-OHP does not increase significantly in response to ACTH.

Infertility

Infertility is a common clinical problem, leading approximately one in six couples in the UK to seek professional advice. Investigation is usually considered appropriate when a couple has been unable to conceive after 18 months of trying, assuming regular, unprotected intercourse. It can be primary (conception has never occurred) or secondary, and due to problems affecting either the male or the female. Ovulatory failure, due most frequently to hyperprolactinaemia or hypothalamic–pituitary dysfunction, is responsible in approximately 20% of cases, and defective sperm production in about one-quarter. Endocrine causes of infertility are rare in males.

The investigation of infertility requires a thorough clinical and laboratory assessment of both partners.

 Case history 10.3

A couple in their late twenties were infertile in spite of regular intercourse over a two-year period. Each partner had a child by previous marriages. The woman's periods had recently become irregular. A semen sample contained a normal count of motile sperm. Physical examination revealed no abnormality. The woman was on steroid replacement treatment for adrenal failure, which had been diagnosed in her late teens.

Investigations (woman)

serum:	prolactin	300 mU/L
	LH	12 U/L
	FSH	25 U/L

Comment

This is secondary infertility. The elevated FSH concentration (due to decreased negative feedback by oestrogens) indicates incipient ovarian failure. FSH is a more sensitive test for this than LH, although, in established ovarian failure (after the menopause), the plasma concentrations of LH and FSH are usually both very high. The adrenal failure in the woman had been shown to be due to autoimmune disease, and there is a recognized association between autoimmune adrenal and ovarian failure (Schmidt's syndrome). Two months later she had not had a period, and a measurement of plasma LH concentration gave a value >100 U/L. It is possible for hCG to cross-react in assays for LH. A pregnancy test was positive. Ovarian failure develops gradually and occasional ovulation may still occur in the early stages.

Anatomical causes, for example damage to the Fallopian tubes, are relatively common. Semen must be examined to ensure that adequate numbers of normal sperm are present. If menstruation is regular, ovulation is probably occurring. Detection of the rise in basal body temperature that follows ovulation is a useful indicator of this. More reliably, the concentration of progesterone (secreted by the corpus luteum) in plasma increases following ovulation. Values greater than 30 nmol/L, seven days before the next period is due, are regarded as diagnostic of ovulation, although lower values do not exclude this. However, a concentration below 10 nmol/L is very suggestive of anovulatory cycles. If cycles are anovulatory but regular, treatment with clomiphene may restore fertility. If not, or if there is oligo- or amenorrhoea, measurements of prolactin and gonadotrophins may indicate a diagnosis (see amenorrhoea, p. 182). Defective sperm production should be investigated by measurements of testosterone and gonadotrophins and, if necessary, by testicular biopsy. The post-coital test, previously used to determine the presence of mobile sperm, is now considered unreliable.

Assisted pregnancy

Numerous treatments for infertility are available, ranging from stimulation of ovulation with clomiphene to *in vitro* fertilization and embryo transfer. Close cooperation between the laboratory staff and the clinical team is essential to maximize the chance of a successful procedure, and to reduce the risk of multiple pregnancy during treatment to induce ovulation for *in vivo* fertilization.

PREGNANCY

Many physiological and metabolic changes take place in the body during pregnancy. These include changes in the concentrations of hormones directly related to pregnancy and resulting secondary metabolic changes.

Specific hormonal changes

Human chorionic gonadotrophin

Fertilization of the ovum prevents the regression of the corpus luteum. Instead, the corpus luteum enlarges, stimulated by the glycoprotein hormone hCG, produced by the trophoblast (the developing placenta). This hormone (assays usually measure the β-subunit) can be detected in maternal blood 7–9 days after conception and may be detectable in urine 1–2 days later. Its detection in the urine provides a highly sensitive and specific test for the diagnosis of pregnancy. The secretion of βhCG begins to fall by 10–12 weeks, although it remains detectable in the urine throughout

pregnancy. hCG is also produced by some tumours; its use as a tumour marker is discussed in *Chapter 18*.

Quantitative measurement of plasma βhCG is valuable in the diagnosis of suspected ectopic pregnancy: if the concentration is greater than 1000 U/L but an intrauterine sac cannot be visualized on transvaginal ultrasound, ectopic pregnancy is likely. Also, plasma βhCG concentrations double every two days in normal pregnancy, but the rate in ectopic pregnancy is usually less.

Oestrogens

The stimulated corpus luteum secretes large amounts of oestrogens and progesterone, but after six weeks the placenta becomes the major source of these hormones. There is a massive increase in the production of oestriol during pregnancy, but production of oestrone and oestradiol increase also. Oestriol is synthesized in the placenta from androgens secreted by the fetal adrenals. Its measurement in maternal plasma or urine was formerly used to assess feto–placental function but now has been superseded by ultrasonography, which can be used to provide direct measurements of fetal growth and placental blood flow. The same applies to measurements of other placental products, e.g. human placental lactogen and placental alkaline phosphatase (a heat-stable isoenzyme), which have been used in the past as indicators of placental function.

Secondary metabolic changes

Many of the metabolic changes that occur in pregnancy are discussed elsewhere in this book. They are summarized in *Fig. 10.9*.

Maternal monitoring

Patients with medical conditions may require close monitoring during pregnancy. For example, strict control of diabetes mellitus is vital, for both maternal and fetal health, and entails frequent monitoring of glycated haemoglobin and blood glucose concentrations. Pregnancy can adversely affect maternal glucose homoeostasis: insulin requirements in patients with type 1 diabetes may increase during pregnancy; patients with type 2 diabetes are usually treated with insulin.

Urine should be tested for proteinuria and glycosuria at all clinic attendances: the renal threshold for glucose is decreased during pregnancy but, if more than a trace

Metabolic changes during pregnancy and use of oral contraceptives

Change	Cause	Pregnancy	Oral contraceptive use
↓ urea	↑ GFR; ↑ plasma volume	*	
↓ albumin	↑ plasma volume	*	
↓ total protein	↑ plasma volume	*	
↑ total thyroxine	↑ TBG	*	*
↑ cortisol	↑ transcortin	*	*
↑ copper	↑ caeruloplasmin	*	*
glycosuria	↓ renal threshold	*	
↓ glucose tolerance (but normal fasting concentrations)		*	
↑ triglyceride (VLDL) ↑ LDL cholesterol ↑ HDL cholesterol	↑ oestrogens (antagonism of actions of insulin)	* * see caption	* variable variable
↑ alkaline phosphatase	placental isoenzyme	*	

Fig. 10.9 Metabolic changes that occur during pregnancy and the use of oral contraceptives. The changes refer to plasma concentrations except where indicated. Low density lipoprotein (LDL) cholesterol concentrations increase during pregnancy; high density lipoprotein (HDL) concentrations increase slightly in early pregnancy but then stabilize or even decline to non-pregnant values. Oestrogens in oral contraceptives may decrease LDL cholesterol and increase HDL cholesterol; progestogens tend to have the opposite effect, the net result depending on the relative amounts of oestrogen and progestogen, and the androgenicity of the progestogen (less androgenic protestogens tending to have lesser effects on LDL and HDL). Effects are concentration dependent: many oral contraceptives contain only low doses of oestrogen, which may have little metabolic effect.

of glycosuria is detected, it is advisable to perform a formal test of glucose tolerance. All pregnant women should have a measurement of blood glucose concentration at 26 or 28 weeks, and, if feasible, at booking. Diabetes (and impaired glucose tolerance, *see p. 197*) diagnosed during pregnancy is termed 'gestational diabetes'. Patients with gestational diabetes are usually treated with insulin during pregnancy, but should have their glucose tolerance reassessed six weeks after delivery since glucose tolerance may revert to normal, although even when it does, the woman is at increased risk of developing diabetes in the future. This condition is discussed further in *Chapter 11*.

The presence of proteinuria may be an early sign of pregnancy-induced hypertension. This condition, previously known as pre-eclampsia, which is peculiar to pregnancy, is characterized by hypertension, proteinuria and oedema. If left untreated, it can lead to severe hypertension and renal failure. An increase in plasma urate concentration can be a sensitive indicator of deteriorating renal function in this condition. Rapid analysis of samples is necessary as pregnancy-induced hypertension can progress very quickly. Liver disease occuring during pregnancy is discussed on *p. 101*. The close cooperation of the laboratory is also requried for the monitoring of patients with thyroid disease during pregnancy: the dose of thyroxine may need to be increased in pregnant women on replacement treatment.

Fetal monitoring

The antenatal diagnosis of inherited metabolic disease in early pregnancy and the use of maternal serum α-fetoprotein measurements to screen for neural tube defects are considered in *Chapter 16*.

Fetal blood can be obtained antenatally by either of two techniques: cordocentesis (aspiration of fetal blood from the umbilical cord under ultrasound control) or fetoscopy (fetal blood sampling under direct vision). Of these, cordocentesis is usually the preferred method. Analysis of fetal blood for blood gases, hydrogen ion concentration and lactate can aid in the assessment of fetal wellbeing when non-invasive studies (e.g. ultrasonic determination of umbilical artery blood flow) suggest that the fetus is at risk. Fetal blood obtained earlier in pregnancy can also be used in the antenatal diagnosis of inherited disease (see *Chapter 16*).

Premature babies are at risk of developing respiratory distress due to lack of surfactant. This is a mixture of phospholipids, including lecithin and sphingomyelin, which lowers the surface tension of the alveoli and facilitates the expansion and aeration of the fetal lungs at birth. The concentration of lecithin in amniotic fluid reflects production by fetal lungs. It increases rapidly after 32–34 weeks of gestation, corresponding to increasing fetal lung maturity and decreasing risk of development of respiratory distress. Surfactant synthesis can be stimulated by giving corticosteroids to the mother, and this is now routine practice when elective premature delivery is planned for any reason. Natural and synthetic surfactants are available for use in the baby immediately after birth. As a result, measurement of the amniotic fluid lecithin:sphingomyelin (L:S) ratio, to provide an indication of fetal lung maturity, is now rarely performed.

During labour, once the cervix is sufficiently dilated, fetal blood hydrogen ion can be measured in capillary samples obtained from the scalp. A concentration of more than 60 nmol/L (pH <7.22) suggests potentially dangerous fetal hypoxaemia. A continuous, direct measurement of fetal P_{O_2} can be obtained using a transcutaneous oxygen electrode.

Metabolic effects of oral contraceptives

Oral contraceptives contain either a combination of an oestrogen and a progestogen or a progestogen alone. In addition to suppressing ovulation, these contraceptives have a number of metabolic effects similar to some of those that occur in normal pregnancy (*Fig. 10.9*).

SUMMARY

- The principal female sex hormone, or **oestrogen**, is **17β-oestradiol**, secreted by the ovaries. The principal male sex hormone, or **androgen**, is **testosterone**, secreted by the testes.

- The secretion of both these hormones is stimulated by pituitary **luteinizing hormone (LH)**. Spermatogenesis and the maturation of ovarian follicles are dependent upon testosterone and oestradiol, respectively, and pituitary **follicle-stimulating hormone (FSH)**. The secretion of LH and FSH is in turn controlled by gonadotrophin-releasing hormone, released from the hypothalamus, and subject to feedback control by the gonadal hormones. Androgens are also produced by the adrenals and in males there is some production of oestrogens by metabolism from androgens.

- Both testosterone and oestradiol are transported in the plasma bound to **sex hormone-binding globulin (SHBG)**, with only about 3% of each hormone being in free solution. Because of the greater avidity of testosterone for SHBG, factors that increase the concentration of SHBG tend to increase oestrogen-dependent effects while those that decrease it increase androgen-dependent effects.

- The secretion of testosterone in men is maintained throughout life but in women oestrogen secretion declines after the **menopause**.

SUMMARY (cont'd)

- Both male and female **hypogonadism** can be either primary or secondary to either pituitary or hypothalamic dysfunction. Measurement of the appropriate gonadal hormone and the gonadotrophins, often after attempted stimulation of their secretion, will usually indicate the correct diagnosis and permit rational treatment.

- Hormone measurements are also valuable in the investigation of **gynaecomastia** in males and **virilism** in females. The commonest feature of excessive androgenization is **hirsutism**, which is most frequently due to **polycystic ovary syndrome**: other features of this condition include menstrual irregularity, infertility and a metabolic syndrome. **Congenital adrenal hyperplasia** can present for the first time in young adults, causing hirsutism, menstrual irregularity and infertility. However, the presence of severe hirsutism and virilism should suggest the possibility of an **androgen-secreting tumour** of the adrenals or ovaries.

- The laboratory investigation of **infertility** also depends heavily upon hormone measurements, though many non-endocrine factors must also be considered. A prime consideration is to establish whether ovulation is taking place: this can be inferred from finding an increase in plasma progesterone concentration on day 21 of the menstrual cycle.

- **Pregnancy** can be diagnosed by the detection of the β-subunit of human chorionic gonadotrophin in the urine. The formerly widely used biochemical tests of fetal well-being during pregnancy have now largely been superseded by fetal ultrasound scanning. Pregnancy causes a number of physiological changes in biochemical variables, including an increase in the plasma concentrations of hormone-binding proteins. As a result, total concentrations of, for example, thyroxine and cortisol, are increased during pregnancy although the free hormone concentrations are normal.

11 Disorders of carbohydrate metabolism

INTRODUCTION

Glucose is a major energy substrate. The body's sources of glucose are dietary carbohydrate and endogenous (principally hepatic) production by glycogenolysis (release of glucose stored as glycogen) and gluco-neogenesis (glucose synthesis from, e.g. lactate, glycerol and most amino acids). Blood glucose concentration depends on the relative rates of influx of glucose into the circulation and of its utilization. Blood glucose concentration is normally subject to rigorous control, rarely falling below 2.5 mmol/L or rising above 8.0 mmol/L in healthy subjects whether fasted or recently fed.

Following a meal, glucose is stored as glycogen, which is mobilized during fasting. Although the blood glucose concentration falls somewhat if fasting continues, and hepatic glycogen stores are used up after about 24 hours, adaptive changes lead to the attainment of a new steady state. After approximately 72 hours, blood glucose concentration stabilizes and can then remain constant for many days. The principal source of glucose becomes gluconeogenesis, from amino acids and glycerol, while ketones, derived from fat, become the major energy substrate (*see p. 194*).

The integration of these various processes, and thus the control of blood glucose concentration, is achieved through the concerted action of various hormones: these are insulin and the 'counter regulatory' hormones, namely glucagon, cortisol, catecholamines and growth hormone. Their effects are summarized in *Fig. 11.1*.

Physiologically, the two most important hormones in glucose homoeostasis are insulin and glucagon. Insulin is a 53 amino acid polypeptide, secreted by the β-cells of the pancreatic islets of Langerhans in response to a rise in blood glucose concentration. It is synthesized as a prohormone, proinsulin. This molecule undergoes cleavage prior to secretion to form insulin and C-peptide (*Fig. 11.2*). Insulin secretion is also stimulated by various gut hormones, including glucagon and gastric inhibitory peptide, GIP (glucose-dependent insulinotrophic peptide). Insulin promotes the removal of glucose from the blood through stimulating the relocation of the insulin-sensitive GLUT-4 glucose transporter from the cytoplasm to cell membranes, particularly in adipose tissue and skeletal muscle. Insulin also stimulates glucose uptake in the liver, but by a different mechanism: it induces the enzyme glucokinase, which phosphorylates glucose to form glucose 6-phosphate, a substrate for glycogen synthesis. This process maintains a low intracellular glucose concentration and thus a con-centration gradient that facilitates glucose uptake. Insulin stimulates glycogen synthesis (and inhibits glycogenolysis) through interaction with an exquisitely coordinated control mechanism that is central to the regulation of blood glucose concentration. In summary, binding of insulin to its receptor leads to activation of protein phosphatase 1. This enzyme dephosphorylates both glycogen synthase (thereby activating it and promoting glycogen synthesis) and phosphorylase kinase (rendering it inactive and thus preventing the activation of glycogen phosphorylase, the key enzyme of glycogenolysis). As a result of these actions, in the fasting state, when insulin secretion is inhibited, hepatic glycogenolysis is stimulated and glucose is liberated into the blood.

Insulin also exerts control over glycolysis and gluco-neogenesis, stimulating the former and reciprocally inhibiting the latter, by stimulating the expression of phosphofructokinase, pyruvate kinase and the enzyme responsible for the synthesis of the key allosteric modifier, fructose 2,6-bisphosphate (*see Fig. 11.3*).

Insulin is also important in the control of fat metabolism: it stimulates lipogenesis and inhibits lipolysis. It also stimulates amino acid uptake into cells and protein synthesis, and intracellular potassium uptake.

Glucagon is a 29 amino acid polypeptide secreted by the α-cells of the pancreatic islets; its secretion is decreased by a rise in the blood glucose concentration. In general, its actions oppose those of insulin: it stimulates hepatic (though not muscle) glycogenolysis through activation of glycogen phosphorylase, gluconeogenesis, lipolysis and ketogenesis. The control of ketogenesis is discussed on *p. 204*. The combined effects of insulin and glucagon are shown diagrammatically in *Fig. 11.4*.

Disordered glucose homoeostasis can lead to hyperglycaemia (often to a degree diagnostic of

Hormones involved in glucose homoeostasis			
Hormone	**Principal actions**		
Insulin	Increases	cellular glucose uptake	M, A
		glycogen synthesis	L, M
		protein synthesis	*L, M*
		fatty acid and triglyceride synthesis	*L, A*
	Decreases	gluconeogenesis	L
		glycogenolysis	L, M
		ketogenesis	*L*
		lipolysis	*A*
		proteolysis	*M*
Glucagon	Increases	glycogenolysis	L
		gluconeogenesis	L
		ketogenesis	*L*
		lipolysis	*A*
Adrenaline	Increases	glycogenolysis	L, M
		lipolysis	*A*
Growth hormone	Increases	glycogenolysis	L
		lipolysis	*A*
Cortisol	Increases	gluconeogenesis	L
		glycogen synthesis	L
		proteolysis	*M*
	Decreases	tissue glucose utilization	L, M, A

Fig. 11.1 Hormones involved in glucose homoeostasis. Letters indicate sites of action: L = liver, M = skeletal muscle, A = adipose tissue. Normal type indicates actions directly affecting glucose; other effects are shown in italics.

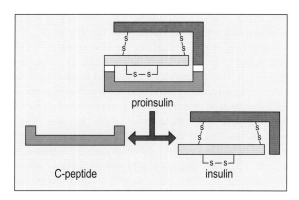

Fig. 11.2 Biosynthesis of insulin. The cleavage of proinsulin produces insulin, consisting of two polypeptide chains linked by disulphide bridges, and C-peptide.

diabetes) or to hypoglycaemia. It is to these conditions that the bulk of this chapter is devoted.

MEASUREMENT OF GLUCOSE CONCENTRATION

Plasma glucose concentration tends to be 10–15% higher than that of whole blood because a given volume of red cells contains less water than the same volume of plasma. The difference is of little significance at normal concentrations except in the interpretation of the results of glucose tolerance tests. However, when glucose concentration is changing rapidly, there may be a considerable discrepancy because of delayed equilibration of glucose across the red cell membranes.

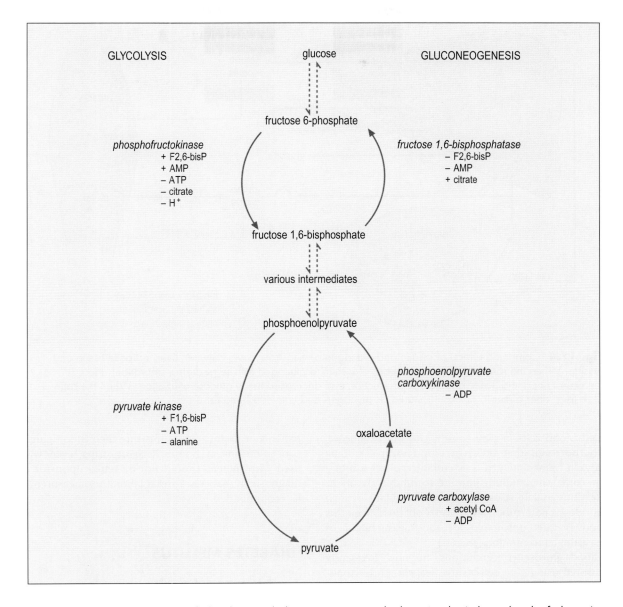

Fig. 11.3 Reciprocal control of glycolysis and gluconeogenesis in the liver. Insulin (released in the fed state) stimulates the expression of phosphofructokinase, pyruvate kinase and the enzyme responsible for the synthesis of fructose 2,6-bisphosphate (F2,6-bisP): glycolysis is promoted and gluconeogenesis is inhibited. Glucagon (released in the fasting state) inhibits expression of these enzymes and stimulates the production of phosphoenolpyruvate carboxykinase and fructose 1,6-bisphosphatase: gluconeogenesis is stimulated and glycolysis is inhibited.

The names of enzymes are given in italics. + Indicates substances that activate enzymes; − indicates substances that inhibit enzymes. ADP = Adenosine diphosphate; AMP = adenosine monophosphate; acetyl CoA = acetyl coenzyme A.

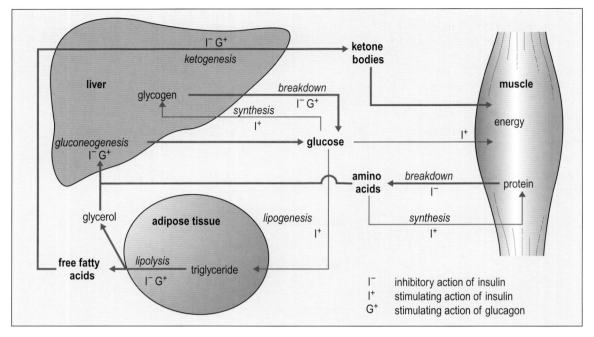

Fig. 11.4 Combined effects of insulin and glucagon on substrate flows between liver, adipose tissue and muscle. When the ratio of the concentrations of insulin to glucagon falls (e.g. during starvation), there is increased hepatic glucose and ketone production and decreased tissue glucose utilization. When the ratio is high (e.g. after a meal), glucose is stored as glycogen and converted into fat.

Red blood cells *in vitro* continue to utilize glucose, with the result that unless a blood sample can be analyzed immediately, it is essential to collect it into a tube containing sodium fluoride to inhibit glycolysis. Potassium oxalate is used as an anticoagulant in such 'fluoride–oxalate' tubes, and plasma obtained from this blood is thus unsuitable for the measurement of potassium concentration (*see p. 3*).

Blood glucose concentrations are now frequently measured using glucose-sensitive reagent strips. Application of (usually capillary) blood to these strips causes a colour change proportional to glucose concentration. After the blood has been washed off, the glucose concentration is read using either a colour comparator or, more accurately, a hand-held electronic instrument ('glucose meter'). Other types of reagent strips generate an electric current proportional to glucose concentration, which is read by a meter. Used carefully, these instruments are robust and produce reliable results. They are often used to monitor blood glucose concentrations in hospital, and have revolutionized the management of diabetes in the community by providing a means for

patients or their carers to measure their blood glucose concentrations at home. Reagent strips, even when used with meters, should not be relied upon for the diagnosis of diabetes: formal laboratory measurement is recommended.

DIABETES MELLITUS

Aetiology and pathogenesis

Diabetes mellitus is a metabolic disorder characterized by chronic hyperglycaemia with disturbances in carbohydrate, fat and protein metabolism arising from a defect in insulin secretion or action or both. It is a common condition, with a prevalence of approximately 1–2% in the western world. Diabetes can occur secondarily to other diseases, for example chronic pancreatitis, following pancreatic surgery and in conditions where there is increased secretion of hormones antagonistic to insulin (e.g. Cushing's syndrome and acromegaly).

Secondary diabetes is, however, uncommon. Most cases of diabetes mellitus (DM) are primary, that is they are not associated with other conditions. There are two distinct types. In type 1 DM, there is destruction of pancreatic cells, leading to a decrease in, and eventually cessation of, insulin secretion. Approximately 10% of all patients with diabetes have type 1. In type 2 DM, insufficient insulin is secreted to prevent hyperglycaemia, often because of resistance to its actions. Most patients with type 2 DM can be treated by diet, with or without oral hypoglycaemic drugs, but some patients, although adequately treated with oral agents initially, eventually require treatment with insulin to achieve adequate glycaemic control.

Type 1 DM usually presents acutely in younger people, with symptoms developing over a period of days or only a few weeks. However, there is evidence that the appearance of symptoms is preceded by a 'prediabetic' period of several months during which growth failure (in children), a fall in insulin response to glucose and various immunological abnormalities can be detected. Type 2 DM tends to present more chronically in the middle-aged and elderly (although it is increasingly being diagnosed in obese young people), with symptoms developing over months or even longer. The prevalence of type 2 DM increases with increasing age and reaches over 10% in people over the age of 75 years.

The previously used terms, 'insulin-dependent' and 'juvenile-onset' diabetes (for type 1) and 'non-insulin-dependent' and 'maturity-onset' diabetes (for type 2) are obsolete. It has become apparent that some young patients with diabetes are not insulin-dependent, while approximately 10% of patients developing diabetes over the age of 25, have 'latent autoimmune diabetes of adulthood' (LADA). Patients with LADA may be misclassified as having type 2 DM. However, in comparison with patients with true type 2 DM, they tend to present younger, are less likely to be overweight, have serum markers of autoimmunity and, although often treated successfully with diet alone or diet and oral agents initially, develop a requirement for insulin, often within a year of diagnosis. Some of the characteristics of type 1 and type 2 DM are shown in *Fig. 11.5*.

The exact pathogenesis of type 2 DM is uncertain. It is undoubtedly a heterogeneous disease. In established cases, β-cell dysfunction and insulin resistance usually coexist but it is not clear which is the primary defect: hyperglycaemia itself causes insulin resistance and β-cell dysfunction.

The condition shows a strong familial incidence. The concordance rate in monozygotic (identical) twins is more than 90% and the risk of an individual developing diabetes is greater than 50% if both parents have the condition. Several single gene defects have been identified

Major characteristics of type 1 DM and type 2 DM		
Feature	**Type 1 DM**	**Type 2 DM**
typical age of onset	children, young adults	middle-aged, elderly
onset	acute	gradual
habitus	lean	often obese
weight loss	usual	uncommon
ketosis-prone	usually	usually not
plasma insulin concentration	low or absent	often normal; may be ↑
family history of diabetes	less common	common
HLA association	DR3, DR4	none

Fig. 11.5 Major characteristics of type 1 (formerly insulin-dependent) and type 2 (formerly non-insulin-dependent) diabetes mellitus.

in specific subsets of patients with type 2 DM, notably in the dominantly inherited forms that typically develop in the young (MODY, maturity-onset diabetes of the young). The commonest mutations responsible for MODY are in the glucokinase gene. Glucokinase is the rate-limiting enzyme of glucose metabolism in pancreatic β-cells and through acting as a 'glucose sensor' is key to the regulation of pancreatic insulin secretion. Such specific mutations are, however, rare in type 2 DM considered overall, where the tendency to develop diabetes is polygenic and there is no clear pattern of inheritance.

Environmental factors are also important. Many patients with type 2 DM are obese, particularly tending to have visceral (intra-abdominal) obesity, which is known to cause insulin resistance (*see p. 360*). Reduced physical activity also causes insulin resistance, and various drugs, including corticosteroids, thiazides in high doses and some β-adrenergic antagonists, are diabetogenic.

The interaction between genetic and environmental factors in the pathogenesis of type 2 DM is exemplified by the high prevalence of the condition in certain ethnic groups (e.g. Pacific islanders) following the adoption of a westernized lifestyle, with good public health facilities and ready access to an assured food supply, in comparison with the prevalence in their aboriginal state. The suggestion is that their genotype evolved to maximize the storage of ingested energy as fat, to provide protection against famine, but that a continuous food supply leads to obesity and insulin intolerance (the 'thrifty genotype' hypothesis). There is also a 'thrifty phenotype' hypothesis, based on the observation that low birth weight is associated with an increased risk of later development of type 2 DM, the putative mechanism being β-cell dysfunction induced by fetal malnutrition.

Type 1 DM is an autoimmune disease. It is much less frequently familial (the concordance rate in monozygotic twins is approximately 40%), but there is a strong association with certain histocompatibility antigens, for example HLA-DR3, DR4 and various DQ alleles. An individual's HLA antigens are genetically determined but it is clear that type 1 DM is a genetically heterogeneous disorder. Environmental factors are also important and there is considerable circumstantial evidence that viral antigens (e.g. Coxsackie B) may initiate the autoimmune process in some genetically susceptible individuals. Proteins in cows' milk have also been implicated.

The pancreatic islets of newly diagnosed patients with type 1 DM show characteristic histological features of autoimmune disease. Islet cell antibodies (ICA) are frequently present in the serum (and may be detectable long before the condition presents clinically), together with antibodies to insulin and glutamic acid decarboxylase (GAD), which, like ICA, are sensitive markers of risk of progression to clinical diabetes in the apparently healthy members of patients' families.

It is thought that β-cell destruction is initiated by activated T-lymphocytes directed against antigens on the cell surface, possibly viral antigens or other antigens that normally are either not expressed or not recognized as 'non-self'. Clinically overt type 1 DM is thought to be a late stage of a process of gradual destruction of islet cells, and there is much interest in the possibility that it may be possible to modify this process in susceptible individuals and prevent or at least retard the development of clinical diabetes.

Pathophysiology and clinical features

There are two aspects to the clinical manifestations of diabetes mellitus: those related directly to the metabolic disturbance and those related to the long-term complications of the condition.

The hyperglycaemia of diabetes mellitus is mainly a result of increased production of glucose by the liver and, to a lesser extent, of decreased removal of glucose from the blood. In the kidneys, filtered glucose is normally completely reabsorbed in the proximal tubules, but at blood glucose concentrations much above 10 mmol/L (the renal threshold), reabsorption becomes saturated and glucose appears in the urine. There is some variation in the threshold between individuals. It is higher in the elderly and lower during pregnancy. Glycosuria results in an osmotic diuresis, increasing water excretion and raising the plasma osmolality, which in turn stimulates the thirst centre. Osmotic diuresis and thirst cause the classic symptoms of polyuria and polydipsia. Other causes of these symptoms include diabetes insipidus, hypercalcaemia, chronic hypokalaemia, chronic renal failure and excessive water intake.

Untreated, the metabolic disturbances may become profound, with the development of life-threatening ketoacidosis, non-ketotic hyperglycaemia or lactic acidosis.

The long-term complications of diabetes fall into two groups: microvascular complications, that is nephropathy, neuropathy and retinopathy, and macrovascular disease related to atherosclerosis. These occur in both type 1 and type 2 DM. The prevalence of all these complications increases with the duration of the disease. The risk of microvascular complications is clearly greater if glycaemic control is poor, but other factors are undoubtedly involved: some patients never develop these complications, even after many years of having diabetes; others develop them rapidly even with seemingly good control. The results of long-term prospective studies indicate that improved glycaemic control significantly reduces the risk of microvascular complications in both type 1 and type 2 DM. For macrovascular disease, there was a trend towards benefit but this was not statistically significant.

The common pathological feature in microvascular disease is narrowing of the lumens of small blood vessels, and this appears to be directly related to prolonged exposure to high glucose concentrations. The processes involved are complex, and still not fully understood: two appear particularly important. One is increased formation of sorbitol (an alcohol derived from glucose) by the action of the enzyme aldose reductase, leading to accumulation of sorbitol in cells. This can cause osmotic damage, alter the redox state and reduce cellular myoinositol concentrations. The other relates to the formation of advanced glycation end-products. Glucose can react with amino groups in proteins to form glycated plasma and tissue proteins (glycated haemoglobin, *see below*, is one example). These can undergo cross-linking and accumulate in vessel walls and tissues, leading to structural and functional damage.

The increased predisposition to atherosclerosis in patients with diabetes is also multifactorial. The abnormalities of lipids that occur as a direct result of diabetes (*see p. 207*) and glycation of lipoproteins leading to altered function are particularly important. Other factors that are implicated include endothelial dysfunction and increased oxidative stress.

The long-term complications of diabetes are a significant source of morbidity and mortality. Their diagnosis, with the exception of nephropathy, is largely clinical, although measurement of plasma lipids is important in the investigation of macrovascular disease. In contrast, the management of the acute metabolic disturbances seen in diabetes requires close collaboration between the physician and laboratory staff.

Diagnosis

The diagnosis of diabetes mellitus depends upon the demonstration of hyperglycaemia. In a patient with classic symptoms and signs, this may be inferred from the presence of glycosuria. Under these circumstances, a random venous plasma or capillary blood glucose concentration ≥ 11.1 mmol/L (venous blood glucose ≥ 10 mmol/L) is diagnostic of diabetes; so, too, is a fasting venous plasma glucose concentration ≥ 7.0 mmol/L (venous or capillary blood glucose ≥ 6.1 mmol/L). In the absence of symptoms, any of these limits must be exceeded on more than one occasion for the diagnosis to be made. Even in symptomatic patients, diabetes is unlikely if a random venous plasma glucose concentration is <5.5 mmol/L (venous or capillary blood glucose <4.4 mmol/L). Individuals who have fasting blood glucose concentrations that are elevated but not in the diabetic range have impaired fasting glycaemia (IFG). Their response to a glucose load should be tested to determine whether they have diabetes. The other indications and the protocol for the oral glucose tolerance test (OGTT) are given in *Fig. 11.6*, and the interpretation of results in *Fig. 11.7*. In the majority of patients suspected of having diabetes, the measurements indicated above will establish the diagnosis, and formal glucose tolerance testing is superfluous: it is only indicated when the diagnosis is in doubt. The OGTT formerly involved blood sampling at 30 minute intervals for 2 hours. Diagnostic criteria are now based only on glucose concentrations fasting and 2 hours after oral glucose: intermediate sampling is of no diagnostic value.

The OGTT also defines a category of hyperglycaemia termed impaired glucose tolerance (IGT), which does not equate to diabetes but represents a stage in the natural history of transition from normal glucose tolerance to frank diabetes. IGT is not a clinical entity in itself, but defines a risk category for progression to diabetes. Impaired fasting glycaemia is a further category of abnormal glucose tolerance: some individuals thus classified are found to be diabetic on formal testing, others have IGT. Patients with IGT should be given dietary and lifestyle advice and reviewed regularly. Some will become frankly diabetic: others revert to normal glucose tolerance. All appear to have a similar predisposition to myocardial infarction and stroke as patients with frank diabetes but they are not at increased risk of microvascular complications.

Gestational diabetes is diabetes or IGT with onset or first recognized during pregnancy. Pregnancy decreases glucose tolerance and patients with gestational diabetes may revert to normal glucose tolerance post partum. This condition is discussed on *p. 188*.

The oral glucose tolerance test	
Indications	**Procedure**
equivocal fasting/random blood glucose concentrations unexplained glycosuria, particularly in pregnancy clinical features of diabetes mellitus or its complications with normal blood glucose concentrations diagnosis of acromegaly (*see p. 133*)	patient should eat normal diet, containing at least 250 g carbohydrate per day for 3 days fast patient overnight take basal blood sample for glucose determination give 75 g glucose in water orally; take further blood samples at 60 and 120 min for glucose determination patient should rest throughout test; smoking not permitted; drinks of water are allowed

Fig. 11.6 The oral glucose tolerance test. For the diagnosis of diabetes, only basal and 120 min samples are required. For the diagnosis of acromegaly, samples should be taken at 30 min intervals.

Diagnostic blood glucose concentrations (mmol/L)				
Diagnosis	**Sample**	**Venous plasma**	**Venous blood**	**Capillary blood**
Normal	fasting	<6.1	<5.6	<5.6
Impaired fasting glycaemia	fasting	≥6.1 & <7.0	≥5.6 & <6.1	≥5.6 & <6.1
	2 h post glucose*	<7.8	<6.7	<7.8
Impaired glucose tolerance	fasting	<7.0 and	<6.1 and	<6.1 and
	2 h post glucose	≥7.8 & <11.1	≥6.7 & <10.0	≥7.8 & <11.1
Diabetes mellitus	fasting	≥7.0 or	≥6.1 or	≥6.1 or
	2 h post glucose	≥11.1	≥10.0	≥11.1

*If measured

Fig. 11.7 Diagnostic blood glucose concentrations. If a patient is asymptomatic, two results in the diabetic range are required to establish a diagnosis of diabetes mellitus.

Management

There are many aspects to the management of diabetes mellitus. Education of patients is vital: they will have diabetes for the rest of their lives and must, to a considerable extent, be responsible for their own treatment, albeit with guidance from a physician. Regular follow-up is essential to monitor treatment and detect early signs of complications, particularly retinopathy, which can in many cases be treated successfully, and nephropathy, since treatment may slow its progression.

The aims of treatment are twofold: to alleviate symptoms and prevent the acute metabolic complications of diabetes, and to prevent long-term complications. The first of these objectives is usually attainable with dietary control (essentially, substitution of complex for simple carbohydrates, an increase in dietary fibre and restriction of energy intake when necessary) with or without oral hypoglycaemic agents (e.g. sulphonylureas and/or metformin) in patients with type 2 DM, and with diet and insulin in patients with type 1 DM. It may sometimes become necessary to treat patients with type 2 diabetes with insulin to achieve adequate glycaemic control.

The demonstration that intensive glycaemic control reduces the risk of microvascular complications in diabetes means that the goal of treatment should be to attempt to maintain the blood glucose concentration within the physiological range. In practice, this may be difficult to achieve and intensification of treatment increases the risk of episodes of hypoglycaemia, particularly in patients treated with insulin. Indeed, some insulin-treated patients prefer to avoid a risk of hypoglycaemia by maintaining a level of glycaemic control that prevents the development of symptomatic acute hyperglycaemia but is less than optimal in terms of reducing the risk of complications long term.

It is sometimes considered that less strict glycaemic control may be acceptable in older patients developing type 2 DM on the basis that their life expectancy is such that they are not at significant risk of developing long-term complications. Such patients may not experience acute symptoms of hyperglycaemia even with persisting blood glucose concentrations of the order of 15 mmol/L and they are not at significant risk of developing ketoacidosis. However, although such a view may sometimes be appropriate, and the targets of treatment should always be assessed on an individual basis, the underlying metabolic abnormality will often have been present for several years before clinical presentation, and indeed patients with type 2 DM sometimes present clinically as a result of complications rather than symptoms of hyperglycaemia.

Whatever the treatment, the fluctuations in blood glucose concentration that occur in most diabetic patients are still greater than those that occur in normal subjects.

Monitoring treatment

The efficacy of treatment in diabetes is monitored clinically, by ensuring that the patient's symptoms are controlled and by measurement of blood glucose concentration and other objective indicators of glycaemic control.

Many patients (or their carers) monitor their own blood glucose concentrations at home using reagent strips and a glucose meter (*see p. 194*). This may be done more or less frequently as circumstances require: exercise, illness or a change of diet may alter insulin requirements and more frequent testing will allow the patient to adjust the dosage accordingly. Urine testing for glucose is being used much less than formerly. Such testing is only semi-quantitative and is of no value in the detection of hypoglycaemia: the urine is virtually free of glucose at normal blood glucose concentrations. Urine glucose excretion also depends on the renal threshold for glucose: if this is low (as, for example, in renal glycosuria, *p. 208*) glucose may be present in the urine at normal blood glucose concentrations. Urine testing for glucose should be used for monitoring diabetes only in patients unable or unwilling to do blood tests, and in older patients in whom control may not need to be so strict, particularly if they are treated with diet alone.

The measurement of glycated haemoglobin provides an important means of monitoring glycaemic control over a longer timespan. Haemoglobin undergoes glycation *in vivo* at a rate proportional to the blood glucose concentration; the reaction proceeds through a reversible stage but, once the major stable product (HbA_{1c}) is formed, it persists in that state for the lifetime of the cell. The proportion of haemoglobin in the glycated form thus effectively 'integrates' the blood glucose concentration over the previous 6–8 weeks. Normal HbA_{1c} is <6%; in uncontrolled diabetes, it may exceed 10%. Caution with interpretation is required in patients with decreased red cell lifespans, for example, due to haemolytic anaemia. In some of the methods used to measure glycated haemoglobin, haemoglobin variants may cross-react and give falsely high results. The measurement and use of glycated haemoglobin is complicated by the varying specificity of the different assays that are available (some also measure the minor glycated haemoglobins in addition to HbA_{1c}) and the lack of a primary standard preparation. Because of this, recommendations for target values for glycated haemoglobin derived from clinical trials may not be strictly applicable to local practice. However, in general, the aim should be to achieve and maintain as low a value (typically <7%) as is possible without unacceptably frequent episodes of hypoglycaemia, especially if they are severe. In practice, however, many patients do not achieve this target.

Since the proportion of glycated haemoglobin reflects the mean blood glucose concentration over the previous few weeks, its measurement is particularly useful

Case history 11.1

A young insulin-dependent diabetic patient attended the outpatient department for his regular follow-up and reported that he had been symptom-free since his last clinic attendance. He had been taught how to measure his own blood glucose concentration but did not do this, because he did not like pricking his finger to obtain capillary blood for testing.

Investigations

blood glucose (2 h after breakfast)	18 mmol/L
urine glucose (early morning)	2%
HbA$_{1c}$	6.5%

Comment

The HbA$_{1c}$ suggests that diabetic control is good, despite the patient's apparent lack of interest, a high blood glucose concentration and glycosuria. It transpired that he had been to a party the night before and had eaten considerably more than usual. He did not want to admit this, since he was, to use his own words, 'fed up with being lectured at'.

whenever there is a discrepancy between the patient's history and blood or urine glucose measurements. It will, for example, be high in patients who are generally poorly controlled but who make a special effort to comply with their treatment before attending a clinic in order to please their doctor by having a normal blood glucose concentration.

Other proteins also undergo glycation. Plasma fructosamine concentration is a measure of the glycation of plasma proteins, particularly albumin, and reflects glycaemic control over a shorter span than HbA$_{1c}$, but is much less widely used than glycated haemoglobin.

Other tests of value in monitoring patients with diabetes include the detection of microalbuminuria (for incipient diabetic nephropathy), plasma creatinine (in established renal disease) and lipids (because of the risk of atherosclerosis), and urine ketones (in patients at risk of ketoacidosis). All these are discussed elsewhere in this chapter.

METABOLIC COMPLICATIONS OF DIABETES

Ketoacidosis

Ketoacidosis may be the presenting feature of type 1 DM, or may develop in a patient known to be diabetic who omits to take his insulin or whose insulin dosage becomes inadequate because of an increased requirement, for example as a result of infection, any acute illness such as myocardial infarction, trauma or emotional disturbance. Newly diagnosed patients account for 20–25% of cases.

Pathogenesis

The sequence of events which leads to hyperglycaemia and the consequences of this are illustrated in *Figs 11.4 and 11.8*. Insulin deficiency, often combined with increased glucagon secretion, causes an increase in the glucagon:insulin ratio in the portal blood which decreases the hepatic concentration of fructose 2,6-bisphosphate, a key regulatory intermediate. This results in inhibition of phosphofructokinase, and thus of glycolysis, and activation of fructose 1,6-bisphosphatase, thus stimulating gluconeogenesis (*see p. 193*). At the same time, glycogen breakdown is promoted and glycogen synthesis is inhibited. Decreased peripheral utilization of glucose, resulting from insulin lack and preferential metabolism of free fatty acids and ketones as energy substrates, contributes to the hyperglycaemia but is less important than the increased rate of glucose production. Increased secretion of catecholamines also contributes to the hyperglycaemia.

Glycosuria causes an osmotic diuresis and hence fluid depletion, which is exacerbated by the hyperventilation and vomiting. The decrease in plasma volume leads to renal hypoperfusion and prerenal uraemia. As the glomerular filtration rate falls, so does the rate of urine production and the patient, initially polyuric, becomes oliguric. The loss of glucose in the urine affords some protection against the development of severe hyperglycaemia, but this is lost once oliguria develops. Established renal failure is an uncommon but recognized consequence of diabetic ketoacidosis.

Insulin lack causes increased lipolysis, with increased release of free fatty acids into the blood from adipose tissue, and decreased lipogenesis. In the liver, fatty acids normally undergo complete oxidation, are re-

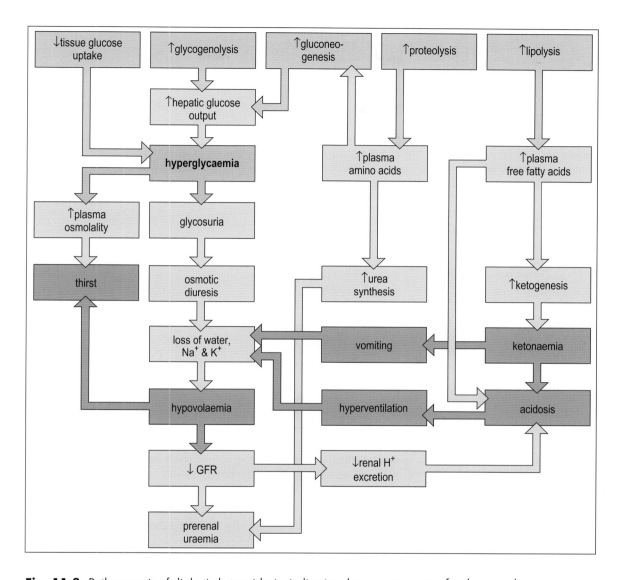

Fig. 11.8 Pathogenesis of diabetic ketoacidosis, indicating the consequences of a decreased insulin:glucagon ratio. Hyperkalaemia is invariably present, in spite of total body potassium depletion, as a result of loss of potassium from the tissues to the ECF and, as the glomerular filtration falls, to decreased renal excretion.

esterified to triglycerides or are converted to acetoacetic and 3-hydroxybutyric acids (ketogenesis). Ketogenesis is promoted in uncontrolled diabetes by the high ratio of glucagon to insulin. The mechanisms involved are shown in *Fig. 11.10*. Some acetoacetate is spontaneously decarboxylated to acetone. Ketones

stimulate the chemoreceptor trigger zone, causing vomiting. Acetoacetic and 3-hydroxybutyric acids are the major acids responsible for the acidosis but free fatty acids and lactic acid also contribute. It should be noted that in severely ill patients a shift in redox state can result in 3-hydroxybutyrate being formed

Case history 11.2

An 18-year-old girl consulted her family doctor because of tiredness and weight loss. On questioning, she admitted to feeling thirsty and had noticed that she had been passing more urine than normal. The doctor tested her urine and found glycosuria. He arranged for her to be seen at the hospital's diabetic clinic the next day. By then, however, she felt too ill to get out of bed, had started vomiting and had become drowsy. Her doctor visited her at home and arranged for immediate admission to hospital. On examination she was found to have a blood pressure of 95/60 mmHg with a pulse rate of 112/min and cold extremities. She had deep, sighing respiration (Kussmaul respiration) and her breath smelt of acetone.

Investigations

serum:	sodium	130 mmol/L
	potassium	5.8 mmol/L
	bicarbonate	5 mmol/L
	urea	18 mmol/L
	creatinine	140 µmol/L
	glucose	32 mmol/L
arterial blood:		
	hydrogen ion	89 nmol/L (pH 7.05)
	$P\text{CO}_2$	2.0 kPa (15 mmHg)

Comment

The clinical and biochemical features are typical of diabetic ketoacidosis (*Fig. 11.9*). She has hypotension, tachycardia and cold extremities, suggesting marked extracellular fluid depletion (sodium depletion). The low bicarbonate and high hydrogen ion concentrations with hyperventilation and thus a decreased $P\text{CO}_2$ indicate a non-respiratory acidosis with partial respiratory compensation. There is renal impairment (raised urea and creatinine) and the disproportionate increase in urea in comparison with creatinine is typical of dehydration compounded by increased urea production due to increased metabolism of amino acids (*see below*).

Hyperkalaemia is commonly present and is a result of the combined effects of decreased renal excretion and a shift of intracellular potassium (due to insulin lack, since insulin promotes cellular potassium uptake, and to acidosis and tissue catabolism). However, in spite of the hyperkalaemia, there is always considerable potassium depletion. The plasma sodium concentration is usually decreased, because of sodium depletion and the osmotically driven shift of water from the intracellular compartment. Although this patient is markedly hyperglycaemic, clinically severe ketoacidosis can sometimes occur with only a moderate increase in the blood glucose concentration (10–15 mmol/L). The presence of ketosis can be confirmed by the detection of ketonuria using a dip-stick test.

The pathogenesis of the acidosis and hyperglycaemia is discussed below. Although the term 'diabetic coma' is often used synonymously with diabetic ketoacidosis, many patients have a normal level of consciousness when they present. Drowsiness is common, but only a minority of patients are actually comatose.

Clinical and metabolic features of diabetic ketoacidosis

Clinical

thirst
polyuria (but oliguria late)
dehydration
hypotension, tachycardia and
   peripheral circulatory failure
ketosis
hyperventilation
vomiting
abdominal pain
drowsiness, coma

Metabolic

hyperglycaemia
glycosuria
non-respiratory acidosis
ketonaemia and ketonuria
uraemia
hyperkalaemia
hypertriglyceridaemia
haemoconcentration

Fig. 11.9 Clinical and metabolic features of diabetic ketoacidosis.

preferentially: this is not detected by conventional tests for ketones.

Management

Diabetic ketoacidosis is a medical emergency. Treatment must be started immediately the diagnosis has been made. The aims of treatment are to maintain tissue perfusion by replacement of lost fluid and minerals, and reverse the metabolic disturbance by providing insulin. Any identifiable precipitating event, for example infection, must also be treated.

Isotonic saline is given intravenously to replace lost fluid. The rate at which it is given will depend upon the precise circumstances, but it should usually be given rapidly, at least initially, to restore the extracellular fluid volume to normal. Careful monitoring of fluid input and output is essential, and it may be necessary to insert a central intravenous catheter to monitor central venous pressure. If there is gastric stasis, the gastric contents must be aspirated. Catheterization of the bladder may be necessary.

Potassium supplements are required: insulin causes rapid potassium uptake into cells with the result that although patients are usually hyperkalaemic at presentation, hypokalaemia will develop during treatment if potassium is not replaced. Regular monitoring of the plasma potassium concentration is essential.

Short-acting insulin should be given, preferably by constant intravenous infusion, at a rate of 6–10 U/h. The blood glucose concentration must be monitored and once it has fallen to near normal levels, the intravenous fluid is changed to 5% dextrose and the rate of insulin infusion decreased to maintain euglycaemia until it is possible to establish oral food and water intake, and a conventional regimen of subcutaneous insulin injections.

It is seldom necessary to give bicarbonate, except in the severest cases, since restoration of normal renal perfusion allows excretion of the hydrogen ion load and regeneration of bicarbonate, while restoration of normal metabolism reduces the production rate. If bicarbonate is used, it should be given in small quantities and the effect monitored by measurements of the arterial hydrogen ion concentration. Rapid correction of an acidosis may impair oxygen delivery to the tissues through an effect on the affinity of haemoglobin for oxygen, lead to later alkalosis as the ketoacid anions are metabolized to bicarbonate and paradoxically increase the cerebrospinal fluid (CSF) hydrogen ion concentration because of delayed equilibration of the bicarbonate between the plasma and the CSF. The response to treatment of a typical patient with diabetic ketoacidosis is shown in *Fig. 11.11*.

The deficits present in a patient with ketoacidosis are considerable and may exceed 5 L of water and 500 mmol each of sodium and potassium. Considerable depletion of other ions, in particular phosphate, may occur in ketoacidosis. The plasma phosphate concentration should be monitored, but specific replacement therapy is not usually required. Other biochemical abnormalities that may be seen include an increase in plasma amylase activity (because of reduced renal excretion), hypertriglyceridaemia and, in severely shocked patients, an increase in aminotransferases (probably related to hypoxic tissue damage).

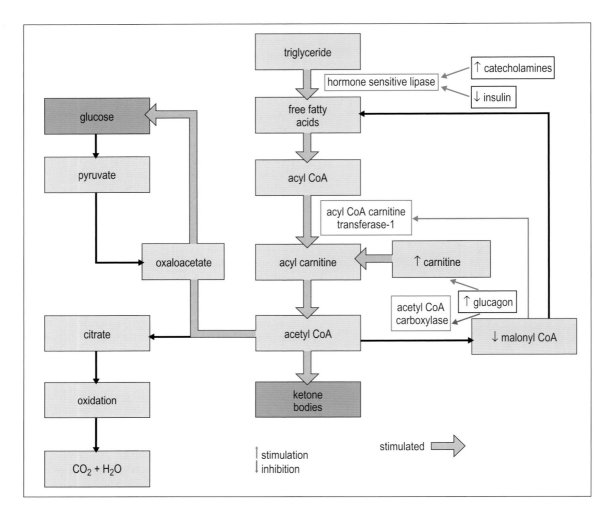

Fig.11.10 Mechanism of increased ketogenesis in diabetic ketoacidosis. Increased concentrations of catecholamines and decreased concentrations of insulin stimulate hormone-sensitive lipase, promoting lipolysis. Glucagon inhibits the synthesis of malonyl CoA, an intermediate in fatty acid synthesis (which thus decreases); malonyl CoA is an inhibitor of acyl CoA carnitine transferase, the activity of which thus increases. Glucagon also promotes the formation of carnitine, by an unknown mechanism. Increased enzyme activity and substrate supply increase the formation of acyl carnitine, which is required for transport of fatty acids into mitochondria, where ketogenesis takes place. Supplies of oxaloacetate necessary for the oxidation of acetyl CoA in the citric acid cycle are diverted instead to gluconeogenesis.

Non-ketotic hyperglycaemia

Not all patients with uncontrolled diabetes develop ketoacidosis. In type 2 DM, severe hyperglycaemia can develop (blood glucose concentration >50 mmol/L) with extreme dehydration and a very high plasma osmolality, but with no ketosis and minimal acidosis. This complication is often referred to as hyperosmolar non-ketotic hyperglycaemia, but patients with ketoacidosis usually also have increased plasma osmolality, although not to the same extent.

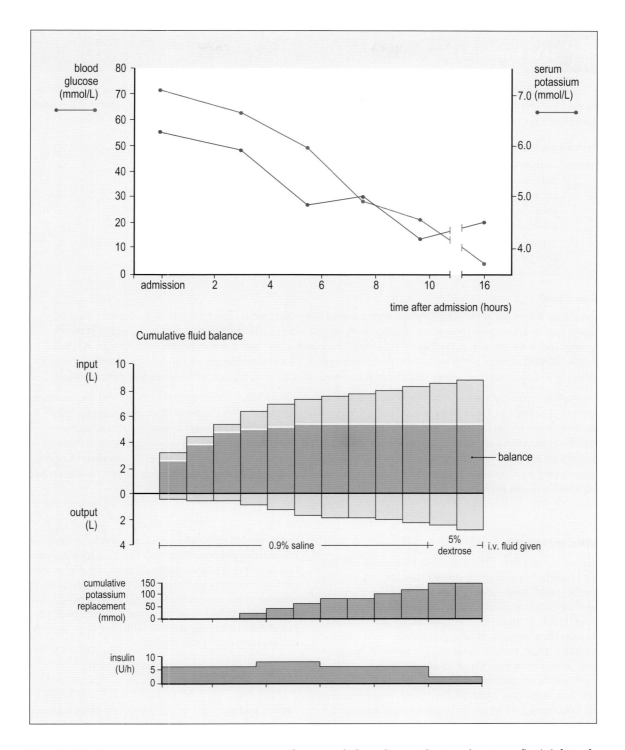

Fig. 11.11 Response to treatment in a patient with severe diabetic ketoacidosis, indicating a fluid deficit of nearly 6 L on admission.

Case history 11.3

A middle-aged widow, who lived alone, was admitted to hospital after her son found her semi-conscious at home. He had not seen her for a week but she had seemed well at their last meeting. On examination, she was extremely dehydrated but not ketotic. Her respiration was normal.

Investigations

serum:		
	sodium	149 mmol/L
	potassium	4.7 mmol/L
	bicarbonate	18 mmol/L
	urea	35 mmol/L
	creatinine	180 µmol/L
	glucose	54 mmol/L
	total protein	90 g/L
	osmolality	370 mmol/kg

Comment

The serum osmolality is very high, reflecting the severe hyperglycaemia. This has caused an osmotic diuresis, resulting in a decrease in glomerular filtration with retention of urea and creatinine and an increase in serum protein concentration due to the loss of water from the plasma. The serum bicarbonate concentration is a little below normal because of the decreased renal hydrogen ion excretion. The plasma sodium concentration is often raised in this condition, reflecting loss of water in excess of sodium as a result of the sustained osmotic diuresis.

Non-ketotic hyperglycaemia occurs only in type 2 DM. There is sufficient insulin secretion to prevent the excessive lipolysis and oppose the ketogenic action of glucagon that are essential for the generation of ketoacidosis (the concentrations of insulin required to do this are lower than those needed to prevent hyperglycaemia). Blood glucose concentrations are in general higher than in ketoacidosis. Perhaps because vomiting is not a feature, patients do not become acutely ill so quickly. A history of thirst and polyuria was subsequently obtained from this patient, who had not been previously diagnosed as having diabetes. She had also been attempting to quench her thirst with copious amounts of sweetened carbonated drinks.

Management

Rehydration and the administration of insulin are the most essential aspects of treatment. Insulin is given by constant intravenous infusion but a satisfactory decrease in glucose concentration is often attainable using a lower rate of infusion than that employed in ketoacidosis. Although these patients have a greatly increased plasma osmolality, fluid replacement should be with isotonic saline, not hypotonic ('half normal') saline, as has sometimes been recommended in the past. Isotonic saline expands the extracellular fluid compartment more effectively and its use helps to prevent too rapid a fall in osmolality and consequent risk of dangerously rapid re-expansion of the intracellular fluid compartment (*see Chapter 2*). Potassium supplements are required, but

less is needed than in ketoacidosis. Careful monitoring of the glucose concentration and fluid balance is essential. Heparin is sometimes given prophylactically in view of the hyperviscosity and attendant danger of thrombosis. In contrast to ketoacidosis, continued treatment with insulin is seldom required once the acute illness is over; patients can usually be managed either with diet alone or with diet and oral hypoglycaemic drugs.

Lactic acidosis

Lactic acidosis is an uncommon complication of diabetes. It was formerly chiefly seen in patients treated with phenformin, a biguanide oral hypoglycaemic drug, but is now more usually associated with severe systemic illness, for example severe shock and pancreatitis. It is discussed in more detail on *p. 48*.

Hypoglycaemia in diabetic patients

Hypoglycaemia can complicate treatment in both type 1 and type 2 DM. It is discussed in more detail on *pp. 210–211*.

 Case history 11.4

A 42-year-old woman, who had been diagnosed as an insulin-dependent diabetic in childhood, complained of frequent episodes of hypoglycaemia, which had continued to occur in spite of reduction of her insulin dosage. She had also developed amenorrhoea. Her diabetes had previously been well-controlled, with only occasional episodes of hypoglycaemia and HbA_{1c} in the range 6.5–7.0%. A review of her history showed that her daily insulin requirement had fallen from 48 to 28 U over the previous 12 months.

Investigations

HbA_{1c}	6.5%
serum LH	1.2 U/L
serum FSH	1.0 U/L

Comment

Occasional hypoglycaemic episodes are common in patients with type 1 DM, and there may be obvious reasons for them, for example a missed meal or an increase in physical activity. Recurrent hypoglycaemia can be due to over-zealous treatment, but a decrease in insulin requirements suggests a change in the activity of counter-regulatory hormones. In this instance, the development of amenorrhoea with low gonadotrophin concentrations suggested that the patient might have developed pituitary failure, with decreased production of growth hormone and ACTH causing increased sensitivity to insulin. This was confirmed by formal pituitary function testing and shown to be due to a non-functioning pituitary tumour.

Diabetic nephropathy

Diabetic nephropathy is a major cause of premature death in patients with diabetes, with deaths related to cardiovascular disease as well as renal failure. It occurs in about 30% of patients with type 1 DM, and 25% of patients with type 2 (more in certain ethnic groups). The earliest detectable abnormality is microalbuminuria. Normal urinary albumin excretion is <20 µg/min (<30 mg/24 h): values between 20 and 200 µg/min (30 and 300 mg/24 h) constitute microalbuminuria. Such amounts are undetectable using conventional urine reagent strips. This progresses through clinical proteinuria (>200 µg/min: >300 mg/24 h) with gradually declining filtration rate and increasing plasma creatinine concentration to frank uraemia. Hyperlipidaemia and hypertension are frequently present.

At the stage of microalbuminuria there is evidence that treatment with angiotensin-converting enzyme inhibitors (even in the absence of hypertension) delays progression. Even in established nephropathy, treatment of hypertension and hyperlipidaemia, and dietary protein restriction may be beneficial. Optimization of glycaemic control is recommended at both stages but has not been proven to influence progression.

Ideally, all diabetic patients (except young children and the very old) should have their urine albumin excretion measured annually. Screening is done on an early morning urine. Precise recommendations vary. One approach is to follow up a positive test (albumin: creatinine ratio >2.5 mg/mmol (males), >3.5 mg/mmol (females)) by timed collections. In the absence of other causes of renal disease, the finding of albumin excretion rates exceeding 20 µg/min in two out of three urine samples tested within 6–12 weeks is indicative of incipient nephropathy; values exceeding 200 µg/min (300 mg/24 h) indicate established nephropathy.

Lipoprotein metabolism in diabetes mellitus

Insulin has a major role in the control of fat metabolism, and both type 1 and type 2 DM are associated with abnormalities of plasma lipids. In type 1 DM, at presentation, or if glycaemic control deteriorates, marked hypertriglyceridaemia (manifest as an increase in very low density lipoprotein (VLDL), and often by chylomicronaemia as well) is often present, as a result of decreased activity of lipoprotein lipase (which insulin stimulates) and increased activity of hormone-sensitive lipase (which insulin inhibits) leading to increased flux of free fatty acids from adipose tissue that act as a substrate for hepatic triglyceride synthesis. Both these effects are reversed by insulin treatment. Indeed, the degree of hypertriglyceridaemia correlates well with glycaemic control. Low density lipoprotein (LDL) concentration can also be increased, and that of high density lipoprotein (HDL) decreased.

In type 2 DM, hypertriglyceridaemia is also common, although it is not usually as severe as in uncontrolled type 1 DM unless there is an additional, genetic, predisposition. It is due mainly to increased hepatic synthesis. The VLDL contains increased triglyceride and cholesteryl ester in relation to the amount of apoprotein and although LDL concentrations are not much increased, the particles tend to be smaller and denser, and are more atherogenic. As in type 1 DM, HDL concentration is often decreased. In both type 1 and type 2 DM, glycation of apolipoprotein B may enhance the atherogenicity of LDL by reducing its affinity for the LDL receptor, so leading to increased uptake by macrophage scavenger receptors.

Plasma lipid concentrations usually become normal in patients with well-controlled type 1 DM; HDL concentrations may even become increased. In contrast, the abnormalities seen in type 2 DM may persist despite adequate glycaemic control. Treatment with lipid-lowering drugs may be appropriate, to reduce the risk of vascular disease.

DIABETES IN PREGNANCY

Maternal diabetes increases the risk of congenital malformations. This risk can be greatly reduced by ensuring excellent glycaemic control at conception and during early pregnancy, to which end women con-templating pregnancy are advised to attend special pre-pregnancy clinics. Maternal hyperglycaemia increases fetal insulin secretion and can cause fetal macrosomia, predisposing to difficult delivery, and neonatal hypo-glycaemia. Maintenance of excellent glycaemic control reduces these risks. Pregnancy reduces glucose tolerance: women previously treated with insulin often have increased insulin requirements during pregnancy; women normally treated with diet alone or diet and oral hypoglycaemic drugs are usually treated with insulin during pregnancy, as are women diagnosed with gestational diabetes (*see p. 188*). Patients with gestational diabetes may revert to normal glucose tolerance after delivery but remain at increased risk of developing diabetes in the future.

GLYCOSURIA

Although diabetes mellitus is the commonest cause of glycosuria, it is also seen in patients with a low renal threshold for glucose. This may occur as an isolated and harmless abnormality (renal glycosuria), can develop during pregnancy and is a feature of congenital and acquired generalized disorders of proximal renal tubular function (the Fanconi syndrome, *see p. 80*).

A positive test for reducing substances in the urine using reagent tablets (Clinitest) is given by a number of substances other than glucose, some of which are indicated in *Fig. 11.12*. Reagent sticks containing glucose oxidase are specific for glucose.

GLUCOSE IN CEREBROSPINAL FLUID

Glucose concentration in the CSF is commonly measured in patients suspected of having bacterial

Substances giving a positive reducing test in urine
glucose
lactose (during lactation and the last trimester of pregnancy)
galactose (in galactosaemia and galactokinase deficiency)
fructose (in hereditary fructose intolerance and essential fructosuria)
pentoses (after eating certain fruits and in essential pentosuria)
homogentisic acid (in alkaptonuria)
glucuronides of drugs
salicylic acid (in aspirin overdose)
ascorbic acid (with high vitamin C intake)
creatinine (only in high concentration)

Fig. 11.12 Substances giving a positive reducing test in urine.

meningitis, since it is usually decreased as a result of bacterial metabolism. If the CSF is frankly purulent, the measurement of CSF glucose provides no useful additional information. The CSF glucose concentration is approximately 65% of the blood glucose concentration and CSF glucose should always be interpreted in the light of the glucose concentration of a blood sample obtained at the same time.

HYPOGLYCAEMIA

Hypoglycaemia is conventionally, though arbitrarily, defined as a blood glucose concentration of less than 2.2 mmol/L.

Causes

It is convenient to divide the causes of hypoglycaemia into those causing a low blood glucose concentration during *fasting* and those in which it follows a stimulus (*reactive* hypoglycaemia), including a meal (post-prandial hypoglycaemia). It is usually possible to distinguish between these categories from the patient's history.

Episodes of reactive hypoglycaemia can occur in patients with fasting hypoglycaemia although fasting hypoglycaemia is virtually never a feature of conditions associated with reactive hypoglycaemia in the absence of the stimulus. The causes of hypoglycaemia are summarized in *Fig. 11.13* and the pathogenesis is indicated in each case. These conditions are discussed further in the following sections.

Clinical features

Glucose is an essential energy substrate for the nervous system, at least in the short term; during starvation, adaptation occurs and ketone bodies can be utilized. The clinical features of hypoglycaemia are the result of dysfunction of the nervous system (neuroglycopenia) and the effects of catecholamines that are released in response to the stimulus provided by the low blood glucose.

The characteristic clinical features of acute hypoglycaemia are summarized in *Fig. 11.13*. Their development is affected by various factors, and the threshold varies between individuals. Typical signs and symptoms are more likely to occur if the blood glucose falls rapidly and if hypoglycaemic episodes are separated by periods of normoglycaemia. If the blood glucose concentration falls rapidly, symptoms can develop at concentrations higher than 2.2 mmol/L. The clinical features of hypoglycaemia are likely to be enhanced if cerebral blood flow is impaired, while they may be attenuated in patients taking β-adrenergic blocking drugs, such as propranolol, and in patients with autonomic nephropathy. In chronic hypoglycaemia, psychiatric manifestations may predominate, and other features may not be present, even with a glucose concentration as low as 1 mmol/L.

Diagnosis

There are two stages in the diagnosis of hypoglycaemia: confirmation of the low blood glucose concentration and elucidation of the cause. Mention has been made of the considerable variation in the blood glucose concentration at which symptoms of hypoglycaemia begin to appear. In children and young adults, symptoms will usually be present only with a concentration of less than 2.2 mmol/L. The elderly tend to be more sensitive to low blood glucose, perhaps because of impaired homoeostatic responses or decreased cerebral perfusion resulting from atheroma. Neonates, however, often develop symptoms only when the blood glucose is less than 1.5 mmol/L. Although reagent strips and glucose meters can be used to confirm a clinical suspicion of hypoglycaemia, they are insufficiently accurate at low blood glucose concentrations to provide a definitive diagnosis and formal laboratory measurements should be used. Blood must be collected into a container with fluoride, to inhibit glycolysis.

That the clinical features are due to hypoglycaemia should be confirmed by giving glucose either by mouth or parenterally, as appropriate. Those that are caused by acute neuroglycopenia and catecholamine release should resolve immediately, but those attributable to chronic hypoglycaemia often persist. The presence of a low blood glucose concentration and symptoms of hypoglycaemia that are abolished by giving glucose constitute 'Whipple's triad'.

The cause of the hypoglycaemia may be obvious from the patient's history, particularly in reactive hypoglycaemia. With fasting hypoglycaemia, many possible causes can be eliminated by simple tests; if this can be done, investigations should be directed towards the detection of possible excessive insulin secretion. In adults, this is often tumour-related, although in infants other causes need to be considered.

Hypoglycaemia	
Causes	**Clinical features**
Reactive hypoglycaemia	**Acute**
post-prandial:	due to neuroglycopenia:
gastric surgery	tiredness
essential (idiopathic)	confusion
drug-induced:	detachment, lack of concentration
insulin	ataxia
sulphonylureas	dizziness
alcohol	paraesthesiae
others	hemiparesis
inherited metabolic disorders:	convulsions
galactosaemia	coma
hereditary fructose intolerance	due to sympathetic stimulation:
	palpitation and tachycardia
Fasting hypoglycaemia	profuse sweating
hepatic and renal disease (rare)	facial flushing
endocrine disease:	tremor
adrenal failure	anxiety
pituitary failure	non-specific:
isolated ACTH or GH deficiency	hunger
inherited metabolic disorders:	weakness
glycogen storage disease type I	blurred vision
hyperinsulinism:	
insulinoma	**Chronic neuroglycopenia**
nesidioblastosis	personality changes
non-pancreatic neoplasms	memory loss
alcohol-induced fasting hypoglycaemia	psychosis
various forms of neonatal hypoglycaemia	dementia
septicaemia	

Fig. 11.13 Major causes and clinical features of hypoglycaemia. Chronic neuroglycopenia is seen mainly in patients with insulin-secreting tumours; the features of acute neuroglycopenia are classically seen in diabetic patients who have taken too much insulin, but may occur with other forms of reactive hypoglycaemia.

HYPOGLYCAEMIC SYNDROMES

Reactive hypoglycaemia

Drug-induced hypoglycaemia

Most patients with type 1 diabetes experience occasional episodes of hypoglycaemia. Disturbed patients sometimes deliberately administer excessive insulin to draw attention to themselves. More frequently, hypoglycaemia is related to a missed meal or some other factor (*see Case History 11.5*). It should be noted that the presence of glycosuria does not exclude a diagnosis of hypoglycaemia, for the renal threshold may have been exceeded since the bladder was last emptied. The diagnosis must rest on the blood glucose concentration, but if there is any doubt it is always safe to give glucose to a confused or unconscious diabetic patient pending the result becoming available. Glucagon can also be used to treat hypoglycaemia: it causes rapid mobilization of hepatic glycogen (and so is not effective in starved individuals). Treatment with β-adrenergic blockers can mask the adrenergic symptoms of hypoglycaemia (except sweating) and delay recovery. Patients treated with insulin, particularly if they are striving to achieve very good glycaemic control, may lose (though reversibly) their awareness of hypoglycaemia.

In patients with type 2 diabetes, hypoglycaemia can complicate treatment with sulphonylureas. Chlorpropamide is most frequently implicated. It has a long plasma half-life and, since it is renally excreted, tends to accumulate in patients with impaired renal function.

Hypoglycaemia caused by drugs other than those used to treat diabetes is uncommon. β-Adrenergic blockers occasionally cause hypoglycaemia, but only when other factors such as starvation, severe exercise or liver disease are involved. Children, but not adults, poisoned with salicylates may develop severe hypoglycaemia. It has also been reported in patients who have taken overdoses of paracetamol and, in these cases, it is probably related to the severe liver damage that this drug can cause.

 Case history 11.5

A young male jogger collapsed during a ten-mile fun run. He was conscious but disorientated and his speech was incoherent. He was taken to hospital where a finger-prick test for blood glucose concentration showed this to be very low. Blood was sent to the laboratory for confirmation of the diagnosis. He was given 25 g glucose i.v. and recovered rapidly. He then admitted that he was an insulin-dependent diabetic; he had injected his normal dose of insulin that morning and eaten his usual breakfast. The laboratory reported a blood glucose concentration on admission of 1.6 mmol/L. He was given further carbohydrate by mouth and was discharged that evening with a normal blood glucose concentration, to be reviewed in the diabetic clinic the next day.

Comment

Insulin requirements in type 1 diabetic patients are reduced by exercise. It is an important part of the education of diabetic patients that they are aware of this and can thus reduce their insulin dose or increase their carbohydrate intake accordingly. Diabetic patients should always carry sugar and a means of identification to facilitate treatment in an emergency.

Post-prandial hypoglycaemia

In patients who have undergone gastric surgery involving either a gastrointestinal anastomosis or a pyloroplasty, hypoglycaemia, developing 90–150 min after a meal, particularly a meal rich in sugar, is common. There is rapid passage of glucose into the small intestine and release of hormones that stimulate insulin secretion. The insulin response is excessive and hypoglycaemia ensues as glucose absorption from the gut falls off rapidly, rather than slowly as it does when gastric emptying is normal.

Symptoms suggestive of hypoglycaemia following meals may be described by people who have not undergone surgery (essential or idiopathic post-prandial hypoglycaemia). Although transient hypoglycaemia is common from 90 to 150 min after taking 75 g glucose orally in a glucose tolerance test, it is often asymptomatic and the relevance of hypoglycaemia after this artificial stimulus is questionable. It is more relevant to examine the blood glucose response to a standard mixed meal, and this diagnosis should not be made unless a low blood glucose concentration is recorded at a time when the patient is symptomatic, and the symptoms are abolished by giving glucose. Thus defined, idiopathic reactive hypoglycaemia is uncommon. Its cause remains uncertain: there is no evidence of any impairment of glucose homoeostasis in these patients.

Alcohol and reactive hypoglycaemia

Insulin- and drug-induced reactive hypoglycaemia are potentiated by alcohol. Alcohol also increases insulin release in response to an oral glucose load and this may enhance any tendency to post-prandial reactive hypoglycaemia. Alcohol-induced fasting hypoglycaemia is considered in *Case History 11.7*.

Other causes of reactive hypoglycaemia

Various inherited metabolic diseases have reactive hypoglycaemia as a feature. Since these are usually first recognized in children, they are considered in the discussion of neonatal and childhood hypoglycaemia (*see p. 214*).

Sudden cessation of a hypertonic dextrose infusion, being given as part of a parenteral feeding regimen, can precipitate hypoglycaemia, especially when insulin has been given concomitantly. Hypoglycaemia can also occur after dialysis against a glucose-rich dialysate.

Fasting hypoglycaemia

Insulinoma

Insulinomas are tumours of the insulin-secreting β-cells of the pancreatic islets. Although uncommon, they are an important cause of fasting hypoglycaemia. The blood glucose concentration should be measured in any patient who experiences a fit, faint, transient ischaemic attack or 'funny turn' in order to exclude hypoglycaemia as a cause, although many patients with an insulinoma present with behavioural changes, rather than with the classic features of acute hypoglycaemia. For this reason, there is often a delay before the diagnosis is considered and appropriate investigations are performed.

Other causes of fasting hypoglycaemia (see below) are usually obvious clinically and, with the exception of insulin- and sulphonylurea-induced hypoglycaemia, and hypoglycaemia caused by sepsis, are associated with low plasma insulin concentrations. The presence of an insulin-secreting tumour can be inferred from the presence of an inappropriately high plasma insulin concentration (>20 pmol/L) at a time when the blood glucose concentration is low (<2.2 mmol/L). C-peptide should also be measured. Although secreted in equimolar amounts with insulin, C-peptide is cleared from the circulation more slowly, so it may be a more reliable marker of endogenous insulin secretion than insulin itself. Measurement of plasma 3-hydroxybutyrate concentration can be informative. Insulin inhibits lipolysis and hence the production of 3-hydroxybutyrate. High concentrations (>600 μmol/L) occur in hypoglycaemia with suppressed insulin secretion (e.g. cortisol deficiency, liver disease). In hyperinsulinaemia and tumour-related hypoglycaemia, 3-hydroxybutyrate concentrations are usually low.

Ideally, blood should be collected for these measurements while the patient is symptomatic. If this cannot be done, or symptoms of acute hypoglycaemia do not occur, blood samples should be collected after an overnight fast on three consecutive mornings: when this is done, biochemical (although often asymptomatic) hypoglycaemia is demonstrable in 90% of patients with an insulinoma. If hypoglycaemia does not occur under these circumstances, patients suspected of having an insulinoma can be fasted for longer. Clinical hypoglycaemia develops in almost all patients during a 72 h fast, and can often be provoked by exercise during this time. Blood samples should be collected every 4–6 h and during any episode of clinical hypoglycaemia;

plasma insulin and C-peptide concentrations are measured in any sample in which the blood glucose concentration is low. Although normal subjects occasionally develop hypoglycaemia during such a fast (women more frequently than men), this is asymptomatic and plasma insulin concentration is low (usually <20 pmol/L).

The 72 h fast is a time-consuming procedure, and as an alternative, when required, an insulin hypoglycaemia test (p. 128) can be performed. Hypoglycaemia is induced with insulin (with the usual strict monitoring mandatory for this test) and plasma C-peptide concentration is measured. C-peptide is not present in insulin produced for therapeutic use. In normal individuals, the induction of hypoglycaemia suppresses endogenous insulin and C-peptide secretion. In patients with an insulinoma, this does not happen; a plasma C-peptide concentration >100 pmol/L implies continuing, autonomous, insulin secretion. Some insulinomas secrete mainly proinsulin, but this is measured as insulin in many insulin assays, and separate measurement of proinsulin is not usually required.

It should be noted that glucose tolerance tests have no role in the investigation of possible insulinomas.

Non-pancreatic neoplasms

Hypoglycaemia can also occur in association with non-pancreatic neoplasms, including hepatocellular and adrenal carcinomas, carcinoid tumours and large mesenchymal tumours such as retroperitoneal sarcomas. Patients are usually not ketotic and, except with some carcinoid tumours, plasma insulin concentrations are not increased. It has been suggested that increased glucose uptake by the tumour may be a factor but this is unlikely ever to be the sole cause. Hepatic glucose output is often reduced although there is a normal glucogenic response to glucagon. It is probable that most such tumour-related hypoglycaemia is related to the secretion of insulin-like growth factors (IGFs). Plasma IGF-1 concentrations are consistently low in such patients but IGF-2 (particularly in the non-protein-bound form) is often increased, and the ratio IGF-1:IGF-2 decreased. Cytokines such as tumour necrosis factor (TNFα) have also been implicated.

Hepatic and renal disease

Although the liver is central to glucose homoeostasis, its functional reserve is so great that hypoglycaemia is a rare feature of hepatic disease. It may occur, however,

Case history 11.6

A woman telephoned for an ambulance when she was unable to rouse her husband one morning; she noticed that his left leg and arm were jerking. In the hospital emergency room, he was seen to be pale and sweaty, with a rapid, poor-volume pulse. His blood glucose concentration was 0.8 mmol/L. He regained consciousness when given a bolus of glucose intravenously, but then became confused and required a continuous glucose infusion for several hours to prevent hypoglycaemia.

His wife revealed that she had been becoming increasingly worried about her husband. Formerly a man of equable temperament, over the past six months he had frequently arrived home in a bad mood, taken little notice of his wife and young child and sat in sullen silence until his evening meal. After eating, he would behave quite normally, apparently with no recollection of his previous behaviour. On the two mornings immediately prior to admission, she had found him sitting up in bed, apparently conscious but staring vacantly at the wall and not speaking; she had managed to get him to drink his usual cup of sweet tea and he had rapidly recovered.

A presumptive diagnosis of insulinoma was made and was confirmed by the finding of a serum insulin concentration of 480 pmol/L at a time when he was hypoglycaemic. He had hepatomegaly, and the serum alkaline phosphatase activity was raised. A coeliac axis angiogram demonstrated a large filling defect in the liver; at laparotomy, the liver was found to have extensive tumour deposits, shown on histological examination to be characteristic of an insulinoma. A single, small tumour was present in the pancreas. No operative treatment was possible; he initially responded well to cytotoxic drugs but relapsed and died six months later.

Comment

This case illustrates the sometimes bizarre symptomatology of patients with insulinomas, who may be chronically hypoglycaemic. A provocative test was clearly not required to establish the diagnosis in this case. When a definitive test is required, the insulin hypoglycaemia test with measurement of C-peptide is preferable to the many other tests that have been described, using, for example, glucagon or alcohol as a secretagogue for insulin. The majority of insulinomas (approximately 90%) are, unlike the tumour in this case, benign. In some 10% of cases there are multiple pancreatic tumours and there may be associated adenomas in other endocrine organs (multiple endocrine neoplasia type 1, *see p. 326*).

The treatment of choice is surgical resection, when possible, and with benign tumours the prognosis is good. Diazoxide may be used to prevent hypoglycaemia pre-operatively. Its main action is to reduce insulin secretion from both normal and neoplastic β-cells. Streptozotocin, a drug which is specifically cytotoxic to β-cells, is valuable in the management of malignant insulinomas when surgical treatment is either not possible or has failed.

with the rapid, massive hepatocellular destruction that can follow poisoning with paracetamol and other toxins. The kidneys are the only organs other than the liver capable of gluconeogenesis; they are also responsible for insulin degradation. These facts may in part explain the severe hypoglycaemia that is occasionally a feature of terminal renal disease.

Endocrine disease

Deficiency of hormones antagonistic to insulin is a recognized but uncommon cause of hypoglycaemia.

Lack of cortisol can be due either to primary adrenal failure or secondary to panhypopituitarism; hypoglycaemia can be a feature of either condition. Mild hypoglycaemia can occur with isolated deficiency of ACTH or growth hormone but in the latter condition it is never symptomatic.

Rather surprisingly, in view of its role in carbohydrate metabolism, lack of adrenaline in patients who have undergone bilateral adrenalectomy and who are maintained on corticoid hormone replacement neither causes hypoglycaemia nor interferes with the ability to recover from artificially induced hypoglycaemia.

Alcohol-induced fasting hypoglycaemia

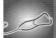 **Case history 11.7**

An elderly man was found to be unrousable one morning by fellow inmates of a derelict house in which they slept. He had been drunk the previous evening and although this was not uncommon he had never before been so stuporous in the morning. An ambulance was called and he was admitted to hospital and found to be profoundly hypoglycaemic. He responded rapidly to intravenous glucose and did not then appear inebriated. He refused further treatment and discharged himself later the same day.

Comment

Alcohol-induced fasting hypoglycaemia is caused mainly by the inhibitory effect of alcohol on gluconeogenesis. However, acquired ACTH deficiency may be present in some alcoholics and poor nutrition and liver disease may also contribute. As in this case, hypoglycaemia characteristically develops several hours after alcohol ingestion (compare alcohol and reactive hypoglycaemia, p. 211), when hepatic glycogen stores become exhausted. Signs of inebriation may not be present at this time and blood alcohol concentrations are unremarkable. Although first described, and most commonly seen, in poorly nourished chronic alcoholics, hypoglycaemia can be readily precipitated by alcohol in healthy subjects whose hepatic glycogen reserves have been depleted by lack of food.

Sepsis

Hypoglycaemia is sometimes seen in patients with septicaemia. It is thought to be a result of the release of cytokines, which may stimulate insulin secretion or have a direct effect on hepatic glucose production. Renal impairment may also be contributory.

Inherited metabolic disease

Fasting hypoglycaemia is an important feature of glycogen storage disease type I, discussed in more detail on p. 297.

HYPOGLYCAEMIA IN CHILDHOOD

Neonatal hypoglycaemia

Although the newborn appear to have a lower threshold for the development of clinical hypoglycaemia, there is good evidence that even asymptomatic hypoglycaemia may be harmful (particularly in relation to the central nervous system). The formerly accepted practice, whereby a lower blood glucose concentration in the newborn than in adults was used for the definition of hypoglycaemia, should, therefore, be abandoned.

Hypoglycaemia may occur transiently in apparently normal babies, but is particularly common in those who have respiratory distress, severe infection, brain damage or who are small-for-dates. Premature and small-for-dates babies are particularly at risk of developing neonatal hypoglycaemia because they are born with low hepatic glycogen stores and are more likely to have feeding problems. Extensive physiological changes occur at birth and, in terms of glucose metabolism, there is a sudden interruption of the maternal glucose supply and glycogenolysis must span the period until feeding becomes established. Babies born to diabetic mothers can have islet cell hyperplasia, which increases the risk of hypoglycaemia developing in the immediate postnatal period, though this does not persist thereafter.

Hypoglycaemia in infancy

Any of the conditions discussed above can cause hypo-glycaemia in infancy. A variety of other conditions may cause hypoglycaemia at this time (Fig. 11.14); these are discussed below. The inherited metabolic diseases associated with hypoglycaemia are particularly likely to present during the first few weeks of life.

Beyond the neonatal period, energy stores are usually sufficient to prevent hypoglycaemia during fasting unless there is a defect in homoeostatic mechanisms (e.g. as a result of endocrine disease). In some children, however, starvation – often in the setting of an intercurrent illness – can lead to hypoglycaemia. Insulin secretion is suppressed and ketosis is present. Such children are often thin and sometimes have a history of being small-for-dates. The hypoglycaemia is thought to be a result of impaired mobilization of glucogenic precursors (particularly alanine) but no specific defect has been described and there is no defining test for this condition, often called idiopathic ketotic hypoglycaemia.

Causes of hypoglycaemia in childhood

Transient neonatal hypoglycaemia

Hyperinsulinaemia
islet cell hyperplasia
insulinoma

Inherited metabolic disorders, including:
glycogen storage diseases
galactosaemia
hereditary fructose intolerance
fatty acid β-oxidation defects

Other causes
prematurity
small-for-dates
endocrine disorders
starvation
drugs
ketotic hypoglycaemia

Fig. 11.14 Causes of hypoglycaemia in childhood.

Affected children usually lose the tendency to hypoglycaemia by the age of five.

Hyperinsulinism can cause persistent neonatal hypoglycaemia. There is often overgrowth of pancreatic ducts and islet cells. This rare condition was formerly known as nesidioblastosis. Many cases have been demonstrated to be the result of genetic mutations, for example in the genes for the sulphonylurea receptor, an ATP-dependent potassium channel in the plasma membrane of islet cells, glucokinase or glutamate dehydrogenase. In infants with glutamate dehydrogenase deficiency, a high protein intake can precipitate the hypoglycaemia, which probably explains what was formerly called 'leucine-induced hypoglycaemia'. The diagnosis is made on the basis of persistent hypoglycaemia without ketosis together with an inappropriate plasma insulin concentration. No tumour is demonstrable. 'Nesidioblastosis' may remit spontaneously in adolescence and should be treated medically (with diazoxide or octreotide), and only surgically, by subtotal pancreatectomy, if medical treatment fails to control the symptoms.

The inherited metabolic diseases associated with hypoglycaemia include galactosaemia, certain glycogen storage diseases, defects of the β-oxidation of fatty acids, hereditary fructose intolerance, and some organic acidaemias and amino acidopathies.

 Case history 11.8

A healthy two-month-old female infant, who had previously been breast-fed, vomited when given supplementary feeds of sweetened cows' milk. She reacted similarly when given fruit juice and sometimes became quiet and sleepy after such a feed. Her mother experimented with various feeds and learnt to avoid those that made her child ill. The child grew up with an aversion to sweet foodstuffs and fruit. Her brother, born three years later, had a similar history.

Later, when both became medical students, they wondered if their aversion was due to hereditary fructose intolerance. Fructose tolerance tests were performed and were found to induce hypoglycaemia, vomiting and other metabolic changes characteristic of this condition.

Comment

If the link between a child's illness and dietary fructose (and sucrose) is not made, there may be serious long-term consequences: failure to thrive, cirrhosis and renal tubular dysfunction, for example. If fructose is avoided and irreversible liver or kidney damage has not occurred, patients with hereditary fructose intolerance remain symptom-free. The cause of the intolerance is a lack of the B isoenzyme of fructose 1-phosphate aldolase, which catalyzes the conversion of fructose 1-phosphate and fructose 1,6-bisphosphate to trioses.

In the absence of the B isoenzyme, the other isoenzymes (A and C), which account for 15% of the catalytic activity, metabolize much less fructose 1-phosphate than normal but are still sufficiently active to convert fructose 1,6-bisphosphate to trioses in the glycolytic pathway. When fructose is ingested, however, it is still converted by fructokinase to fructose 1-phosphate in the normal way, but because the A and C isoenzymes have insufficient activity to metabolize it, the fructose 1-phosphate accumulates. The clinical manifestations stem from this accumulation, which inhibits glucose synthesis, and the depletion of ATP and phosphate as fructose is phosphorylated but not further metabolized.

SUMMARY

- **In health**, homoeostatic mechanisms ensure the maintenance of blood glucose concentrations within a narrow range, whether an individual is fed or fasting.

- **Diabetes mellitus** is a condition characterized by **abnormal glucose tolerance with a tendency to hyperglycaemia** and is due to a relative or absolute deficiency of insulin. It can occur secondarily to other pancreatic disease but the majority of cases are idiopathic. **Type 1** typically affects younger patients. It is an autoimmune disease and usually has an acute onset. **Type 2** typically affects middle-aged and elderly people and has a more gradual onset. Genetic and environmental factors are important in its pathogenesis.

- **Hyperglycaemia** leads to glycosuria and causes an osmotic diuresis, producing the classical clinical features of polyuria and thirst. If inadequately treated, patients with type 1 DM may develop **diabetic ketoacidosis**. In this condition, hyperglycaemia, together with increased lipolysis, proteolysis and ketogenesis, leads to severe dehydration, mineral loss, prerenal uraemia and a profound non-respiratory acidosis. Patients with type 2 DM appear to have sufficient insulin secretion to prevent the excessive lipolysis and ketogenesis that are essential to the production of ketoacidosis. Instead, inadequate treatment may lead to the development of very severe hyperglycaemia and dehydration, producing a **non-ketotic, hyperosmolar state**. Both ketoacidosis and non-ketotic hyperosmolar coma are medical emergencies; their management involves provision of fluid and insulin, with general supportive measures and treatment of any specific pre-existing or complicating factors.

- In the longer term, patients with diabetes are at risk of developing **microvascular complications** (retinopathy, neuropathy and nephropathy) and **atherosclerosis**. The presence of **microalbuminuria** may indicate early (and potentially treatable) nephropathy. Diabetes is associated with various perturbations of lipid metabolism that predispose to atherosclerosis.

- The **treatment** of diabetes is aimed at relieving symptoms and preventing both short- and long-term complications. The efficacy of treatment, whether with insulin, oral hypoglycaemic drugs or dietary modification alone, can be assessed clinically and by measurements of blood glucose concentration, both in the clinic and by patients themselves. Measurements of **glycated haemoglobin** (**HbA_{1c}**) provide a valuable index of glycaemic control over a period of several weeks.

- **The causes of hypoglycaemia** can be divided into two groups according to whether the condition occurs in the fasting state (fasting hypoglycaemia) or is provoked by a specific stimulus, which can include food intake (reactive hypoglycaemia). Causes of **fasting hypoglycaemia** include insulin-secreting tumours (**insulinomas**) and certain other tumours producing insulin-like substances, pituitary and adrenal failure, severe liver disease and glycogen storage diseases, notably type I (glucose 6-phosphatase deficiency). Except in patients with insulinomas, clinical features due to hypoglycaemia are rarely the only feature of any of these conditions. The diagnosis of an insulinoma depends upon the finding of inappropriately high insulin (and C-peptide) concentrations in the blood at a time when the patient is hypoglycaemic. This is often demonstrable after an overnight fast, precipitated if necessary by exercise. Provocation tests to stimulate insulin secretion are rarely required in patients with an insulinoma.

SUMMARY (cont'd)

- **Reactive hypoglycaemia** can be caused by drugs, including insulin and some oral hypoglycaemic agents. Hypoglycaemia can occur following alcohol ingestion; several distinct syndromes of alcohol-related hypoglycaemia have been described. Following gastric surgery, rapid transit of food into the small intestine can cause inappropriate insulin secretion and lead to hypoglycaemia.

- Hypoglycaemia is particularly common in **neonates** who are small-for-dates and is a risk in those born to diabetic mothers. It is also a feature of several inherited metabolic diseases.

- Acutely, hypoglycaemia causes **clinical features** related to increased activity of the sympathetic nervous system and decreased substrate supply to the central nervous system. These usually respond rapidly to the administration of glucose. Patients who are chronically hypoglycaemic, for example due to an insulinoma, often present with behavioural disturbance or frank psychosis and the acute manifestations of hypoglycaemia may be absent.

Calcium, phosphate and magnesium

INTRODUCTION

Calcium is the most abundant mineral in the human body. The average adult body contains approximately 25,000 mmol (1 kg), of which 99% is bound in the skeleton. The total calcium content of the extracellular fluid (ECF) is only 22.5 mmol, of which about 9 mmol is in the plasma (*Fig. 12.1*). Bone is not metabolically inert.

Most of the calcium in bone is stable but approximately 500 mmol/24 h moves between bone and the ECF to support calcium homoeostasis. Approximately 7.5 mmol/24 h moves between the stable pool and the ECF in the course of bone remodelling (*see below*). In the kidneys, ionized calcium is filtered by the glomeruli (240 mmol/24 h). Most of this is reabsorbed in the tubules and normal renal calcium excretion is 2.5–7.5 mmol/24 h. Obligatory renal calcium excretion

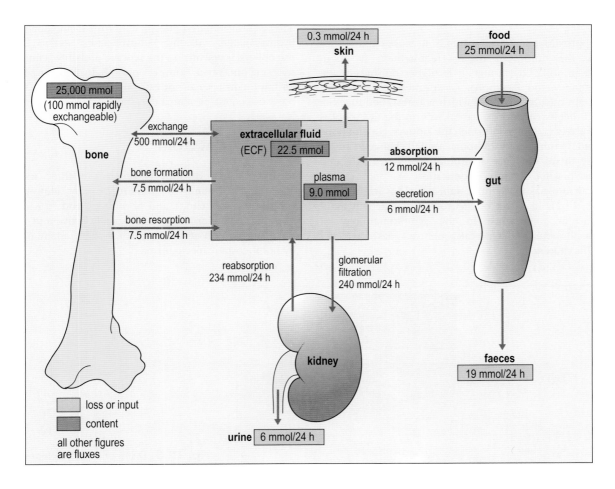

Fig. 12.1 Calcium exchange in the body.

Functions of calcium	
Function	**Example**
structural	bone teeth
neuromuscular	control of excitability release of neurotransmitters initiation of muscle contraction
enzymic	coenzyme for coagulation factors
signalling	intracellular second messenger

Fig. 12.2 Functions of calcium.

is approximately 2.5 mmol/24 h. Because of the faecal loss, the minimum dietary requirement is about 12.5 mmol/24 h (though it is higher during growth, pregnancy and lactation). Gastrointestinal secretions contain calcium, some of which is reabsorbed together with dietary calcium. Since calcium in the ECF pool is effectively exchanged through the kidneys, gut and bone about 33 times every 24 hours, a small change in any of these fluxes can have a profound effect on ECF, and hence plasma, calcium concentration.

Calcium has many important functions in the body (*Fig. 12.2*). Its effect on neuromuscular activity is of particular importance in the symptomatology of hypocalcaemia and hypercalcaemia, as is described later in this chapter.

BONE

Bone consists of osteoid, a collagenous organic matrix, on which is deposited complex inorganic hydrated calcium salts known as hydroxyapatites. These have the general formula:

$$Ca_{10}(PO_4)_6(OH)_2$$

Even when growth has ceased, bone remains biologically active. Continuous turnover ('remodelling') occurs with bone resorption (mediated by osteoclasts) being followed by new bone formation (mediated by osteoblasts) (*see Fig. 15.1*). At any one time, about 5% of bone mass in adults is subject to remodelling. This process is controlled and coordinated by hormones, growth factors and cytokines. Bone formation requires osteoid synthesis and adequate calcium and phosphate for the laying down of hydroxyapatite. Alkaline phosphatase, secreted by osteoblasts, is essential to the process, probably acting by releasing phosphate from pyrophosphate. Bone provides an important reservoir of calcium, phosphate and, to a lesser extent, magnesium and sodium.

PLASMA CALCIUM

In the plasma, calcium is present in three forms (*Fig. 12.3*): bound to protein (mainly albumin), complexed with citrate and phosphate, and free ions. Only the latter form is physiologically active and it is the concentration of ionized calcium that is maintained by homoeostatic mechanisms.

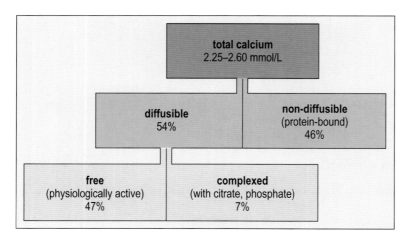

Fig. 12.3 Distribution of calcium in human plasma. Some 80% of the amount bound to protein is bound to albumin, the remainder to γ-globulins.

In alkalosis, hydrogen ions dissociate from albumin, and calcium binding to albumin increases. There is also an increase in calcium complex formation. As a result, the concentration of ionized calcium falls, and this may be sufficient to produce clinical symptoms and signs of hypocalcaemia although total plasma calcium concentration is unchanged. In an acute acidosis, the reverse effect is observed, i.e. the ionized calcium concentration is increased.

The most frequently used methods for determining plasma calcium concentration measure total calcium, although ionized calcium can be measured using an ion-selective electrode. However, accurate measurements of ionized calcium require the exclusion of air from the sample; this is inconvenient other than for point-of-care testing. Fortunately, measurements of total calcium are satisfactory for most clinical purposes. One undoubted advantage of ionized calcium measurements over conventional measurements of total calcium is the speed with which results are available. They may thus be useful to monitor calcium in circumstances when rapid changes in concentration can occur, for example during exchange blood transfusion and during surgery with extracorporeal bypass.

Changes in plasma albumin concentration will affect total calcium concentration independently of the ionized calcium concentration, leading to possible misinterpretation of results in both hypoproteinaemic and hyperproteinaemic states. Various formulae have been devised to indicate the total calcium concentration to be expected if the albumin concentration were normal. One widely used formula is given in *Fig. 12.4*,

but such estimates of 'corrected' calcium concentration should be interpreted with caution, especially when blood hydrogen ion concentration is abnormal. This is another instance where a direct measurement of ionized calcium may be helpful.

A common cause of apparent hyperproteinaemia, and hence hypercalcaemia, is venous stasis during blood sampling; this must be avoided when determinations of plasma calcium are to be made. For example, a tourniquet should not be used. Although globulins bind calcium to a lesser extent than albumin, the increase in γ-globulin in patients with myeloma can also increase the total plasma calcium concentration. In myeloma, however, hypercalcaemia is frequently present with an increased ionized calcium concentration because of the secretion of calcium-mobilizing substances by the tumour cells.

CALCIUM-REGULATING HORMONES

Calcium concentration in the ECF is normally maintained within narrow limits by a control system involving two hormones: parathyroid hormone (PTH) and calcitriol (1,25-dihydroxycholecalciferol). These hormones also control the inorganic phosphate concentration of the ECF. Calcitonin probably has only a minor role in calcium homoeostasis.

Parathyroid hormone

This hormone is a polypeptide, comprising 84 amino acids; as with many peptide hormones, it is synthesized as a larger precursor, pre-pro-PTH (115 amino acids). Prior to secretion, two amino acid sequences are lost; the removal of a 25 amino acid chain produces pro-PTH, a further six amino acids being removed to form PTH itself. The pre- and pro-sequences are thought to be involved in the intracellular transport of the hormone. The biological activity of PTH resides in the N-terminal 1–34 amino acid sequence of the hormone. PTH is secreted by the parathyroid glands in response to a fall in plasma (ionized) calcium concentration. Hypercalcaemia and calcitriol (*see below*) inhibit PTH secretion and synthesis, respectively. PTH acts on bone and the kidneys, tending to increase the plasma concentration of calcium and reduce that of phosphate (*Fig. 12.5*).

PTH mobilizes calcium from bone: this action is biphasic, a rapid phase involving existing cells (probably osteocytes) and a longer-term response dependent on the

---

Calculation of 'corrected' plasma calcium concentration
if plasma albumin concentration is [alb] g/L and measured total calcium is [Ca] mmol/L
for [alb] <40, corrected calcium = [Ca] + 0.02 × {40 − [alb]} mmol/L
for [alb] >45, corrected calcium = [Ca] − 0.02 × {[alb] − 45} mmol/L
for example: [Ca] = 1.82 mmol/L [alb] = 28 g/L 'corrected' calcium = 2.06 mmol/L

Fig. 12.4 Correction of plasma total calcium concentration for changes in albumin concentration.

Actions of parathyroid hormone			
	Target organ	**Action**	**Effect**
PTH	bone	rapid release of calcium ↑ osteoclastic resorption	↑ plasma [Ca⁺]
	kidney	↑ calcium reabsorption ↓ phosphate reabsorption ↑ 1α-hydroxylation of 25-hydroxycholecalciferol	↑ plasma [Ca⁺] ↓ plasma [Pi] ↑ calcium and phosphate absorption from gut
		↓ bicarbonate reabsorption	acidosis

Fig. 12.5 Actions of parathyroid hormone. In bone, PTH causes rapid release of calcium to the ECF mediated by osteocytes; calcitriol has a permissive effect on this process. PTH also stimulates osteoclastic bone resorption. Although it increases renal tubular reabsorption of calcium, the amount filtered is greatly increased as a result of hypercalcaemia, and hypercalciuria is usual. The phosphaturic action of PTH causes hypophosphataemia if renal function is normal.

proliferation of osteoclasts. In the kidneys, PTH increases the fraction of the filtered load that is reabsorbed. However, because increased resorption of bone increases the amount of calcium that is filtered, there is hypercalciuria despite the increased reabsorption. Also in the kidneys, PTH promotes phosphaturia by decreasing the reabsorption of filtered phosphate and stimulates the formation of calcitriol (*see Fig. 12.7*), the calcium-regulating hormone derived from vitamin D.

Despite the importance of PTH in the control of phosphate excretion, changes in phosphate concentration do not directly affect secretion of the hormone. Mild hypomagnesaemia stimulates PTH secretion, but more severe hypomagnesaemia reduces it, as the secretion of PTH is magnesium-dependent.

Intact PTH has a half-life in the blood of only 3–4 minutes. It is rapidly metabolized in liver and kidney, undergoing cleavage in the region of amino acids 33–37 and elsewhere. As a result, various fragments of the hormone are present in the blood as well as the intact hormone; these include an N-terminal fragment, with a similar half-life to that of the intact hormone, a C-terminal fragment (half-life: 2–3 hours) and others (*Fig. 12.6*). Previously used PTH immunoassays suffered from a lack of specificity for the biologically active moieties; even the now widely used immunometric assays for 'intact PTH' may detect an inactive fragment missing only the N-terminal six amino acids (PTH 7–84)

in addition to intact (1–84) PTH; assays that measure only PTH 1–84 are being introduced and appear to perform even better.

Calcitriol

This hormone is derived from vitamin D by successive hydroxylation in the liver (25-hydroxylation) and kidney (1α-hydroxylation). Hydroxylation in the liver is not subject to feedback control, but that in the kidney is closely regulated (*Fig. 12.7*). When the 1α-hydroxylation of 25-hydroxycholecalciferol is inhibited, there is an increase in 24-hydroxylation. The product of this reaction, 24,25-dihydroxycholecalciferol, has no known physiological function. Both this metabolite and calcitriol undergo further metabolism in the kidney to physiologically inactive products.

The principal actions of calcitriol are indicated in *Fig. 12.7*. In the gut, it stimulates absorption of dietary calcium and phosphate; this process involves the synthesis of a calcium-binding protein (calbindin D) in enterocytes. This protein is one of a widely distributed group of calcium-binding proteins that are present in many other tissues. In bone, calcitriol promotes mineralization largely indirectly, through its role in the maintenance of ECF calcium and phosphate concentrations. The binding of calcitriol to osteoblasts increases

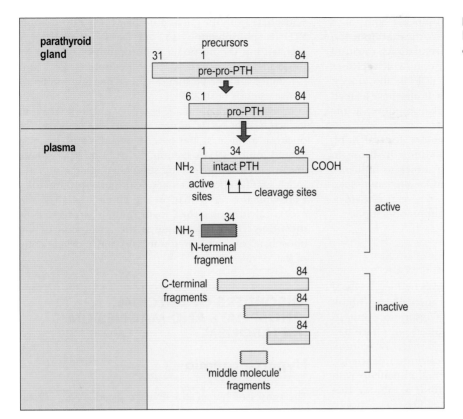

Fig. 12.6 Parathyroid hormone: precursors and cleavage products.

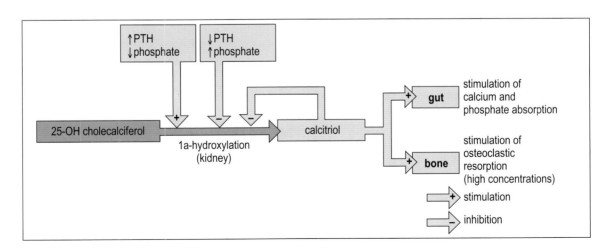

Fig 12.7 Calcitriol (1,25-dihydroxycholecalciferol): principal actions and control of renal synthesis. These actions increase the extracellular concentrations of calcium and phosphate. Other hormones, including growth hormone, prolactin and oestrogens, have a longer term stimulatory effect on calcitriol synthesis (25-OH cholecalciferol = 25-hydroxycholecalciferol).

the production of alkaline phosphatase and of a calcium-binding protein, osteocalcin, the exact function of which is uncertain. At high concentrations, calcitriol stimulates osteoclastic bone resorption, which releases calcium and phosphate into the ECF. In the kidney, calcitriol inhibits its own synthesis. It may have a small stimulatory effect on calcium reabsorption, acting permissively with PTH.

Many other tissues have receptors for calcitriol, suggesting that it has roles in addition to those in calcium homoeostasis. It has been shown to influence cellular differentiation in normal and malignant tissues; it also stimulates the production of several cytokines, suggesting that it has a role in immunomodulation.

Calcitonin

This polypeptide hormone, produced by the C-cells of the thyroid, can be shown experimentally to inhibit osteoclast activity, and thus bone resorption, but its physiological role is uncertain. Subjects who have had a total thyroidectomy do not develop a clinical syndrome that can be ascribed to calcitonin deficiency. Also, calcium homoeostasis is normal in patients with medullary carcinoma of the thyroid, a tumour that secretes large quantities of calcitonin. Plasma calcitonin concentration is elevated during pregnancy and lactation. So, too, is calcitriol concentration, and calcitonin may block the action of calcitriol on bone and permit increased calcium uptake from the gut to take place to satisfy increased requirements without loss of mineral from bone.

Calcitonin has been detected in many other sites, including the gut and the central nervous system, where it may act as a neurotransmitter. In some tissues, calcitonin m-RNA is translated to peptides other than calcitonin (calcitonin gene-related peptides). The function of these peptides is unknown.

CALCIUM AND PHOSPHATE HOMOEOSTASIS

The response of the body to a fall in plasma calcium concentration, provided that this is not due to disordered homoeostasis in the first instance, is illustrated in *Fig. 12.8*. Hypocalcaemia stimulates the secretion of PTH and, through this, increases the production of calcitriol. There is an increase in the uptake of both calcium and phosphate from the gut and in their release from bone. PTH is phosphaturic, so the excess phosphate is excreted but the fractional reabsorption of calcium by the kidney is increased, some of the mobilized calcium is retained and the plasma calcium concentration tends to rise towards normal.

In hypophosphataemia (*Fig. 12.9*), calcitriol secretion is increased but PTH is not. Indeed, any tendency for calcitriol to increase the plasma calcium concentration should inhibit PTH secretion. Calcium and phosphate absorption from the gut are stimulated. Calcitriol has a much smaller effect on renal calcium reabsorption than PTH with the result that, in the absence of PTH, the excess calcium absorbed from the gut is excreted in the urine. The net outcome is the restoration of the phosphate concentration towards normal, independently of that of calcium.

DISORDERS OF CALCIUM, PHOSPHATE AND MAGNESIUM METABOLISM

Hypercalcaemia

The causes of hypercalcaemia are listed in *Fig. 12.10*. Two conditions account for up to 90% of cases: primary hyperparathyroidism and malignancy. Hypercalcaemia may be discovered during the investigation of an illness in which it is known to be a potential complication or during the investigation of clinical features suggestive of hypercalcaemia (*Fig. 12.10*). However, hypercalcaemia is often clinically silent and discovered incidentally when calcium is measured as part of a biochemical profile.

Malignant disease

This is a very common cause of hypercalcaemia, particularly in patients in hospital. There may or may not be obvious metastases in bone. Patients with hypercalcaemia and malignant disease are usually symptomatic, owing to the malignancy, the hypercalcaemia or both. Non-metastatic hypercalcaemia is discussed on *p. 322*; with most solid tumours, it is due to the secretion by the tumour of PTH-related peptide (PTHrP). This is a peptide having some N-terminal amino acid sequence homology with PTH. It acts as a growth factor in the fetus but is not detectable in significant amounts in adults except in the breast during

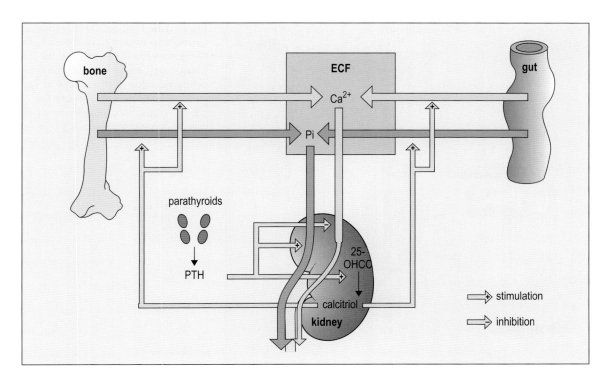

Fig. 12.8 Homoeostatic responses to hypocalcaemia. Hypocalcaemia stimulates the release of PTH, which in turn stimulates calcitriol synthesis. These hormones act together to restore plasma calcium concentration to normal, independently of phosphate concentration (25-OHCC = 25-hydroxycholecalciferol).

lactation. It is secreted in breast milk but its function in this fluid is unknown. In patients with metastases in bone there is often no relationship between the extent of metastasis and the severity of the hypercalcaemia, suggesting that humoral factors may be involved in the pathogenesis of hypercalcaemia in malignant disease whether or not osseous metastases are present. Other humoral factors that have been implicated include transforming growth factors, prostaglandins and, particularly in haematological malignancies, osteoclast-activating cytokines (*see Case History 13.1*).

Primary hyperparathyroidism

The prevalence of this condition is of the order of one case per thousand persons. It can occur at any age and affects both men and women but is most common in post-menopausal women. It is usually due to a parathyroid adenoma, less often to diffuse hyperplasia of the glands, and only rarely to parathyroid carcinoma.

Adenomas may be multiple and the condition is sometimes familial; it may occur as part of one of the syndromes of multiple endocrine neoplasia.

The definitive treatment for hyperparathyroidism is surgery. Patients with mild (<3.00 mmol/L) asymptomatic hypercalcaemia may stay healthy for many years without an operation, but are at increased risk of developing osteoporosis and renal impairment and should be reassessed regularly. A high fluid intake should be maintained to discourage renal calculus formation. Surgery is recommended even for asymptomatic patients if plasma calcium concentrations exceed 3.00 mmol/L, there is marked hypercalciuria (*see Case History 12.1*), complications (e.g. calculus formation, osteoporosis or renal impairment) are present, and in patients below the age of 50. Parathyroid adenomas are usually small and rarely palpable. Imaging techniques may help to localize the tumour preoperatively but are usually reserved for patients who have had previous surgery to the neck, in whom the normal anatomical

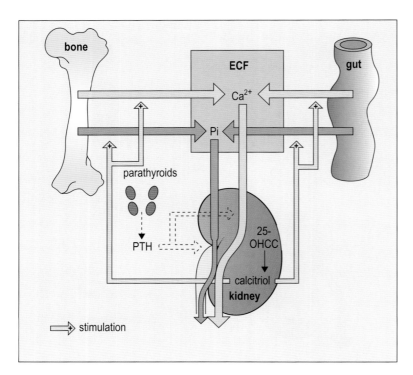

Fig. 12.9 Homoeostatic responses in hypophosphataemia. In the absence of PTH (secretion is not affected by phosphate), an increase in calcitriol production due to stimulation of 1α-hydroxylase tends to increase the plasma phosphate independently of calcium concentration.

relationships may have been distorted. ^{99m}Tc-sestamibi scanning is the most widely used localization technique. Selective cannulation of neck veins with measurement of PTH may also be helpful in localizing a tumour.

Secondary and tertiary hyperparathyroidism

Plasma PTH concentrations are also raised in many patients with chronic renal disease and with vitamin D deficiency. Both these conditions are associated with decreased synthesis of calcitriol, which causes hypocalcaemia, and the increase in PTH secretion is an appropriate physiological response. This is termed secondary hyperparathyroidism. The increase in PTH may not normalize the plasma calcium. In the absence of adequate calcitriol there is resistance to the calcium-mobilizing effect of PTH on bone. Occasionally, patients with end-stage renal failure become hypercalcaemic, owing to the development of autonomous PTH secretion, presumably as a result of the prolonged hypocalcaemic stimulus. Such hypercalcaemia may manifest for the first time in a patient given a renal transplant, who becomes able to metabolize vitamin D normally. This is termed tertiary hyperparathyroidism.

Parathyroid hormone is, in part, metabolized and excreted by the kidneys. Increased plasma concentrations of PTH in renal failure reflect impairment of these processes as well as increased secretion. Much of the excess consists of C-terminal fragments, which are inactive in calcium homoeostasis. Measurement of PTH is essential to the monitoring of patients with chronic renal failure.

Other causes of hypercalcaemia

Malignancy and hyperparathyroidism account for the majority of cases of hypercalcaemia but other conditions can be responsible. It is sometimes seen in patients with thyrotoxicosis, although thyroid hormones have no specific role in calcium homoeostasis, hypercalcaemia being due to the increased osteoclastic activity that may be present in this condition. Coincidental thyrotoxicosis may provoke symptomatic hypercalcaemia in a patient with mild, sub-clinical hyperparathyroidism. Thyrotoxicosis can also cause osteoporosis (see p. 280).

Excessive intake of vitamin D itself is a rare cause of hypercalcaemia, but the 1-hydroxylated derivatives (calcitriol, alfacalcidol) are extremely potent and may cause hypercalcaemia. Plasma calcium concentration

Hypercalcaemia	
Causes	**Clinical features**
Common	weakness, tiredness, lassitude, weight loss and
malignant disease, with or without	muscle weakness
metastasis to bone	
	mental changes (impaired concentration,
primary hyperparathyroidism	drowsiness, personality changes, coma)
	anorexia, nausea, vomiting and constipation
Less common	
thyrotoxicosis	abdominal pain (rarely peptic ulceration and
	pancreatitis)
vitamin D intoxication	
	polyuria, dehydration and renal failure
thiazide diuretics	
	renal calculi and nephrocalcinosis (mainly
sarcoidosis	associated with primary hyperparathyroidism)
familial hypocalciuric hypercalcaemia	short QT interval on ECG
renal transplantation (tertiary	cardiac arrhythmias and hypertension
hyperparathyroidism)	
	corneal calcification and vascular calcification
Uncommon	
milk–alkali syndrome	there may also be features of the underlying
	disorder, such as bone pain in malignant
lithium treatment	disease and hyperparathyroidism
tuberculosis	
immobilization (especially in Paget's disease)	
acute adrenal failure	
idiopathic hypercalcaemia of infancy	
diuretic phase of acute renal failure	

Fig. 12.10 Causes and clinical features of hypercalcaemia. Mild hypercalcaemia is often asymptomatic.

should be monitored regularly in patients treated with these agents.

In the milk–alkali syndrome, hypercalcaemia is associated with the ingestion of milk and antacids for the control of dyspeptic symptoms. The ingestion of alkali is important in the pathogenesis of the hypercalcaemia: it increases the renal reabsorption of filtered calcium but the precise mechanism is unknown. This syndrome is uncommon, and becoming more so since the introduction of drugs which inhibit gastric acid secretion for the treatment and prevention of peptic ulceration. It should also be remembered that dyspepsia itself may be a feature of hyperparathyroidism since calcium stimulates gastrin release. Occasionally, patients

Case history 12.1

A 51-year-old woman was investigated after two episodes of ureteric colic, shown on radiological examination to be due to calcium-containing calculi. She also complained of constipation, although she previously had normal bowel movements, but was otherwise well. No abnormality was found on physical examination.

Investigations

serum:	calcium	2.95 mmol/L
	phosphate	0.70 mmol/L
	total CO_2	19 mmol/L
	PTH (intact hormone assay)	150 ng/L
		(reference range 10–65 ng/L)
bone radiographs		normal
serum urea, albumin and alkaline phosphatase		all normal

Comment

Hyperparathyroidism may present in many ways (*see Fig. 12.10*), including renal or ureteric colic due to calculi which are themselves a result of hypercalciuria. Only about 10% of patients have clinical evidence of bone disease at presentation, although biochemical and radiological evidence is present in more than 20%. Many patients with hyperparathyroidism have no or few symptoms and are detected as a result of biochemical screening. Indeed, hyperparathyroidism is by far the most common cause of asymptomatic hypercalcaemia.

The plasma calcium concentration is nearly always raised. Exceptions to this occur if there is concomitant renal disease, vitamin D deficiency or hypothyroidism; occasionally the calcium is only raised intermittently. The phosphaturic action of PTH causes hypophosphataemia but this is not invariable; the plasma phosphate concentration may be normal or raised, particularly if there is renal damage. The plasma alkaline phosphatase is raised in only 20–30% of cases. Hypercalciuria is a reflection of the hypercalcaemia and is not usually of diagnostic importance. However, an excretion of >9 mmol/24 h is a risk factor for nephrolithiasis and should prompt a consideration of surgical intervention even in an asymptomatic patient. A low urine calcium excretion in a patient with hypercalcaemia is suggestive of familial hypocalciuric hypercalcaemia (*see p. 229*).

The plasma PTH concentration is usually elevated but may be high–normal. Measurements of PTH should be interpreted in relation to the plasma calcium concentration. If this is elevated by any mechanism that does not involve PTH, parathyroid activity should be suppressed. Although PTH secretion does not cease completely under these circumstances, the hormone will be undetectable in plasma or present only at a low concentration.

with parathyroid adenomas may have associated gastrin-secreting tumours (multiple endocrine neoplasia type 1).

Thiazide diuretics sometimes cause mild hypercalcaemia, owing to an effect on renal calcium excretion. Chronic lithium therapy can cause increased PTH secretion and is an occasional cause of hypercalcaemia. Approximately 10% of patients with sarcoidosis develop hypercalcaemia, as a result of 1-hydroxylation of 25-hydroxycholecalciferol by macrophages in the sarcoid granulomas. Hypercalcaemia can also complicate other granulomatous disorders (e.g. tuberculosis) for a similar reason. Hypercalcaemia is a rare feature of acute adrenal failure, possibly related to the sudden fall in cortisol concentration.

During a period of immobilization, there is a decreased stimulus to bone formation and continued resorption (a part of normal bone turnover) results in hypercalciuria. Hypercalcaemia is usually only seen in immobilized patients if there is pre-existing increased bone turnover, as occurs during puberty and in patients with Paget's disease.

Case history 12.2

A 38-year-old man developed thirst and polyuria while on holiday in Spain. He had no other symptoms. He consulted his family doctor when he arrived home. The urine was tested but there was no glycosuria. Blood was taken for biochemical investigations.

Investigations

serum:		
	calcium	3.24 mmol/L
	phosphate	1.20 mmol/L
	alkaline phosphatase	90 U/L
	urea	10.0 mmol/L
	creatinine	150 μmol/L

The patient, a non-smoker, was admitted to hospital for investigation. He had previously been well, apart from some joint pain and a painful rash on his legs several months before which had resolved spontaneously. The chest radiograph showed some increased hilar shadowing but was otherwise normal. No bony abnormality was seen on skeletal radiographs. He was slightly dehydrated and was given an intravenous saline infusion. Despite a good diuresis, the serum calcium remained elevated. He was then given hydrocortisone, 40 mg three times daily, and a week later the serum calcium was 2.80 mmol/L. At this time, the result of the PTH assay on blood taken on admission became available: no PTH was detected.

Comment

The patient presents with acute, symptomatic hypercalcaemia. The diagnosis could be hyperparathyroidism, an occult malignancy or some other condition. In view of the slight renal impairment, the normal serum phosphate is not helpful. PTH is undetectable, implying suppression of the parathyroids by hypercalcaemia, rather than autonomous PTH secretion, and the dramatic response to hydrocortisone also militates against hyperparathyroidism. The hypercalcaemia of malignancy responds unpredictably to steroids. The clue to the diagnosis is provided by the chest radiograph and the previous history, which are suggestive of sarcoidosis. The hypercalcaemia in this condition is characteristically sensitive to steroids and is often more severe in summer, owing to increased synthesis of vitamin D by the action of ultraviolet light on the skin. The diagnosis of sarcoidosis was further supported by the finding of a raised serum angiotensin-converting enzyme activity.

Familial hypocalciuric hypercalcaemia is inherited as an autosomal dominant trait. It is a result of mutation in the calcium-sensor gene, which leads to an increase in the parathyroids' set point for calcium. Chronic hypercalcaemia develops from childhood and is usually asymptomatic. Hypophosphataemia is sometimes present; PTH concentrations are usually normal but may be slightly elevated. The diagnosis may be made only when hypercalcaemia persists after parathyroidectomy, but it may be inferred from finding a low rate of calcium excretion in the urine of a patient with hypercalcaemia (the ratio of calcium clearance to creatinine clearance is typically less than 0.01: in primary hyperparathyroidism it is usually greater than 0.02), or from the presence of hypercalcaemia in an infant relative.

The cause of idiopathic hypercalcaemia of infancy is unknown. It is associated with characteristic elfin facies and supravalvar aortic stenosis (Williams' syndrome). The hypercalcaemia usually resolves by the age of four years.

Investigation

The way in which hypercalcaemia is investigated is dependent on the clinical setting. In hospital patients, malignancy is much commoner than hyperparathyroidism;

the reverse is true in asymptomatic individuals with hypercalcaemia. In any patient, clinical features of the causative disorder may be present. The plasma phosphate concentration is of limited diagnostic value: although low in most uncomplicated cases of primary hyperparathyroidism, it can also be decreased in hypercalcaemia due to malignancy and can be raised in either condition if there is renal impairment. Plasma alkaline phosphatase activity can be elevated in either condition, although is more frequently so in malignant disease.

Radiographic examination may occasionally reveal the characteristic subperiosteal bone reabsorption and bone cysts of hyperparathyroidism, but these are only present in a minority of cases. A primary lung tumour or bony metastases will often, but not always, be revealed by radiography, but other tumours may not be so easily detected.

Measurement of PTH, using an assay for the intact hormone, is essential. Even if there is clear evidence of malignant disease or some other cause of hypercalcaemia, hyperparathyroidism is sufficiently common for there to be a real possibility of it being present coincidentally. The measurement of urinary calcium excretion is of no diagnostic value, except in the diagnosis of familial hypocalciuric hypercalcaemia.

If hyperparathyroidism and malignancy are excluded, reassessment of the history, for both drugs and features of other conditions associated with hypercalcaemia, may prompt appropriate further investigations.

Management

When possible, the underlying cause should be treated but the hypercalcaemia itself may require treatment in the short term. Dehydrated patients should be rehydrated with intravenous saline. Once this has been achieved, an intravenous infusion of a bisphosphonate can be given to lower the calcium. Furosemide (frusemide) is sometimes recommended (it inhibits renal calcium reabsorption) but can worsen any dehydration. If hypercalcaemia does not respond to a bisphosphonate, calcitonin or high-dose corticosteroids may be effective. Intravenous infusion of sodium phosphate has been recommended in the past but is potentially very dangerous, particularly in patients with renal impairment, since it may cause extensive metastatic calcification. Life-threatening resistant hypercalcaemia may require treatment by dialysis or, exceptionally, emergency parathyroidectomy.

Hypocalcaemia

The causes of hypocalcaemia are listed in *Fig. 12.11*. Deficiency or impaired metabolism of vitamin D, renal failure, hypoparathyroidism and hypomagnesaemia account for the majority of cases. The importance of interpreting a low plasma calcium concentration in relation to the albumin concentration has already been stressed. The clinical features relate to increased neural and muscular excitability (*Fig. 12.11*). Mild hypocalcaemia may be asymptomatic: in severe cases the condition can be life-threatening.

Vitamin D deficiency

The causes of this condition, which causes osteomalacia in adults and rickets in children, are discussed in *Chapter 15*. Deficiency may be due to inadequate endogenous synthesis or dietary supply of vitamin D, or to malabsorption. Whatever the cause, the effect is to decrease the amount of 25-hydroxycholecalciferol available for calcitriol synthesis, leading to decreased absorption of calcium and phosphate from the gut (see *Case History 6.3*). Although the 1α-hydroxylation of 25-hydroxycholecalciferol is stimulated in hypocalcaemia, with severe deficiency of the vitamin, lack of the substrate will prevent sufficient calcitriol being formed.

Vitamin D deficiency is a cause of secondary hyperparathyroidism. This further lowers the plasma phosphate concentration and patients with vitamin D deficiency usually have hypocalcaemia, hypophosphataemia and a raised plasma alkaline phosphatase activity. The plasma concentration of 25-hydroxycholecalciferol is low.

Impaired vitamin D metabolism

The formation of calcitriol requires the successive hydroxylation of vitamin D in the liver and kidneys. Renal disease as a cause of hypocalcaemia is discussed below.

Hypocalcaemia and bone disease are occasionally seen in epileptic patients treated with phenobarbital or phenytoin. Both drugs are inducers of hepatic microsomal hydroxylating enzymes and are thought to alter the metabolism of vitamin D in the liver. They probably also directly inhibit intestinal calcium absorption. In some forms of chronic liver disease, particularly primary biliary cirrhosis, hypocalcaemia and a metabolic bone disease with some features of osteomalacia develop. Mechanisms include malabsorp-

Hypocalcaemia	
Causes	**Clinical features**
Artefactual (blood collected into EDTA tube)	behavioural disturbance and stupor
	numbness and paraesthesiae
Associated with low PTH concentration	muscle cramps and spasms (tetany)
hypoparathyroidism	laryngeal stridor
hypomagnesaemia	convulsions
hungry bone syndrome (*see p. 232*)	cataracts (chronic hypocalcaemia)
neonatal hypocalcaemia	basal ganglia calcification (chronic hypocalcaemia)
	papilloedema
Associated with high PTH concentration	Trousseau's sign positive
vitamin D deficiency:	Chvostek's sign positive
dietary	prolonged QT interval on ECG
malabsorption	
inadequate exposure to ultraviolet light	
disordered vitamin D metabolism:	
renal failure	
anticonvulsant treatment	
1α-hydroxylase deficiency	
pseudohypoparathyroidism	
acute pancreatitis	
high phosphate intake (rare)	
massive transfusion with citrated blood	
acute rhabdomyolysis	

Fig. 12.11 Causes and clinical features of hypocalcaemia. Chvostek's sign (contraction of facial muscles on tapping facial nerve) and Trousseau's sign (carpal spasm when sphygmomanometer cuff applied to upper arm is inflated to midway between systolic and diastolic blood pressures for 3 min) may be positive before other signs are present (latent tetany). Additional features in patients with vitamin D deficiency include myopathy and bone pain.

tion of vitamin D, decreased 25-hydroxylation and decreased synthesis of vitamin D-binding protein.

Inherited disorders of vitamin D metabolism are discussed on *p. 82*.

Renal disease

Hypocalcaemia is common in patients with end-stage renal disease (see *Case History 4.3*) but is rarely symptomatic. It is often associated with a complex metabolic bone disease known as renal osteodystrophy. This condition is discussed in *Chapter 4*.

Hypoparathyroidism

This can be congenital or acquired. Acquired causes are listed in *Fig. 12.12*. The congenital form may be associated with thymic aplasia and immune deficiency, the DiGeorge syndrome.

Pseudohypoparathyroidism superficially resembles hypoparathyroidism, but plasma concentrations of PTH are elevated. There are two types: both are hereditary disorders. The effects of PTH are mediated through the formation of cyclic 3,5-AMP. In type 1, activation of adenyl cyclase is defective and cyclic AMP is not formed in response to the binding of PTH to its receptor. In type 2, cyclic AMP is formed, but the responses to it are blocked. The two types can be distinguished by measuring urinary cyclic AMP after administration of PTH. In normal individuals, and in patients with type 2 pseudohypoparathyroidism, there is an increase; in type 1, this does not occur. Patients with type 1 pseudohypoparathyroidism have characteristic skeletal abnormalities, including a rounded face, short stature, shortening of the fourth and fifth metacarpals and metatarsals, and a tendency for exostoses to form. Patients may have learning difficulties. In

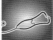

Case history 12.3

A 56-year-old woman was admitted to hospital for cataract extraction, in good health apart from her failing vision. She had undergone thyroidectomy for a multinodular goitre 20 years earlier. Routine preoperative investigations were carried out.

Investigations

serum:		
	calcium	1.60 mmol/L
	phosphate	2.53 mmol/L
	albumin	44 g/L
	alkaline phosphatase	76 U/L

Comment

The combination of hypocalcaemia, hyperphosphataemia and a normal alkaline phosphatase is typical of hypoparathyroidism, probably due in this case to inadvertent removal of the glands. It is not uncommon for patients with chronic hypocalcaemia to be symptom free. In this patient, both Chvostek's and Trousseau's signs (*see Fig. 12.11*) were positive. Cataracts are a recognized complication of hypoparathyroidism, presumably because the high phosphate concentration leads to precipitation of calcium phosphate in the lens.

Causes of hypoparathyroidism
Congenital (may be associated with immune deficiency)
Acquired idiopathic autoimmune (may be associated with other organ-specific endocrine disease) surgery (thyroidectomy) haemochromatosis infiltrative conditions

Fig. 12.12 Causes of hypoparathyroidism.

---

pseudohypoparathyroidism, similar skeletal abnormalities are present but the plasma calcium concentration is normal. All these conditions are rare.

Hungry bone syndrome

This term is used to describe the hypocalcaemia (often severe and symptomatic) that can follow the treatment of conditions in which hypercalcaemia has been caused by increased bone resorption. It is particularly associated with the surgical treatment of primary hyperparathyroidism and thyrotoxicosis. Removal of the stimulus to bone resorption results in rapid uptake of calcium by bone, leading to hypocalcaemia. With parathyroid adenomas and in hypercalcaemic thyrotoxicosis, continuing suppression of normal PTH production may contribute to the hypocalcaemia. Hungry bone syndrome should be anticipated, and should be preventable by the

provision of vitamin D and calcium pre- and post-operatively; this is the treatment if the condition does occur.

Magnesium deficiency

Since magnesium is required for both PTH secretion and its action on target tissues, magnesium deficiency can cause hypocalcaemia or render patients insensitive to the treatment of hypocalcaemia with vitamin D or calcium, or both.

Pancreatitis

The causes of hypocalcaemia in acute pancreatitis are discussed in *Chapter 6*.

Management

Patients with symptomatic hypocalcaemia are usually treated with intravenous calcium gluconate at least until their symptoms are controlled. Any coexisting magnesium deficiency must also be corrected. Persistent hypocalcaemia is usually treated with calcium supplements, vitamin D (or its hydroxylated derivatives) or both, according to the cause.

Hyperphosphataemia

By far the most common cause of hyperphosphataemia is renal insufficiency; other causes are listed in *Fig. 12.13*. Hyperphosphataemia is a hazard if infants are fed undiluted cows' milk but excessive intake is an uncommon cause in adults, only occurring if excessive

Causes of hyperphosphataemia

renal failure
hypoparathyroidism
pseudohypoparathyroidism
acromegaly
excessive phosphate intake/administration
vitamin D intoxication
catabolic states, e.g. tumour lysis syndrome

Fig. 12.13 Causes of hyperphosphataemia. This can develop *in vitro* if there is a delay in separating serum from cells prior to analysis.

 Case history 12.4

An elderly woman who presented with weight loss and malabsorption due to amyloidosis of the small intestine was found to have osteomalacia and was hypocalcaemic. She was given parenteral nutritional support but despite what was considered to be adequate calcium and vitamin D supplementation, she remained hypocalcaemic.

Investigations

serum magnesium   0.35 mmol/L

Comments

Patients with malabsorption may develop magnesium deficiency and while this patient's parenteral feeds contained magnesium, there was presumably an insufficient amount to correct her deficit. When she was given additional magnesium supplements, her serum calcium rapidly returned to normal.

Causes of hypophosphataemia

vitamin D deficiency
primary hyperparathyroidism
enteral/parenteral nutrition with inadequate
    phosphate (particularly in malnourished
    patients); intravenous glucose
    therapy
diabetic ketoacidosis (recovery phase)
alcohol withdrawal
renal tubular disease
phosphate binding agents, such as magnesium
    and aluminium salts (rare)
respiratory alkalosis

Fig. 12.14 Causes of hypophosphataemia.

hydroxycholecalciferol in the kidney; phosphate may also combine with calcium, resulting in metastatic calcium deposits in the tissues and hypocalcaemia.

Management

Management should be directed at the underlying cause but, in practice, the most effective treatment is to give calcium or aluminium salts by mouth to bind phosphate in the gut and reduce its absorption.

Hypophosphataemia

This is a common biochemical finding. When mild it is probably of little consequence, but severe hypophosphataemia (<0.3 mmol/L) can have important consequences on the function of all cells, particularly muscle cells (causing muscle weakness or even rhabdomyolysis), red and white blood cells, and platelets, by limiting the formation of essential phosphate-containing compounds such as adenosine triphosphate (ATP) and 2,3-diphosphoglycerate (2,3-DPG). Chronic hypophosphataemia is a cause of rickets and osteomalacia.

Hypophosphataemia can be due to decreased intestinal absorption, increased renal excretion or redistribution. Specific causes are given in *Fig. 12.14*. Although hyperphosphataemia is usual in diabetic ketoacidosis, hypophosphataemia is seen during the recovery phase when there is increased uptake of phosphate into depleted tissues. This is also the mechanism of hypophosphataemia seen in patients with

phosphate is given intravenously, for example during parenteral feeding. Increased tissue catabolism, for example in the treatment of malignant disease (particularly haematological malignancy), can cause hyperphosphataemia. Tissue catabolism is also one of its causes in diabetic ketoacidosis, but in these patients renal impairment is often also present.

Hyperphosphataemia is important clinically because it results in inhibition of the 1-hydroxylation of 25-

malnutrition who are given a high calorie intake either enterally or parenterally (see Case History 20.3). Hypophosphataemia is common during alcohol withdrawal and is multifactorial in origin. The causes include decreased intake, alkalosis and refeeding. Respiratory alkalosis can cause hypophosphataemia by stimulating phosphofructokinase and the formation of phosphorylated glycolytic intermediates.

Management

Hypophosphataemia should be anticipated, and prevented, in conditions where it may occur. It is treated by the administration of phosphate, either enterally or parenterally as appropriate, but intravenous phosphate should not be given to a patient who is hypercalcaemic or oliguric.

Magnesium

Magnesium is the fourth most abundant cation in the body. The adult human body contains approximately 1000 mmol, with about half in bone and the remainder distributed equally between muscle and other soft tissues. Only 11–17 mmol is found in the ECF, the plasma concentration being 0.8–1.2 mmol/L. The normal daily intake of magnesium (10–12 mmol) is greater than is necessary to maintain magnesium balance (approximately 8 mmol/24 h) and the excess is excreted through the kidneys.

Urinary magnesium excretion is increased by ECF volume expansion, hypercalcaemia and hypermagnesaemia, and decreased in the opposite of these states. There is no one specific homoeostatic mechanism for magnesium. Various hormones, including PTH and aldosterone, affect the renal handling of magnesium; the effects of aldosterone are probably secondary to changes in ECF volume but PTH, which increases the tubular reabsorption of filtered magnesium, appears to act directly.

Magnesium acts as a cofactor for some 300 enzymes, including enzymes involved in protein synthesis, glycolysis and the transmembrane transport of ions. A magnesium–ATP complex is the substrate for many ATP-requiring enzymes. Magnesium is important in the maintenance of the structure of ribosomes, nucleic acids and some proteins. It interacts with calcium in several ways and affects the permeability of excitable membranes and their electrical properties

such that extracellular magnesium depletion causes hyperexcitability.

Hypermagnesaemia

Significant hypermagnesaemia is uncommon. Cardiac conduction is affected at concentrations of 2.5–5.0 mmol/L; very high concentrations (>7.5 mmol/L) cause respiratory paralysis and cardiac arrest. Such extreme hypermagnesaemia may occasionally be seen in renal failure.

Intravenous calcium may give short-term protection against the adverse effects of hypermagnesaemia but in renal failure dialysis may be necessary.

Hypomagnesaemia

Hypomagnesaemia almost always indicates magnesium deficiency. Surveys have shown that it may be present in up to 10% of hospital patients; it occurs more frequently than hypermagnesaemia. The causes and clinical features are summarized in Fig. 12.15. Hypocalcaemia, due to decreased PTH secretion, is a clinically important consequence of hypomagnesaemia (see Case History 12.4). Hypophosphataemia and hypokalaemia may also be present, but all these abnormalities usually respond to magnesium supplementation. Plasma

Magnesium deficiency
Causes
malabsorption, malnutrition and fistulae
alcoholism (chronic alcoholism and alcohol withdrawal)
cirrhosis
diuretic therapy (especially loop diuretics)
renal tubular disorders (in advanced renal disease hypermagnesaemia is usual)
chronic mineralocorticoid excess
Clinical features
tetany (with normal or decreased calcium)
agitation, delirium
ataxia, tremor, choreiform movements and convulsions
muscle weakness, cardiac arrhythmias

Fig. 12.15 Causes and clinical features of magnesium deficiency.

Case history 12.5

A young man presented with a short history of severe diarrhoea, abdominal pain, weight loss and rectal bleeding. He had had several previous episodes of diarrhoea and abdominal pain, but these had been much milder and he had not sought medical advice. He also complained of cramp in his arms and legs, and on testing had latent tetany.

Investigations

serum:		
	sodium	142 mmol/L
	potassium	3.1 mmol/L
	urea	5.4 mmol/L
	creatinine	96 μmol/L
	calcium	2.42 mmol/L
	phosphate	0.9 mmol/L
	albumin	44 g/L

Comment

The low potassium concentration was thought to reflect potassium loss in the stool. In view of the normal calcium, his serum magnesium was measured and found to be 0.38 mmol/L. He was given parenteral magnesium replacement (not oral, in view of his diarrhoea) and the cramps resolved. Crohn's disease was diagnosed from the appearances of a rectal biopsy.

When symptoms of hypocalcaemia occur in patients whose serum calcium concentration is normal, hypomagnesaemia should be considered as a cause. Low concentrations of magnesium are often found in association with low concentrations of calcium, phosphate and potassium but hypomagnesaemia can occur in isolation. Other manifestations include cardiac arrhythmias and delirium.

magnesium concentration should always be measured in patients with hypocalcaemia, or clinical features suggestive of hypocalcaemia, when these do not respond to calcium supplementation, and also in patients with refractory hypokalaemia. Other indications for its measurement include parenteral nutrition, chronic diarrhoea and other conditions listed in *Fig. 12.15*.

Mild magnesium deficiency is treated by oral supplementation; in severe deficiency, and with malabsorption, magnesium may be given by slow intravenous infusion.

SUMMARY

- **Calcium** has many functions in the body in addition to its **structural role** in bones and teeth. It is essential for **muscle contraction**, affects the **excitability of nerves**, is a **second messenger**, involved in the action of several hormones, and is required for **blood coagulation**.

- About half the calcium in the plasma is bound to protein; it is the unbound fraction that is physiologically active and whose concentration is closely regulated.

SUMMARY (cont'd)

- Two hormones have a central role in **calcium homoeostasis**. The main action of **calcitriol**, the hormone derived from vitamin D by successive hydroxylations in liver and kidney, is to stimulate calcium (and phosphate) uptake from the gut. **Parathyroid hormone (PTH)**, secreted in response to a fall in plasma ionized calcium concentration, stimulates calcitriol formation, stimulates calcium resorption from bone and reabsorption by the renal tubules, and has a powerful phosphaturic action. These two hormones also regulate extracellular phosphate concentration. **Calcitonin** has only a minor role in calcium homoeostasis.

- The common causes of **hypercalcaemia** are **primary hyperparathyroidism**, due to parathyroid adenomas or hyperplasia, and **malignant disease**, with or without metastasis to bone, including myeloma. Less common causes include sarcoidosis and overdosage with vitamin D or its derivatives. Mild hypercalcaemia is often asymptomatic; when more severe, clinical features may include bone and abdominal pain, renal calculi, polyuria, thirst and behavioural disturbances.

- **Hypocalcaemia** causes hyperexcitability of nerve and muscle, leading to muscle spasm (tetany) and, in severe cases, to convulsions. Causes include **vitamin D deficiency** and **hypoparathyroidism**. Vitamin D deficiency may be either dietary in origin, often exacerbated by poor exposure to sunlight (and hence reduced endogenous synthesis), or due to malabsorption.

- **Hyperphosphataemia** is particularly associated with renal failure; it inhibits vitamin D metabolism and can cause hypocalcaemia. Severe **hypophosphataemia**, such as can occur with inadequate phosphate provision during intravenous feeding, has potentially harmful effects on many body tissues, particularly blood cells and skeletal muscle.

- **Magnesium** is an essential cofactor for many enzymes. Its concentration in the extracellular fluid is controlled primarily through regulation of its urinary excretion. **Hypomagnesaemia** can cause clinical features similar to those of hypocalcaemia and indeed can cause hypocalcaemia, since the secretion of parathyroid hormone is magnesium-dependent. Deficiency of magnesium can occur with prolonged diarrhoea and malabsorption. **Hypermagnesaemia** is common in renal failure, but it appears to be tolerated well by the body and increased concentrations rarely give rise to obvious clinical disturbances.

Plasma proteins and enzymes

INTRODUCTION

Proteins are present in all body fluids, but it is the proteins of the blood plasma that are examined most frequently for diagnostic purposes. Over 100 individual proteins have a physiological function in the plasma. Their principal functions, and some of the proteins, are indicated in *Fig. 13.1*. Quantitatively, the single most important protein is albumin. With the exception of fibrinogen, the other proteins are known collectively as globulins. Changes in the concentrations of individual proteins occur in many conditions and their measurement can provide useful diagnostic information.

Some plasma proteins are enzymes (e.g. renin, coagulation factors). In addition to these, many primarily intracellular enzymes are detectable in plasma as a result of their loss from cells during normal cell turnover. The measurement of such enzymes provides a sensitive (though often relatively non-specific) indicator of tissue damage. Most of these enzymes are described in chapters of this book describing conditions in which their measurement is of particular value, but some general principles of the use of enzyme measurements are discussed in this chapter.

MEASUREMENT OF PLASMA PROTEINS

Total plasma protein

In very general terms, variations in plasma protein concentrations can be due to any of three changes: in the rate of protein synthesis, the rate of removal, and in the volume of distribution.

The concentration of proteins in plasma is affected by posture: an increase in concentration of 10–20% occurs within 30 minutes of becoming upright after a period of recumbency. Also, if a tourniquet is applied before venepuncture, a significant rise in protein concentration can occur within a few minutes. In both cases, the change in protein concentration is caused by increased diffusion of fluid from the vascular into the interstitial

Functions of plasma proteins	
Function	**Example**
transport	thyroxine-binding globulin (thyroid hormones) apolipoproteins (cholesterol, triglyceride) transferrin (iron)
humoral immunity	immunoglobulins
maintenance of oncotic pressure	all proteins, particularly albumin
enzymes	renin coagulation factors complement proteins
protease inhibitors	α_1-antitrypsin (acts on proteases)
buffering	all proteins

Fig. 13.1 Functions of plasma proteins.

compartment. These effects must be borne in mind when blood is being drawn for the determination of protein concentration.

Only changes in the more abundant plasma proteins (i.e. albumin or immunoglobulins) will have a significant effect on the total protein concentration.

Except when patients have been given blood or proteins intravenously, a rapid increase in total plasma protein concentration is always due to a decrease in the volume of distribution (in effect, to dehydration). A rapid decrease is often the result of an increase in plasma volume. Thus, changes in plasma protein concentration can provide a valuable aid to the assessment of a patient's state of hydration.

The total protein concentration of plasma can also fall rapidly if capillary permeability increases, since protein will diffuse out into the interstitial space. This can be seen, for example, in patients with septicaemia or generalized inflammatory conditions. Causes of increased

Causes of changes in total plasma protein concentration			
Increase		**Decrease**	
hypergammaglobulinaemia paraproteinaemia	↑ protein synthesis	malnutrition and malabsorption liver disease humoral immunodeficiency	↓ protein synthesis
artefactual	haemoconcentration due to stasis of blood during venepuncture	over-hydration increased capillary permeability	↑ volume of distribution
		protein-losing states catabolic states	↑ excretion/ catabolism
dehydration	↓ volume of distribution		

Fig.13.2 Causes of changes in total plasma protein concentration.

and decreased total plasma protein concentration are summarized in *Fig. 13.2*.

Protein electrophoresis

This technique was formerly widely used for the semi-quantitative assessment of plasma proteins but now that specific assays are available for all the important proteins, it only remains essential for the detection of paraproteins (monoclonal proteins produced by tumours of B-cell origin, particularly myeloma). Electrophoresis is usually performed on serum rather than plasma since the fibrinogen present in plasma produces a band in the β_2 region that might be mistaken for a paraprotein.

Electrophoresis, on cellulose acetate or agarose gel, separates the proteins into distinct bands: albumin, α_1- and α_2-globulins, β-globulins and γ-globulins. Plasma proteins are often still classified into groups according to their electrophoretic mobility (*Fig. 13.3*) although this classification has no relevance in relation to their function, with the exception that the normal immuno-globulins migrate (and are still often referred to) as γ-globulins.

Fig. 13.4 shows diagrammatically the appearance of normal serum (a) and serum containing a paraprotein (b) after electrophoresis on agarose gel and staining with a protein-sensitive stain. Note that in (b) there is a decrease in normal immunoglobulins, as characteristically occurs in patients with paraproteinaemia due to myeloma (*see p. 244*). Paraproteins typically migrate in the γ-region but (especially the IgA class) may migrate more anodally. Pattern (c) shows a polyclonal increase in immunoglobulins (as may occur in some auto-immune diseases and chronic infections).

SPECIFIC PLASMA PROTEINS

Albumin

Albumin, the most abundant plasma protein, makes the major contribution (about 80%) to the oncotic pressure of plasma. Oncotic pressure is the osmotic pressure due to the presence of proteins and is an important determinant of the distribution of extracellular fluid (ECF) between the intravascular and extravascular compartments.

In hypoalbuminaemic states, the decreased plasma oncotic pressure disturbs the equilibrium between plasma and interstitial fluid with the result that there is a decrease in the movement of the interstitial fluid back into the blood at the venular end of the capillaries (*Fig. 13.5*). The accumulation of interstitial fluid is seen clinically as oedema. The relative decrease in plasma volume results in a fall in renal blood flow. This stimulates the secretion of renin, and hence of aldosterone, through the formation of angiotensin (secondary aldosteronism, *see p. 22*). This results in sodium retention and thus an increase in ECF volume, which potentiates the oedema.

There are many possible causes of hypoalbuminaemia (*Fig. 13.6*), a combination of which may be important in individual cases. For example, in a patient with malabsorption due to Crohn's disease, a low albumin

Principal plasma proteins		
Class	**Protein**	**Approximate mean serum concentration (g/L)**
	prealbumin	0.25
	albumin	40
α_1-globulin	α_1-antitrypsin α_1-acid glycoprotein	2.9 1.0
α_2-globulin	haptoglobins α_2-macroglobulin caeruloplasmin	2.0 2.6 0.35
β-globulin	transferrin low density lipoprotein complement components (C3)	3.0 1.0 1.0
γ-globulins	IgG IgA IgM IgD IgE	14.0 3.5 1.5 0.03 trace

Fig. 13.3 Principal plasma proteins. Many other important proteins are present in only very low concentrations, for example thyroxine-binding globulin, transcortin and vitamin-D binding globulin.

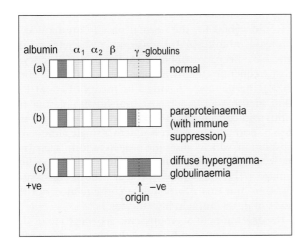

Fig. 13.4 Some typical serum electrophoretic abnormalities.

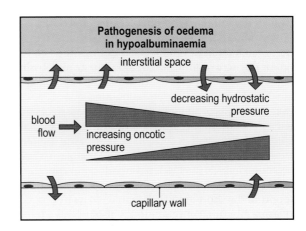

Fig. 13.5 Pathogenesis of oedema in hypoalbuminaemia. The normal balance of hydrostatic and oncotic pressures is such that there is net movement of fluid out of the capillaries at their arteriolar ends and net movement in at their venular ends (indicated here by arrows). Oedema can thus be due to an increase in capillary hydrostatic pressure, a decrease in plasma oncotic pressure, or an increase in capillary permeability.

Causes of hypoalbuminaemia
Decreased synthesis
malnutrition
malabsorption
liver disease
Increased volume of distribution
over-hydration
increased capillary permeability:
septicaemia
hypoxia
Increased excretion/degradation
nephrotic syndrome
protein-losing enteropathies
burns
haemorrhage
catabolic states:
severe sepsis
fever
trauma
malignant disease

Fig. 13.6 Causes of hypoalbuminaemia.

may reflect both decreased synthesis (decreased supply of amino acids due to malabsorption) and increased loss (directly into the gut from ulcerated mucosa).

Hyperalbuminaemia can be either an artefact, for instance as a result of venous stasis during blood collection, or due to over-infusion of albumin or to dehydration. Albumin synthesis is increased in some pathological states but this never causes hyperalbuminaemia.

Measurements of albumin concentration are frequently used in relation to the provision of nutritional support. This topic is discussed in detail in *Chapter 20* but it should be noted that, because of its relatively long plasma half-life (approximately 20 days), plasma albumin concentration is not a useful marker of the response to nutritional support in the short term (less than ten days).

Plasma albumin concentration is also used as a test of liver function. Because of its relatively long half-life in the plasma, albumin concentration is usually normal in acute hepatitis. Low concentrations are characteristic of chronic liver disease, being due to both decreased synthesis and an increase in the volume of distribution as a result of fluid retention and the formation of ascites.

Albumin is a high capacity, low affinity transport protein for many substances, such as thyroid hormones,

calcium and fatty acids. The influence of low plasma albumin concentration on measurements of thyroid hormones and calcium is considered on *pp. 162* and *220*, respectively. Albumin binds unconjugated bilirubin, and hypoalbuminaemia increases the risk of kernicterus in infants with unconjugated hyperbilirubinaemia. Salicylates, which displace bilirubin from albumin, can have a similar effect.

Many drugs are bound to albumin in the blood and a decrease in albumin concentration can have important pharmacokinetic consequences, for example increasing the concentration of free drug and thus the risk of toxicity.

A number of molecular variants of albumin exist. In bisalbuminaemia, the variant protein has a slightly different electrophoretic mobility from normal albumin and a pair of albumin bands is seen on electrophoresis: there are no clinical consequences. Analbuminaemia is a rare, inherited condition in which the plasma albumin concentration is 250 mg/L or less. People with this condition tend to suffer episodic mild oedema but are otherwise well.

α_1-Antitrypsin

This α_1-globulin is a naturally occurring inhibitor of proteases. Its significance is related to the clinical consequences of inherited disorders of α_1-antitrypsin synthesis. These can cause emphysema, occurring at a younger age (third and fourth decades) than is usual for this condition, and neonatal hepatitis, which can progress to cirrhosis.

Homozygotes for the normal protein are termed Pi (protease inhibitor) MM. Over seventy alleles of the gene have been described. α_1-Antitrypsin deficiency is most frequently due to homozygosity for the Z allele (PiZZ), this genotype having a frequency of about 1 in 3000 in the UK. In affected individuals, plasma α_1-antitrypsin concentration is reduced to between 10 and 15% of normal. The defect is due to a single amino acid substitution, which causes the protein to form aggregates that cannot be secreted from the liver and cause liver damage. The abnormal protein shows decreased glycation, but this is probably a consequence, not the cause, of its retention in hepatocytes.

The development of emphysema is believed to be due to a lack of natural inhibition of the enzyme neutrophil elastase, which results in destructive changes in the lung. Not all PiZZ homozygotes develop liver or lung disease. The risk of developing emphysema is greatly increased by smoking; cigarette smoke oxidizes a thiol group at the active site of α_1-antitrypsin, decreasing the inhibitory activity of what small amounts of the protein are present.

PiMZ heterozygotes have plasma α_1-antitrypsin concentrations that are about 60% of normal; there is probably only a very slightly increased tendency for these individuals to develop lung disease when compared with normal PiMM homozygotes. The relatively common S allele is not a cause of α_1-antitrypsin deficiency: some studies have suggested that PiSZ heterozygotes have a slightly increased susceptibility to liver disease, but others have not confirmed this finding.

Accurate phenotyping is required for the screening of an affected individual's family members. This involves the use of special techniques, such as isoelectric focusing, to allow identification of individual proteins. Genotypic antenatal screening is possible, using the polymerase chain reaction (PCR) to amplify fetal DNA obtained by chorionic villus sampling.

α_1-Antitrypsin is an acute phase protein. Its concentration increases in acute inflammatory states and this may be sufficient to bring a genetically determined low concentration of the protein, for example in a PiMZ heterozygote, into the normal range. However, even with an acute phase response, the α_1-antitrypsin concentration in PiZZ homozygotes never rises above 50% of the lower limit of the normal range.

Haptoglobin

Haptoglobin is an α_2-globulin. Its function is to bind free haemoglobin released into the plasma during intravascular haemolysis. The haemoglobin–haptoglobin complexes formed are removed by the reticuloendothelial system and the concentration of haptoglobin falls correspondingly. Thus, a low plasma haptoglobin concentration can be indicative of intravascular haemolysis. However, low concentrations due to decreased synthesis are seen in chronic liver disease, metastatic disease and severe sepsis.

Haptoglobin is an acute phase protein and its concentration also increases in hypoalbuminaemic states such as the nephrotic syndrome. It demonstrates considerable genetic polymorphism: the molecule consists of pairs of two types of subunit, α and β, and whilst the β-chain is constant, there are three alleles for the α-chain. However, as far as is known, these different proteins are functionally similar and their existence is not known to be of clinical significance.

α_2-Macroglobulin

α_2-Macroglobulin is a high molecular weight protein (820 kDa) that constitutes approximately one-third of the α_2-globulins. Its plasma concentration is increased in the nephrotic syndrome. Like α_1-antitrypsin, α_2-macroglobulin is an inhibitor of proteases, though it has a broader spectrum of activity.

Caeruloplasmin

This is a copper-carrying protein, which functions as a ferroxidase and superoxide scavenger. Its synthesis and plasma concentration are greatly reduced in Wilson's disease. Its concentration is increased in pregnancy (an oestrogen-related effect). It is an acute phase protein.

Transferrin

This β-globulin is the major iron-transporting protein in the plasma; normally about 30% saturated with iron, it is characteristically 100% saturated in haemochromatosis. Its measurement as an index of nutritional status is discussed in *Chapter 20*. Transferrin and ferritin are discussed in more detail in *Chapter 17*. Ferritin is also an iron-carrying protein and measurement of its plasma concentration is used as a test for assessing body iron stores.

Acute phase proteins and the acute phase response

The term 'acute phase response' encompasses a complex range of physiological changes that occur following trauma and in burns, infection, inflammation and other related conditions. It comprises haemodynamic changes, increases in the activity of the coagulation and fibrinolytic systems, leucocytosis, changes in the concentration of many plasma proteins and systemic effects, particularly pyrexia. It is mediated by a host of cytokines, tumour necrosis factor and vasoactive substances.

Increases occur in the plasma concentrations of C-reactive protein and procalcitonin (*see below*), protease inhibitors, caeruloplasmin, α_1-acid glycoprotein, fibrinogen and haptoglobins: these are a result of increased synthesis, mediated primarily by interleukin-6 (IL-6) and other cytokines. At the same time there are decreases in the concentration of albumin, prealbumin and transferrin: these are mainly a result of increased vascular permeability, mediated by prostaglandins, histamine, etc.

C-reactive protein is so called because of its property to bind to a polysaccharide (fraction C) from the cell wall of pneumococci. It may have a general function in defence against bacteria and foreign substances. Its concentration can increase 30-fold from a normal value of less than 5 mg/L during the acute phase response and it is a valuable marker for this, particularly in the context of monitoring patients with inflammatory conditions such as rheumatoid arthritis and Crohn's disease. Its measurement appears to be both more sensitive and more specific than measurements of the erythrocyte sedimentation rate (ESR) and plasma viscosity in this respect. C-reactive protein concentration begins to rise at about 8 hours after the precipitation of an acute phase response and reaches a peak after about 48 hours before beginning to fall. The concentrations of α_1-acid glycoprotein and fibrinogen rise and fall more slowly: peak concentrations occur at about 70 and 90 hours, respectively.

Procalcitonin is a 116 amino acid protein that undergoes cleavage in the C-cells of the thyroid to produce calcitonin. Procalcitonin is another acute phase protein; its plasma concentration increases to particularly high levels in the acute phase response to infection. Neither the function of procalcitonin in the acute phase response, nor its origin (it is not secreted by C-cells) is certain. It is not a substitute for C-peptide as a marker of acute phase response, but its measurement may provide additional information, since it appears to have greater sensitivity and specificity for infection than C-reactive protein, and to be a better prognostic indicator.

Other plasma proteins

Measurements of other plasma proteins may provide useful information in particular circumstances. Measurement of coagulation factors (fibrinogen, factor VIII and others) is usually carried out in haematology laboratories and is essential in the investigation of some bleeding disorders. Measurement of the proteins of the complement system is of considerable value in the investigation of some diseases with an immunological

basis. The apolipoproteins are considered in detail in *Chapter 14*. The importance of hormone-binding proteins, such as cortisol-binding globulin and sex hormone-binding globulin, is considered in *Chapters 8 and 10*, respectively. Plasma proteins used in the assessment of nutritional status are discussed in *Chapter 20*. Measurement of the plasma concentration of β_2-microglobulin is of value in monitoring patients with myeloma (*see p. 245*). The measurement of plasma proteins derived from tumours (tumour markers) is discussed in *Chapter 18*.

IMMUNOGLOBULINS

The immunoglobulins are a group of plasma proteins that function as antibodies, recognizing and binding foreign antigens. This facilitates the destruction of these antigens by elements of the cellular immune system.

Since every immunoglobulin molecule is specific for one antigenic determinant, or epitope, there are vast numbers of different immunoglobulins. All share a similar basic structure (*Fig. 13.7*), consisting of two identical 'heavy' polypeptide chains and two identical 'light' chains, linked by disulphide bridges. There are five types of heavy chain (γ, α, μ, δ, ε) and two types of light chain (κ, λ), the immunoglobulin class being determined by the type of heavy chain that the molecule contains (*Fig. 13.8*).

The N-terminal amino acid sequences of both the heavy and light chains show considerable variation between individual immunoglobulin molecules; these form the part of the immunoglobulin molecule responsible for recognition of the antigen (the antigen binding site). The amino acid sequence of the rest of the chains varies little within one immunoglobulin class; this constant part of the molecule is concerned with complement activation and interaction with the cellular elements of the immune system. The characteristics and functions of the immunoglobulins are summarized in *Fig. 13.8*.

On electrophoresis, immunoglobulins behave mainly as γ-globulins, but IgA and IgM may migrate with the β- or α_2-globulins. Because the normal plasma concentration of IgG is much higher than that of the other immunoglobulins, the γ-globulin band seen on electrophoresis of normal serum is largely due to IgG.

Increases and decreases of plasma immunoglobulin concentrations can be either physiological or pathological in origin.

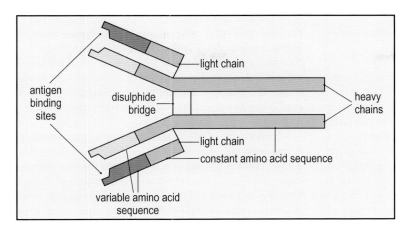

Fig. 13.7 Structure of immunoglobulins. All immunoglobulins have the same basic structure. IgM consists of a pentamer of the basic structure. IgA is secreted as a dimer.

Characteristics of the immunoglobulins				
Class	**Heavy chain**	**Mean plasma concentration (g/L)**	**Molecular weight (kDa)**	**Function**
IgG	γ	14.0	146	the major antibody of secondary immune responses
IgA	α	3.5	160	secreted as a dimer (molecular weight 385 kDa) the major antibody in seromucous secretions, e.g. saliva, bronchial mucus
IgM	μ	1.5	970	a pentamer, confined to the vascular spaces the major antibody of the primary immune response
IgD	δ	0.03	184	present on the surface of B-lymphocytes, involved in antigen recognition
IgE	ε	trace	188	present on surface of mast cells and basophils probable role in immunity to helminths and associated with immediate hypersensitivity reactions

Fig. 13.8 Characteristics of the immunoglobulins. Immunoglobulins of each class contain either κ- or λ-light chains. In IgA and IgG, slight variations in the structure of the constant regions of the heavy chains give rise to different subclasses.

Hypogammaglobulinaemia

Physiological causes

At birth, IgA and IgM concentrations are low and they rise steadily thereafter (*Fig. 13.9*), although IgA may not reach the normal adult concentration until the end of the first decade. IgG is transported across the placenta, mainly during the last trimester of pregnancy, and concentrations are high at birth (except in premature infants). IgG concentration then declines, as maternal IgG is cleared from the body, before rising again as it is slowly replaced by the infant's own IgG.

Physiological hypogammaglobulinaemia is one of the reasons for the susceptibility of infants (especially the premature) to infection.

Pathological causes

Various inherited disorders of immunoglobulin synthesis are known, ranging in severity from X-linked agamma-globulinaemia (Bruton's disease), in which there is a complete absence of immunoglobulins and affected children develop recurrent bacterial infections, to milder dysgammaglobulinaemias, in which there is a defect or partial defect of only one or two immunoglobulins. The commonest of these, IgA deficiency, has an incidence of about 1 in 400 in the UK.

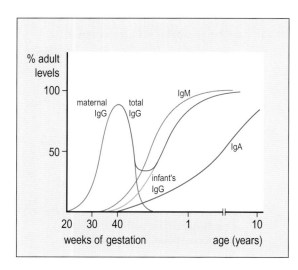

Fig. 13.9 Changes in plasma immunoglobulin concentrations with age.

Hypogammaglobulinaemia may also be acquired. It commonly occurs in haematological malignancies, such as chronic lymphatic leukaemia, multiple myeloma and Hodgkin's disease. It can be a complication of the use of cytotoxic drugs and is a feature of severe protein-losing states, for example the nephrotic syndrome. Increased catabolism also contributes to hypogammaglobulinaemia in protein-losing states.

Measurement of the specific class of immunoglobulin is essential for the diagnosis of hypogammaglobulin-aemia. Electrophoresis is not sufficient for this purpose since the normal concentrations of the immunoglobulins, with the exception of IgG, are relatively low and the effect of any decrease on the γ-globulin peak is too small to be detectable. IgG deficiency can be inferred if the γ-globulin band is faint, but possible coexistent deficiencies of other immunoglobulins will not be apparent.

Hypergammaglobulinaemia

Physiological causes

Increased concentrations of immunoglobulins are seen in both acute and chronic infections. Serological inves-tigations, involving the measurement of antibodies against specific antigens (e.g. hepatitis B surface antigen), are widely used in the diagnosis of infectious diseases.

Pathological causes

Increases in plasma immunoglobulin concentrations are common in autoimmune diseases, for example rheumatoid disease and systemic lupus erythematosus (SLE), and in chronic liver diseases, some of which have an autoimmune basis.

The measurement of specific autoantibodies is of great value in the diagnosis of autoimmune disease. Many examples are described elsewhere in this book. Many different immunoglobulins are produced in these conditions and they give rise to a diffuse (polyclonal) increase in the γ-globulin band on electrophoresis (*see Fig. 13.4*, pattern c). Occasionally, several discrete ('oligoclonal') bands are seen.

Paraproteins

A paraprotein is an immunoglobulin produced by a single clone of cells of the B-lymphocyte series, most frequently plasma cells. Since all the molecules are identical, the paraprotein is seen on electrophoresis of serum as a discrete band, usually in the γ-region (*see Fig. 13.4*, pattern b). The band may migrate elsewhere, particularly if the protein is an IgA or IgM, or if complex formation with another plasma protein has occurred. More than one paraprotein band may occasionally be seen: this may be due to dimerization, as frequently occurs with IgA paraproteins, or to the presence of complexes or fragments of paraproteins in addition to the intact molecule.

If plasma is electrophoresed, the presence of a fibrinogen band may mimic or mask a paraprotein. Even with serum, a paraprotein may be missed on electrophoresis if, as occasionally happens, it coincides exactly with a normal band, for example α_2-globulin.

Paraproteins (usually IgG or IgA) occur most frequently in multiple myeloma (disseminated malignant proliferation of plasma cells) and solitary plasmacytoma, and in Waldenström's macro-globulinaemia (IgM). Paraprotein secretion (usually IgM) occurs less frequently and, to a lesser extent, in chronic lymphatic leukaemia and B-cell lymphomas.

Serum protein electrophoresis is essential for the detection of paraproteins but the urine must be examined too. In 20% of cases of myeloma, the tumour secretes only immunoglobulin light chains. These are of low molecular weight and are rapidly cleared from (and undetectable in) the plasma. They are, however, detectable in urine; immunoglobulin light chains found in the urine are known as Bence Jones protein and are present in some 75% of all cases of myeloma.

Paraproteins are not always associated with malignant disease. The incidence of such 'benign' paraproteinaemias increases with age and has been reported to be as high as 3% in people over the age of 70. This diagnosis should not be made without vigorous investigation to exclude malignancy (*Fig. 13.10*). The most definitive diagnostic criterion is a failure of the paraprotein concentration to increase with time and this necessitates regular follow-up of the patient. There are no absolute criteria: the diagnosis is essentially one of exclusion. Because there have been reports of patients with apparently benign paraproteins developing myeloma 20 years after their discovery, the term 'monoclonal gammopathy of uncertain significance (MGUS)' is preferred to 'benign paraprotein'.

The presence of paraprotein causes red cells to adhere to each other (rouleaux formation) and may be sufficient to cause an increase in the background staining of the blood film. Hyponatraemia can occur in patients with paraproteinaemia, owing to replacement of plasma water with protein ('pseudohyponatraemia', (*see p. 24*).

Renal failure is the cause of death in approximately one-third of patients with myeloma. It is often multifactorial in origin: contributory factors include obstruction of nephrons by protein, hypercalcaemia, pyelonephritis and amyloid. Hypercalcaemia is common in myeloma; its cause is discussed elsewhere (*see pp. 224 and 322*).

Despite the extensive lytic lesions of bone, there is no increase in osteoblastic activity and plasma alkaline phosphatase activity is usually normal. The laboratory findings in myeloma are summarized in *Fig. 13.12*. It should be appreciated that metabolic abnormalities may not be present when the condition is first diagnosed; they may develop subsequently and so patients should be periodically monitored for these complications. Serum β_2-microglobulin concentration is a good prognostic indicator in myeloma because it reflects both the activity of the tumour and renal function: an increased concentration (>6 mg/L) implies a poor prognosis. Other features correlated with a poor prognosis include anaemia, renal impairment, hyper-calcaemia, hypoalbuminaemia and tumour bulk as indicated by the amount of paraprotein (e.g. IgG >70 g/L, IgA >50 g/L, Bence Jones protein >12 g/24 h), which acts as a tumour marker (*see p. 330*).

Myeloma is treated using cytotoxic drugs but the prognosis is generally poor and the disease usually becomes refractory to treatment. Local radiotherapy may be useful for isolated lesions (plasmacytomas) and for localized bone pain. Some patients have been treated successfully by bone marrow transplantation.

Waldenström's macroglobulinaemia is also a B-cell tumour. The paraprotein is an IgM, and a hyperviscosity syndrome, causing sludging of red cells in capillaries and predisposing to thrombus formation, is a prominent feature. It is much less common than myeloma.

Rarer still is Franklin's (heavy chain) disease, in which the paraprotein produced is immunoglobulin heavy chain only. This is usually an α-chain, but may also be a γ- or μ-chain. Patients with α-chain disease typically present with malabsorption due to infiltration of the gut by malignant cells.

Some paraproteins precipitate out of solution when cooled to 4°C and redissolve on warming. These proteins are known as cryoglobulins and are asso-ciated with Raynaud's phenomenon, although the majority of patients with this condition do not have cryoglobulinaemia. Cryoglobulins can also occur in

Case history 13.1

A 70-year-old man presented with back pain and loss of weight. Although a non-smoker, he had had several recent chest infections and was increasingly short of breath on exercise. On examination, he was anaemic but there were no other obvious abnormalities.

Investigations

serum:
sodium	130 mmol/L
urea	15.3 mmol/L
creatinine	212 µmol/L
calcium	2.75 mmol/L
total protein	85 g/L
albumin	30 g/L
urate	0.51 mmol/L
ESR	>100 mm/h
haemoglobin	8.5 g/dL

A blood film showed normochromic, normocytic anaemia; rouleaux were present on the blood film and there was increased background staining.

Serum protein electrophoresis revealed a paraprotein in the γ-globulin region (*Fig. 13.4*, pattern b); this was typed by immunofixation and shown to be IgG-κ. There was a decrease in the normal γ-globulin band. Bence Jones protein was present in the urine and identified as κ in type.

Radiological examination showed the typical punched-out lytic lesions of myeloma in the lumbar vertebrae, ribs and pelvis.

Comment

This is a typical presentation of multiple myeloma. The paraprotein is an IgG in 55% of cases (*Fig. 13.11*). Replacement of normal bone marrow by malignant plasma cells frequently results in anaemia and in decreased synthesis of normal immunoglobulins.

The diagnosis rests on the demonstration of any two of the following: the presence of a paraprotein, typical radiological appearances, and the presence of increased numbers of abnormal plasma cells in the bone marrow. However, it is normal practice to confirm the diagnosis by examination of a bone marrow smear, even if the diagnosis is already obvious. Occasionally, if the marrow involvement is not widespread, an aspirate may not contain any abnormal cells.

other conditions in which high concentrations of immunoglobulins occur, for instance systemic lupus erythematosus.

CYTOKINES

Cytokines are low molecular weight (<80 kDa) peptides secreted by cells involved in inflammation and immunity, which control the activity and growth of these cells. Most of their functions are local, either on nearby cells (paracrine) or on the cells that secrete the peptide (autocrine), but some have remote (endocrine) effects. They show some functional overlap with peptide growth factors, which influence the growth of non-immune cells. The two groups of factors are collectively known as peptide regulatory factors.

Four classes of cytokines are recognized:

- interleukins (IL), which are regulators of inflammation
- interferons (IF), naturally occurring anti-viral agents,

Diagnostic criteria for benign paraproteinaemia

no clinical features of myeloma or associated disorder (e.g. no anaemia or hypercalcaemia, normal renal function)

no suppression of normal immunoglobulins

no lytic lesions in bone on radiography

normal bone marrow

paraprotein concentration: IgG <20 g/L, IgA <10 g/L

no Bence Jones proteinuria

no increase in paraprotein concentration with age

no positive evidence of malignancy on follow-up (at least three years)

Fig. 13.10 Diagnostic criteria for benign paraproteinaemia.

Paraproteins in myeloma

Protein	Incidence (%)
IgG	55
IgA	22
IgD	1.5
Bence Jones	75
Bence Jones only	20

Fig. 13.11 Paraproteins in myeloma. IgE and IgM myelomas occur, but are very rare. In about 1% of all cases, no paraprotein can be detected.

which in general have an inhibitory effect on cell growth
- colony-stimulating factors (CF), which stimulate the growth of macrophages and white blood cells
- tumour necrosis factors (TNF), which stimulate the proliferation of many cells, including cytolytic T-cells.

Typical laboratory findings in multiple myeloma

Biochemical
serum: paraprotein
 $\downarrow$ normal immunoglobulins
 $\uparrow$ urea
 $\uparrow$ creatinine
 $\uparrow$ β_2-microglobulin
 $\uparrow$ calcium
 $\uparrow$ urate
 normal alkaline phosphatase
urine: Bence Jones protein

Haematological
$\uparrow$ erythrocyte sedimentation rate (ESR)
anaemia (usually normochromic, normocytic)
rouleaux formation

Fig. 13.12 Typical laboratory findings in multiple myeloma.

Transudates and exudates

The protein concentration of pleural fluid or abdominal ascites is occasionally measured to determine whether the sample is a transudate (fluid with a low protein content derived by filtration across capillary endothelium) or an exudate (fluid with a high protein content actively secreted in response to inflammation). A value of 30 g/L is often taken as the dividing line between the two types of fluid, but this is not a reliable criterion as the protein content of both is very variable.

The critical question is more often whether the ascites or pleural fluid is infected or if it is related to the presence of a tumour. This can only be determined by microbiological and cytological examination, so protein measurement is of little value.

Many cytokines have multiple properties and some cytokine-mediated responses can be brought about by more than one cytokine. Cytokines interact with each other, with the result that the effect of an individual cytokine depends upon which other cytokines are present. They are also capable of inducing and inhibiting each other's secretion.

Cytokines are of considerable importance in the coordination of the immune and inflammatory responses, and in the control of myelopoiesis. Some cytokines are secreted by tumours and can contribute to the effects of those tumours. They can be measured in serum by sensitive and specific assays, although as yet there are no clear clinical indications for doing so. Possible applications for cytokine measurements include the early diagnosis of sepsis and graft reaction, for which TNFα and IL-6 show promise.

Growth factors (GF) include epidermal GF, platelet-derived GF, transforming GF and the insulin-like GFs. Secretion of the latter by mesenchymal tumours is a cause of tumour-associated hypoglycaemia.

PLASMA ENZYMES

Measurements of the activity of enzymes in plasma are of value in the diagnosis and management of a wide variety of diseases. Most enzymes measured in plasma are primarily intracellular, being released into the blood when there is damage to cell membranes, but many enzymes, for example renin, complement factors and coagulation factors, are actively secreted into the blood, where they fulfil their physiological functions. The use of enzyme measurements in tissue for the diagnosis of inherited metabolic diseases is discussed in *Chapter 16*.

Small amounts of intracellular enzymes are present in the blood as a result of normal cell turnover. When damage to cells occurs, increased amounts of enzymes will be released and their concentrations in the blood will rise. However, such increases are not always due to tissue damage. Other possible causes include:

- increased cell turnover
- cellular proliferation (e.g. neoplasia)
- increased enzyme synthesis (enzyme induction)
- obstruction to secretion
- decreased clearance.

Little is known about the mechanisms by which enzymes are removed from the circulation. Small molecules, such as amylase, are filtered by the glomeruli but most enzymes are probably removed by reticulo-endothelial cells. Plasma amylase activity rises in acute renal failure but, in general, changes in clearance rates are not known to be important as causes of changes in plasma enzyme levels.

Enzyme activity

Enzyme assays usually depend on the measurement of the catalytic *activity* of the enzyme, rather than the *concentration* of the enzyme protein itself. Since each enzyme molecule can catalyze the reaction of many molecules of substrate, measurement of activity provides great sensitivity. It is, however, important that the conditions of the assay are optimized and standardized to give reliable and reproducible results.

Reference ranges for plasma enzymes are dependent on assay conditions, for example temperature, and may also be subject to physiological influences. It is thus important to be aware of both the reference range for the laboratory providing the assay and the physiological circumstances when interpreting the results of enzyme assays. Ranges quoted in this book (*see p. 375*) are from the first author's laboratory and may not necessarily be the same as those of the reader's.

Disadvantages of enzyme assays

A major disadvantage in the use of enzymes for the diagnosis of tissue damage is their lack of specificity to a particular tissue or cell type. Many enzymes are common to more than one tissue, with the result that an increase in the plasma activity of a particular enzyme could reflect damage to any one of these tissues. This problem may be obviated to some extent in two ways: first, different tissues may contain (and thus release when they are damaged) two or more enzymes in different proportions; thus alanine and aspartate aminotransferases are both present in cardiac and skeletal muscle and hepatocytes, but there is only a very little alanine aminotransferase in either type of muscle; second, some enzymes exist in different forms (isoforms), colloquially termed isoenzymes (although, strictly, the term 'isoenzyme' refers only to a genetically determined isoform). Individual isoforms are often characteristic of a particular tissue: although they may have similar catalytic activities, they often differ in some other measurable property, such as heat stability or sensitivity to inhibitors.

After a single insult to a tissue, the activity of intracellular enzymes in the plasma rises as they are released from the damaged cells, and then falls as the enzymes are cleared. It is thus important to consider the time at which the blood sample is taken in relation to the insult. If taken too soon, there may have been insufficient time for the enzyme to reach the blood-stream and if too late, it may have been completely cleared (*see Case History 21.1*). As with all diagnostic techniques, data acquired from measurements of enzymes in plasma must always be assessed in the light of whatever clinical and other information is available, and their limitations borne in mind.

In the tables that follow, typical plasma activities of enzymes in various conditions are given. Higher (or lower) levels may of course occur in more (or less) severe cases.

Alkaline phosphatase (ALP)

This enzyme is present in high concentrations in the liver, bone (osteoblasts), placenta and intestinal epithelium. These tissues each contain specific isoenzymes (strictly, isoforms) of ALP. Pathological increases in ALP activity are most frequently seen in cholestatic liver disease and in bone diseases in which there is an increase in osteoblastic activity (e.g. Paget's disease and osteomalacia).

The causes of an increase in plasma ALP activity are summarized in *Fig. 13.13*. Physiological increases are seen in pregnancy, due to the placental isoenzyme, and in childhood (when bones are growing), due to the bone isoenzyme. Plasma ALP activity is high at birth but falls rapidly thereafter. However, it remains two to three times the normal adult level and rises again during the adolescent growth spurt before falling to the adult level as bone growth ceases (*Fig. 13.14*). Plasma ALP activity is slightly higher than normal in apparently healthy elderly people. This may reflect the high incidence of mild, sub-clinical Paget's disease in the elderly. Levels of ALP as high as ten times the upper limit of normal (10 × ULN) may be seen in severe Paget's disease of bone, rickets and osteomalacia and occasionally in cholestatic liver disease. Lesser increases are, however, more common in these conditions (*see Fig. 13.13*). Note that ALP activity is not increased in uncomplicated osteoporosis, unless the condition has been complicated by a fracture.

Plasma ALP is frequently elevated in malignant disease: it may be of bony or hepatic origin and associated with the presence of either primary or secondary tumours in these tissues. A number of apparently tumour-specific ALPs, secreted by tumour cells themselves, have also been described. The best known of these is the Regan isoenzyme, which has similar heat stability to placental ALP and is found in some patients with bronchial carcinoma.

Causes of an increased plasma alkaline phosphatase

Physiological
pregnancy (last trimester)
childhood

Pathological
often >5 × ULN
    Paget's disease of bone
    osteomalacia, rickets
    cholestasis (intra- and extrahepatic)
    cirrhosis

usually <5 × ULN
    bone tumours (primary and secondary)
    renal bone disease
    primary hyperparathyroidism with bone
       involvement
    healing fractures
    osteomyelitis
    hepatic space-occupying lesions (tumour,
       abscess)
    infiltrative hepatic disease
    hepatitis
    inflammatory bowel disease

Fig. 13.13 Causes of an increased plasma alkaline phosphatase activity. ULN = upper limit of normal.

ALP is frequently measured as part of a biochemical profile and it is not uncommon to find a raised activity in the absence of clinical evidence of bone or liver disease, and in the absence of other biochemical abnormalities. In establishing the cause of such an increase it is clearly helpful to determine the tissue of origin. This can be done by measuring tissue-specific isoenzymes of ALP. These can be separated and quantitated using various techniques, including electrophoresis and differential heat inactivation. A simpler but less reliable alternative is to measure plasma γ-glutamyl transferase. This enzyme is found in the liver but not in bone. Its plasma activity is often (but not always) increased when there is an excess of hepatic ALP in the plasma.

Aminotransferases

Two aminotransferases are used in diagnosis and management: aspartate aminotransferase (AST) and

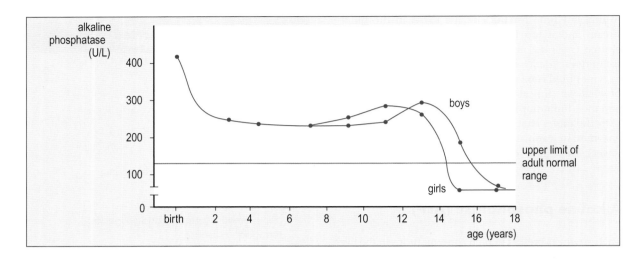

Fig. 13.14 Serum alkaline phosphatase activity as a function of age in childhood. Mean values are shown; the peaks between 10 and 16 years correspond to the pubertal growth spurt, and levels of up to three times the upper limit of the adult normal range may be seen at this time.

alanine aminotransferase (ALT)*. Both enzymes are widely distributed in body tissues, but ALT is present in only small amounts except in the liver. Even here, there is more than three times as much AST; in cardiac and skeletal muscle, there is twenty times as much AST as ALT.

The causes of increased plasma AST activity are shown in *Fig. 13.15*. Very high levels, sometimes in excess of $100 \times$ ULN, are seen with severe tissue damage, such as in acute hepatitis, crush injuries and tissue hypoxia. More usually in hepatitis, the peak level is only $10–20 \times$ ULN. In myocardial infarction, plasma AST begins to rise some 12 h after the infarct, reaching a peak of up to $10 \times$ ULN at 24–36 h and then declining over two to three days providing that there is no further cardiac damage (*see p. 270*).

In most conditions in which AST is elevated there is a concurrent, though proportionally smaller, rise in ALT. In hepatitis, however, plasma activities of ALT may exceed those of AST. AST is often measured as part of a biochemical profile in multichannel auto-analyzers. It is very uncommon to find levels greater than $20 \times$ ULN unexpectedly; this is most likely to occur in the prodromal phase of viral hepatitis. Levels of up to $2 \times$

---

*The 'T' in the abbreviation stands for 'transaminase'; this term has now been replaced by 'aminotransferase' although the abbreviation has not been changed and indeed the term 'transaminase' remains colloquial.

Causes of an increased plasma aspartate aminotransferase
often >10 × ULN
acute hepatitis and liver necrosis
major crush injuries
severe tissue hypoxaemia
(levels may sometimes exceed
100 × ULN in these conditions)
5–10 × ULN
myocardial infarction
following surgery or trauma
skeletal muscle disease
cholestasis
chronic hepatitis
usually <5 × ULN
physiological (neonates)
other liver diseases
pancreatitis
haemolysis (*in vivo and in vitro*)

Fig. 13.15 Causes of an increased plasma aspartate aminotransferase activity. Plasma alanine aminotransferase is raised to a similar extent in liver diseases but to a lesser degree, if at all, in the other conditions. ULN = upper limit of normal.

ULN are sometimes found in patients who have no clinical evidence of tissue damage. Alcohol abuse and non-alcoholic steatohepatitis should be considered as possible causes in such cases. There are no tissue-specific isoenzymes of AST and if there are no other biochemical changes, nor any readily apparent cause of the raised level, the wisest procedure is to repeat the analysis after an interval of one or two weeks.

γ-Glutamyl transferase (GGT)

This enzyme is present in high concentrations in the liver, kidney and pancreas. Measurement of its plasma activity provides a sensitive indicator of hepatobiliary disease although it is of no value in distinguishing *between* cholestatic and hepatocellular disease. In biliary obstruction, plasma GGT activity may increase before that of alkaline phosphatase.

Plasma GGT is raised in the absence of liver disease in many patients taking the anticonvulsant drugs phenytoin and phenobarbital; rifampicin, used in the treatment of tuberculosis, can have a similar effect. This is an example of enzyme induction. The increased plasma GGT is not due to cell damage but to an increase in enzyme production within cells with the result that an increased amount is released during normal cell turnover.

Plasma GGT activity is frequently very high in patients with alcoholic liver disease but can be elevated, due to enzyme induction, in heavy alcohol drinkers in the absence of other evidence of liver damage. Up to 70% of such people may have elevated levels of the enzyme but it should be appreciated both that similar increases may be seen in other conditions (*see Fig. 13.16*) and that a significant number of people who abuse alcohol have a normal plasma enzyme activity. Plasma GGT activity can remain elevated for up to 3–4 weeks following abstinence from alcohol, even in the absence of liver damage.

Lactate dehydrogenase (LD)

This enzyme exists in body tissues as a tetramer. Two monomers, H and M, can combine in various proportions with the result that five isoenzymes of LD are known.

Increases in plasma LD activity are seen in a wide variety of conditions including acute damage to the liver, skeletal muscle and kidneys, and also in megaloblastic

Some causes of an increased plasma γ-glutamyl transferase

often >10 × ULN
  cholestasis
  alcoholic liver disease

5–10 × ULN
  hepatitis (acute and chronic)
  cirrhosis (without cholestasis)
  other liver diseases
  pancreatitis

usually <5 × ULN
  excessive alcohol ingestion
  enzyme-inducing drugs
  congestive cardiac failure

Fig.13.16 Causes of an increased plasma γ-glutamyl transferase activity. Increases of less than 5 × ULN are seen in many conditions and probably reflect secondary effects on the liver. γ-Glutamyl transferase is not usually increased with hepatic space-occupying lesions provided that liver function is normal.

and haemolytic anaemias. In patients with lymphoma, a high plasma LD activity indicates a poor prognosis. There is a correlation between enzyme activity and tumour bulk and so serial measurements may be useful in following response to treatment.

In both cardiac muscle and red blood cells LD_1 (H_4) is the predominant isoenzyme. This shows much greater catalytic activity with α-hydroxybutyrate (rather than lactate) as a substrate than the other isoenzymes and is also known as α-hydroxybutyrate dehydrogenase (HBD). HBD/LD_1 increases later after myocardial infarction (*see Fig. 14.14*), but its measurement is of no practical value in the management of this condition. An increased plasma activity (due to release from red blood cells) occurs in haemolytic crises in sickle cell anaemia, and measurement of the enzyme may be of value when this diagnosis is suspected.

Creatine kinase (CK)

The enzymatically active CK molecule is a dimer; there are two monomers, M and B. Three isoenzymes, BB, MM and MB, occur. BB is confined mainly to the brain. The CK normally present in plasma is mainly the MM isoenzyme. Even in severe brain damage, the contribution of the BB isoenzyme to plasma activity is minimal. Increases in plasma CK activity are usually the result of skeletal or cardiac muscle damage (*see Fig. 13.17*). The CK in skeletal muscle is almost entirely MM; in cardiac muscle, up to 30% is the MB isoenzyme. When plasma CK activity is increased, the demonstration that more than 5% of the total CK is due to the MB isoenzyme is highly suggestive of its being cardiac in origin. The diagnostic uses of CK measurements are discussed in *Chapters 14 and 15*.

CK-MB can be measured either by measurement of enzyme activity in the presence of an antibody that inhibits the M subunit, or by measurement of enzyme mass using an immunoassay. In the plasma, the terminal lysine residue of the CK-M polypeptide is removed by a carboxypeptidase. This does not affect enzyme activity but alters the charge on the polypeptide and hence the electrophoretic mobility of the enzyme. The three possible forms of CK-MM are termed isoforms: CK-MM3 is composed of two intact CK-M polypeptides; in CK-MM1, both polypeptides have had their terminal lysines removed; CK-MM2 has one polypeptide of each type. An increase in the ratio CK-MM3:CK-MM1 occurs earlier than other enzyme changes following myocardial infarction (2–5 h after the onset of chest pain). However, the measurement of CK isoforms is technically demanding and few laboratories offer it routinely.

Amylase

This enzyme is found in the salivary glands and exocrine pancreas, and tissue-specific isoenzymes can be distinguished by means of electrophoresis or the use of inhibitors.

Plasma amylase activity is usually increased, often to 5 × or even to more than 10 × ULN, in acute pancreatitis. Its use in the diagnosis of patients presenting with an acute abdomen, and the other causes of an increase in plasma amylase activity, are discussed in *Chapter 6*.

Cholinesterase

This enzyme is secreted by the liver into the bloodstream and low plasma activities occur in chronic hepatic dysfunction. It is, however, rarely measured for this reason. Plasma cholinesterase activity also falls in organophosphate poisoning. Low activities occur physiologically during pregnancy.

Interest in this enzyme derives largely from the fact that it hydrolyzes a muscle-relaxant drug, widely used in anaesthesia, called succinylcholine (scoline). Occasionally, patients are found in whom the effect of this drug, which paralyzes respiration, persists for several hours after it has been administered (scoline apnoea). Many of these patients have an abnormal cholinesterase activity.

Four enzyme variants have been recognized on the basis of the activity of the enzyme in the presence of inhibitors: normal, dibucaine resistant, fluoride resistant and inactive. Normal homozygotes (genotype $E_1^u E_1^u$) account for 95% of the population, and heterozygotes for dibucaine resistance ($E_1^u E_1^a$) 4%. Such individuals do not usually react abnormally to succinylcholine, but homozygotes for dibucaine resistance ($E_1^a E_1^a$) (0.05%) are at risk of developing scoline apnoea as are patients who produce an inactive enzyme ($E_1^s E_1^s$). Individuals having an adverse reaction to scoline, and their relatives, should be screened to identify those who have an abnormal cholinesterase so that scoline can be avoided should they need to undergo anaesthesia.

Causes of an increased plasma creatine kinase

often >10 × ULN
  polymyositis
  rhabdomyolysis (e.g. trauma, malignant hyperpyrexia)
  Duchenne muscular dystrophy
  myocardial infarction

5–10 × ULN
  following surgery
  skeletal muscle trauma
  severe exercise
  grand mal convulsions
  myositis
  carriers of Duchenne muscular dystrophy

usually <5 × ULN
  physiological (Afro-Caribbeans)
  hypothyroidism
  drug (statin) treatment

Fig. 13.17 Causes of an increased plasma creatine kinase activity. Concentrations as high as 100 × ULN may be seen in rhabdomyolysis.

SUMMARY

- The most abundant protein in plasma is **albumin**, which is synthesized in the liver. Through its contribution to the **colloid osmotic pressure**, albumin has an important role in determining the distribution of the extracellular fluid between the vascular and extravascular spaces. It is also an important **transport protein** for several hormones, drugs, free fatty acids, unconjugated bilirubin and various ions. Its concentration is, however, affected by so many pathological processes (decreases occur in chronic liver disease, protein-losing states, malabsorption, following trauma and when capillary permeability is increased) that measurements must be interpreted with caution.

- Most of the other plasma proteins are classified as globulins. The **immunoglobulins** are synthesized by plasma cells and constitute the **humoral arm of the immune system**. Five main classes are known of which the most abundant are IgG, IgM and IgA. IgM is the main antibody of the primary immune response and is largely confined to the vascular compartment; IgG is involved in the secondary response and is distributed throughout the extracellular fluid; IgA is secreted onto mucosal surfaces. An increase in total immunoglobulins is characteristic of chronic inflammatory conditions and autoimmune diseases. Measurement of immunoglobulins is of value in the investigation of immunodeficiency syndromes. Measurement of **specific antibodies** is of value in the investigation of autoimmune and infectious diseases.

- **Myelomas** are malignant tumours of plasma cells, which produce large amounts of identical, monoclonal, immunoglobulin molecules or fragments thereof, known as **paraproteins**. Serum and urine protein electrophoresis is essential for the detection of paraproteins but other abnormalities of plasma proteins are better investigated by specific measurement of the protein, or proteins, in question. **Metabolic features of myeloma** include renal impairment, hypercalcaemia and hyperuricaemia. Patients are frequently anaemic and may have an immune paresis. Causes of death include infection and renal disease.

- **Other plasma proteins** include the coagulation factors, complement components and various transport proteins, for example thyroxine-binding globulin, transcortin, sex hormone-binding globulin, transferrin and caeruloplasmin. Increases in the concentration of certain proteins occur in association with acute inflammatory reactions. These **acute phase proteins** include α_1-antitrypsin, **C-reactive protein** and haptoglobins. Measurement of C-reactive protein is valuable in following the course of conditions characterized by episodes of acute inflammation, such as rheumatoid arthritis and Crohn's disease. α_1-**Antitrypsin** is a protease inhibitor; inherited deficiency of the protein can cause neonatal hepatitis, which may progress to cirrhosis, and emphysema in adults, particularly those who smoke.

- The **cytokines** are a large group of autocrine and paracrine regulatory peptides, which modulate the activity of the immune system and are involved in the coordination of acute inflammation and the immune response.

SUMMARY (cont'd)

- The **enzymes** present in the plasma include those that have a physiological function there, for example renin and the blood clotting factors, and those that have been released from cells as a result of damage or normal cell turnover. Diagnostic enzymology is principally concerned with the latter; the measurement of enzyme activity in the plasma can give useful diagnostic information concerning the site and extent of tissue damage. Examples of such enzymes include **creatine kinase**, which is released from cardiac muscle following myocardial infarction and damage to skeletal muscle, and the **aminotransferases**, which are widely distributed and are released into the blood in a variety of conditions, including hepatitis, myocardial infarction and skeletal muscle injury.

- Few enzymes that are measured for diagnostic purposes in plasma are tissue specific, but when the origin of increased plasma activity is not obvious either clinically or for other reasons, measurement of the **isoenzymes** (molecular variants of the enzymes that have similar catalytic activity but a different chemical structure, rendering them distinguishable, for example immunochemically or by electrophoresis) can often provide this information. Thus the measurement of ALP isoenzymes will distinguish between a hepatic, osseous or other source for increased plasma activity of this enzyme, and the measurement of isoenzymes of creatine kinase will distinguish between a cardiac or skeletal muscle origin. Another method to improve specificity involves measuring more than one enzyme, since the concentration of different enzymes, and thus the amount released when cells are damaged, varies between different tissues.

- Though tending to lack specificity, the measurement of plasma enzyme activity can provide a very sensitive means of detecting tissue damage and can be invaluable in following the course of an illness such as hepatitis or Paget's disease of bone, even though the diagnosis may have been established using another technique.

Lipids, lipoproteins and cardiovascular disease

INTRODUCTION

The major lipids present in the plasma are fatty acids, triglycerides, cholesterol and phospholipids. Other lipid-soluble substances, present in much smaller amounts but of considerable physiological importance, include steroid hormones and fat-soluble vitamins; these are discussed in *Chapters 8 and 20*, respectively.

Elevated plasma concentrations of lipids, particularly cholesterol, are causally related to the pathogenesis of atherosclerosis, the process responsible for the majority of cardiovascular disease (coronary, cerebrovascular and peripheral vascular disease). Cardiovascular disease is the commonest cause of death in the UK: about a quarter of all deaths (more in women than in men) are due to coronary heart disease (CHD). Many of these are in people under the age of 60. Effective management of hypercholesterolaemia and other risk factors is of proven benefit in reducing cardiovascular disease mortality.

TRIGLYCERIDES, CHOLESTEROL AND PHOSPHOLIPIDS

Triglycerides are more correctly called triacylglycerols, but this term is not in general use in clinical medicine, and the more colloquial term is used in this book to avoid confusion. They consist of glycerol esterified with three long-chain fatty acids, such as stearic (18 carbon atoms) or palmitic (16 carbon atoms) acids. Triglyceride is present in dietary fat, and can be synthesized in the liver and adipose tissue to provide a source of stored energy; this can be mobilized when required, for example during starvation. Although the majority of fatty acids in the body are saturated, certain unsaturated fatty acids are important as precursors of prostaglandins and in the esterification of cholesterol. Triglycerides containing both saturated and unsaturated fatty acids are important components of cell membranes.

Cholesterol is also important in membrane structure and is the precursor of steroid hormones and bile acids. Cholesterol is present in dietary fat, and can be synthesized in the liver by a mechanism that is under close metabolic regulation. Cholesterol can be excreted in the bile either *per se*, or after metabolism to bile acids.

Phospholipids are compounds similar to the triglycerides but with one fatty acid residue replaced by phosphate and a nitrogenous base.

Because they are not water soluble, lipids are transported in the plasma in association with proteins. Albumin is the principal carrier of free fatty acids (FFA); the other lipids circulate in complexes known as lipoproteins. These consist of a non-polar core of triglyceride and cholesteryl esters surrounded by a surface layer of phospholipids, cholesterol and proteins known as apolipoproteins (*Fig. 14.1*). The latter are important both structurally and in the metabolism of lipoproteins (*Fig. 14.2*).

CLASSIFICATION OF LIPOPROTEINS

Lipoproteins are classified on the basis of their densities as demonstrated by their ultracentrifugal separation. Density increases from chylomicrons (CM, of lowest density) through lipoproteins of very low density

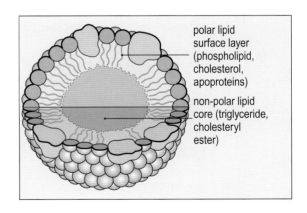

polar lipid surface layer (phospholipid, cholesterol, apoproteins)

non-polar lipid core (triglyceride, cholesteryl ester)

Fig. 14.1 Diagram showing the composition of a lipoprotein particle. A segment has been removed to reveal the non-polar core of cholesteryl ester and triglyceride surrounded by phospholipids and apoprotein.

Apolipoprotein	Function
A-I	activates LCAT structural (in HDL)
A-II	inhibits HTGL at high concentration structural (in HDL)
B-100	structural (in LDL and VLDL) receptor binding
B-48	structural (in chylomicrons)
C-I	cofactor for LCAT
C-II	activator of LPL
C-III	inhibits LPL inhibits clearance of CM and VLDL remnant particles
E	binding to LDL and remnant receptors

Fig. 14.2 Functions of the major apolipoproteins. Abbreviations are explained in the text.

(VLDL), intermediate density (IDL) and low density (LDL) to high density lipoproteins (HDL). HDL can be separated, on the basis of density, into two metabolically distinct subtypes, HDL2 (density 1.064–1.125) and HDL3 (density 1.126–1.21). Distinct sub-types of LDL (LDL-I, II and III, in increasing order of density) are also recognized. IDL are normally present in the blood-stream in only small amounts but can accumulate in pathological disturbances of lipoprotein metabolism. This classification is illustrated in *Fig. 14.3* and the approximate lipid and apolipoprotein content in *Fig. 14.4*. However, it is important to appreciate that the composition of the circulating lipoproteins is not static. They are in a dynamic state with continuous exchange of components between the various types. Their principal functions are summarized in *Fig. 14.3* and discussed in greater detail in the next section.

Lipoprotein(a), or Lp(a), is an atypical lipoprotein of unknown function. It is larger and more dense than LDL but has a similar composition, except that it contains in addition one molecule of apo(a) for every molecule of apo B-100. Apo(a) shows considerable homology with plasminogen. The concentration of Lp(a) in the plasma varies considerably between individuals, ranging from 0 to 1000 mg/L. An elevated concentration of Lp(a) appears to be an independent

Classification and characteristics of lipoproteins					
lipoprotein	density (g/mL)	mean diameter (nm)	electrophoretic mobility	source	principal function
CM	<0.95	500	remains at origin	intestine	transport of exogenous triglyceride
VLDL	0.96–1.006	43	pre-β	liver	transport of endogenous triglyceride
IDL	1.007–1.019	27	'broad β'	catabolism of VLDL	precursor of LDL
LDL	1.02–1.063	22	β	catabolism of VLDL, via IDL	cholesterol transport
HDL	1.064–1.21	8	α	liver, intestine; catabolism of CM & VLDL	reverse cholesterol transport

Fig. 14.3 Classification and characteristics of lipoproteins.

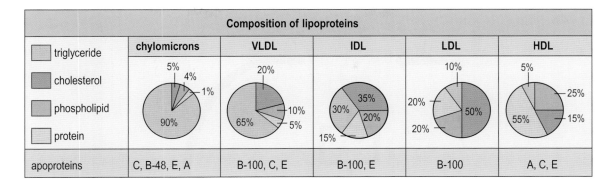

Fig. 14.4 Composition of lipoproteins; although the composition in each class is similar, the particles are heterogeneous so the percentages given are approximate. Figures shown for HDL are for HDL3; HDL2 contains less protein and more lipid. Only the principal apoproteins are shown.

risk factor for CHD. Conventional drug treatments that lower LDL have little effect on Lp(a) concentration.

LIPOPROTEIN METABOLISM

Chylomicrons

Chylomicrons (*Fig. 14.5*) are formed from dietary fat (principally triglycerides, but also cholesterol) in enterocytes; they enter the lymphatics and reach the systemic circulation via the thoracic duct. Chylomicrons are the major transport form of exogenous (dietary) fat. Triglycerides constitute about 90% of the lipid. Triglycerides are removed from chylomicrons by the action of the enzyme lipoprotein lipase (LPL), located on the luminal surface of the capillary endothelium of adipose tissue, skeletal and cardiac muscle and lactating breast, with the result that free fatty acids are delivered to these tissues to be used either as energy substrates or, after re-esterification to triglyceride, for energy storage. LPL is activated by apo C-II.

Apo A and apo B-48 are synthesized in the gut and are present in newly formed chylomicrons; apo C-II and apo E are transferred to chylomicrons from HDL. As triglycerides are removed from chylomicrons by the action of lipoprotein lipase, these become smaller; cholesterol, phospholipids, apo A and apo C-II are released from the surface of the particles and taken up by HDL. Esterified cholesterol is transferred to the chylomicron remnants from HDL, in exchange for triglyceride, by cholesteryl ester transfer protein. The chylomicron remnants, depleted of triglyceride and enriched in cholesteryl ester, are cleared from the circulation by hepatic parenchymal cells. This hepatic uptake depends on the recognition of apo E by hepatic remnant receptors (also known as LDL-related receptor protein).

Although their major function is the transport of dietary triglyceride, chylomicrons also transport dietary cholesterol and fat-soluble vitamins to the liver. Under normal circumstances, chylomicrons cannot be detected in plasma in the fasting state (>12 h after a meal).

Very low density lipoproteins

VLDL (*Fig. 14.6*) are formed from triglycerides synthesized in the liver either *de novo* or by re-esterification of free fatty acids. VLDL also contain some cholesterol, apo B, apo C and apo E; the apo E and some of the apo C is transferred from circulating HDL.

VLDL are the principal transport form of endogenous triglycerides and initially share a similar fate to chylomicrons, triglycerides being removed by the action of LPL. As the VLDL particles become smaller, phospholipids, free cholesterol and apolipoproteins are released from their surfaces and taken up by HDL, thus converting the VLDL to denser particles, IDL. Cholesterol that has been transferred to HDL is esterified and the cholesteryl ester is transferred back to IDL by cholesteryl ester transfer protein in exchange for triglyceride. More triglycerides are removed by hepatic triglyceride lipase, located on hepatic endothelial cells, and IDL are thereby converted to LDL, composed mainly of cholesteryl esters,

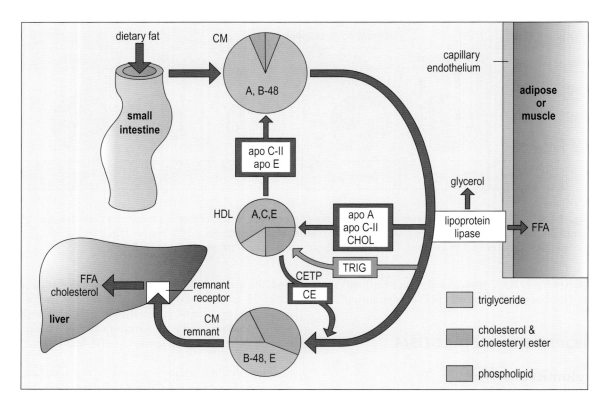

Fig. 14.5 Chylomicrons transport dietary triglycerides to tissue where they are removed by the action of lipoprotein lipase. The resulting remnant particles are removed by the liver. They bind to remnant receptors (which recognize apo E) on hepatic cells, are internalized and catabolized. Apolipoproteins A and B-48 are synthesized in intestinal cells; apo C and apo E are acquired, together with cholesteryl esters (CE), from HDL. Apolipoprotein C-II activates lipoprotein lipase. As triglycerides are removed from chylomicrons, apo A, apo C, cholesterol and phospholipids are released from their surfaces and transferred to HDL where the cholesterol is esterified. Cholesteryl ester is transferred back to the remnant particles in exchange for triglycerides by cholesteryl ester transport protein (CETP).

apo B-100 and phospholipid. Some IDL are taken up by the liver via LDL receptors. These receptors, also known as B, E receptors, are capable of binding apo B-100 and apo E. Under normal circumstances, there are very few IDL in the circulation because of their rapid removal or conversion to LDL.

Low density lipoproteins

LDL are the principal carriers of cholesterol, mainly in the form of cholesteryl esters. LDL are formed from VLDL via IDL (*Fig. 14.6*). LDL can pass through the junctions between capillary endothelial cells and attach to LDL receptors on cell membranes that recognize apo B-100. This is followed by internalization and lysosomal degradation with release of free cholesterol (*Fig. 14.7*). Cholesterol can also be synthesized in these tissues, but the rate-limiting enzyme, HMG-CoA reductase (hydroxymethylglutaryl CoA reductase), is inhibited by cholesterol with the result that, in the average adult, cholesterol synthesis in peripheral cells probably does not occur. Free cholesterol also stimulates its own esterification to cholesteryl ester by stimulating the enzyme acyl CoA:cholesterol acyl transferase (ACAT).

LDL receptors are saturable and subject to down regulation by an increase in intracellular cholesterol. Macrophages derived from circulating monocytes can

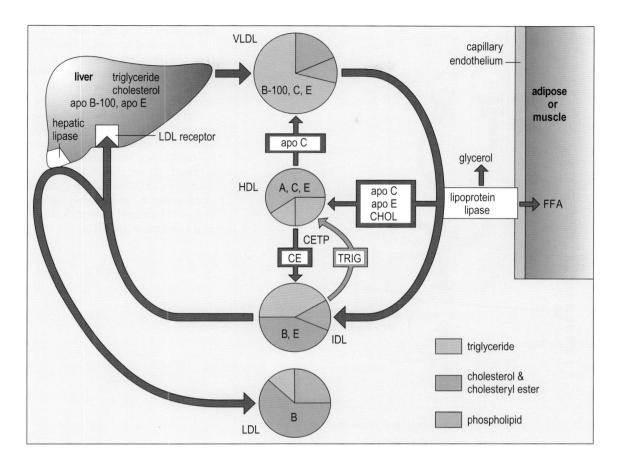

Fig. 14.6 VLDL are synthesized in the liver and transport endogenous triglyceride from the liver to other tissues where it is removed by the action of lipoprotein lipase. At the same time, cholesterol, phospholipids and apo C and apo E are released and transferred to HDL. By this process VLDL are converted to IDL. Cholesterol is esterified in HDL and cholesteryl ester is transferred to IDL by cholesteryl ester transfer protein. Some IDL is removed by the liver but most has more triglyceride removed by hepatic triglyceride lipase and is thereby converted into LDL. Thus the triglyceride-rich VLDL are precursors of LDL, which comprise mainly cholesteryl ester and apo B-100.

take up LDL via scavenger receptors. This process occurs at normal LDL concentrations but is enhanced when LDL concentrations are increased and by modification (e.g. oxidation) of LDL. Uptake of LDL by macrophages in the arterial wall is an important event in the pathogenesis of atherosclerosis. When macrophages become overloaded with cholesteryl esters, they are converted to 'foam cells', the classic components of atheromatous plaques. In human neonates, plasma LDL concentrations are much lower than in adults and cellular cholesterol uptake is probably all receptor mediated and controlled.

LDL concentrations increase during childhood and reach adult levels after puberty.

High density lipoproteins

HDL (*Fig. 14.8*) are synthesized primarily in the liver and, to a lesser extent, in small intestinal cells, as a

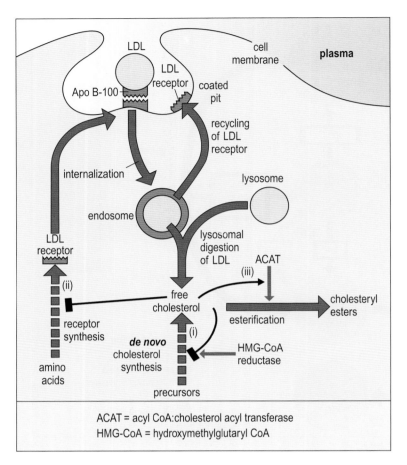

Fig. 14.7 LDL uptake and catabolism. LDL are derived from VLDL, via IDL. They are removed by the liver and other tissues by a receptor-dependent process involving the recognition of apo B-100 by the LDL receptor. The LDL particles are hydrolyzed by lysosomal enzymes, releasing free cholesterol which (i) inhibits HMG-CoA reductase, the rate-limiting step in cholesterol synthesis, (ii) inhibits LDL receptor synthesis and (iii) stimulates cholesterol esterification by augmenting the activity of the enzyme acyl CoA:cholesterol acyl transferase (ACAT).

ACAT = acyl CoA:cholesterol acyl transferase
HMG-CoA = hydroxymethylglutaryl CoA

precursor ('nascent HDL') comprising phospholipid, cholesterol, apo E and apo A. Nascent HDL is disc-shaped; in the circulation, it acquires apo C and apo A from other lipoproteins and from extrahepatic tissues, and in doing so assumes a spherical conformation. The free cholesterol is esterified by the enzyme lecithin-cholesterol acyltransferase (LCAT), which is present in nascent HDL and activated by its cofactor, apo A-I. This increases the density of the HDL particles, which are thus converted from HDL3 to HDL2.

Cholesteryl esters are transferred from HDL2 to remnant particles in exchange for triglycerides, this process being mediated by cholesteryl ester transfer protein. Cholesteryl esters are taken up by the liver in chylomicron remnants and IDL and excreted in bile, partly after metabolism to bile acids.

The triglyceride-enriched HDL2 is converted back to HDL3 by the removal of triglycerides by the enzyme

hepatic triglyceride lipase, located on the hepatic capillary endothelium. Some HDL2 is probably removed from the circulation by the liver, through receptors that recognize apo A-I.

Thus HDL has two important functions: it is a source of apoproteins for chylomicrons and VLDL, and it mediates reverse cholesterol transport, taking up cholesterol from senescent cells and other lipoproteins and transferring it to remnant particles, which are taken up by the liver. Cholesterol is excreted by the liver in bile, both as free and esterified cholesterol and after metabolism to bile acids.

The essential features of lipoprotein metabolism are as follows.

- Dietary triglycerides are transported in chylomicrons to tissues where they can be used as an energy source or stored.

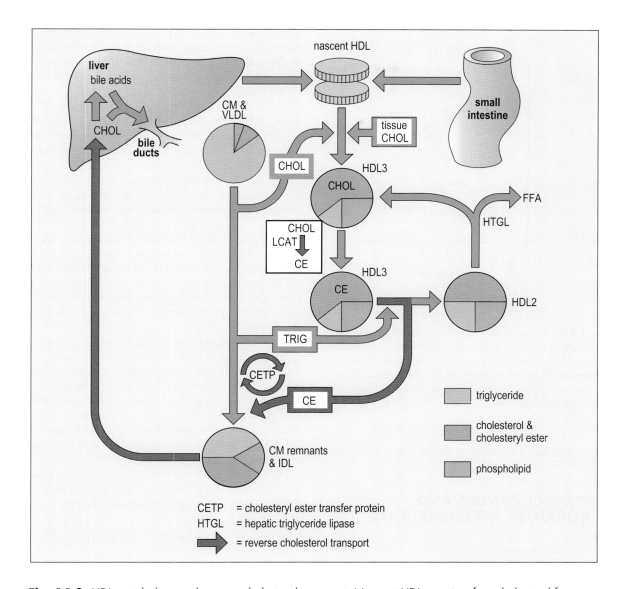

Fig. 14.8 HDL metabolism and reverse cholesterol transport. Nascent HDL acquires free cholesterol from extrahepatic cells, chylomicrons and VLDL and is thereby converted to HDL3. The cholesterol is esterified by the enzyme LCAT and cholesteryl ester is transferred to remnant lipoproteins by CETP in exchange for triglyceride. Remnant particles are removed from the circulation by the liver whence the cholesterol is excreted in bile both *per se* and as bile acids. Much HDL is recycled although some is probably taken up by the liver and catabolized. Apoprotein transfers have been omitted for clarity.

- Endogenous triglycerides, synthesized in the liver, are transported in VLDL and are also available to tissues as an energy source or for storage.
- Cholesterol synthesized in the liver is transported to tissues in LDL, derived from VLDL; dietary

cholesterol reaches the liver in chylomicron remnants.
- HDL acquire cholesterol from peripheral cells and other lipoproteins and this is esterified by LCAT. Cholesteryl esters are transferred to remnant

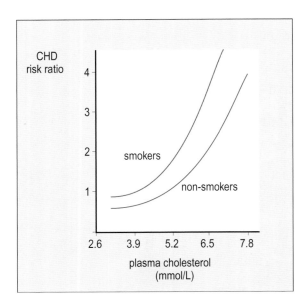

Fig. 14.9 Mortality from coronary heart disease (CHD) and plasma cholesterol concentration. Mortality is expressed as risk relative to that associated with a concentration of 5.2 mmol/L. With additional risk factors (e.g. cigarette smoking) the curve is shifted upwards and is steeper.

particles, which are taken up by the liver, whence the cholesterol is excreted.

REFERENCE RANGES AND LABORATORY INVESTIGATIONS

At birth, the plasma cholesterol concentration is very low (total cholesterol less than 2.6 mmol/L, LDL cholesterol less than 1.0 mmol/L). There is a rapid increase in concentration in the first year of life; the mean value in childhood is approximately 4.2 mmol/L. In affluent societies particularly, concentrations rise further in early adulthood. Elevated plasma cholesterol concentrations are a major risk factor for CHD. The relationship between cholesterol concentration and CHD mortality is curvilinear (see Fig. 14.9). The curve becomes increasingly steep as cholesterol concentration increases: CHD mortality doubles between concentrations of 5.2 and 6.5 mmol/L, and quadruples between 5.2 and 7.8 mmol/L. Approximately two-thirds of adults in the UK have a plasma cholesterol

concentration >5.2 mmol/L and a quarter >6.5 mmol/L. While at a concentration <5.2 mmol/L, the curve becomes shallow, it does not become flat. In individuals with other risk factors, e.g. cigarette smoking (see below), the curve is moved upwards and is steeper.

Because of the gradation of CHD risk even within the range of cholesterol concentrations found in the bulk of the adult population, it is inappropriate to define a reference range for plasma cholesterol concentration. Rather, it is preferable to consider an individual person's concentration in terms of what is ideal or desirable for that individual: this will depend on many factors, including the presence or absence of other CHD risk factors.

While there is an undoubted association between plasma cholesterol concentration (and, in particular, LDL cholesterol) and an increased risk of CHD, there is an inverse correlation between HDL cholesterol and CHD risk. Many physiological factors influence LDL and HDL cholesterol, some of which are indicated in Fig. 14.10.

Hypertriglyceridaemia is also a risk factor for CHD (probably more so in women than in men), albeit a less important one. Hypertriglyceridaemia due to small, dense, triglyceride-rich LDL-particles (LDL-III), which are particularly associated with type 2 diabetes mellitus, is of particular significance, since these particles appear to be more atherogenic than other LDL sub-types. Plasma triglyceride concentrations >10 mmol/L carry an increasing risk of pancreatitis.

Triglyceride, and total and HDL cholesterol concentrations can easily be measured in the laboratory. LDL cholesterol can be calculated using the formula:

$$LDL\ CHOL = TOTAL\ CHOL - \left(HDL\ CHOL + \frac{TRIG}{2.2} \right)$$

where all quantities are expressed in mmol/L. This formula is invalid if the triglyceride concentration exceeds 4.5 mmol/L.

Separation of lipoproteins by ultracentrifugation is not a convenient technique for routine use and is primarily a research tool. Formerly, separation of lipoproteins by electrophoresis was widely used, but this only provides qualitative information and is now obsolete. Genotyping, or phenotyping, of apo E is required to confirm the diagnosis of remnant hyperlipidaemia (see p. 267). Assays for lipoprotein lipase and apo C-II are required for the diagnosis of the cause of fasting chylomicronaemia. Assays for other apoproteins

Influences on plasma lipoproteins			
Variable	HDL cholesterol	LDL cholesterol	Triglyceride
sex	F > M	M = F	F < M
age	slight ↑ in F	↑	↑
high P:S ratio	N or ↓	↓	N or ↓
exercise	↑	↓	↓
obesity	↓	N	↑
alcohol	↑	N	↑
exogenous oestrogens	↑	↓	↑*

Fig. 14.10 Some physiological and external influences on plasma lipoproteins. P:S is the ratio of polyunsaturated to saturated fats in the diet. *In susceptible individuals. N = no significant effect.

are available but are not of proven value in routine practice.

The appearance of the plasma in the laboratory may provide the first clue that a patient has hyperlipidaemia. In health, in the fasting state, plasma is clear. Following a meal, it often becomes opalescent due to the light-scattering properties of chylomicrons and VLDL. At triglyceride concentrations above about 4 mmol/L, the plasma becomes increasingly turbid; with severe hypertriglyceridaemia it appears milky (lipaemic). If plasma is left undisturbed, chylomicrons float to the surface, leaving a clear infranatant layer; VLDL remain in suspension. LDL do not scatter light and even at high plasma cholesterol concentrations the plasma remains clear.

Blood for lipid studies

Blood for lipid studies should be drawn after an overnight fast (12–14 h), when chylomicrons, being derived from dietary fat, should normally have been cleared; a pathological disturbance may thus be inferred if they are present. The patient should have kept to his or her own normal diet for two weeks before the blood is taken. Alcohol should not have been taken on the evening before blood sampling. This is a common cause of hypertriglyceridaemia even in patients who have otherwise fasted. When lipid studies are done on a patient who has had a myocardial infarction or stroke, blood should either be taken within 24 h or after an interval of three months, since the metabolism of

lipoproteins is disturbed during the convalescent period and analytical results may be misleading.

Selection of patients for investigation

There is conclusive evidence from clinical trials that lowering plasma cholesterol concentration reduces mortality from CHD and decreases overall mortality. This has been demonstrated both in the context of secondary prevention (treatment of individuals with pre-existing disease) and primary prevention (treatment of individuals in whom there is no evidence of disease). Lowering cholesterol also reduces the risk of stroke. Lowering cholesterol is not associated with an increase in mortality from other diseases (e.g. cancer) with the exception that there is some evidence that it may increase the risk of haemorrhagic stroke, albeit to an extent that is far outweighed by the potential benefits.

It is therefore clear that lipid measurements should be made in all patients known to have vascular disease, and in those at increased risk (see p. 268). Thus plasma lipids should be measured in the individuals with the following:

- CHD (and cerebrovascular and peripheral vascular disease)
- a family history of premature coronary disease (occurring at age <60 years)
- other major risk factors for CHD (e.g. diabetes mellitus, hypertension)

- patients with clinical features of hyperlipidaemia (*see below*)
- patients whose plasma is seen to be lipaemic.

Given the high prevalence of cardiovascular disease, there is an increasing tendency to screen all adults (more especially males) above the age of 20 for risk factors, including hyperlipidaemia.

DISORDERS OF LIPID METABOLISM

There are several rare, inherited metabolic diseases associated with the accumulation of lipids in tissues and others in which plasma lipoprotein concentrations are reduced. By far the commonest disorders, however, are the hyperlipidaemias, both primary (genetic) and secondary.

Classification

Hyperlipidaemias are classified as either primary, comprising a group of genetically determined disorders, or secondary, in which the abnormalities are the result of an acquired condition.

Hyperlipidaemias used to be classified using the WHO system, based on the work of Fredrickson. This is a phenotypic classification, based on the observed pattern of lipoprotein abnormality. Although widely used for many years, several flaws became apparent: with some inherited hyperlipidaemias, the same genotype can be expressed as more than one phenotype in different individuals; similarly, the phenotypes associated with individual secondary hyperlipidaemias can vary; in both inherited and secondary hyperlipidaemias, drug treatment can alter the phenotype, and finally, the classification takes no account of HDL cholesterol.

Secondary hyperlipidaemias

These are common (*see Fig. 14.11*) and, since resolution of the lipid abnormality should follow successful treatment of the underlying condition, management should be directed towards the cause. Although the presence of a primary disorder may be inferred from a relevant family history, it is always important to exclude secondary causes in the investigation of patients with hyperlipidaemias. Occasionally, such a cause may coexist with a primary hyperlipidaemia and exacerbate its manifestations.

Several drugs can also cause or exacerbate hyperlipidaemia, including thiazides, β-blockers lacking intrinsic sympathomimetic activity (ISA) and corticosteroids. Ideally, calcium antagonists, angiotensin-converting enzyme (ACE) inhibitors, β-blockers with ISA or α-blockers should be used for treating hypertension in patients with hyperlipidaemia. Oestrogens, especially when given to post-menopausal women, may lower

Condition	HDL cholesterol	Lipid abnormality LDL cholesterol	Triglyceride
obesity	↓	N	↑
excessive alcohol intake	↑	N	↑
diabetes mellitus	N/sl ↓	N	↑↑
hypothyroidism	N	↑↑	N/↑
nephrotic syndrome	↓	↑↑	↑↑
chronic renal failure	↓	N/↑	↑
cholestasis	N	↑	N

Fig. 14.11 Common causes of secondary hyperlipidaemia. In cholestasis, much of the hypercholesterolaemia is due to the accumulation of lipoprotein X, an aggregate of free cholesterol, lecithin, albumin and apo C. The changes shown for diabetes are for untreated disease. Abnormalities can persist with treatment and are discussed further in *Chapter 11*. N = normal; sl = slight.

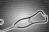

Case history 14.1

A 55-year-old man presented with a history of lethargy, loss of concentration and constipation. He had suffered from angina for two years, but this had become less of a problem recently, since he had become much less active. On examination, he appeared myxoedematous.

Investigations

serum: TSH   >100 mU/L
       cholesterol   12.2 mmol/L
       triglyceride   1.5 mmol/L

He was treated cautiously with thyroxine, starting with a low dose; his angina was controlled effectively with nitrates and a calcium antagonist. His serum cholesterol fell to 8.2 mmol/L on treatment, with an LDL cholesterol of 6.4 mmol/L.

Comment

Hypothyroidism frequently causes hypercholesterolaemia, owing to decreased removal of LDL from the circulation. The persistence of a raised cholesterol despite adequate treatment of the hypothyroidism is suggestive of the presence of an additional, genetically determined, predisposition to hypercholesterolaemia.

In view of his ischaemic heart disease, this man's target cholesterol concentration should be <5.0 mmol/L (*see p. 269*). Statin treatment would be indicated, but only when he was biochemically euthyroid: there is a theoretically increased risk of myopathy if statins are given to hypothyroid patients.

Note that hypothyroidism should be treated under close medical supervision in patients with ischaemic heart disease. The increase in metabolic rate increases the body's oxygen requirements and can exacerbate angina or precipitate myocardial infarction.

Case history 14.2

A 45-year-old obese barman who complained of recurrent epigastric pain underwent endoscopy. Because he admitted to heavy alcohol ingestion, blood was taken for liver function tests prior to the procedure. Endoscopy revealed a duodenal ulcer.

In the laboratory, the technician noticed that the serum looked opalescent and analyzed it for lipids.

Investigations

serum: cholesterol   7.5 mmol/L
        triglyceride   8.4 mmol/L

Comment

Alcohol causes hypertriglyceridaemia by increasing triglyceride synthesis and the insulin resistance seen in obesity has a similar effect. Massive hypertriglyceridaemia (more than 20 mmol/L) may occur in patients with a high alcohol intake when there is an additional, inherited tendency to hypertriglyceridaemia. Moderate alcohol intake increases HDL cholesterol concentration and is cardioprotective but, with a high intake, although HDL concentrations remain elevated, this protection is lost.

plasma cholesterol concentrations but may cause, or exacerbate, hypertriglyceridaemia. Certain progestogens used in oral contraceptives also have an adverse effect on plasma lipids.

Primary hyperlipidaemias

Familial hypercholesterolaemia (FH)

This condition is characterized by high plasma cholesterol concentrations that are present from early childhood and do not depend upon the presence of environmental factors (*see polygenic hypercholesterolaemia, below*). It is inherited as an autosomal dominant characteristic, with a prevalence in the population in the UK of about 1 in 500. Different mutations can affect LDL synthesis, transport, ligand binding, clustering in

Case history 14.3

An obese 44-year-old woman with type 1 diabetes was found to have a blood glucose concentration of 32 mmol/L at the outpatient clinic and was admitted to hospital. Blood was taken for further biochemical analysis and the serum was seen to be grossly lipaemic.

Investigations

serum: cholesterol   53 mmol/L
        triglyceride   150 mmol/L

The sample was inspected after standing overnight and had a creamy, supernatant layer, although the infranatant remained lipaemic.

Comment

The appearance of the serum indicates the presence of both chylomicrons and VLDL. Hyperlipidaemia can complicate uncontrolled type 1 and type 2 diabetes and is due to a combination of decreased lipoprotein lipase activity and increased hepatic triglyceride synthesis. It may exacerbate a coexisting familial hyperlipidaemia. This patient was treated with an intravenous insulin infusion. Her blood glucose concentration fell rapidly and she was restabilized on an appropriate regimen of subcutaneous insulin injections. After a week her serum cholesterol and triglycerides were 8.0 and 11 mmol/L, respectively. Thereafter diabetes remained well controlled and follow-up lipid analysis showed cholesterol 6.0 mmol/L and triglycerides 5.3 mmol/L. Her immediate family had normal serum lipids and it was concluded that her persistently elevated triglyceride was related at least in part to her obesity.

coated pits and recycling but all cause a similar phenotype. Familial defective apo B-100, in which a mutation in the apo B gene decreases the avidity of LDL for its receptor, causes a similar phenotype. In all cases there is a defect in the uptake and catabolism of LDL, and its plasma concentration is increased. In heterozygotes, total cholesterol is typically in the range 7.5–12 mmol/L.

 Case history 14.4

A 36-year-old man consulted an optician to obtain a prescription for reading glasses. The optician noticed that the patient had bilateral arcus senilis, and recommended that he consult his GP. The GP found that he also had tendon xanthomata, arising from the Achilles tendons. Blood pressure was normal; he was a non-smoker and not overweight. His father had died of a heart attack at the age of 40. An ECG taken at rest was normal but ischaemic changes developed on exercise. Analysis of fasting blood for lipids showed the following.

Investigations

serum: cholesterol   13.2 mmol/L
        triglyceride   1.3 mmol/L
        LDL cholesterol 11.4 mmol/L
        HDL cholesterol 1.2 mmol/L

Comment

This is a characteristic picture of familial hypercholesterolaemia. Tendon xanthomata, although not an invariable finding, are virtually pathognomonic of FH. Their development is age related. They are accumulations of cholesterol, but deep-seated, with the result that the overlying skin has a normal colour. Arcus senilis and xanthelasmata are frequently present but, unlike tendon xanthomata, may occur in the absence of an obvious disturbance of lipid metabolism, although usually only in older people (>60 years). Even though this patient is normotensive and a non-smoker, the hypercholesterolaemia alone considerably increases his risk of dying of ischaemic heart disease and indeed he has an abnormal exercise ECG. Familial hypercholesterolaemia is ten times more common in victims of myocardial infarctions than in the rest of the population. Patients with FH require rigorous treatment, invariably requiring lipid-lowering drugs as well as diet (*see below*) and, if other risk factors are present these, of course, must also be tackled.

The diagnosis is based on the presence of hyper-cholesterolaemia (>7.5 mmol/L in adults (LDL cholesterol >4.5 mmol/L)) together with tendon xanthomata in the subject or tendon xanthomata or hypercholesterolaemia in a close relative.

In the very rare homozygotes (1 in 1,000,000), no receptors are present. Plasma cholesterol concentrations can be as high as 20 mmol/L. These individuals develop coronary artery disease in childhood and, if untreated, rarely survive into adult life; heterozygotes tend to develop coronary artery disease some 20 years earlier than the general population; more than half of those untreated die before the age of 60.

'Common' (polygenic) hypercholesterolaemia

In FH, the distribution of plasma cholesterol concentrations in relatives of the proband is bimodal, with a clear distinction between heterozygotes and normals. More frequently, when the family of an individual with hypercholesterolaemia is studied, a continuous distribution is found, consistent with the plasma cholesterol being influenced by several genes. This entity has been termed 'common' or polygenic hypercholesterolaemia. Plasma cholesterol is not as high as in FH, and is influenced to a greater extent by environmental factors (e.g. diet).

The significance of this condition again lies in its relationship to the risk of coronary artery disease and the principles of management are similar to those for FH. In polygenic hypercholesterolaemia, however, dietary treatment alone may sometimes be adequate to lower the cholesterol concentration to acceptable levels.

Familial dysbetalipoproteinaemia

This condition is characterized clinically by the presence of fat deposits in the palmar creases and by tuberous xanthomata; the latter tend to occur over bony prominences and, unlike tendon xanthomata, are reddish in colour. However, neither of these cutaneous stigmata is invariably present. In some patients eruptive xanthomata are present. Biochemically, the condition is characterized by the presence of an excess of IDL and chylomicron remnants; chylomicrons are sometimes also present. An alternative name is remnant hyper-lipoproteinaemia. Total cholesterol and triglyceride concentrations are elevated, typically to approximately equal values. This condition used to be called 'broad

 Case history 14.5

A middle-aged man was referred by his family doctor to a dermatologist because of extensive yellowish papules, with erythematous bases, on his buttocks and elbows. The dermatologist recognized these as eruptive xanthomata and noticed that there were yellow, fatty streaks in the palmar creases. Blood was drawn after an overnight fast for lipid analysis and the serum was seen to be slightly turbid.

Investigations

serum: cholesterol 8.5 mmol/L
          triglyceride 6.4 mmol/L

Apo E genotyping indicated that the patient was homozygous for the apo E e2 gene.

Comment

This patient was treated with a low-fat diet and bezafibrate and after three months serum lipid concentrations had become normal. There was also considerable regression of the xanthomata. When the bezafibrate was stopped, the lipid abnormalities recurred but resolved again on restarting the drug. Familial dysbetalipoproteinaemia characteristically responds very well to treatment.

beta disease', because the remnant particles give rise to a broad band extending between the pre-β (corresponding to VLDL) and β (LDL) positions on serum lipoprotein electrophoresis. Patients with remnant hyperlipo-proteinaemia have an increased risk not only of coronary artery disease but also of peripheral and cerebral vascular disease.

Apo E shows polymorphism. The commonest phenotype is termed E-3/E-3. Familial dysbetalipopro-teinaemia is associated with the E-2/E-2 phenotype, which can result in impaired IDL uptake by the liver. However, the fact that this phenotype is present in 1 in 100 of the normal population, while dysbetalipopro-teinaemia is an uncommon disorder (prevalence approximately 1 in 10,000), implies a role for other factors in its expression, and in this context it is noteworthy that although the variant apoprotein is present from birth, the condition does not appear clinically until adult life. Such factors include obesity, alcohol, hypothyroidism and diabetes.

Although the diagnosis can be inferred from the clinical and biochemical findings, it should ideally be confirmed by apo E genotyping.

The significance of apo E polymorphism is not limited to lipid metabolism. Increased frequency of the e4 allele has been demonstrated in patients with familial Alzheimer's disease.

Familial chylomicronaemia

Fasting chylomicronaemia is a feature of two rare hyperlipidaemias, both having an autosomal recessive inheritance: in one there is a deficiency of the enzyme lipoprotein lipase and in the other a deficiency of apo C-II, which is required for activation of this enzyme. The result in each case is a failure of chylomicron clearance from the bloodstream. Presentation is usually in childhood, with eruptive xanthomata, recurrent abdominal pain due to pancreatitis and sometimes hepatosplenomegaly.

Chylomicronaemia may also be seen in other patients with a genetic predisposition to hypertriglyceridaemia when this is exacerbated by obesity, diabetes mellitus, hyperuricaemia or alcohol ingestion; some drugs, for example thiazides, may also have this effect.

Management involves giving a low fat diet, with substitution of some fat by triglycerides based on medium-chain fatty acids: these are absorbed directly from the gut into the bloodstream and therefore do not produce chylomicrons. The major complication of the chylomicronaemic syndromes is recurrent pancreatitis and since this is uncommon with triglyceride concentrations below 10 mmol/L, it is not usually considered necessary to achieve normalization of plasma triglyceride concentration.

Familial hypertriglyceridaemia

This condition, which has a prevalence of approximately 1 in 600, is usually associated with an excess of VLDL in plasma. The molecular basis is uncertain; there is increased hepatic synthesis of VLDL. Inheritance is autosomal dominant. Triglyceride concentrations are not usually higher than 5 mmol/L but in severe cases, in which other factors (e.g. obesity and alcohol) are often implicated, they can be much higher; chylomi-

cronaemia can occur and only then are physical signs (e.g. eruptive xanthomata and lipaemia retinalis) usually present.

It is uncertain whether there is an increased risk of CHD in patients with familial hypertriglyceridaemia, though HDL concentration is often reduced; in severe cases there is a risk of pancreatitis.

Familial combined hyperlipidaemia

This is due to hepatic overproduction of apo B, leading to increased VLDL secretion and increased production of LDL from VLDL. Either plasma cholesterol or triglyceride, or both, may be elevated; typically, in affected relatives, one-third have an increase in LDL, one-third in VLDL and one-third have an excess of both lipoproteins. Cutaneous manifestations of hyperlipidaemia may be present and in all cases there is an increased risk of coronary artery disease.

The prevalence is approximately 1 in 200; inheritance is probably autosomal dominant. There are no distinctive clinical features and the diagnosis is often presumptive, based on the increase in both cholesterol and triglyceride in the absence of tendon xanthomata or a secondary cause of hyperlipidaemia.

Familial hyperalphalipoproteinaemia

In this condition, there is hypercholesterolaemia due to an increase in only the HDL fraction, which may be present in other members of the family. CHD risk is decreased, and no treatment is required. The existence of this condition underlines the need to measure HDL cholesterol in patients with hypercholesterolaemia. Generally, if total cholesterol is greater than 7 mmol/L, there will always be an increase in LDL, but, even then, measurement of HDL helps in the assessment of CHD risk.

THE MANAGEMENT OF LIPID DISORDERS

Risk factors for vascular disease and the rationale for treatment

The major reason for treating hyperlipidaemia is to decrease the risk of cardiovascular disease. In patients with severe hypertriglyceridaemia, treatment may be necessary to reduce the risk of pancreatitis. It cannot be overemphasized that hyperlipidaemia is only one of many risk factors for cardiovascular disease: over 200 have been identified. The decision to treat a patient with hyperlipidaemia must be based on an adequate assessment of risk: with the exception of patients with very high lipid concentrations and those known to have arterial disease, the decision to prescribe lipid-lowering treatment should not be based on measurements of lipids alone. Some of the more important risk factors are indicated in *Fig. 14.12*.

These risk factors tend to be multiplicative: in people in the lowest quintile of cholesterol concentrations, hypertension increases CHD risk by approximately twice and cigarette smoking by a factor of about 1.6; a combination of hypertension and smoking increases risk by a factor of about 3.4.

Cigarette smoking, hypertension and diabetes are all major risk factors that are susceptible to intervention. A family history of premature vascular disease, age and being male clearly are not, but may require a more aggressive approach to the management of those factors, including hyperlipidaemia, that are. It should be appreciated that the single most important risk factor for symptomatic coronary disease is a history of previous myocardial infarction or coronary revascularization, or of angina. This has major implications for treatment (*see below*).

There is currently much interest in risk factors that have been recognized relatively recently, including hyperfibrinogenaemia, a high plasma Lp(a) and an increased plasma concentration of homocysteine. The latter has long been known to occur in the inherited metabolic disease homocystinuria (classically a result of a deficiency of the enzyme cystathionine β-synthase); patients with this disease have a tendency to die from premature vascular disease. However, numerous studies have implicated lesser elevations of homocysteine (than are characteristic of homocystinuria) as a risk factor for vascular disease. Possible mechanisms include promotion of the oxidation of LDL and a direct toxic action of homocysteine on the vascular endothelium. Vitamins B_6, B_{12} and folate act as cofactors in homocysteine metabolism: there is an association between elevated plasma homocysteine concentrations and low folate, raising the possibility that folate supplementation may be of therapeutic benefit in the prevention of vascular disease. Although the results of some clinical trials appear to support this idea, others have been negative and the case for folate supplementation of the diet to reduce the risk of CHD remains unproven.

All patients at risk of CHD should be encouraged to make appropriate changes to their diet and lifestyle. The diet should be designed to achieve/maintain an ideal body weight and not more than 30% of energy should be provided by fat, of which not more than one-third should be saturated. The effects of dietary intervention on lipid concentrations are more apparent in clinical trials than in free-living subjects. Other risk factors should be managed appropriately.

Target lipid concentrations recommended on the basis of clinical trials should be a total plasma cholesterol concentration of no more than 5.0 mmol/L or LDL cholesterol of no more than 3.0 mmol/L, although it can be argued on the basis of epidemiological evidence that even lower targets may be appropriate in patients at very high risk. The benefits of prescribing cholesterol-lowering drugs to achieve target concentrations in the context of secondary prevention (patients with established coronary heart disease) are well established. Such treatment clearly reduces mortality: it is effective and cost-effective. It must of course be combined with other appropriate intervention, including both adoption of a healthier lifestyle (improved diet, increased exercise, cessation of smoking, etc.) and drugs (e.g. aspirin, and ß-blockers and ACE inhibitors in patients in whom they are indicated, and additional hypotensive medication when required). Patients with cerebrovascular disease and peripheral vascular disease should be treated similarly.

Risk factors for cardiovascular disease	
modifiable	**not modifiable**
hypercholesterolaemia*	personal history of
hypertension*	cardiovascular
cigarette smoking*	disease*
diabetes mellitus*	family history of
hyperfibrinogenaemia	premature
hyperhomocysteinaemia	cardiovascular
low HDL cholesterol	disease*
hypertriglyceridaemia	male sex*
overweight	age*
etc.	

Fig. 14.12 Risk factors for cardiovascular disease. Major risk factors are indicated with an asterisk.

In the context of primary prevention, however, the situation is less clear-cut. Because the absolute risks of CHD are lower, the benefits of intervention (in terms, for example, of the numbers of patients treated in relation to numbers of lives saved) are lower, and the cost-effectiveness is also lower. Guidelines for the prescription of lipid-lowering drugs in primary prevention take such factors into account and are usually set around specific levels of risk. Some guidelines recommend treatment if the cumulative risk of myocardial infarction over ten years is 30% or more; others set the cut-off at 20%. It cannot, however, be overemphasized that such guidelines are only guidelines: they should not be regarded as proscriptive, and are not a substitute for the exercise of clinical judgement in individual patients. In practice, lipid-lowering medication is likely to be indicated in all individuals whose total cholesterol concentration remains more than 7.8 mmol/L after an adequate trial of dietary modification. It will be indicated at lower concentrations if other risk factors are present. At any given cholesterol concentration, the indication for intervention will be strengthened by the presence of hypertriglyceridaemia or a low HDL cholesterol concentration.

In the context of primary prevention, patients with diabetes constitute a special case: the risk of CHD associated with diabetes is so great that it is increasingly recommended that they should be considered as if they were subjects for secondary prevention.

Hypercholesterolaemia

The drugs of choice for the treatment of hyper-cholesterolaemia are the statins, inhibitors of HMG-CoA reductase, the rate-limiting step in cholesterol synthesis. These decrease intracellular cholesterol concentrations and thus increase LDL receptor expression and decrease plasma LDL. Statins lower triglycerides slightly and tend to increase HDL. Bile acid sequestrants are also effective, though often less well tolerated. They act by binding bile acids in the gut, preventing their absorption and thus interrupting their enterohepatic circulation. This depletes the hepatic bile acid pool and causes increased conversion of cholesterol into bile acids. Bile acid sequestrants tend to increase triglyceride concentrations. Ezetimibe is a new, more specific and better tolerated inhibitor of cholesterol absorption. Fibrates have various effects on lipid metabolism, but work primarily by stimulating lipoprotein lipase. They tend to be less effective than statins at lowering cholesterol but more effective at lowering triglycerides; they increase HDL concentrations.

Patients with homozygous FH tend to respond poorly to drugs and are usually treated by repeated LDL apheresis, a process that physically removes LDL from the circulation. Ileal bypass has been used in the past: it is effective, but has major long-term adverse side effects. Liver transplantation has also been used successfully.

Hypertriglyceridaemia

This may respond well to control of body weight and any coexistent exacerbating factors (e.g. excessive alcohol intake). The main classes of drug used for treating hypertriglyceridaemia are the fibrates, nicotinic acid derivatives and fish oils. Nicotinic acid derivatives decrease VLDL synthesis and may also decrease LDL and increase HDL. Fish oils, rich in ω-3 polyunsaturated fatty acids, also decrease VLDL synthesis.

LIPOPROTEIN DEFICIENCY

There are three rare inherited lipoprotein deficiencies.

Abetalipoproteinaemia

In abetalipoproteinaemia there is a defect in the synthesis of apo B; CM, VLDL and LDL are absent from the plasma. Clinically, there is malabsorption of fat, acanthocytosis, retinitis pigmentosa and an ataxic neuropathy.

Hypobetalipoproteinaemia

In this condition there is partial deficiency of apo B; CM, VLDL and LDL are present, but in low concentrations.

Tangier disease

In Tangier disease HDL levels are reduced; clinically, the condition is characterized by hyperplastic, orange tonsils and the accumulation of cholesteryl esters in other reticuloendothelial tissues. The condition is due to accelerated catabolism of apo A-I.

MYOCARDIAL INFARCTION

Many patients with myocardial infarction have a typical history of crushing central chest pain, perhaps radiating to the arm or jaw, associated with typical ECG changes. Myocardial infarction can, however, present atypically, or even be clinically silent, particularly in the elderly (*see Case History 21.1*). The ECG changes may not always be typical, particularly with partial thickness infarcts, where there has been previous infarction, or in left bundle branch block. Also, even apparently typical chest pain is not always due to myocardial infarction.

Measurements of plasma enzymes have long been used to assist in the diagnosis of myocardial infarction. The first enzyme to increase is the MB isoenzyme of creatine kinase (CK-MB), followed by total CK, aspartate aminotransferase (AST) and hydroxybutyrate dehydrogenase (HBD, the cardiac isoenzyme of lactate dehydrogenase) (*see Fig. 14.13*). CK-MB has long been regarded as the gold standard. Cardiac muscle contains

about 30% of its CK as CK-MB; the proportion in healthy skeletal muscle is about 1%. Thus, even if total plasma CK is elevated (for example as a result of trauma or vigorous exercise), the presence of more than about 5% of the total as CK-MB (this value is dependent on the assay used and applies to measurements of activity, not CK mass) suggests cardiac muscle damage (*see Case History 14.6*).

In patients with a typical history and ECG changes of myocardial infarction, enzyme measurements do not contribute to the initial management. Thrombolytic therapy is usually given unless specifically contra-indicated; this should be done as soon as possible, yet an increase in CK-MB in the plasma may not be seen until 4–8 h after the onset of chest pain. When the diagnosis is not obvious, an elevated CK-MB or an increase in CK-MB of more than 15% over a 4-h period, even if both values are within the reference range, are suggestive of myocardial infarction. As so often with biochemical measurements, the detection of a trend by serial measurements, if feasible, may provide more information than single measurements. If CK does not increase in a patient with chest pain, myocardial infarction is unlikely; a failure of an elevated CK to fall suggests that extension of the infarct has occurred.

AST and HBD measurements are rarely of practical value in the management of patients with suspected myocardial infarction. Exceptionally, when a patient with chest pain presents late, measurement of HBD may be helpful as this enzyme remains elevated in the plasma for several days following myocardial infarction. However, plasma troponin (*see below*) also remains elevated for up to a week.

The lack of specificity and sensitivity of CK-MB measurements for myocardial infarction, particularly in the first few hours after the onset of chest pain, has prompted the investigation of many other potential cardiac markers, including myoglobin and the troponins. Troponin I and troponin T are component proteins of the contractile apparatus in muscle cells. Cardiac-specific isoforms of both have been identified. Neither increases in plasma sufficiently early after the onset of chest pain to inform the use of thrombolysis, but both are highly specific and sensitive for myocardial damage. Troponin T (and to a lesser extent troponin I) can also increase in plasma in unstable angina. Their greatest use is to exclude cardiac damage in patients with chest pain: myocardial infarction is highly unlikely if there is no increase in troponins. Myoglobin is also a

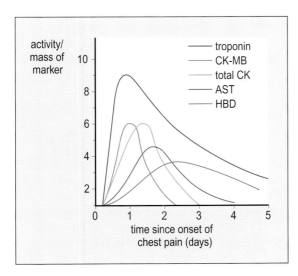

Fig. 14.13 Plasma enzyme activities* and troponin concentration following myocardial infarction. Values are shown as multiples of the upper limit of normal. The extent to which the various markers rise relative to one another is not constant but the time courses of the increases and subsequent decreases are characteristic. *Measurement of CK mass is more sensitive than activity.

sensitive early indicator of cardiac damage (and may increase before CK-MB), but is non-specific, being present in skeletal muscle as well.

If thrombolytic therapy is successful in restoring perfusion, there is a rapid rise in plasma markers of myocardial damage (wash-out phenomenon). The rises are slower if perfusion remains compromised.

In patients who have sustained a myocardial infarction, biochemical monitoring is important. Measurements of plasma potassium, glucose and arterial 'blood gases' may be vital to appropriate management. Plasma lipids should be measured either on presentation, or three months later (*see p. 263*).

Case history 14.6

A recently retired lawyer was admitted to hospital with chest pain which had developed during the evening after a day spent digging in the garden.

There were no specific signs of myocardial infarction on the ECG. He was monitored in the acute coronary unit for 24 h and then transferred to a general ward. His pain subsided rapidly and he was discharged after five days.

Investigations

	on admission	48 h	72 h
serum:			
creatine kinase (total)	300 U/L	80 U/L	40 U/L
creatine kinase CK-MB)	5 U/L	–	–
hydroxybutyrate dehydrogenase	–	–	70 U/L

Comment

Although the total CK activity was raised, the MB isoenzyme was normal. It was concluded that no myocardial infarction had taken place and that the chest pain was musculoskeletal in origin, related to the unaccustomed exercise. Total CK may reach a peak of greater than 20 × ULN after severe exercise, especially if the individual is unaccustomed to this. The normal HBD supported these conclusions.

Case history 14.7

Two days after sustaining myocardial infarction, confirmed by ECG changes and the finding of a raised total CK, a 54-year-old social worker complained of discomfort in the right epigastrum. On examination, the jugular venous pressure was elevated and the liver was slightly enlarged and tender.

Investigations

serum:	bilirubin	60 μmol/L
	alkaline phosphatase	130 U/L
	aspartate phosphatase	125 U/L
	creatine kinase	80 U/L
		(280 U/L on admission)

Comment

The serum ALP is not usually increased after uncomplicated myocardial infarction but this patient has clinical evidence of right heart failure. Hepatic venous congestion is a consequence of this and can cause a mild, usually transient, cholestatic jaundice, reflected here by the increase in ALP and bilirubin. If it is measured, the ALT is often elevated to an extent commensurate with AST, whereas in uncomplicated myocardial infarction the ALT is usually normal. In pulmonary embolism, which may mimic myocardial infarction clinically, AST (from an infarcted area of lung) and HBD (from lysis of red blood cells in the embolus and infarct) may be elevated, but the CK is not. Note that the CK has become normal by 48 h (*see Fig. 14.13*).

HEART FAILURE

Heart failure has been defined as a failure of the cardiac output to meet the needs of the tissues (excluding situations where this is caused by volume depletion, e.g. haemorrhage). However, it is probably more useful to regard it as a clinical syndrome with a variety of causes. It may present as a medical emergency (acute pulmonary oedema) or be asymptomatic in the early stages. It is relatively common, with an overall prevalence in the UK of about 1%, although this rises to 8% in those aged over 65. The condition is chronic and progressive, and patients with heart failure have a shortened life-expectancy and impaired quality of life. The prognosis can be improved by appropriate treatment, but since, particularly in the early stages, the symptoms and signs are non-specific, the diagnosis is not easy.

This problem has prompted interest in a biochemical test for heart failure. As discussed in *Chapter 2*, the heart secretes two natriuretic peptides, ANP and BNP. ANP is produced mainly in the atria and BNP (although first isolated in brain) comes mainly from the cardiac ventricles. Release of both is increased in heart failure, although it would appear that BNP is better for assessing ventricular function and as a prognostic indicator. It is synthesized as a prohormone, which is cleaved on release from the cardiac muscle cell to produce BNP itself and an N-terminal fragment of the prohormone called NT-proBNP. Both can be measured in plasma, and a normal value virtually excludes heart failure, although a raised concentration may occur in other conditions. NT-proBNP has a longer half-life and is less sensitive to short-term stimuli for secretion than BNP, so may prove more useful as a 'rule-out' test for heart failure, and reduce the need for echocardiography for definitive diagnosis. However, with a shorter half-life, BNP may also prove useful in tailoring the response to treatment.

Laboratory investigations are also important in the general assessment of patients with heart failure: some examples are given in *Fig. 14.14*.

HYPERTENSION

Hypertension is a common condition affecting, on the basis of widely accepted criteria for normality, approximately 15% of the population. Though usually itself asymptomatic, it is an important cause of morbidity and mortality, particularly from stroke and coronary heart disease. In approximately 95% of patients, a specific cause for raised blood pressure cannot be demonstrated. Such hypertension is termed 'essential': its pathogenesis is not clear, although in some 70% of cases, at least one other member of the family also has hypertension. There are several rare inherited conditions that cause hypertension. They are listed in *Fig. 14.15*, not because of their individual importance, but because of the clinicopathological correlations that they demonstrate. *Fig. 14.15* also includes inherited conditions associated with hypotension, for the same reason.

Laboratory investigations in patients with heart failure	
investigation	**explanation**
full blood count	anaemia is a cause of 'high output' heart failure
plasma albumin	hypoalbuminaemia is another cause of oedema
plasma creatinine	renal impairment
plasma potassium	diuretic-induced hypokalaemia
thyroid function tests*	thyrotoxicosis
plasma ferritin*	haemochromatosis
serum and urine electrophoresis*	myeloma-related amyloid
endocrine causes of hypertension*	*see Fig.14.16*

Fig. 14.14 Laboratory investigations in patients with heart failure.
*Indicates investigations only appropriate if indicated clinically.

Inherited conditions associated with hypertension and hypotension					
Condition	**Inheritance**	**Plasma**		**Cause**	**Other features**
		Aldo	**Renin**		
Hypertension					
glucocorticoid-remediable aldosteronism	AD	N/↓	↓	mutation causes fusing of regulatory sequence of steroid-11β-hydroxylase with coding sequence of aldosterone synthase	variable hypokalaemic alkalosis ↑ plasma 18-hydroxycortisol
Liddle's syndrome	AD	↓	↓	activating mutation in distal tubular sodium transporter	variable hypokalaemic alkalosis
syndrome of apparent mineralocorticoid excess	AR	↓	↓	steroid-11β-hydroxysteroid dehydrogenase deficiency, causing decreased metabolism of cortisol to cortisone	hypokalaemic alkalosis
pseudohypoaldosteronism type II (Gordon's syndrome)	AD	↓	↓	unknown	hyperkalaemia, renal tubular acidosis; responds to salt restriction and thiazides
steroid 11β-hydroxylase deficiency	AR	↓	↓		hypokalaemic alkalosis virilization ↑ plasma 11-deoxycorticosterone and 11-deoxycortisol
steroid 17α-hydroxylase deficiency	AR	↓	↓		hypokalaemic alkalosis feminization (males); lack of normal maturation (females) ↑ plasma 11-deoxycorticosterone and 11-deoxycortisol
Hypotension					
pseudohypoaldosteronism type I	AR	↑	↑	loss of function mutation in distal tubular sodium transporter	salt wasting, hyperkalaemia, metabolic acidosis
	AD	↑	↑	deficiency of mineralocorticoid receptor	
steroid-21-hydroxylase deficiency	AR	↓	↑		salt wasting, hyperkalaemia, metabolic acidosis

Fig. 14.15 Inherited conditions associated with hypertension and hypotension. Aldo = aldosterone; N = normal, sl = slight.

Inherited conditions associated with hypertension and hypotension (cont'd)					
Condition	Inheritance	Plasma Aldo	Renin	Cause	Other features
Gitelman's syndrome	AR	↑	↑	deficiency of thiazide-sensitive sodium transporter	salt wasting, hypokalaemic alkalosis
Bartter's syndrome	AR	↑	↑	deficiency in sodium reabsorption in loop of Henle	salt wasting, hypokalaemic alkalosis

Causes of secondary hypertension
coarctation of the aorta
renal disease
endocrine disease
Conn's syndrome
Cushing's syndrome
phaeochromocytoma
hyperparathyroidism*
pregnancy-associated hypertension

Fig. 14.16 Causes of secondary hypertension. *There is an association between hyperparathyroidism and hypertension but the hypertension often persists after parathyroidectomy.

Biochemical investigations in patients with hypertension	
Investigation	Explanation
urine analysis	for protein (renal disease) and glucose (diabetes, a cardiovascular risk factor)
plasma creatinine	renal disease
plasma potassium	mineralocorticoid excess (primary or secondary)
plasma calcium	hyperparathyroidism
plasma cholesterol and triglycerides	cardiovascular risk assessment
plasma renin and aldosterone*	Conn's syndrome
overnight dexamethasone suppression test*	Cushing's syndrome
urinary catecholamines/ metabolites*	phaeochromocytoma

Fig. 14.17 Biochemical investigations in patients with hypertension. *Indicates investigations only appropriate if indicated clinically or if simple investigations suggest a specific cause.

Biochemical investigations play no part in the diagnosis of essential hypertension, although they are important in assessing possible adverse effects of medication (e.g. diuretic-induced hypokalaemia) and complications of hypertension (particularly renal impairment). They are, however, of value in diagnosing some causes of secondary hypertension, particularly renal and endocrine disease (see Fig. 14.16 and the rare inherited causes).

Because it is so common, it is clearly impractical to investigate all patients with hypertension for these conditions. All patients should have simple investigations performed (see Fig. 14.17), either for the diagnosis of a specific cause or as part of overall cardiovascular risk assessment. More complex investigations, particularly to diagnose Conn's syndrome, phaeochromocytoma or Cushing's syndrome, should be reserved for patients in whom the simple testing suggests a specific cause (e.g. hypokalaemia in an untreated patient should raise a suspicion of excessive mineralocorticoid secretion), those with clinical features suggestive of an underlying cause, and patients with more severe hypertension, particularly if it is difficult to control with conventional treatment.

SUMMARY

- The main lipids in the blood are **triglycerides**, an important energy substrate, and **cholesterol**, a component of the membranes of cells and their organelles. Cholesterol and triglycerides are insoluble in water and are transported in the blood in **lipoproteins**, complexes of lipids with specific proteins known as apolipoproteins.

- There are four major classes of lipoprotein: (i) **chylomicrons**, which carry exogenous, that is dietary, fat (mainly triglyceride) from the gut to peripheral tissues; (ii) **very low density lipoproteins (VLDL)**, which carry endogenous triglyceride from the liver to those tissues; (iii) **low density lipoproteins (LDL)**, which transport cholesterol from the liver to peripheral tissues, and (iv) **high density lipoproteins (HDL)**, involved in reverse cholesterol transport from peripheral tissues to the liver whence it can be excreted. These particles are in a dynamic state and there is considerable exchange of lipid and proteins between them.

- **Hypercholesterolaemia**, when due to an increase in LDL, is an important risk factor for **coronary heart disease**; an excess of cholesterol in HDL confers some protection against this condition. **Hypertriglyceridaemia** is a less important risk factor for coronary heart disease but, when very severe, can cause pancreatitis. Both hypercholesterolaemia and hypertriglyceridaemia are associated with various types of cutaneous fat deposition, or xanthomata.

- **Hyperlipidaemia may be either primary**, that is genetically determined, **or occur secondarily to a variety of other conditions**, including diabetes mellitus, hypothyroidism, obesity, alcoholism, renal disease and certain drugs. The diagnosis of a primary hyperlipidaemia is supported when such conditions can be excluded, especially if there is a family history; often, however, an underlying genetic tendency to hyperlipoproteinaemia is exacerbated by the presence of one of these conditions.

- The most important primary hyperlipidaemia is **familial hypercholesterolaemia**. The molecular basis of this condition is a functional defect in, or a decrease in the number of, LDL receptors, which leads to decreased clearance of these lipoproteins from the blood and an increase in cholesterol synthesis. Heterozygotes for the condition occur with a frequency of approximately 0.2% and have a greatly increased risk of coronary heart disease. Homozygotes are very rare; affected patients develop coronary heart disease in their teens. Other inherited hyperlipidaemias include familial hypertriglyceridaemia, familial combined hyperlipidaemia and dysbetalipoproteinaemia, in which particles with a density intermediate between the low and very low density lipoproteins accumulate.

- **Screening for hypercholesterolaemia** is essential in patients with cardiovascular disease or a strong family history of this condition or of hyperlipidaemia, and in patients with other major cardiovascular disease risk factors, xanthomata or lipaemic plasma. Screening all adults is desirable.

- The rationale for the **treatment of hyperlipidaemias** is largely related to their role in causing cardiovascular disease. The management of secondary hyperlipidaemias should be directed towards the underlying cause. Primary hyperlipidaemias that do not respond adequately to dietary and lifestyle measures require drug treatment but (with the exception of isolated hypertriglyceridaemia, a risk factor for pancreatitis) this must always be done in the context of overall cardiovascular disease risk management, e.g. identification and management of other risk factors, especially hypertension and cigarette smoking.

SUMMARY (cont'd)

- Biochemical tests can be helpful in the diagnosis of **myocardial infarction**, although in practice they may be more useful to exclude the condition than to confirm the diagnosis prior to thrombolysis.

- Measurements of **natriuretic peptides** are of value in the investigation of **heart failure**.

- **Hypertension** is a common clinical problem. It is usually 'essential', but investigations for treatable causes (mainly endocrine) may be appropriate. Simple tests should be performed on all patients, but the more complex reserved for those in whom the results of simple tests are abnormal, hypertension is particularly severe or difficult to control, or in whom there are clinical features suggestive of an underlying cause.

15 The locomotor and nervous systems

INTRODUCTION

It is convenient to consider these systems in the same chapter. Although the diseases that affect them may show little or no overlap, there are obvious functional links. This chapter is mainly devoted to the clinical biochemistry of metabolic bone disease, articular disease and muscle disease. Numerous conditions with a biochemical basis affect the central and peripheral nervous systems: many are rare and beyond the scope of this book, but biochemical investigations have an important, albeit limited, role in a few of the more common conditions.

METABOLIC BONE DISEASE

Bone has three important functions: it provides structural support to the body, it houses the haemopoietic bone marrow, and it is metabolically active, being essential for calcium and phosphate homoeostasis (*see Chapter 12*). Bone consists of a proteinaceous matrix, 90% of which is formed by type I collagen fibres, the remainder being glycoprotein and proteoglycan ground substance. This provides the support for the mineral component, which consists of spindle-shaped crystals of calcium hydroxyapatite. Bone has two structurally distinct components: compact cortical bone and spongy trabecular bone, which supports the bone marrow.

Mature bone undergoes constant remodelling, a process that involves approximately 5% of the skeleton at any one time. This process involves the resorption of small volumes of bone by osteoclasts and their replacement by new bone generated by osteoblasts (*Fig. 15.1*). The osteoblasts become trapped in the new bone and are transformed into osteocytes. The whole process is coordinated by hormones, growth factors and cytokines. Metabolic bone diseases are a result of a disruption of this normally orderly process. The corresponding changes in plasma calcium and phosphate concentrations, and alkaline phosphatase activity (a marker of osteoblastic activity) are summarized in *Fig. 15.2*.

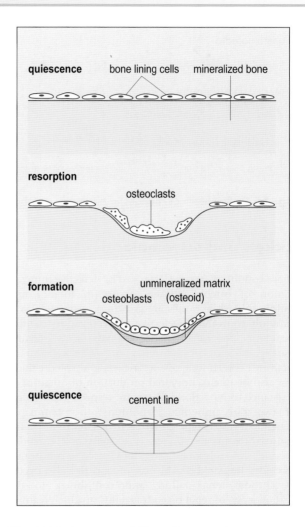

Fig. 15.1 Bone remodelling. Quiescent bone surfaces are covered by osteoblast-related bone lining cells. Remodelling begins with the replacement of these cells by osteoclast precursor cells from blood, perhaps in response to cytokines released from areas of microdamage. These cells differentiate into osteoclasts, which excavate resorption pits. When resorption is complete, the osteoclasts undergo apoptosis and are replaced by osteoblasts, which lay down new osteoid. This becomes mineralized and a new quiescent phase begins. The whole process takes 6–12 months.

Plasma concentration				
Condition	**Calcium**	**Phosphate**	**Alkaline phosphatase**	**Other**
osteoporosis	N	N	N	–
osteomalacia	↓ or N	↓	↑ (↑↑)†	–
Paget's disease	N(↑*)	N	↑↑↑	–
renal osteodystrophy	↓ or N	↑	↑	↑ creatinine
primary hyperparathyroidism	↑	N or ↓	N or ↑	–
secondary tumour deposits	N or ↑	↓ N or ↑	↑	–
* during immobilization	† during early phase of recovery			

Fig. 15.2 Biochemical changes in plasma in metabolic bone disease. N = normal.

Rickets and osteomalacia

These conditions are characterized by defective mineralization of osteoid. Rickets occurs in infancy and childhood (while bones are growing); osteomalacia is its adult equivalent. Defective mineralization is most frequently due to an inadequate supply of calcium, usually because of deficiency or malabsorption of vitamin D. Such 'calciopenic' rickets and osteomalacia can also be due to impaired production of calcitriol or resistance to its actions. These are respectively features of two rare, inherited conditions: in vitamin D-dependent rickets type I, there is deficiency of renal 1α-hydroxylase; in type II, there is resistance to the actions of calcitriol. Inheritance in both cases is autosomal recessive. Impaired production of calcitriol also occurs in chronic renal failure and contributes to the pathogenesis of renal osteodystrophy, in which features of osteomalacia are usually present.

Defective bone mineralization can also be due to an inadequate supply of phosphate. The cause is usually a renal tubular phosphate leak, such as occurs in the Fanconi syndrome, renal tubular acidosis type 1 and, as an isolated phenomenon, in familial X-linked hypophosphataemic rickets.

The clinical features of rickets and osteomalacia include bone pain and tenderness, and (particularly in rickets) skeletal deformities. Proximal muscle weakness is frequently present; hypocalcaemia is occasionally symptomatic but in about 50% of patients with privational disease, calcium concentration is maintained just within the normal range by secondary hyperparathyrodism. Osteomalacia can coexist with osteoporosis.

Both rickets and osteomalacia give rise to characteristic radiological appearances, although these may not always be apparent in osteomalacia, and bone biopsy is sometimes required to confirm the diagnosis. Treatment is with vitamin D or one of its hydroxylated derivatives, together with supplements of calcium or phosphate as appropriate.

Osteoporosis

Osteoporosis is characterized by reduced bone mass and abnormalities of bone micro-architecture, which render it more fragile and susceptible to fracture. Fractures are particularly likely to occur in the vertebral bodies, wrist and proximal femur: they are a considerable source of morbidity and mortality. The lifetime risk of fracture due to osteoporosis is about 40% in women and 15% in men.

The two most frequent causes are post-menopausal oestrogen deficiency and ageing. Post-menopausal osteoporosis results from accelerated bone loss and primarily affects trabecular bone. It typically leads to compression fractures of the vertebral bodies (leading to deformity and loss of height). Age-related osteoporosis occurs in men

Causes of osteoporosis

Primary
ageing
post-menopausal oestrogen deficiency

Secondary
endocrine:
    premature ovarian failure
    thyrotoxicosis
    Cushing's syndrome
    diabetes mellitus
    hypogonadism
drugs:
    prolonged heparin treatment
    glucocorticoids
    alcoholism
others:
    immobilization
    malabsorption of calcium
    weightlessness

Fig. 15.3 Causes of osteoporosis.

and women. It is a result of loss of bone (about 1% of mass per year) because of the decrease in osteoblastic activity in relation to osteoclastic activity that occurs in the remodelling process with ageing. It affects both trabecular and cortical bone and is particularly associated with femoral neck fractures.

These types of osteoporosis are classified as primary. Osteoporosis can also occur secondarily to a variety of conditions (*see Fig. 15.3*), often in younger people. These conditions can also exacerbate primary osteoporosis.

The diagnosis of osteoporosis is based on measurements of bone density, for example by dual-energy X-ray absorptiometry (DEXA). Quantitative ultrasonography appears a promising, though not yet established, technique. Plasma calcium and phosphate concentrations are normal in uncomplicated osteoporosis; so too is alkaline phosphatase activity (unless a fracture has occurred or osteomalacia is also present).

There is considerable interest in the development of markers of bone turnover that could be used to identify patients at risk of developing osteoporosis (fast bone-losers) and to monitor the effects of treatment. Several markers are available for the assessment of both bone resorption and bone formation. Markers of bone resorption include various substances derived from collagen, e.g. pyridinium cross-links of collagen (deoxy-pyridinoline and pyridinoline, both measured in urine) and cross-linking telopeptides of type I collagen (measured in serum). Markers of bone formation include plasma osteocalcin, bone-specific alkaline phosphatase and procollagen type I terminal peptides (N-terminal and C-terminal). These all show promise but no one substance in either class has yet been shown conclusively to be superior to any other. Their value in guiding clinical practice has yet to be fully established but suppression of markers of resorption during treatment with bisphosphonates and oestrogens becomes maximal sooner (approximately three months) than changes in bone density can reliably be detected (up to two years); furthermore, a failure to respond is suggestive of non-compliance with treatment.

Osteoporosis is associated with high morbidity and mortality. Valuable preventative measures include moderate regular weight-bearing exercise and an adequate dietary calcium intake, particularly during growth, to optimize peak bone mass, and continuation of these measures, reduction of alcohol intake and cessation of smoking to reduce the rate of bone loss. In women with premature menopause, hormone replacement treatment (HRT) is the most effective preventative measure. Bisphosphonates (drugs that reduce osteoclastic activity) are regarded as the treatment of choice. HRT is also effective, even in elderly women, but the benefits have to be balanced against the increased risks of certain malignancies. Calcium and vitamin D supplements, calcitonin and calcitriol may be valuable in particular circumstances. Testosterone is effective in hypogonadal men but should not be used in men with normal testicular function since it increases the risk of prostatic cancer. Treatment with intermittent parathyroid hormone is currently being evaluated. In patients with established osteoporosis, it is important to identify and manage appropriately risk factors for falls (e.g. postural hypotension).

Paget's disease of bone

This is a condition of unknown aetiology (though there is some evidence that paramyxovirus infection in genetically predisposed individuals is responsible), characterized by increased osteoclastic activity, which engenders increased osteoblastic activity and thus new bone formation. The new bone that is formed is abnormal and laid down in a disorganized fashion. As a result, bones become thickened, deformed and painful. The most frequently affected bones are those of the pelvis, spine and skull, and the femora.

Case history 15.1

An elderly man who complained of severe pain in his pelvis and thighs was diagnosed on radiological evidence as having Paget's disease of bone. The serum alkaline phosphatase was 750 U/L. He was treated with oral bisphosphonates and made a good clinical recovery, though when his medication was stopped his thighs became painful again.

Investigations
The serum alkaline phosphatase activities are shown in *Fig. 15.4*.

Comment
The primary defect in Paget's disease is an increase in osteoclastic activity, but this causes increased osteoblastic activity, reflected by high serum alkaline phosphatase activities. Serial measurements can be used, as in this case, to monitor the disease and its response to treatment.

Paget's disease can also be monitored by serial measurements of the urinary excretion of hydroxyproline. This amino acid, a component of collagen, is not reutilized in the body and once released from bone by osteoclastic activity is excreted in the urine. Hydroxyproline is present in certain foodstuffs, for example gravies and jellies, and such substances must be avoided before and during urine collections. Other sources of collagen, notably the skin, also contribute to urinary hydroxyproline excretion.

Paget's disease is a disease of the elderly. It is frequently asymptomatic: only about 5% of patients have symptoms, of which the most frequent (80%) is pain. Others features include deformity, pathological fracture, compression of adjacent tissues (e.g. the auditory nerve, causing deafness) and a steal syndrome in which the increased vascularity of the abnormal bone diverts blood flow away from adjacent tissues, causing ischaemia. Osteosarcoma is a feared, but rare (<1%) complication.

Plasma alkaline phosphatase activity is increased and reflects disease activity; plasma calcium and phosphate concentrations are usually normal, although hypercalcaemia may develop if a patient with Paget's disease is immobilized. Treatment involves analgesics and, in more severe cases, the use of bisphosphonates or other agents to reduce osteoclastic activity.

Renal osteodystrophy

Patients with end-stage renal failure develop a complex bone disease, primarily as a result of decreased renal synthesis of calcitriol. This condition is discussed in detail in *Chapter 4*.

Hyperparathyroid bone disease

Clinical evidence of bone involvement used to be a common feature of primary hyperparathyroidism (*see Chapter 12*) but most patients with hyperparathyroidism are now are identified when hypercalcaemia is found incidentally. They are usually asymptomatic and have no abnormal physical signs or radiographic findings. Plasma alkaline phosphatase activity is normal unless there is significant bone involvement.

The characteristic features of hyperparathyroid bone disease include bone pain and evidence of localized areas of bone resorption on radiography, e.g. subperiosteal bone resorption, small, widespread lucencies in the skull ('pepper-pot skull') and bone cysts (brown tumours, composed of osteoclasts and fibrous tissue). These features are due to increased osteoclastic activity, and any increase in plasma alkaline phosphatase is due to an associated increase in osteoblastic activity.

ARTICULAR DISEASE

Joints can be affected by a wide variety of diseases, both specifically and as part of multi-system disease. Osteoarthritis and rheumatoid and other inflammatory arthritides are a major source of pain and disability. For most, the role of the biochemical laboratory in management is limited: one example is the measurement of C-reactive protein (*see p. 241*) to monitor inflammatory conditions. For one group, however, biochemical tests are important in both diagnosis and management: these are the crystalline arthritides, in particular, gout.

Many biochemistry laboratories also provide a service for the measurement of autoantibodies. Rheumatoid

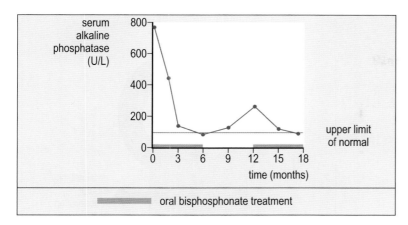

Fig. 15.4 Serum alkaline phosphatase activities in a patient with Paget's disease of bone. Periods of treatment with oral bisphosphonates are indicated. After a good response to the first period of treatment the serum alkaline phosphatase begins to rise, indicating recrudescence of the disease; a good response was again achieved when treatment was restarted.

factor (an IgM antibody against the Fc portion of the IgG molecule) is present in patients with rheumatoid disease. Approximately 30% of patients with this condition are also positive for antinuclear antibodies, but these are particularly associated with systemic lupus erythematosus (SLE). Both these conditions (particularly SLE) can affect many tissues other than joints.

Gout and hyperuricaemia

Clinical gout is the result of the deposition of crystals of monosodium urate in the cartilage, synovium and synovial fluid of joints as a consequence of hyperuricaemia. Uric acid is the end-product of purine metabolism in humans. At physiological pH, uric acid is 98% ionized and is therefore present mainly as the urate ion. In the extracellular fluid (ECF), where sodium is the major cation, uric acid effectively exists as a solution of its sodium salt, monosodium urate. This salt has low solubility, and the ECF becomes saturated at concentrations a little above those that normally prevail. In patients with hyperuricaemia, there is thus a tendency for crystals of monosodium urate to form. In addition to acute gout, other manifestations of crystal formation include renal calculi and tophi (accretions of sodium urate in soft tissues). A sudden increase in urate production, typically seen as a consequence of treatment of haematological malignancy, can lead to widespread crystallization in the renal tubules, causing obstruction and acute renal failure (acute urate nephropathy).

Uric acid metabolism

Purine nucleotides are essential components of nucleic acids: they are intimately involved in energy transformation and phosphorylation reactions and act as intracellular messengers. There are three sources of purines in humans: the diet, degradation of endogenous nucleotides and *de novo* synthesis (*Fig. 15.5*). Since purines are metabolized to uric acid, the body urate pool (and hence plasma concentration) depends on the relative rates of both urate formation from these sources and urate excretion. Urate is excreted by both the kidneys and the gut, renal excretion accounting for approximately two-thirds of the total. Urate secreted into the gut is metabolized to carbon dioxide and ammonia by bacterial action (uricolysis).

Urate handling by the kidney is complex (*Fig. 15.6*). It is filtered at the glomeruli and almost totally absorbed in the proximal convoluted tubules; distally, both secretion and reabsorption occur. Normal urate clearance is about 10% of the filtered load. In normal subjects, urate excretion increases if the filtered load is increased. In chronic renal failure, the plasma concentration rises only when the glomerular filtration rate falls below about 20 mL/min.

Dietary purines account for about 30% of excreted urate. The introduction of a purine-free diet typically reduces plasma urate concentrations by only 10–20%.

The metabolic pathways leading to uric acid synthesis are shown in outline in *Fig. 15.7*. *De novo* synthesis leads to the formation of inosine monophosphate (IMP), which can be converted to the nucleotides adenosine monophosphate (AMP) and guanosine monophosphate

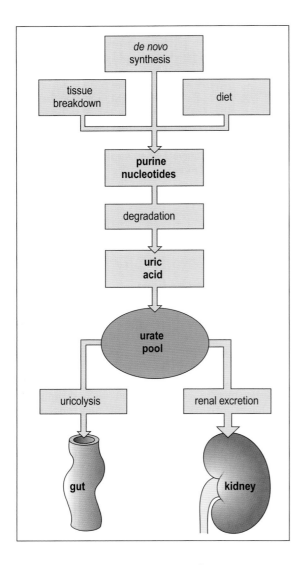

Fig. 15.5 Sources and excretion of urate.

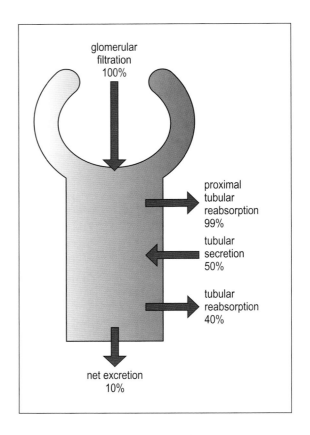

Fig. 15.6 Urate excretion in the kidney.

(GMP). Nucleotide degradation involves the formation of the respective nucleosides (inosine, adenosine and guanosine); these are then metabolized to purines. The purine derived from IMP is hypoxanthine, which is converted by the enzyme xanthine oxidase first to xanthine and then to uric acid. Guanine can be metabolized to xanthine (and so to uric acid) directly, but adenine cannot. However, AMP can be converted to IMP by the enzyme AMP deaminase and, at the nucleoside level, adenosine can be converted to inosine. Thus,

surplus GMP and AMP can be converted to uric acid and excreted.

However, the excretion of uric acid represents the waste of a metabolic investment since purine synthesis requires considerable energy expenditure. Pathways exist whereby purines can be salvaged and converted back to their parent nucleotides. For guanine and hypoxanthine, this is accomplished by the enzyme, hypoxanthine–guanine phosphoribosyl transferase (HGPRT), and for adenine by adenine phosphoribosyl transferase (APRT).

Plasma urate concentrations are, in general, higher in men than in women. Marked increases occur at puberty in males (there is a lesser increase in females at this time) and perimenopausally in women (*Fig. 15.8*). Urate concentrations tend to be higher in people in the higher socioeconomic groups and in the obese. There is considerable, genetically determined, variation in plasma urate concentrations between different ethnic groups.

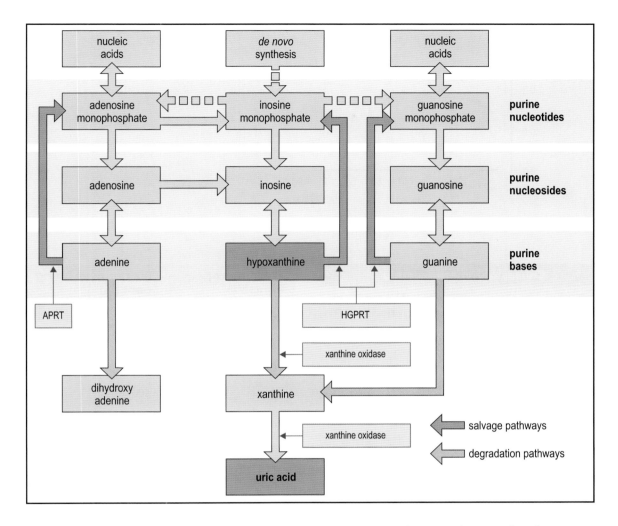

Fig. 15.7 Simplified diagram of the pathways of purine nucleotide metabolism and uric acid synthesis in humans. APRT = adenine phosphoribosyl transferase; HGPRT = hypoxanthine–guanine phosphoribosyl transferase.

In adult males in the UK, the upper limit of the reference range is usually taken as 0.42 mmol/L (0.36 mmol/L in females). In an aqueous solution of pH 7.4 ([H^+] 40 nmol/L), at 37°C, and with an ionic strength similar to that of plasma, the solubility of monosodium urate is 0.57 mmol/L; in plasma, the presence of protein appears to reduce this somewhat.

Hyperuricaemia

Hyperuricaemia may occur because of increased formation of uric acid, decreased excretion, or a combination of both. Some causes of increased formation are given in *Fig. 15.9*.

When hyperuricaemia is due to decreased excretion, it is renal excretion that is usually affected. Indeed, in hyperuricaemia the total amount of urate removed by uricolysis in the gut is increased. Reference to *Fig. 15.6* will show that decreased renal urate excretion could result from decreased filtration or tubular secretion. Plasma urate concentration only rises late in chronic renal failure, but many factors can affect tubular function and thereby cause hyperuricaemia: the more important of these are given in *Fig. 15.9*. Excessive alcohol probably

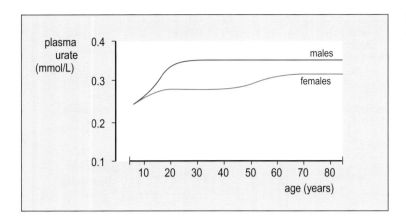

Fig. 15.8 Mean plasma urate concentrations in men and women.

Causes of hyperuricaemia	
Increased urate formation	**Decreased renal urate excretion**
Primary increased purine synthesis: idiopathic inherited metabolic disease	**Primary** idiopathic
	Secondary chronic renal disease increased renal reabsorption/ decreased secretion: thiazide diuretics salicylates (low doses) organic acids (e.g. lactic acid, hence alcohol) lead
Secondary excessive dietary purine intake disordered ATP metabolism: alcohol tissue hypoxia increased nucleic acid turnover: malignant disease psoriasis cytotoxic drugs	

Fig. 15.9 Causes of increased formation of uric acid and reduced uric acid excretion by the kidneys. Note that salicylates reduce uric acid excretion at low doses only; at high doses (>4 g/24 h) aspirin is uricosuric as it blocks the tubular reabsorption of uric acid.

Plasma urate (mmol/L)	Risk of developing gout (%)
<0.41	1
0.42–0.47	1
0.48–0.53	4
>0.54	50

Fig. 15.10 Risk of developing gout in relation to plasma urate concentration. The figures are the incidences per year per 1000 men. A similar trend is apparent in women but few women have plasma urate concentrations >0.48 mmol/L.

increases adenine nucleotide degradation (and some alcoholic beverages contain high concentrations of purines), but any increase in lactate production due to alcohol may also impair urate excretion.

Gout

Acute gout is characterized by severe joint pain of rapid onset associated with swelling and redness. The risk of gout increases with increasing plasma urate concentrations (*Fig. 15.10*). At any particular urate concentration, the risk is similar in males and females. However, although hyperuricaemia is a prerequisite for the development of gout, gout by no means always complicates hyperuricaemia. Indeed, some 85% of people with hyperuricaemia remain asymptomatic throughout life.

Gout can be precipitated by a sudden change (either increase or decrease) in urate concentration. When urate concentration has fallen rapidly in a hyperuricaemic individual (for example, as a result of a change in diet, decrease in alcohol consumption or treatment with a hypouricaemic drug), the plasma urate concentration may not be elevated when the patient presents with gout. The solubility of monosodium urate declines rapidly with decreasing temperature and this may, to some extent, explain the tendency for the more peripheral joints, which have lower intra-articular temperatures, to be more frequently affected.

Gout is customarily defined as primary (idiopathic) or secondary (when a condition known to cause hyper-uricaemia is present). However, gout is uncommon when hyperuricaemia develops secondarily to other conditions. The tendency for hyperuricaemia and gout to be familial has led to investigation for a causal inherited metabolic defect. Although there are a few rare conditions in which such a defect does lead to hyperuricaemia, none has been found in the great majority of cases of primary gout. Some 90% of patients appear to excrete urate at a rate inappropriately low for the plasma concentration, while about 10% have excessive urate production. Dietary factors and alcohol ingestion exacerbate hyperuricaemia in about half the cases, but while their amelioration may reduce the plasma urate concentrations somewhat, these usually remain elevated. Gout is rare in premenopausal women, in whom mean plasma concentrations of urate are much lower than in men of corresponding age (*see* Fig. 15.8), but the incidence increases markedly after the menopause.

Patients with gout frequently have hyperlipidaemia (particularly hypertriglyceridaemia). The cause of the link is uncertain: it may be genetic or related to causal factors common to both conditions, such as alcohol, or both.

Diagnosis

The diagnosis of gout is primarily clinical but is supported by the demonstration of hyperuricaemia. The diagnosis is confirmed by the presence of tophi or of monosodium urate crystals in the synovial fluid. These crystals are typically needle-shaped, 2–10 μm long and are seen within neutrophils. They show strong negative birefringence when viewed with polarized light.

The differential diagnosis includes other crystalline arthropathies and septic arthritis.

Pathogenesis

Monosodium urate crystals forming in joints are engulfed by neutrophil leucocytes but damage the lysosomal

Case history 15.2

An obese 55-year-old male was awoken from sleep after spending the evening at a business dinner, by excruciating pain in his left first metatarsophalangeal joint. He was unable to put his foot to the floor. The affected joint was hot, swollen, red and extremely tender. He was treated with indometacin and the symptoms resolved rapidly. One year previously he had had an episode of renal colic but had declared himself to be too busy to be investigated in connection with this.

Investigations

serum: urate   0.78 mmol/L

Comment

This is the classic presentation of gout. The onset is often sudden, nocturnal and monoarticular. In 70% of cases the metatarsophalangeal joint of the great toe is the first to be affected. The classic signs of inflammation were present and hyperuricaemia was confirmed. In this case, the previous episode of renal colic may well have been due to a renal urate stone. Gout is more common in men than in women and is associated with higher social class, driving (type A) personality, obesity, hypertriglyceridaemia, hypertension and excessive food and alcohol intake.

membranes of these cells, so causing cellular disruption. The generation of superoxide free radicals and release of lysosomal enzymes into the joint precipitates an acute inflammatory reaction. The release of interleukins and other inflammatory mediators from monocytes and tissue macrophages also provides an inflammatory stimulus.

Management

Non-steroidal anti-inflammatory drugs (of which indometacin is the most widely used for the purpose) are used to treat acute gout. Colchicine is also effective. Steroids are sometimes required.

None of these agents affects the hyperuricaemia. This can be treated by dietary measures, avoidance of alcohol and, if possible, of relevant drugs (especially diuretics).

Urate-lowering drugs, of which the most widely used is allopurinol, are used for long-term treatment when there have been recurrent acute attacks of gout, when there is renal damage or renal calculi with hyperuricaemia, in tophaceous gout, or after an attack of gout associated with hyperuricaemia. Allopurinol is an inhibitor of xanthine oxidase and thus inhibits the synthesis of urate from xanthine. It decreases plasma urate concentration and urinary urate excretion; urinary xanthine excretion is increased, but xanthine is more water soluble than urate. Allopurinol is also used prophylactically to prevent hyperuricaemia in the treatment of haematological malignancies (*see pp. 324–325*).

Starting treatment with hypouricaemic drugs may precipitate an acute attack of gout and they must not be taken during or for several weeks after an acute episode. Colchicine is effective for prophylaxis if recurrent acute attacks occur or attacks occur during treatment to lower urate concentrations.

Stages of gout

Four stages in the natural history of gout have been described (*Fig. 15.11*). Asymptomatic hyperuricaemia (i) can be present for years before an acute attack (ii) is precipitated by, for example, trauma or dietary indiscretion. Symptom-free periods of months or years follow ('intercritical gout') (iii), punctuated by acute attacks leading, if untreated, to chronic tophaceous gout (iv). Since the introduction of allopurinol, tophaceous gout, once common, is now rarely seen. It tends to occur mainly in elderly women treated with diuretics for many years (in particular thiazides, which inhibit renal tubular secretion of urate) rather than as a sequel to recurrent attacks of acute gout.

Rare causes of hyperuricaemia

There are a number of rare, inherited metabolic diseases associated with hyperuricaemia and gout (*Fig. 15.12*). In all of them, hyperuricaemia results from increased uric acid synthesis.

Hypouricaemia

This is uncommon and in itself clinically inconsequential. It may be due to either decreased urate

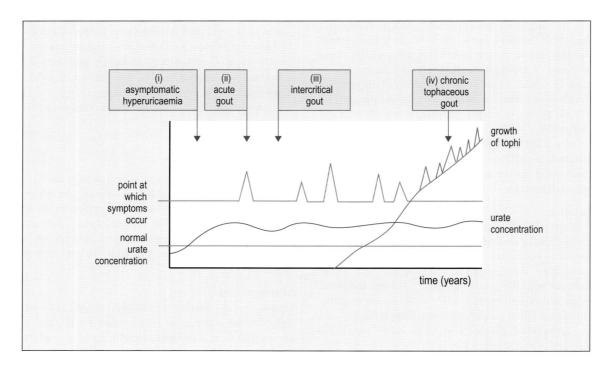

Fig. 15.11 The natural history of gout. Modified from Dieppe & Calvert (1983) *Crystals and Joint Disease*, London: Chapman & Hall.

Major inherited metabolic diseases associated with hyperuricaemia	
Enzyme abnormality	**Consequence**
hypoxanthine–guanine phosphoribosyl transferase deficiency (Lesch–Nyhan syndrome and less severe variants)	decreased activity of salvage pathway decreases purine reutilization and thus increases uric acid synthesis
glucose 6-phosphatase deficiency (glycogen storage disease type I)	(i) increased metabolism of glucose 6-phosphate through pentose phosphate pathway increases formation of ribose 5-phosphate, a substrate for purine nucleotide synthesis
	(ii) hyperlactataemia decreases uric acid secretion in renal tubules
phosphoribosyl pyrophosphate synthetase (PRPP synthetase) variant (with increased activity)	PRPP is a substrate for purine nucleotide synthesis and also activates the rate-limiting enzyme

Fig. 15.12 Inherited metabolic diseases associated with hyperuricaemia.

synthesis or increased excretion and so is seen in congenital xanthine oxidase deficiency (xanthinuria), severe liver disease and renal tubular disorders such as the Fanconi syndrome. It can also result from excessive medication with allopurinol and the use of uricosuric drugs such as probenecid.

Other crystalline arthropathies

Gout is not the only crystalline arthropathy. The deposition of calcium pyrophosphate in joints may mimic gout clinically (pseudogout). It can also cause a chronic arthropathy that mimics and overlaps with osteoarthritis. Calcium pyrophosphate crystals may be demonstrable in synovial fluid. They are characteristically rhomboid or rod-shaped and show weak positive birefringence when viewed with polarized light. Chondrocalcinosis (calcium deposition in articular cartilage) may also be present. Calcium pyrophosphate arthropathy is predominantly a disease of the elderly. The condition may be familial but most cases occur in association with hyperparathyroidism, haemochromatosis or other metabolic disorders.

Hydroxyapatite crystals can occur in joints. This is often asymptomatic but can occasionally cause an acute synovitis clinically resembling gout. Very rarely, other crystals occur in joints, for example calcium oxalate in patients with type 1 hyperoxaluria.

MUSCLE DISEASE

Skeletal muscle can be affected by several disease processes, including trauma, inflammation, metabolic myopathies (both genetic and acquired) and non-metabolic genetically determined myopathies. Some of the more important causes of myopathy are indicated in *Fig. 15.13*. Biochemical investigations in traumatic and inflammatory muscle disease are limited to the detection of muscle damage and its consequences, but investigation of suspected myopathies may involve highly specialized biochemical investigations, together with histological and histochemical examination.

Markers of muscle damage

The most widely used marker of muscle damage is the enzyme creatine kinase (CK). Human tissues contain three forms of CK, comprising dimers of the muscle (M) and brain (B) subunits. Skeletal muscle contains mainly CK-MM, with about 1% CK-MB, this proportion being higher in type I (aerobic, slow twitch) fibres and in

Some causes of skeletal muscle disease	
physical damage	crush syndrome
	ischaemia
inflammation	polymyositis
	dermatomyositis
	viral myositis
metabolic	endocrine disease:
	hypo-, hyperthyroidism
	hyperadrenalism
	alcohol
genetic	phosphorylase deficiency
	fatty acid oxidation disorders
	respiratory chain disorders
	muscular dystrophies
	malignant hyperpyrexia

Fig. 15.13 Some causes of skeletal muscle disease.

regenerating fibres. Normal plasma CK activity is almost entirely due to CK-MM, and is derived from skeletal muscle. Cardiac muscle contains about 30% CK-MB: the use of CK measurements in the management of patients with chest pain is discussed in *Chapter 14*. Although it is usually considered that a high plasma CK activity with more than 5% due to CK-MB is characteristic of cardiac muscle damage, it should be appreciated that the contribution from skeletal muscle alone can be this high following acute muscle injury, in patients with chronic muscle disease and in children.

The activity of CK in the plasma varies considerably in healthy individuals and is higher in certain racial groups, particularly Afro-Caribbeans. Conditions causing an increase in plasma CK activity are indicated in *Fig. 13.17*. The highest activities are seen in association with severe muscle necrosis, for example in polymyositis and rhabdomyolysis, and Duchenne muscular dystrophy. The elevation in CK following severe exercise can be up to $10 \times$ ULN and tends to be greater in untrained subjects. The rise begins immediately and reaches a peak after 1–2 days. Serial plasma CK measurements are of value in following the progress of myopathic disorders and their response to treatment.

Other enzymes that have been used as markers of muscle damage include aldolase and lactate dehydrogenase, but CK offers better sensitivity than either. Myoglobin is also released from damaged muscle but its measurement provides no more information than CK. In severe muscle damage, myoglobinuria can occur and cause a brown coloration of the urine. Myoglobin can precipitate out in the renal tubules and cause an obstructive nephropathy: the renal failure associated with crush injuries is in part due to this. Other metabolic consequences of severe muscle damage include hyperkalaemia, due to release of intracellular potassium, and hypocalcaemia, due to calcium becoming bound by damaged tissue.

Muscular dystrophies

The muscular dystrophies are inherited disorders characterized clinically by progressive muscular weakness due to muscle degeneration. The commonest type is Duchenne muscular dystrophy, an X-linked condition with a prevalence of approximately 1 in 3000 live male births in the UK. It usually presents in the first decade; most patients die within ten years of diagnosis.

Duchenne muscular dystrophy is a result of a mutation in the dystrophin gene, dystrophin being an intracellular muscle protein. Perhaps because the gene is unusually large, about a third of all cases arise from new mutations. The clinical diagnosis of the condition can be confirmed by direct analysis of a muscle biopsy for dystrophin content. Molecular genetic analysis can be used for prenatal diagnosis. Plasma CK activity can be $50–100 \times$ ULN in patients with Duchenne muscular dystrophy. Female carriers are usually asymptomatic but most have moderate elevations in CK; symptoms occur in only 2–3% of females ('manifesting carriers', presumably due to genetic mosaicism).

Becker muscular dystrophy, a less severe condition, usually presenting later in childhood, is about ten times less common. It is also due to a mutation in the dystrophin gene but, whereas in Duchenne the protein is undetectable in muscle biopsies, in Becker it is present either in reduced amounts or is structurally altered.

Other non-metabolic myopathies

Hypo- and hyperkalaemic periodic paralyses are muscle membrane disorders. Redistribution of potassium causes abnormal plasma concentrations and patients experience episodes of generalized or localized muscle weakness. They are usually familial, but can be acquired. Malignant hyperpyrexia is a rare condition in which certain inhalation anaesthetics or suxamethonium trigger

Case history 15.3

An 18-year-old man was investigated for pain in his muscles associated with exercise. He said that he had experienced occasional muscle pain for years, but it had recently become more noticeable since he had started working out in a gym. Physical examination at rest was unremarkable. Plasma creatine kinase activity was twice the upper limit of normal.

Investigation

Ischaemic exercise test:
    plasma lactate pre-exercise   0.9 mmol/L

He developed pain in his arm and the test was stopped after 45 seconds.
    plasma lactate post-exercise   1.1 mmol/L

Comment

In this test, a sphygmomanometer cuff is placed around the upper arm and inflated to just above systolic blood pressure. The subject squeezes a spare sphygmomanometer bulb rapidly for a minute. Blood samples are taken prior to exercise and at intervals up to 10 min thereafter. A normal subject can exercise without discomfort and plasma lactate concentration in the ischaemic arm increases three- to fivefold. A failure to increase is characteristic of either abnormal glycogen metabolism or glycolysis. Analysis of a muscle biopsy showed low phosphorylase activity (McArdle's disease, glycogen storage disease type V).

---

a rapid rise in body temperature, lactic acidosis and rhabdomyolysis with hyperkalaemia and hundred-fold elevations of plasma CK activity.

Metabolic myopathies

This group of muscle diseases includes two main groupings: acquired, for example secondary to alcohol abuse or endocrine disease, and genetic, due to an inherited defect of an enzyme involved in muscle metabolism. There are several of these; all are rare, but biochemical investigations are essential to their diagnosis.

NERVOUS SYSTEM DISEASE

Biochemical investigations have a limited role in the investigation of nervous system diseases although tests on cerebrospinal fluid are valuable in certain conditions (*see below*).

Coma

There are numerous causes of coma or decreased consciousness. The history, careful physical examination and imaging will often reveal the cause. Biochemical investigations that may be helpful include measurement of drugs, including alcohol, and glucose (for hypo- or hyperglycaemia). The possibility of alcohol ingestion should be considered in patients with head injuries and patients who have taken drug overdoses. Routine biochemical tests will detect hyponatraemia and uraemia. Arterial blood gases should be measured in all unconscious patients: the clinical circumstances may indicate a need for specific tests (e.g. for endocrine dysfunction).

Dementia

Dementia is characterized by a loss of intellectual function in the absence of impairment of consciousness. The most frequent causes are Alzheimer's disease and cerebrovascular disease. Both are primarily diseases of the elderly, although Alzheimer's disease can have its onset in middle age (pre-senile dementia). There is a strong genetic component to the pre-senile type. Huntington's disease is a rare, inherited (autosomal dominant) cause of dementia, often accompanied by chorea: it is caused by a repeating base-triplet sequence of variable length. There is no effective treatment. Dementia can also be a feature of endocrine disorders (e.g. hypothyroidism), hepatic and renal failure, chronic alcohol misuse, heavy metal poisoning, carbon monoxide poisoning and vitamin deficiency. Simple laboratory investigations that should be performed in dementia, either to identify the small number of patients with treatable causes, or conditions that increase the morbidity of the condition, are shown in *Fig. 15.14*.

Routine laboratory investigations in dementia
full blood count and ESR
calcium
folate and vitamin B_{12}
glucose
liver function tests
sodium, potassium, creatinine
thyroid function tests

Fig. 15.14 Routine laboratory investigations on blood or serum in patients with dementia; additional investigations, e.g. CSF examination, measurement of heavy metal concentrations, may be appropriate according to the clinical circumstances.

The development of acetylcholinesterase inhibitors to treat patients with early Alzheimer's disease has stimulated research to identify biochemical markers of the condition. Two CSF proteins, α-protein and β-amyloid peptide 42, have been investigated to this end, but neither is sufficiently sensitive or specific for diagnosis; however, some studies have suggested that the latter reflects disease activity and so might have potential in monitoring the response to treatment.

Epilepsy

The importance of monitoring plasma concentrations of certain anticonvulsants is discussed in *Chapter 19*.

Peripheral neuropathies

These conditions are diagnosed clinically and on the basis of neurophysiological studies. When caused by a metabolic or endocrine disease (particularly diabetes mellitus), the cause is usually obvious, but peripheral neuropathy can be the presenting feature of lead poisoning and acute intermittent porphyria.

Stroke

In stroke, there is damage to brain tissue, due either to ischaemia (80–85% cases) or haemorrhage (15–20%). Ischaemic stroke is usually due to cerebrovascular atherosclerosis. The diagnosis of stroke is clinical; distinction between ischaemic and haemorrhagic stroke can only be made reliably by CT or MRI. Although clinical trials of cholesterol-lowering drugs have tended to concentrate on cardiovascular disease, there is evidence that treatment with statins to lower cholesterol can reduce the risk of stroke; furthermore, most patients with cerebrovascular disease will also have cardiovascular disease. For these reasons, the target cholesterol concentrations in patients with stroke should be a total of <5.0 mmol/L and LDL <3.0 mmol/L, as it is for patients with cardiovascular disease.

Other neurological disorders

Numerous very rare inherited disorders can affect the central nervous system and cause developmental delay and poor intellectual attainment. Many are incurable, and lead to death in early childhood. These conditions include lysosomal storage disorders, in which lysosomal enzyme defects lead to the accumulation of macro-molecules in the brain, amino acidopathies, and others. Phenylketonuria is an example of a treatable condition, but treatment must begin very soon after birth. Neonatal screening for this condition is discussed in *Chapter 16*.

Examination of the cerebrospinal fluid

Cerebrospinal fluid (CSF) is usually obtained for diagnostic purposes by lumbar puncture. The protein concentration is normally 0.1–0.4 g/L and the protein is predominantly albumin; higher concentrations are found in neonates (up to 0.9 g/L) and the elderly. It is important that the CSF is not contaminated with blood since the presence of plasma proteins will completely invalidate the results of CSF protein measurement.

Examination of the CSF is most often performed in cases of suspected meningitis. The diagnosis of this condition is primarily the concern of the medical microbiologist, but it is usual also to request biochemical analysis for glucose and protein. The significance of the CSF glucose concentration is considered in *Chapter 11*. In meningitis, there is secretion of IgG into the CSF but this has little effect on the total amount of protein. However, meningeal inflammation may lead to an increase in capillary permeability and, therefore, a marked increase in CSF protein content. It is important to note that, in suspected meningitis, a normal CSF protein does not exclude the diagnosis.

CSF protein concentration is increased in patients with tumours of the central nervous system and may exceed 5 g/L in patients with tumours that obstruct the normal circulation of the CSF (spinal block or Froin's syndrome).

Examination of the CSF can be of great value in the diagnosis of multiple sclerosis. Although the total protein concentration is usually only slightly raised, there is increased local synthesis of IgG and the ratio of IgG to albumin is increased from less than 10% to as much as 50%. Greater sensitivity is provided if the IgG:albumin ratio of the CSF is compared with that of plasma. The ratio is abnormal in approximately 80% of cases of multiple sclerosis but may also be abnormal in neurosyphilis, with tumours of the central nervous system and after cerebrovascular accidents.

An even more sensitive test is provided by electrophoresis of CSF on polyacrylamide gel. In multiple sclerosis, only a small number of clones of B-cells produce IgG, which is seen as discrete 'oligoclonal' bands when CSF is electrophoresed. The methodology is technically demanding and considerable experience is necessary for interpretation of the results. Oligoclonal bands can be detected in over 95% of cases of multiple sclerosis, although they may also be seen in other, less common, demyelinating diseases, such as subacute sclerosing panencephalitis and in neurosyphilis.

Examination of the CSF can also be useful in patients with suspected subarachnoid haemorrhage (SAH). SAH is spontaneous arterial bleeding into the subarachnoid space, usually from a berry aneurysm. There is a high mortality rate and a high risk of re-bleeding, so it is important to make the diagnosis and refer patients to a neurosurgical centre for their management. In most patients, a CT scan will demonstrate blood in the subarachnoid space. However, if there is a suggestive clinical history and the CT is negative (approximately 10% of cases of SAH), examination of the CSF may help. Three consecutive samples of CSF are collected into separate containers and a cell count is carried out. In SAH, each sample has approximately the same raised red blood cell count. If blood has been introduced into the CSF during the lumbar puncture (a 'traumatic tap'), the red cell count is higher in the first sample than in the second and third.

Following haemorrhage into the CSF, red cells undergo lysis and phagocytosis, and the oxyhaemoglobin that is released is slowly converted into bilirubin (and sometimes methaemoglobin). In some cases, the bilirubin imparts a yellow colour (xanthochromia) to the CSF that is visible to the naked eye. However, visual inspection is not an effective way of detecting small amounts of bilirubin: spectrophotometric scanning is far more sensitive and, in equivocal cases, scanning of apparently colourless CSF for xanthochromia may help to distinguish SAH from a traumatic tap. The spectrophotometric scan detects oxyhaemoglobin as well as bilirubin, but it is safer to take only the presence of bilirubin to indicate SAH, as oxyhaemoglobin may be present as a result of either SAH or *in vitro* haemolysis of red cells introduced during a traumatic tap. It is important that the lumbar puncture be performed at least 12 hours after the onset of symptoms, so that there is time for bilirubin to have been formed.

PSYCHIATRIC DISEASE

Although many psychiatric disorders are considered to have a biochemical basis, measurements of analytes in plasma play no part in the diagnosis of psychiatric disease with the exception of acute confusional states (delirium), which can be caused by endocrine and metabolic disease, by hypoxia and by toxins. The importance of the measurement of plasma lithium concentrations in patients treated with this drug for affective disorders is discussed in *Chapter 19*.

SUMMARY

- The **metabolic bone diseases** include osteoporosis, osteomalacia, Paget's disease, hyperparathyroid bone disease and renal osteodystrophy. Characteristic biochemical changes in plasma occur in all of them with the exception of osteoporosis.

- **Osteomalacia** is usually due to deficiency or abnormal metabolism of vitamin D; **rickets** is its childhood equivalent. In **osteoporosis**, a decrease in osteoid and mineral reduces the strength of bone and predisposes it to fracture. It is a major cause of morbidity and mortality in the elderly, particularly in women. **Paget's disease** is also primarily a condition of the elderly; increased osteoclastic activity and abnormal new bone formation cause bone pain and, in severe cases, deformity.

- **Gout** is an arthropathy caused by the precipitation of monosodium urate crystals in synovial joints. This occurs when plasma urate concentrations are elevated. Secondary causes of **hyperuricaemia** include renal disease, thiazide diuretics, increased cell turnover and a high intake of purine-rich foods. Gout and hyperuricaemia show a strong familial incidence. Some very rare inherited defects in purine metabolism that cause hyperuricaemia have been described but in the majority of patients there is no such defect, and hyperuricaemia is thought to be due to decreased renal urate excretion. Gout usually presents as an acute arthritis, but can lead to chronic joint disease, and crystals of monosodium urate can be deposited in tissues and in the renal tubules, causing an obstructive uropathy.

- Plasma creatine kinase activity is a valuable test for the presence of **damage to skeletal muscle**, and serial measurements can be used to monitor the progress of response to treatment of patients with muscle diseases. Many muscle diseases have a metabolic basis, including the **muscular dystrophies** and inherited **metabolic myopathies**. Highly specialized biochemical investigations are used, together with histological and histochemical investigations, in their diagnosis.

- Biochemical investigations are of limited value in the diagnosis and management of **neurological and psychiatric disease**. Important applications include the investigation and management of the unconscious patient, examination of the cerebrospinal fluid in patients suspected of having multiple sclerosis and subarachnoid haemorrhage, and therapeutic monitoring of the plasma concentrations of certain anticonvulsant drugs used in the treatment of epilepsy, and of lithium, used in the treatment of some affective disorders.

16 Inherited metabolic diseases

INTRODUCTION

Many inherited diseases are known to be due to the genetically determined absence or modification of specific proteins. For example, in sickle cell anaemia the protein is haemoglobin; in agammaglobulinaemia, antibody production is defective. However, in the majority of such diseases, the protein in question is an enzyme and the effect is to cause a metabolic disorder. Other inherited metabolic diseases may be due to defective receptor synthesis (for example, familial hyper-cholesterolaemia, which affects the receptor for low density lipoprotein), or to defects involving carrier proteins (for example, cystinuria, in which renal tubular reabsorption of cystine is impaired). Whatever the cause, the clinical features of inherited metabolic diseases stem directly from the metabolic abnormalities to which they give rise. Although individually these conditions are rare (*see Fig. 16.1*), they are of considerable signifi-

Approximate incidences of some inherited metabolic diseases	
Condition	**Incidence**
familial hypercholesterolaemia	1:500
cystic fibrosis	1:2500
steroid 21-hydroxylase deficiency	1:5000
α_1-antitrypsin deficiency	1:3500
phenylketonuria	1:10,000
glycogen storage disease (all types combined)	1:50,000
classical galactosaemia	1:60,000
tyrosinaemia type 1	1:100,000
hereditary fructose intolerance	1:200–250,000
maple syrup urine disease	1:250,000

Fig. 16.1 Approximate incidences of some inherited metabolic diseases. Note that there is considerable variation in the incidence of these conditions in different countries and in different ethnic groups.

cance; the consequences of many of them are potentially severe but may in some cases be ameliorated if an early diagnosis is made and the appropriate treatment instituted.

In recent years, application of the techniques of molecular genetic analysis has massively increased our understanding of these conditions. Whereas it used to be thought that each condition was the result of a single mutation, it is now clear that many inherited metabolic diseases can arise because of one of a number of genetic defects. Furthermore, it is clear that the concept of 'one gene, one enzyme' is no longer generally applicable. Many inherited metabolic diseases are a consequence of a mutation in a single gene affecting the synthesis of one enzyme: classical phenylketonuria is an example. However, there are many exceptions. For example, one polypeptide chain can occur in more than one enzyme: an example is the β-subunit of hexosaminidase A (one α-, one β-chain) and B (two β-chains), deficiency of which causes Sandhoff disease, one of the gangliosidoses; inherited deficiency of the α-chain affects only hexos-aminidase A, and causes a related but distinct disorder, Tay–Sachs disease. Or the active form of an enzyme may consist of sub-units coded by different genes, an example being propionyl CoA carboxylase: mutations in either gene can lead to deficiency of the enzyme, causing propionic acidaemia. Another variant is that one polypeptide chain may have more than one enzyme activity, as is the case with two enzymes involved in pyrimidine metabolism, orotate phospho-ribosyltransferase and orotidine 5'-monophosphate decarboxylase, deficiency of which causes orotic aciduria.

Because they are individually rare, it is important for the clinician to have a high index of suspicion and actively consider the possibility that an illness may be caused by an inherited metabolic disease. Common clinical presentations of inherited metabolic diseases are indicated in *Fig. 16.2*. Screening tests for these conditions are discussed in *Chapter 21*. Most inherited metabolic diseases present in infancy and childhood, and their diagnosis and management is the province of the paediatrician, albeit often in close collaboration

Common clinical features of inherited metabolic diseases presenting in childhood

acidosis
central nervous system dysfunction: irritability, coma, hypotonia, seizures, etc.
failure to thrive
frequent vomiting, other gastrointestinal abnormalities
hypoglycaemia
unusual odour

Fig. 16.2 Common clinical features of inherited metabolic diseases presenting in childhood. Features may be provoked by a specific stimulus, e.g. feeding or a lack of feeding.

Inherited metabolic diseases discussed in other chapters of this book

Inherited metabolic disease	Page
Bartter's syndrome	274
congenital adrenal hyperplasia	157
Crigler–Najjar disease types 1 and 2	99
cystinosis	81
cystinuria	82
Dubin–Johnson syndrome	99
Duchenne muscular dystrophy	290
familial combined hyperlipidaemia	268
familial dysbetalipoproteinaemia	267
familial hypercholesterolaemia	265
Gilbert's syndrome	97
haemochromatosis	317
hereditary fructose intolerance	215
hyperoxaluria types 1 and 2	82
Huntington's disease	291
Lesch–Nyhan syndrome	289
Liddle's syndrome	273
muscle phosphorylase deficiency (glycogen storage disease type V)	291
porphyrias	311
renal glycosuria	81
Rotor syndrome	99
urea cycle defects	370
vitamin D-dependent rickets	280
vitamin D-resistant rickets	82
Wilson's disease	99

Fig. 16.3 Inherited metabolic diseases discussed in other chapters of this book.

with the laboratory staff, although with improving treatment, affected children with some conditions that hitherto were usually fatal in childhood are surviving into adulthood. Some inherited metabolic diseases only present clinically in adults, an important example being familial hypercholesterolaemia (*see* p. 265) although homozygotes for this dominantly inherited condition tend to present in their late teenage years and early twenties.

Most inherited metabolic diseases show autosomal recessive inheritance; heterozygotes are usually phenotypically normal. Familial hypercholesterolaemia and most of the porphyrias are important exceptions, being inherited as autosomal dominants.

The techniques of molecular genetic analysis are now also being increasingly used in the screening and diagnosis of inherited metabolic diseases (although with genetically heterogeneous diseases, phenotypic diagnosis may still be more reliable). These techniques, for example mutational analysis using the polymerase chain reaction, and the detection of restriction fragment length polymorphisms, are discussed in detail in textbooks of basic biochemistry and molecular biology and are not discussed further here.

In a book of this size, it is only possible to discuss a selection of the many hundreds of inherited metabolic diseases that have been described. The ones that have been chosen are either among the more common, or illustrate important general principles, or both. Many others are discussed in other chapters of this book (*see* Fig. 16.3).

EFFECTS OF ENZYME DEFECTS

Fig. 16.4a shows a hypothetical metabolic pathway involving the synthesis of product D from substrate A by successive, enzyme-catalyzed reactions through intermediates B and C. If the formation of B from A, catalyzed by enzyme a, is rate limiting, as the first step unique to a metabolic pathway frequently is, then the concentrations of intermediates B and C will normally be low. The formation of product E from C, catalyzed by enzyme c', is normally a minor pathway, only a small amount of E being formed.

Three distinct sequelae of a lack of enzyme c, which could occur alone or in combination, can be envisaged.

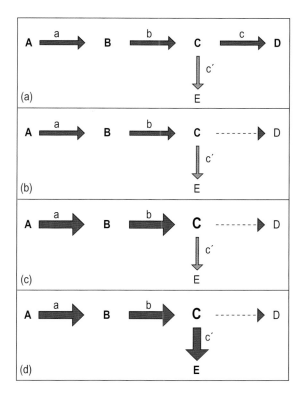

Fig. 16.4 Effects of enzyme defects. (a) Product D is synthesized from A by a series of reactions catalyzed by enzymes a, b and c. Enzyme c' catalyzes the formation of a small amount of product E in a minor pathway. (b) In the absence of the enzyme c, no D is synthesized. (c) If the conversion of C to D is blocked, the concentration of the intermediate C, and possibly other precursors, may increase. (d) Increased formation of E may occur if the concentration of C increases and conversion of C to D is blocked.

Decreased formation of the product

Decreased formation of the product of a reaction is the most obvious consequence of a lack of enzyme c (*Fig. 16.4b*). If enzyme c is defective, D cannot be synthesized. Clinical features will arise due to a lack of D if it is an essential product with no alternative pathway for its synthesis.

Accumulation of the substrate

Accumulation of the substrate (C) of the missing enzyme would also be expected (*Fig. 16.4c*). If this is biologically active, clinical manifestations will result. Other, earlier substrates may also accumulate if the reactions prior to the one blocked are reversible. This will occur particularly if there is negative feedback by the product on an early reaction in the pathway, with the result that, with decreased formation of the product, feedback is lost, thus reversing the inhibition and stimulating the formation of the intermediate substrates.

Increased formation of other metabolites

Increased formation of E, the product of a minor pathway, may occur if the concentration of C is increased as a result of the enzyme deficiency, the reaction being promoted by a mass action effect (*Fig. 16.4d*). Again, if E is biologically active, a clinical syndrome will result.

INHERITED METABOLIC DISORDERS

Glucose 6-phosphatase deficiency

Glucose 6-phosphatase deficiency (glycogen storage disease type IA) exemplifies the production of a clinical syndrome due to lack of formation of the product of an enzyme-catalyzed reaction. Glucose synthesis from glycogen or by gluconeogenesis is blocked (*Fig. 16.5*). Children with this disorder are prone to severe fasting hypoglycaemia since their only source of glucose is dietary carbohydrate.

Acute hypoglycaemia is treated with intravenous glucose infusion. Maintenance treatment is with frequent daytime feeding and overnight constant intragastric infusion with a glucose/glucose polymer feed. Older children are given uncooked corn starch, from which glucose is released only slowly in the gut.

Glucose 6-phosphatase deficiency also exemplifies the consequences of accumulation of a precursor other than the immediate substrate of the defective enzyme. Glycogen accumulates in the liver, causing hepatomegaly. The block in gluconeogenesis results in an accumulation of lactate, and lactic acidosis is a common

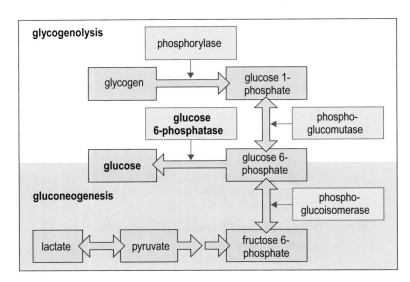

Fig. 16.5 Glucose production by glycogenolysis and gluconeogenesis. Glucose 6-phosphate is an essential intermediate in the production of glucose by either glycogenolysis or gluconeogenesis. In the absence of glucose 6-phosphatase, glucose cannot be formed from glucose 6-phosphate.

finding. Hyperlipidaemia results from increased fat synthesis and hyperuricaemia is also frequently present. Accumulation of glycogen in platelets leads to disordered platelet function and a bleeding tendency. Due to the enzyme block, neither glucagon nor adrenaline increases the blood glucose in glucose 6-phosphatase deficiency but the definitive diagnosis is made by demonstrating lack of enzyme activity in a sample of liver obtained by biopsy. In glycogen storage diseases types IB and IC, similar clinical and metabolic abnormalities occur (with an additional impairment of immune function) as a result of defects in the translocases involved in the transport of glucose 1-phosphate (type IB) and phosphate (IC) in the endoplasmic reticulum.

At least seven other glycogen storage diseases are known, each due to the deficiency of an enzyme related to glycogen metabolism.

Galactosaemia

Three enzyme defects can cause galactosaemia, and exemplify the production of a clinical syndrome due to the accumulation of a substrate of the missing enzyme. In classic galactosaemia, the absence of the enzyme galactose 1-phosphate uridyl transferase, which is required for the conversion of galactose to glucose 1-phosphate (*Fig. 16.6*) (thereby allowing galactose to be incorporated into glycogen, converted into glucose or undergo glycolysis), results in the accumulation of galactose 1-phosphate, and the clinical features of the

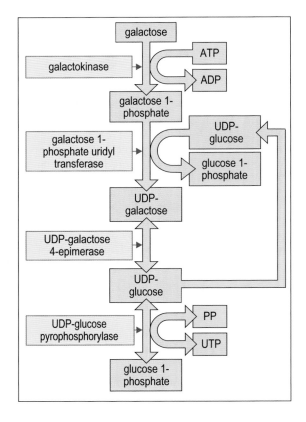

Fig. 16.6 Metabolic pathway for the conversion of galactose to glucose. UDP = uridine diphosphate.

condition are thought to be due directly to the toxicity of this metabolite. In addition, the plasma concentration of galactose is increased and galactose is excreted in the urine. Infants with galactosaemia present with failure to thrive, vomiting, hepatomegaly and jaundice. Septicaemia, particularly due to *E. coli*, is also common. Cataracts may be present as a result of the conversion of excess galactose to galacticol in the lens. There may also be hypoglycaemia and impairment of renal tubular function. Galactose is a reducing sugar and a positive test for urinary reducing substances in a child, diagnosed as galactosaemia on clinical grounds, merits withdrawal of galactose (and lactose) from the diet pending a definitive diagnosis, based on measurements of galactose 1-phosphate uridyl transferase in erythrocytes. The response to treatment is monitored by measuring galactose 1-phosphate in erythrocytes. A case of classic galactosaemia is presented in *Case History 21.5*. Deficiency of the enzyme UDP-galactose 4-epimerase causes a similar clinical syndrome, but is much less common. Deficiency of the enzyme galactokinase prevents the phosphorylation of galactose and leads to an increase in the plasma concentration of galactose and thus to galactosuria. Because galactose 1-phosphate

formation is blocked, this metabolite does not accumulate and, although cataracts may occur, the other clinical features of classical galactosaemia are not seen in galactokinase deficiency.

Phenylketonuria

Phenylketonuria (PKU) is another condition in which the accumulation of the substrate of the missing enzyme gives rise to a clinical syndrome. The enzyme concerned is phenylalanine hydroxylase, which hydroxylates phenylalanine to form tyrosine (*Fig. 16.7*).

Phenylalanine accumulates in the blood and if the condition is untreated it results in severe learning difficulties, thought to be due directly to the effect of excess phenylalanine on the developing brain. The name of the condition derives from the urinary excretion of phenylpyruvic acid, a phenylketone. This is normally a minor metabolite of phenylalanine but is produced in excess when the normal, major metabolic pathway is blocked. Many children with PKU have fair hair and blue eyes, owing to defective melanin synthesis: tyrosine, the formation of which is blocked, is a precursor of this

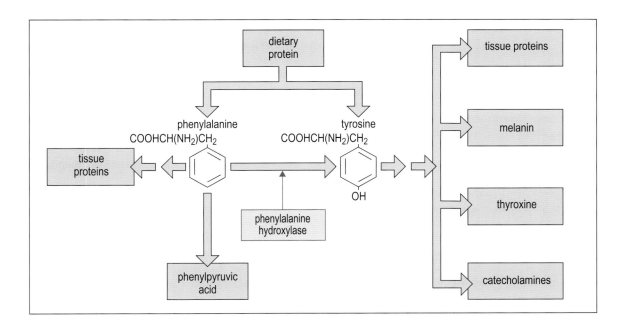

Fig. 16.7 Metabolic pathway for the conversion of phenylalanine to tyrosine. The site of action of phenylalanine hydroxylase, the enzyme deficient in PKU, is shown.

pigment. The diagnosis depends on the demonstration of an abnormally high concentration of phenylalanine in the blood: neonatal screening for the condition is discussed below.

The management involves restricting the dietary intake of phenylalanine using diets based on special proteins and pure amino acids. The plasma concentration of phenylalanine should not be allowed to exceed 0.3 mmol/L in the first year of life, when there is rapid brain development, but may, without detriment, be allowed to rise to 0.5 mmol/L by the age of four. The diet is unpalatable, and compliance can be a major problem. Although there has been a tendency to allow less rigorous dietary restriction after the age of ten, most paediatricians now advocate a policy of 'diet for life'. Strict dietary control is essential when a woman with PKU becomes pregnant, since maternal hyperphenyl-alaninaemia has been shown to affect the fetus *in utero* even if it does not itself have PKU.

Since phenylalanine is an essential amino acid, a certain amount must be provided in the diet and while tyrosine is not normally an essential amino acid, it becomes so when the intake of phenylalanine is limited: adequate quantities must therefore be provided. Thus treated, children in whom a diagnosis of PKU is made shortly after birth will grow and develop normally. Untreated, they rarely achieve an IQ of above 70, and usually require life-long institutional care.

Variants

The enzyme phenylalanine hydroxylase has tetrahydro-biopterin as a coenzyme. A number of variant forms of PKU have been described, some involving a defect in the metabolism of this coenzyme. Several other inherited metabolic diseases are associated with abnormalities of phenylalanine and tyrosine metabolism, including tyrosinaemia and alkaptonuria.

Tyrosinaemia type 1 (due to deficiency of fumarylaceto-acetate hydrolase, a late enzyme in tyrosine degradation) causes liver damage leading to cirrhosis, and renal tubular damage resulting in Fanconi syndrome. Alkaptonuria (due to deficiency of homogentisic acid oxidase) causes accumulation of homogentisic acid (a metabolite of phenylalanine and tyrosine). This polymerizes in skin and sclerae, causing brown–black discoloration (ochronosis), and in fibrous tissue and cartilage, including articular cartilage, where it can cause arthritis. Homogentisic acid is colourless but it becomes oxidized in urine and causes it to become brown–black on standing.

Steroid 21-hydroxylase deficiency

Steroid 21-hydroxylase deficiency, the commonest cause of congenital adrenal hyperplasia, exemplifies the effects of increased activity of a normally minor metabolic pathway, in this case the synthesis of adrenal androgens (*Fig. 16.8*). Due to the defective synthesis of cortisol, there is a decreased negative feedback to the pituitary and thus increased secretion of ACTH, which stimulates the synthesis of adrenal androgens. It is discussed in more detail in *Chapter 8*.

Cystic fibrosis

Cystic fibrosis is a common inherited metabolic disease, with an incidence of approximately 1 in 2500 live births in the UK. It is a generalized disorder of exocrine secretion, in which the secretions have greatly increased viscosity. The functional defect is impaired chloride transport. Affected children develop recurrent respiratory infections leading to irreversible lung disease, and pancreatic insufficiency leading to malabsorption. Intestinal obstruction may occur in the neonatal period ('meconium ileus'), owing to the increased viscosity of faecal material.

In contrast to most inherited metabolic diseases, the basis of the functional defect in cystic fibrosis was not understood until the gene responsible had been identified, cloned and sequenced. This allowed the amino acid sequence and hence the three-dimensional structure of the gene product to be predicted. This protein, known as the 'cystic fibrosis transmembrane conductance regulator', is involved in the control of transmembrane chloride transport.

Sweat chloride concentration is increased in cystic fibrosis and its measurement provides the definitive test for the condition (a concentration of >60 mmol/L or more being diagnostic). This is too time-consuming to be a practical screening test. The value of neonatal screening has been in doubt because of a lack of clear evidence that early diagnosis (before the condition presents clinically) is of any benefit. However, such evidence is now accumulating, and neonatal screening for cystic fibrosis may become routine. The screening test is based on the detection of the high neonatal plasma concentrations of immunoreactive trypsin that are characteristic of cystic fibrosis. When the test is positive, molecular genetic analysis for the common mutations in the cystic fibrosis gene can be used to confirm the diagnosis.

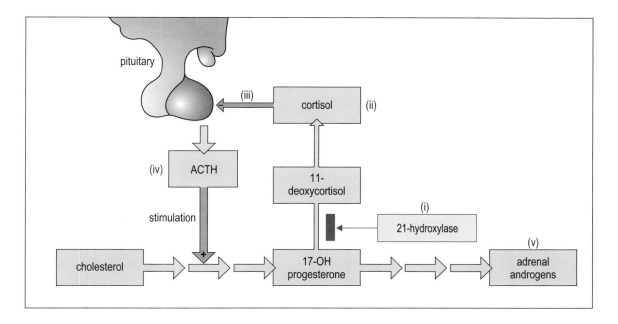

Fig. 16.8 Adrenal steroid hormone synthesis, showing the increased synthesis of androgens when cortisol synthesis is blocked. Decreased 21-hydroxylase activity (i) leads to decreased cortisol synthesis (ii). Negative feedback to the pituitary (iii) is decreased leading to increased secretion of ACTH (iv). The conversion of cholesterol to 17-hydroxyprogesterone is stimulated, leading to increased synthesis of androgens (v).

Management is directed towards the prevention of respiratory infections by regular physiotherapy and prophylactic antibiotic treatment, and maintenance of adequate nutrition with a good diet; pancreatic enzymes can be added to food to counter the effects of pancreatic insufficiency.

Although the prognosis for children with cystic fibrosis has greatly improved with modern methods of treatment, this is not achieved without cost to patient and parents. Many patients still die in early adult life.

Antenatal screening for cystic fibrosis and screening of prospective parents for carrier status are discussed on *p. 303.*

DIAGNOSIS

The diagnosis of an inherited metabolic disease may be suggested by clinical features and the results of simple tests. However, the diagnosis will not be made if a possible metabolic origin of the symptoms is not considered. Although most inherited metabolic diseases are rare, as a group they are an important cause of

illness in neonates and infants. Effective treatment is now available for many of these conditions and thus it would be tragic if treatment were not given because of a missed diagnosis.

The definitive diagnosis usually depends on the demonstration of decreased activity of the enzyme or concentration of the protein responsible in an appropriate tissue. This may involve biopsy of an affected organ but in some cases the enzyme can be assayed in red or white blood cells. The identification of probable cases by neonatal or prenatal screening merits special consideration. Contrasting examples of the clinical presentation and management of two inherited metabolic diseases are provided by *Case Histories 11.8* and *21.5.*

NEONATAL SCREENING

Screening is designed to detect individuals affected with a condition before it is apparent clinically. This may be done prenatally, during the neonatal period or later, according to the nature of the condition. The criteria for an effective neonatal screening programme are indicated in *Fig. 16.9*. Neonatal screening is exemplified by the programme for the detection of phenylketonuria.

Phenylketonuria

In many countries, including the UK and USA, all babies are screened at birth for PKU, which has an incidence of approximately 1 in 10,000. The screening test involves measurement of the concentration of phenylalanine in a sample of capillary blood taken from a heel-prick six to ten days after birth. The delay after birth is to allow sufficient time for feeding (and hence protein intake) to become established, and for the effect of maternal metabolism on fetal metabolism to subside. Formerly, the Guthrie test, a microbiological test using a strain of *Bacillus subtilis* in conditions such that growth is only seen if excess phenylalanine is present, was used to detect high concentrations of phenylalanine, but most laboratories now use a chromatographic technique. If the screening test is found to be positive, further, definitive tests are then performed. Screening for congenital hypothyroidism (incidence of 1 in 3500) is also widely practised. Economic considerations dictate that a screening test should be cost-effective. Even though it may be technically feasible, it is not economic to screen whole populations for very rare diseases, although this may change with the development of new technology.

In screening for PKU, the concentration of phenylalanine taken as positive is set such that the sensitivity of the test is virtually 100% (all cases are detected). The specificity is greater than 99% (there are very few false positives). However, because the condition is rare, the predictive value of a positive test is low (*see p. 11*); thus most positive screening tests are found not to be due to PKU. This means that some children will be subjected to further investigation and subsequently shown not to have the disease, but this is acceptable if it ensures that genuine cases are not missed.

PRENATAL DIAGNOSIS

When an inherited disease cannot be successfully treated, or the treatment imposes harsh restrictions on the patient, early prenatal diagnosis will allow parents the option of having the pregnancy terminated. The indications for undertaking prenatal diagnosis are set out in *Fig. 16.10*.

Satisfactory diagnostic tests are available for many inherited metabolic diseases but whether an attempt at prenatal diagnosis is justified depends upon the risk of the procedure. Most of these conditions have a recessive mode of inheritance, and thus prenatal diagnosis should usually be considered only if there is an affected child from a previous pregnancy, if one parent is affected, or if there is a strong family history of the disease. Screening of selected populations may be justified if a disease has a high incidence in a particular population, for example, the lipid storage disorder Tay–Sachs disease in Ashkenazi Jews.

Maternal and fetal screening

The introduction of the technique of chorionic villus biopsy, to obtain samples of fetal tissue very early in pregnancy, together with the development of techniques of molecular genetic analysis, has revolutionized prenatal diagnosis. The number of inherited disorders

---

Indications for neonatal screening tests

- condition is fatal or leads to severe disability if untreated
- condition is treatable
- condition is relatively common
- reliable, cheap screening test available (no false negatives; some false positives acceptable)

Fig. 16.9 Indications for neonatal screening tests.

Indications for prenatal diagnosis

- disease sufficiently serious to justify termination of pregnancy if present
- disease not amenable to treatment
- reliable, safe diagnostic test available for use in early pregnancy
- significant risk of disease occurring
- parents are willing to consider termination of the pregnancy should the fetus be shown to be affected

Fig. 16.10 Indications for prenatal diagnosis.

that can be diagnosed using these techniques is increasing and will no doubt continue to do so.

The techniques available for prenatal diagnosis are summarized in *Fig. 16.11*.

Maternal screening is not diagnostic, but may point to the need to proceed to a more invasive, but definitive test. Although the diseases are not metabolic in origin, a method of screening for open neural tube defects (spina bifida and anencephaly) exemplifies this type of procedure. The screening test involves measurement of α-fetoprotein in maternal blood. If the concentration is raised in relation to the expected value for gestational age and no other cause is found, for example wrong dates, twins or spurious results, the woman is then offered diagnostic ultrasound examination. In many centres, ultrasound scanning has replaced measurement of α-fetoprotein. It is also a valuable technique for the detection of other structural abnormalities. In Down's syndrome (trisomy 21, a chromosomal disorder), maternal α-fetoprotein concentration is decreased in relation to gestational age; unconjugated oestriol concentration also tends to be decreased, and that of chorionic gonadotrophin increased. Fetuses affected by Down's syndrome show a characteristic ultrasound sign (nuchal translucency) and the detection of this and/or a positive maternal biochemical screen indicates a need for definitive diagnosis by amniocentesis (sampling of amniotic fluid) and chromosomal analysis of cultured amniotic cells. Amniocentesis can be performed from approximately the tenth week of gestation. The risk of miscarriage following the procedure is approximately 1%.

An inherited metabolic defect may be reflected by the presence of an abnormally high concentration of a metabolite in maternal blood as, for example, in some organic acidaemias, but such metabolites, derived from the fetus, would normally be cleared by maternal enzymes. However, analysis of amniotic fluid, or cultures of amniotic cells obtained by amniocentesis, will give a more accurate reflection of fetal metabolism.

Direct inspection of the fetus is possible by fetoscopy, using a fibreoptic endoscope, during the second trimester of pregnancy. At the same time, a fetal blood sample can be obtained for analysis. If only a fetal blood sample is required, this can be obtained by cordocentesis – transabdominal aspiration from the umbilical cord under ultrasound control.

Chorionic villus sampling allows the collection of fetal tissue earlier in pregnancy, at 11–12 weeks of gestation. Placental tissue, which is of fetal origin and so contains fetal chromosomes, is removed transabdominally or transcervically and can be used for examination of fetal chromosomes or analysis of fetal DNA. In experienced hands this is a safe procedure, the excess rate of fetal loss being less than 1%. As is the case with all screening procedures, this risk must be considered in relation to the risk that a severe defect is present and will not be diagnosed.

Some of the issues relating to prenatal diagnosis are exemplified by a consideration of screening for cystic fibrosis.

Cystic fibrosis

Cystic fibrosis is a serious disorder which, despite considerable improvements in treatment, still has a poor prognosis.

Cystic fibrosis is a genetically heterogeneous disease. Several hundred mutations in the cystic fibrosis gene have been described in families with the condition. Many of these are private – that is, they occur only in one family – but approximately 70% of mutations causing cystic fibrosis in the UK involve the deletion of a single codon. This mutation is designated ΔF508. It is now possible to screen for this and several of the other more common mutations simultaneously. Screening can be performed on fetal tissue obtained by chorionic biopsy when a couple has already had one affected child, and on prospective parents from families in which the condition occurs. Such screening is capable of detecting up to 90% of carriers, and given the frequency of the heterozygous carrier state in the UK (approximately 1 in 25), there has been discussion as to whether a programme for carrier screening in the

Techniques available for prenatal diagnosis
maternal plasma screening
ultrasonography
amniocentesis
fetoscopy
chorionic villus sampling
cordocentesis

Fig. 16.11 Techniques available for prenatal diagnosis.

population as a whole should be established. This is a complex matter, involving financial, ethical and practical issues. The availability of adequate genetic counselling would be important: a positive result would indicate that an individual was a carrier but an apparently negative result would not exclude the possibility of carriage of a mutation that had not been screened for.

DNA ANALYSIS

DNA analysis is now a standard technique for the investigation of an increasing number of inherited disorders. When appropriate, it can be used to genotype fetal tissue for prenatal diagnosis, and to aid genetic counselling by genotyping of individuals in families in which a particular condition occurs. The index case may have been diagnosed by conventional means, but if the condition is one that is amenable to genetic analysis, other members of the family can then be studied. In some cases, notably cystic fibrosis and Duchenne muscular dystrophy, genetic analysis has led to the identification of the gene product.

It is beyond the scope of this book to discuss genetic analysis in detail. The techniques involved have many applications in medicine and science and are explained in numerous textbooks of general biochemistry and molecular biology.

Direct detection of mutant genes is particularly suited to the diagnosis of homogeneous genetic disorders, that is, ones that are always due to the same mutation. As discussed for cystic fibrosis, when a disease can be due to any one of several mutations in the same gene, 100% sensitivity in diagnosis would require the use of a battery of probes, which between them could detect all the mutations. If these are not available, diagnosis and screening must continue to depend at least in part on the detection of the effects of the mutation, usually by measurement of the gene product. This technique, or, if applicable, the detection of linkage through RFLP (restriction fragment length polymorphism) analysis, will continue to be used for conditions where the responsible gene has not yet been identified.

It would be wrong to give the impression that the techniques of molecular genetics are applicable only to comparatively rare inherited metabolic diseases caused by single gene defects. Genetic factors play an important part in the aetiology of many common conditions, including hypertension, some cancers and coronary heart disease. For example, mutations in the p53 tumour suppressor gene have been detected in more than half of some groups of patients with cancer. Identification of the genes involved in such conditions will make it possible to screen for them, and thus for susceptibility to the conditions. Such knowledge would potentially be a powerful tool in preventative medicine, but its application poses considerable ethical questions.

TREATMENT

Possible approaches to the treatment of inherited metabolic diseases are given in *Fig. 16.12*.

Restriction of substrate intake

This is exemplified in the treatment of galactosaemia. If all foodstuffs containing galactose and lactose are removed from the diet, clinical symptoms regress. Similarly, hereditary fructose intolerance (*see p. 215*) is asymptomatic if fructose is avoided. The management is less straightforward, however, if the substrate is essential for life. In PKU, the metabolism of phenylalanine to tyrosine is blocked (*see p. 299*), but phenylalanine is an essential amino acid and must therefore be provided in the diet to allow normal growth and development.

Supply of missing product

Congenital adrenal hyperplasia is managed by giving cortisol, production of which is impaired in this condition. In salt-losing types, a mineralocorticoid must also be given.

Addition of vitamin cofactors

If the defective enzyme has a vitamin cofactor, the supply of large amounts of the vitamin may, by a mass action effect, increase cofactor binding and thus enzyme activity. Many enzymes have separate catalytic and regulatory sites, and amino acid substitution due to a mutant gene may affect either of such sites, or alter the way in which they interact. Homocystinuria is a condition in which the conversion of homocysteine to cystathionine is blocked. The enzyme involved, cystathionine β-synthase, requires pyridoxal phosphate as a cofactor, and giving large amounts of this vitamin may be of therapeutic benefit in some cases. Some organic

Treatment strategies for inherited metabolic diseases	
Treatment	**Example**
restriction of substrate intake	galactose in galactosaemia
supply of missing product	cortisol in congenital adrenal hyperplasia
supply of vitamin cofactors	pyridoxal phosphate in homocystinuria
increased excretion of toxic substances	copper in Wilson's disease
replacement of missing protein	factor VIII in haemophilia
replacement of mutant gene	organ grafting

Fig. 16.12 Treatment strategies for inherited metabolic diseases.

acidaemias may similarly respond to high-dose vitamin supplementation.

Increased excretion of toxic substances

This approach is used in the treatment of Wilson's disease (*see p. 99*) to remove the excess copper, which is responsible for the tissue damage in this condition. D-Penicillamine forms a soluble complex with copper, which is then readily excreted in the urine. This drug is also used in the treatment of cystinuria, an inherited disorder characterized by defective renal tubular reabsorption of cystine and the dibasic amino acids lysine, ornithine and arginine. Cystine is relatively insoluble and there is a marked tendency to urinary stone (calculus) formation. Cystine may be kept in solution if the urine is kept sufficiently dilute and alkaline. If calculi continue to form, penicillamine may be used; the drug complexes with cysteine (from which cystine is derived) and reduces the urinary excretion of cystine.

Replacement of missing protein

If the replacement of a missing protein were to be a feasible method of treatment it would need to be repeated at regular intervals, as there is a continuous turnover of proteins in the body. Replacement of gamma-globulins is the mainstay of treatment of agamma-globulinaemia and, when necessary, factor VIII can be given in haemophilia. With the great majority of inherited metabolic diseases, the defective protein is intracellular and thus replacement is not feasible. Attempts have been made to treat some disorders involving lysosomal enzymes by infusing liposomes (lipid droplets) containing the missing enzyme into the bloodstream. Unfortunately, the potential of this novel approach to treatment is limited.

Replacement of the defective gene

This should allow normal synthesis of the product of the gene, for example an enzyme. The technical problems are considerable, including not only the engineering of the gene but also its insertion into a sufficient number of the appropriate somatic cells in such a way that its activity is subject to normal regulation. Over-expression of a normal gene might be as harmful as the effect of the abnormal gene. Nevertheless, this technique is now the subject of clinical trials.

Organ grafting may be appropriate in some conditions; liver transplantation has been used successfully in patients with Wilson's disease and α_1-antitrypsin deficiency who have developed hepatic failure, and patients with renal failure caused by cystinuria have been treated by kidney transplantation. Homozygous familial hypercholesterolaemia has also been treated successfully by liver transplantation. Organ grafting effectively replaces the missing or mutant gene and the engrafted organ synthesizes the normal gene product.

SUMMARY

- **Inherited metabolic diseases are the result of gene mutations** that either prevent the synthesis of a protein or cause the production of an abnormal protein molecule. **In the majority of these disorders, the protein is an enzyme** and the result is a decrease in catalytic activity. In some, the defective or missing protein is a receptor (e.g. familial hypercholesterolaemia) or a transport protein (e.g. cystinuria).

- Hundreds of these disorders have been described: most of them are rare, some to the extent that only a handful of cases have been documented world wide. Their effects vary in severity from the completely benign (e.g. renal glycosuria) to the invariably fatal (e.g. Tay–Sachs disease).

- Most inherited metabolic diseases have an **autosomal recessive mode of inheritance**; heterozygotes are usually phenotypically normal. Most of the porphyrias (*see Chapter 17*) are unusual in having an autosomal dominant mode of inheritance.

- **A decrease in catalytic activity can have a number of consequences**. In the case of an enzyme involved in a synthetic pathway, there could be decreased synthesis of the product of the enzyme or pathway, accumulation of the substrate and other precursor metabolites, or increased activity in a usually minor pathway which has, as its starting point, one of the intermediates that accumulates. Thus the clinical effects may relate to decreased quantities of a product of the pathway or increased quantities of other metabolites (which may be toxic in excess), or to a combination of these.

- The **definitive diagnosis** of an inherited metabolic disease requires either measurement of the activity of the relevant enzyme, a procedure that may necessitate tissue biopsy unless the enzyme is present in blood cells, or detection of the defective gene. The diagnosis can, however, often be inferred from the clinical features and measurements of the concentrations of metabolites or precursors of the enzyme, and may then be confirmed by the response to treatment.

- **Prenatal screening** for inherited metabolic diseases may be appropriate when there is a significant risk of a fetus being affected, for instance when a previous child is known to have had the condition or when there is a strong family history of the disorder. **Neonatal screening**, though technically feasible for many inherited metabolic disorders, is widely practised in the general population only for phenylketonuria; congenital hypothyroidism is also screened for in the newborn. **Screening tests must be highly sensitive and specific**; the condition in question should have severe consequences that can be ameliorated by early treatment (or avoided by termination of the pregnancy in the case of prenatal screening); and the condition must occur sufficiently frequently in the population being screened for the exercise to be worthwhile.

SUMMARY (cont'd)

- There is no **treatment** for many inherited metabolic diseases: others can be treated relatively simply. Congenital adrenal hyperplasia, a group of conditions in each of which one of the enzymes involved in the synthesis of cortisol is defective, can be treated by **replacing the missing product**, cortisol. Others, such as galactosaemia and phenylketonuria, can be treated by **dietary modifications**, which prevent the accumulation of toxic metabolites. A few metabolic disorders are due to decreased ability of the enzyme to bind a coenzyme; **giving large amounts of the coenzyme** may overcome this by a mass action effect and restore catalytic activity to normal.

- The **definitive treatment** for an inherited metabolic disease would be **replacement of the defective protein or gene**. Attempts have been made to treat some lysosomal enzyme deficiencies by enzyme replacement, but such treatment needs to be repeated frequently and has other disadvantages. Organ transplantation for the renal failure that can occur in cystinuria or the liver failure in Wilson's disease effectively replaces the defective gene; considerable research is taking place into techniques to allow modification or replacement of specific genes in patients with inherited metabolic diseases.

17 Disorders of haemoproteins, porphyrins and iron

INTRODUCTION

Haemoglobin, the oxygen-carrying pigment of blood, consists of a protein, globin, and four haem molecules (*Fig. 17.1*). Globin comprises two pairs of polypeptide chains (the principal haemoglobin in adults, haemoglobin A, HbA, has two α- and two β-chains); each polypeptide binds one haem molecule. Haem consists of a tetrapyrrole ring, protoporphyrin IXα, linked to an iron II ion (Fe^{2+}) to which oxygen becomes reversibly bound during oxygen transport. Other haemoproteins include myoglobin, which binds oxygen in skeletal muscle, and the cytochromes, enzymes responsible for catalyzing many oxidative processes in the body.

The major part of the body's iron is present in haemoglobin and the major product of porphyrin metabolism is haem. It is thus convenient to discuss the chemical pathology of the haemoproteins, the porphyrins and iron together, although disorders affecting any one of these do not necessarily (indeed do not often) involve the others.

HAEMOPROTEINS

Haemoglobin and haemoglobinopathies

Haemoglobin is a very accessible protein and has been extensively studied. The haemoglobinopathies (genetically determined abnormalities of haemoglobin synthesis) fall into two groups: qualitative, involving amino acid substitutions, and quantitative disorders, known as thalassaemias.

Amino acid substitutions

Here there is a single amino acid substitution in one of the polypeptide chains. Over 200 such variants have been described. Some of these involve amino acids that are not structurally or functionally vital, and are clinically silent; others have important consequences including

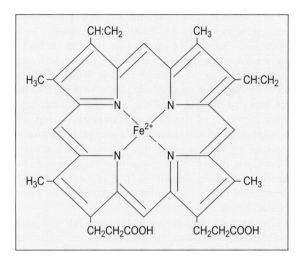

Fig. 17.1 The structure of haem.

effects on haemoglobin solubility (for example, HbS, the haemoglobin of sickle cell disease), stability and oxygen-carrying capacity.

Thalassaemias

In the thalassaemias there is an inherited defect in the rate of synthesis of one of the globin chains. This can involve the α-chains (α-thalassaemia) or the β-chains (β-thalassaemia). The consequences include ineffective erythropoiesis, haemolysis and a variable degree of anaemia. The clinical severity varies between the different thalassaemias. Some are clinically silent except during periods of stress, such as severe infection or pregnancy, when anaemia may develop, while others cause severe, persistent anaemia. When α-chain synthesis is totally absent, affected infants are either stillborn or die shortly after birth.

The investigation and management of the haemoglobinopathies is the province of the haematologist, and these disorders are not considered further in this book.

Abnormal derivatives of haemoglobin

Methaemoglobin

Methaemoglobin is oxidized haemoglobin, with iron in the Fe^{3+} form. It is incapable of carrying oxygen. A small amount is normally produced spontaneously in red blood cells but can be enzymatically reduced back to haemoglobin. Excessive methaemoglobin (methaemoglobinaemia) can be congenital or acquired. It can occur in some haemoglobinopathies, with an inherited deficiency of the reductase enzyme, and also as a result of the ingestion of large amounts of certain drugs, such as sulphonamides. In toxic methaemoglobinaemia, the presence of methaemalbumin (formed as a result of haemolysis of red cells containing methaemoglobin) imparts a brown colour to the plasma, while the presence of free methaemoglobin may give the urine a similar colour.

The major clinical manifestation of congenital methaemoglobinaemia is cyanosis. Acute toxic methaemoglobinaemia causes symptoms of anaemia and may lead to vascular collapse and death. Methaemoglobinaemia, except when due to a haemoglobinopathy, can be treated with methylene blue or ascorbic acid, agents that reduce the abnormal derivative back to haemoglobin.

Sulphaemoglobin

Sulphaemoglobin, a group of poorly characterized derivatives of haemoglobin, is often formed together with methaemoglobin. It is also incapable of carrying oxygen but cannot be converted back to haemoglobin.

Carboxyhaemoglobin

Carboxyhaemoglobin (COHb) is formed from haemoglobin in the presence of carbon monoxide, the affinity of the pigment for this gas being some 200 times greater than for oxygen. Because of this, only small quantities of carbon monoxide in the inspired air can result in the formation of large amounts of COHb and hence greatly reduce the oxygen-carrying capacity of the blood. The binding of carbon monoxide to haemoglobin also causes a left shift in the oxyhaemoglobin dissociation curve (*see p. 59*), decreasing the availability of oxygen to tissues. Small amounts of COHb (less than 2%) are commonly present in the blood of urban dwellers and greater amounts (up to 10%) may be found in the blood of tobacco smokers.

Haematin

Haematin is oxidized (Fe^{3+}) haem. It is released from methaemoglobin when red cells containing this pigment are haemolyzed but can be formed from free haem in severe intravascular haemolysis. Haematin combines with albumin in the bloodstream to form methaemalbumin. Methaemalbuminaemia is sometimes a feature of acute haemorrhagic pancreatitis.

Detection

These various derivatives of haemoglobin can be detected by their spectral characteristics, and quantified when necessary.

PORPHYRINS

Protoporphyrin IXα, which combines with iron to form haem, is the end-product of a series of complex reactions. The first step that is unique to this pathway is the combination of glycine and succinyl CoA to form δ-aminolaevulinic acid (ALA), a reaction catalyzed by the enzyme ALA synthase (*Fig. 17.2*). Two molecules of ALA then condense to form porphobilinogen (PBG), in a reaction catalyzed by PBG synthase (also known as ALA dehydratase).

The first porphyrins (strictly, porphyrinogens, *see below*) are formed when four molecules of PBG condense together. The initial product of this reaction, catalyzed by hydroxymethylbilane synthase (PBG deaminase) is hydroxymethylbilane. In the presence of uroporphyrinogen III cosynthase, this is converted to uroporphyrinogen III. In the absence of this enzyme, hydroxymethylbilane is converted non-enzymatically to uroporphyrinogen I. A series of enzyme-catalyzed reactions through isomers of the III series leads to the formation of protoporphyrin IXα. Haem is formed when iron is incorporated into this molecule in a reaction catalyzed by ferrochelatase.

The porphyrinogens are themselves unstable and become oxidized to their corresponding porphyrins when they are excreted in faeces or urine. Porphyrinogens and porphyrin precursors are colourless. Porphyrins are dark red in colour and intensely fluorescent. The major sites of porphyrin synthesis are the liver and the erythroid bone marrow.

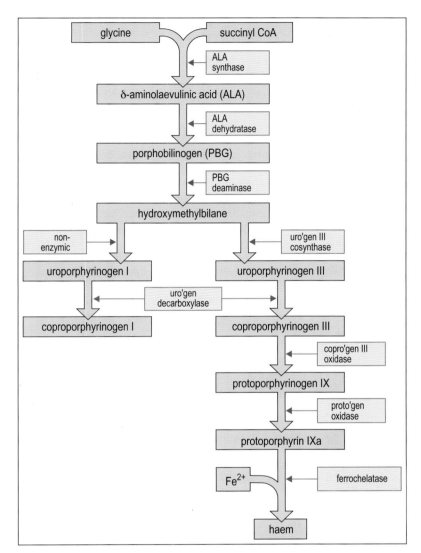

Fig. 17.2 The biosynthesis of porphyrins. PBG deaminase is also known as hydroxymethylbilane synthase and ALA dehydratase as PBG synthase.

The rate-limiting step in this sequence of reactions is the first, catalyzed by ALA synthase, which is susceptible to inhibition by the end-product, haem.

The porphyrias

These are a group of inherited diseases in which a partial deficiency of one of the enzymes of porphyrin synthesis leads to decreased formation of haem and thus, by releasing ALA synthase from inhibition, results in the formation of excessive quantities of porphyrin precursors (ALA and PBG) or porphyrins. When precursors are produced in excess, the clinical manifestations are primarily neurological (the precursors are neurotoxins). When porphyrins themselves are the major product, the predominant feature is photosensitivity; the porphyrins absorb light and become excited, inducing the formation of toxic free radicals. The porphyrias are diagnosed on the basis of their clinical features and the pattern of porphyrins and precursors present in blood and excreted in faeces and urine.

The porphyrias are classified as acute or non-acute, according to their clinical presentation, and hepatic or erythropoietic, depending on the major site of abnormal metabolism (*Fig. 17.3*). All the porphyrias are rare. Cutaneous hepatic porphyria is the most common but many cases are not inherited. Of the purely genetic types, acute intermittent porphyria is the most common, with a prevalence in the UK, where it occurs more frequently than in many countries, of only 1–2 cases per 100,000 of the population. Unusually for inherited metabolic diseases, the mode of inheritance of most porphyrias is autosomal dominant, the exceptions being congenital erythropoietic porphyria, ALA dehydratase deficiency porphyria and hepatoerythropoietic porphyria (autosomal recessive). The features of the porphyrias are summarized in *Fig. 17.4*. The genes for the enzymes involved in porphyrin synthesis have been identified and cloned but the porphyrias are genetically heterogeneous; this hinders the application of molecular biological techniques to the identification of carriers and to screening for porphyrias.

Acute porphyrias

Acute intermittent porphyria (AIP) is the commonest of these. Photosensitivity is never a feature of AIP although it may occur in patients with hereditary coproporphyria and variegate porphyria.

Classification of the porphyrias		
acute	acute intermittent porphyria	**hepatic**
	hereditary coproporphyria	
	variegate porphyria	
chronic	cutaneous hepatic porphyria	
	congenital erythropoietic porphyria	**erythropoietic**
	erythropoietic protoporphyria	

Fig. 17.3 Classification of the porphyrias. In addition to these conditions, two very rare porphyrias have been described: aminolaevulinic dehydratase deficiency porphyria (acute) and hepatoerythropoietic porphyria (chronic).

Clinical features

These conditions are characterized by a tendency to acute attacks, separated by long periods of complete remission. The clinical features of acute attacks are summarized in *Fig. 17.5*. Abdominal pain and psychiatric disturbances are nearly always present; peripheral neuropathy occurs in some 60% of patients. They can be precipitated by various factors, including many drugs (*Fig. 17.5*); most frequently implicated are barbiturates, oral contraceptives and alcohol. These probably act by increasing the activity of ALA synthase, in many cases by increasing the synthesis of hepatic cytochrome P450 and hence the demand for haem, thereby decreasing intrahepatic haem concentration and releasing the enzyme from inhibition. Some drugs, notably the sulphonamides, inhibit PBG deaminase directly. Whatever the cause, the resulting increased activity of the metabolic pathway increases the formation of metabolites before the enzyme block.

Hormonal factors are also extremely important; symptoms rarely occur before puberty and may fluctuate in relation to menstruation or pregnancy. Women are affected more commonly than men. In some 90% of individuals who inherit the defective gene for AIP, the disease remains clinically latent throughout adult life.

Diagnosis

In the acute porphyrias, excessive ALA and PBG are excreted in the urine during an acute attack. In suspicious circumstances, such as unexplained acute abdominal pain, peripheral neuropathy or psychosis, the urine can be tested for PBG by a simple screening test, which, if positive, will indicate the need to carry out further investigations (*see Fig. 17.4*) to establish the precise diagnosis. When an acute porphyria has been diagnosed, blood relatives should be screened for latent disease, and if necessary advised concerning the avoidance of precipitating factors. It is important to appreciate that the concentrations of porphyrins and their precursors in the blood, urine and faeces may be normal except during an attack, with the result that it may be necessary to measure the defective enzyme itself to establish who is at risk.

Classification and characteristics of the porphyrias

Condition	Deficient enzyme	Inheritance	Course	Erythroid/hepatic	Sympto-matology	Abnormal porphyrin concentrations		
						Red cells	Urine	Stools
ALA dehydratase deficiency porphyria	ALA dehydratase	AR	acute	E	N	Zn-proto	**ALA**	
acute intermittent porphyria	PBG deaminase	AD	acute	H	N		ALA, **PBG**	
hereditary copropor-phyria	copro'gen oxidase	AD	acute	H	N, P		ALA, PBG **copro-**	copro-
variegate porphyria	proto'gen oxidase	AD	acute	H	N, P		ALA, PBG **copro-**	copro- **proto-**
cutaneous hepatic porphyria	uro'gen decarboxylase	variable†	chronic	H	P		**uro-**	**isocopro-**
hepatoerythro-poietic porphyria	uro'gen decarboxylase	AR	chronic	both	P	Zn-proto	uro-	isocopro-
congenital erythropoietic porphyria	uro'gen III cosynthase	AR	chronic	E	P	uro-* copro-*	**uro-*** copro-*	copro-*
erythropoietic protopor-phyria	ferrochelatase	AD	chronic	E	P	**proto**		proto

* type I isomers †AD in some families N = neurological P = photosensitizing

Fig. 17.4 Features of the porphyrias. The most important abnormalities are in bold; the changes shown for the acute porphyrias may only be present during an attack.

Management

Once the diagnosis of acute porphyria has been made, every effort must be made to prevent attacks by the avoidance of precipitating factors. During an attack, any such features must be identified and treated appropriately. General supportive measures include maintenance of fluid and electrolyte balance, adequate carbohydrate intake (intravenous glucose is often beneficial), and physiotherapy. Pain can be safely relieved with narcotic analgesics. The specific treatment of choice for acute attacks is intravenous haem arginate, which decreases the activity of ALA synthase.

Acute attacks of porphyrias		
Clinical features		**Factors involved**
Gastrointestinal abdominal pain vomiting constipation	**Central nervous system** seizures depression hysteria psychosis	anaesthesia drugs pregnancy premenstrual infection stress starvation alcohol

Peripheral neuropathy
pain, stiffness and muscle weakness
   (limb and girdle muscles > trunk;
   upper limbs > lower;
   proximal > distal)
paraesthesiae, numbness
	Cardiovascular
	sinus tachycardia
	systemic hypertension	

Fig. 17.5 Clinical features and factors involved in acute attacks of porphyria; gastrointestinal, neuropsychiatric and cardiovascular derangements are all common.

Non-acute porphyrias

Erythropoietic protoporphyria and congenital erythropoietic porphyria are both very rare. Photosensitivity occurs with both but is much more severe with the latter, causing extensive blistering and leading to tissue destruction and scarring.

Cutaneous hepatic porphyria (also known as porphyria cutanea tarda and symptomatic porphyria) also presents with photosensitivity. The initial lesion is just erythema but this progresses to the formation of vesicles and bullae, and eventually to scarring and pigmentation. This porphyria can be inherited (familial, type II) (15–20% of cases) or acquired (sporadic, type I). In both types, there is an approximately 50% reduction in hepatic uroporphyrinogen decarboxylase activity in the liver; in type II, this deficiency occurs in all tissues. Although the acquired type can develop spontaneously, it is more frequently seen in association with excessive alcohol ingestion (often with liver disease) (90% of cases) or as a consequence of exposure to hepatotoxins or drugs. The very rare hepato-erythropoietic porphyria is the homozygous form of cutaneous hepatic porphyria.

Management

Management involves the identification and removal of precipitating factors; venesection to remove excess iron from the liver (iron inhibits uroporphyrinogen III cosynthase and uroporphyrinogen decarboxylase); avoidance of direct sunlight, and the use of barrier creams to protect the skin.

Other causes of porphyrinuria

Increased urinary porphyrin excretion can occur in conditions other than the porphyrias. In patients with liver disease, particularly with cholestasis, the normal biliary excretion of porphyrins is impaired and there is increased urinary excretion – just as occurs with bilirubin. Porphyrinuria can also result from acquired defects in haem synthesis, as for example in lead poisoning. Lead inhibits ALA dehydratase (*see* Fig. 17.2) and, to a lesser extent, coproporphyrinogen oxidase and ferrochelatase. As a result, the urinary excretion of ALA and coproporphyrin, and red cell zinc protoporphyrin content, may all be increased in lead poisoning. However, the measurement of blood lead concentration is to be preferred for the diagnosis of both lead poisoning and occupational overexposure to lead (*see* Chapter 19).

IRON

The total iron content of the adult body is approximately 4 g (70 mmol), of which some two-thirds is in haemoglobin. Iron stores (mainly spleen, liver and bone marrow) contain about one-quarter of the body's

Case history 17.1

A 19-year-old woman was admitted to hospital with colicky abdominal pain, which had started suddenly 12 h before. She had vomited several times but had not opened her bowels since the pain started. Her abdomen was tender on examination but was otherwise normal. Her pulse was 140/min and her blood pressure was 160/100 mmHg. After she had been taken to the ward for observation, a nurse in the emergency room noticed that a specimen of the patient's urine, which had been collected for routine testing, had become a deep red colour although it had been normal when first passed. On being informed of this, the admitting doctor questioned the patient further and examined her more carefully. She said that she had also noticed cramping pains in her arms and was found to have bilateral wrist drop.

Investigations

screening test for urinary
    porphobilinogen: strongly positive

quantitative analysis of urine:
    porphobilinogen   very high
    δ-aminolaevulinic acid   very high
    uroporphyrin   slightly raised
    coproporphyrin   slightly raised

Comment

Acute porphyrias may present as an acute abdomen; systemic hypertension and sinus tachycardia are often present. They are of course a very uncommon cause of abdominal pain and the diagnosis may be missed, at least initially. In this case the nurse's observation of the changed colour of the urine was crucial and led to the presumptive diagnosis of an acute porphyria being made, supported clinically by the evidence of neuropathy and also by the positive screening test for PBG. There was no evidence of photosensitivity and the very high urinary excretion of porphyrin precursors, with only slightly increased excretion of intact porphyrins, favours a diagnosis of acute intermittent porphyria rather than variegate or hereditary coproporphyria, both of which are anyway much less common.

The patient's symptoms and signs resolved rapidly with appropriate treatment. It transpired that she had started taking an oral contraceptive pill a few days before. The diagnosis was later confirmed by the demonstration of a reduced red cell hydroxymethylbilane synthase activity; she was advised to use an alternative method of contraception and told which drugs she should avoid. She remained well thereafter and no problems arose when she underwent elective surgery (cholecystectomy) three years later, nor even during a subsequent pregnancy.

iron. Most of the remainder is in myoglobin and other haemoproteins; only 0.1% of the total body iron is in the plasma, where it is almost all bound to a transport protein, transferrin.

Iron absorption and transport

The mean daily intake of iron is about 20 mg (0.36 mmol), but less than 10% of this is absorbed. The regulation of iron absorption is not fully understood. It is determined by the state of the body's iron stores, being increased when they are depleted and decreased when they are adequate. It is also increased when erythropoiesis is increased, irrespective of the state of the iron stores.

The main site of iron absorption is the proximal small bowel. Iron is more readily absorbed in the Fe^{2+} form but dietary iron is mainly in the Fe^{3+} form. Gastric secretions are important in iron absorption in that they liberate iron from food (although haem can be absorbed intact) and promote the conversion of Fe^{3+} to Fe^{2+}. Ascorbic acid and other reducing substances facilitate iron absorption while phytic acid (in cereals), phosphates and oxalates form insoluble complexes with iron and decrease its absorption.

Once absorbed into the intestinal mucosal cells, iron is either transported directly into the bloodstream, or else combines with apoferritin, a complex iron-binding protein, to form ferritin. This iron is lost into the lumen of the gut when mucosal cells are shed. In iron deficiency, the apoferritin content of mucosal cells decreases and a greater proportion of absorbed iron reaches the bloodstream.

In the blood, iron is transported mainly bound to transferrin, each molecule of which binds two Fe^{2+} ions. Transferrin is normally about one-third saturated with iron. In tissues, iron is bound in ferritin and haemo-siderin. Free iron is very toxic and protein binding allows iron to be transported and stored in a non-toxic form.

Iron is lost from the body in faeces (non-absorbed and shed mucosal iron), by desquamation of skin and, in women, by menstrual blood loss. Endogenous iron loss in males is about 1 mg (18 μmol)/24 h. Very little iron is excreted in the urine.

Diagnostic tests for iron status

Iron status may require assessment when iron deficiency or overload is suspected or when the distribution or metabolism of iron is thought to be abnormal. Haematological tests used in this context include measurement of haemoglobin and red cell indices. Iron stores can be assessed directly by examination of the bone marrow, but measurement of plasma ferritin concentration is the best non-invasive test for iron deficiency. It is rarely necessary to use biochemical tests merely to substantiate a diagnosis of iron deficiency, since this is by far the commonest cause of microcytic, hypochromic anaemia and the diagnosis is confirmed by a response to iron therapy.

Plasma iron

Normal plasma iron concentration in men is 9–29 μmol/L; it is marginally lower in women. However, measurement of plasma iron concentration is of little value in the investigation of iron metabolism, except in relation to haemochromatosis and in the diagnosis and management of iron poisoning. A fall in plasma iron concentration is a late feature of iron deficiency, although a raised plasma iron is usually present in iron overload. However, the concentration of iron in the plasma of normal individuals fluctuates considerably; differences of more than 20% can occur within a few minutes, and of 100% from one day to the next. Considerable catamenial variation occurs in women. Many conditions, including infection, trauma, chronic inflammatory disorders (especially rheumatoid arthritis) and neoplasia, are associated with low plasma iron concentrations (but normal iron stores), while others, for example hepatitis, cause an increase in concentration.

Plasma total iron-binding capacity

Measurement of iron-binding capacity is effectively a functional measurement of transferrin concentration. Knowing the plasma iron concentration, the transferrin saturation can then be calculated: it is normally about 33%. Although plasma total iron-binding capacity is increased in iron deficiency, many other factors can affect it, while the saturation, dependent as it is upon the (highly variable) plasma iron concentration, is itself highly variable. While a low saturation is characteristic of iron deficiency, it also occurs in other conditions, such as pregnancy and chronic disease, in the absence of iron deficiency. Transferrin saturation is consistently increased in iron overload.

Plasma ferritin

Measurement of plasma ferritin concentration is superior to plasma iron and iron-binding capacity for the assessment of body iron stores. In healthy individuals, plasma ferritin concentrations are usually within the range 20–300 μg/L. The only known cause of a low concentration is a decrease in body iron stores; concentrations below 20 μg/L indicate depletion, and below 12 μg/L suggest a complete absence of stored iron. However, ferritin is an acute phase protein and patients with iron deficiency may have plasma ferritin concentrations within the reference range (e.g. up to 50–60 μg/L) when they are acutely ill. The same applies to patients with chronic inflammatory conditions (e.g. rheumatoid disease). Patients with chronic disease frequently develop chronic anaemia, as a result of impaired utilization of stored iron. This can coexist with iron deficiency, but iron deficiency is unlikely if plasma ferritin concentration is >60 μg/L.

Plasma ferritin concentration is increased in iron overload, for example in haemochromatosis, but may also be increased in some patients with liver disease and certain types of cancer, owing to release of the protein from tissues. Elevated concentrations should thus be interpreted with caution, although iron overload is excluded if plasma ferritin concentration is normal.

Transferrin receptor

Measurement of plasma soluble transferrin receptor concentration is a recent addition to the tests available for the investigation of iron status. Transferrin has a very high affinity for iron at normal hydrogen ion concentrations. The uptake of iron into cells is facilitated by a receptor that is present on the surface of all iron-requiring cells in the body, with the highest number on the surface of erythrocyte precursors in the bone marrow. Binding of transferrin to receptors leads to internalization and uptake into vesicles where the high hydrogen ion concentration allows the iron to be released. Transferrin receptor synthesis is controlled by iron: it is increased in iron deficiency. The plasma concentration increases to two to three times normal when anaemia is present, but the rise occurs only after iron stores become functionally depleted, whereas ferritin concentrations rise earlier, as iron stores fall. The concentration is also increased in conditions in which there is chronically increased erythroid proliferation, for example sickle cell disease and hereditary spherocytosis. Transferrin receptor concentration does not increase significantly in patients with the anaemia of chronic disease.

Iron deficiency

This may be due to inadequate intake, impaired absorption, excessive loss or a combination of these. The anaemia that develops is hypochromic and microcytic, and if there is an obvious cause of iron deficiency, further investigation of the anaemia is not required. If the cause of an anaemia is in doubt, the finding of a low plasma ferritin concentration and/or an increase in transferrin receptor concentration will indicate iron deficiency.

Iron overload

This can occur with increased intestinal absorption of iron, either acutely, as in iron poisoning, or chronically, as occurs, for example, in some peoples in southern Africa who brew a beer using iron vessels (Bantu siderosis). Increased parenteral iron administration occurs unavoidably in patients given repeated blood transfusions for the treatment of refractory anaemias and can also lead to overloading of the body's iron stores (haemosiderosis or acquired haemochromatosis). The excess iron is deposited mainly as haemosiderin in reticuloendothelial cells in the liver and spleen, where it is relatively innocuous, but with time parenchymal deposition may lead to hepatic fibrosis and myocardial damage.

Hereditary (primary) haemochromatosis

The most severe iron overload is seen in patients with hereditary or primary haemochromatosis. This condition is characterized by excessive intestinal iron absorption. Its precise molecular basis remains uncertain, although it is known that the gene product (HFE protein) binds to the transferrin receptor and that the most frequent mutation (C282Y) prevents the formation of a disulphide bond required for the transport of the protein to the cell surface. The mode of inheritance is autosomal recessive. The haemochromatosis gene (the HFE gene) is located on chromosome 6, closely linked to the class 1 HLA locus. In the UK, 90% of patients with haemochromatosis are homozygous for C282Y mutation and most of the remainder for the H63D mutation: detection of these mutations can be used to screen for the condition. It is thought that the prevalence of the homozygous state for haemochromatosis is about 5 in 1000 in northern European populations, making it possibly the most common of the inherited metabolic diseases.

The phenotypic expression in homozygotes depends upon the availability of dietary iron and overall iron turnover. Thus the condition occurs clinically in men more frequently than in women (because of menstrual iron loss), and when it does occur in women, does so on average at a later age. Even in men it is uncommon before the age of 40; although the defect is present from birth, it is only when the body becomes massively overloaded with iron that clinical features develop. Furthermore, the prevalence in homozygotes in countries with a high dietary content of available iron is greater than where the dietary content is low.

Haemochromatosis is probably underdiagnosed, and it should be considered in all patients with chronic liver

Case history 17.2

A 45-year-old man presented with weight loss, lassitude and weakness. His skin was noticeably bronzed, although it was winter and he had not been out of the country. On examination, he was found to have hepatosplenomegaly, rather sparse body hair and small testes. On further questioning, he admitted that he had lost his libido and become impotent.

Investigations

urine	positive for glucose
blood glucose (fasting)	10 mmol/L
serum: iron	70 µmol/L
iron-binding capacity	67 µmol/L
ferritin	5000 µg/L
testosterone	9 nmol/L
luteinizing hormone	2 U/L

Comment

The high percentage saturation of transferrin and massively elevated ferritin concentrations are typical of severe haemochromatosis. Skin pigmentation is virtually always present in idiopathic haemochromatosis, although it develops insidiously and may go unnoticed by the patient. It is a result of increased melanin deposition (and haemosiderin in advanced cases). Deposition of iron in the pancreas causes islet cell destruction and diabetes. Parenchymal iron deposition in the liver leads to cirrhosis, which may be complicated by hepatoma formation; the liver disease is often exacerbated by excessive alcohol ingestion. Both primary and secondary hypogonadism can occur; in this case, the low luteinizing hormone concentration suggests that the hypogonadism is secondary to pituitary damage. The joints are often involved and deposition of iron in the myocardium can cause arrhythmias and cardiac failure.

The families of patients with haemochromatosis should be screened to detect homozygotes for the defective gene, who are at risk of developing the condition and can be given prophylactic treatment. Treatment of homozygotes before the onset of overt disease has been shown to prevent the development of cirrhosis and reduce the (otherwise considerable) risk of hepatocellular carcinoma. Screening has previously been by measurement of percentage saturation of iron-binding capacity but molecular genetic techniques to detect mutations in the haemochromatosis gene are increasingly being used. Heterozygotes have increased plasma ferritin concentrations but are not at risk of developing tissue damage.

disease (unless some other obvious cause is apparent) and in males developing diabetes in middle life, particularly if they are not obese or require insulin.

The diagnosis is suggested by a transferrin saturation >60% together with elevated plasma ferritin concentration (typically >700 µg/L in symptomatic patients and often much higher). It can be confirmed by molecular genetic analysis. Liver biopsy is recommended, particularly if there is biochemical evidence of liver damage (increased plasma aspartate aminotransferase activity), to detect possible fibrosis or cirrhosis. Biopsy also per-

mits demonstration of the massive excess of parenchymal iron: in other forms of iron overload, the excess iron is typically present in the Kupffer (reticuloendothelial) cells.

Management and prognosis

The mainstay of treatment of idiopathic haemochromatosis is repeated venesection; with each 500 mL of blood, 200–250 mg of iron is removed from the body. It is often possible to do this as frequently as once a week without rendering the patient anaemic. Plasma iron and ferritin concentrations are used to monitor treatment and, once the excess iron has been removed, further accumulation can be prevented by less frequent (two- to three-monthly) venesection. Diabetes and heart failure are treated by conventional means, and hormonal deficiencies by appropriate replacement. Untreated, the prognosis is poor, but it is considerably improved by removal of the excess iron. There is often an improvement in cardiac and hepatic function, but the diabetes, hypogonadism and joint disease are not affected.

Desferrioxamine, an iron-chelating agent, is valuable in patients receiving multiple blood transfusions for refractory anaemia, who are at risk of developing iron overload. Desferrioxamine has to be infused intra-venously: unless this is performed daily, the rate of removal of iron is much slower than with venesection.

SUMMARY

- **Haemoproteins** consist of a haem molecule (a tetrapyrrole ring linked to an Fe^{2+}) bound to a protein. In **haemoglobin**, the protein consists of two pairs of identical polypeptide chains and four haem molecules; it is the latter that are responsible for binding oxygen. **Haemoglobin contains two-thirds of the body's iron**. Iron is essential for normal haemopoiesis and iron deficiency is an important cause of anaemia. Many genetically determined variants of haemoglobin are known, including haemoglobin S, responsible for **sickle cell anaemia**; some of these variants are of no clinical consequence, but others, like HbS, can cause severe disease. Haemoglobin can undergo chemical changes in the blood, for example binding carbon monoxide and forming carboxyhaemoglobin, which is incapable of transporting oxygen.

- The synthesis of the tetrapyrrole ring of haem involves a complex metabolic pathway from glycine and succinyl CoA through intermediates known as porphyrinogens. Inherited metabolic disorders are known affecting each of the enzymes of the haem synthetic pathway and are collectively called **porphyrias**. These conditions are classified into the **acute** porphyrias (whose effects are primarily neurological), for example acute intermittent porphyria, and the **chronic** porphyrias (with primarily cutaneous manifestations) such as cutaneous hepatic porphyria. The neurological features are due to the accumulation of porphyrin precursors, whereas the accumulation of porphyrins themselves causes photosensitivity and hence leads to skin damage.

- The **porphyrias are also classified into hepatic and erythropoietic porphyrias**, according to the major site of the enzyme abnormality. With the exceptions of congenital erythropoietic porphyria and ALA dehydratase deficiency porphyria, which are autosomal recessive, the porphyrias are unusual among inherited metabolic disorders in having an autosomal dominant mode of inheritance. Although cutaneous hepatic porphyria may be inherited, it is often acquired, such as when it occurs with excessive alcohol intake. Each porphyria gives rise to a characteristic pattern of porphyrins and metabolites in blood, urine and faeces, which can be used to make the diagnosis.

- **Dietary iron is absorbed in the proximal small intestine**, more readily in the Fe^{2+} form. Almost all the iron in the plasma is protein-bound to transferrin. Iron deficiency can be due to inadequate intake or malabsorption, or to excessive loss of iron, and gives rise to a microcytic, hypochromic anaemia. The plasma iron concentration is an unreliable guide to the body's iron status; measurement of plasma **ferritin** concentration (ferritin is primarily an intracellular iron-binding protein) is the best biochemical test of iron status.

- **Free iron is highly toxic** and iron poisoning, particularly in children, can be fatal.

SUMMARY (cont'd)

- **Chronic iron overload occurs in haemochromatosis**, a genetically determined disorder characterized by excessive absorption of dietary iron, which becomes deposited in many tissues of the body, including cardiac muscle, endocrine organs and parenchymal cells of the liver. Clinical features of haemochromatosis include skin pigmentation, cirrhosis, cardiomyopathy and impaired endocrine function. The condition is best treated by repeated venesection to remove iron from the body. In **haemosiderosis**, in which iron accumulates, for example as a result of repeated blood transfusion for refractory anaemia, the excess iron is deposited in reticuloendothelial cells and there is much less tissue damage.

Metabolic aspects of malignant disease

INTRODUCTION

The clinical signs and symptoms in patients suffering from cancer are often directly related to the physical presence of the tumour. For example, the tumour may destroy essential normal tissue, cause obstruction of ducts or exert pressure on nerves. Systemic manifestations, including cachexia and pyrexia, are also frequently present and indeed may be the only evidence of the presence of a tumour. In some patients, the clinical features may be those of an endocrine syndrome. This would be expected with a tumour of endocrine tissue such as a malignant insulinoma (producing hypoglycaemia) or an adrenal carcinoma (producing Cushing's syndrome), but often occurs with tumours not obviously of endocrine origin.

In many cases, these syndromes are caused by the secretion of a hormone by the tumour. This has been termed *ectopic* hormone secretion since the hormone is not secreted from its normal site, while *eutopic* hormone secretion describes secretion from the endocrine gland. However, it seems likely that in many cases these tumours arise from cells normally capable of hormone secretion, but which are present in only very small numbers in the non-neoplastic tissue. 'Aberrant' rather than 'ectopic' hormone secretion may be a more accurate term for this phenomenon. Tumours can be associated with other systemic manifestations, for example a cerebellar syndrome, arthropathy, etc. The term 'paraneoplastic syndromes' encompasses all the systemic manifestations of cancer not directly related to the physical presence of the primary tumour, whether or not they are due to a hormone.

This chapter discusses paraneoplastic endocrine syndromes, certain familial endocrine syndromes and also tumour markers, substances whose presence is a reflection of the presence of tumours, and whose concentrations can be measured as an aid to the diagnosis or monitoring of malignant disease.

PARANEOPLASTIC ENDOCRINE SYNDROMES

Origins and classification

These syndromes are due to the secretion of peptide hormones or other humoral factors, which are coded for by genes and translated from m-RNA. All somatic cells contain a full complement of genes, and aberrant hormone secretion could be explained either by novel expression of a gene that is not normally expressed in the cells from which the tumour arises, or by re-expression of a gene that is expressed during development in a stem cell from which the tumour cells are derived. The fact that these syndromes tend to be associated with certain tumours, notably small cell carcinoma of bronchus, and that some tumours give rise to predominantly only one syndrome, favours the second explanation.

Small cell carcinoma of bronchus is an example of an APUD tumour. This term, derived from 'amine precursor uptake and decarboxylation', was originally used to describe tumours of neuroectodermal origin sharing similar amine-handling characteristics. In fact, the principal products of most of these tumours are low molecular weight peptides (many of them hormones). However, paraneoplastic endocrine syndromes also occur in association with tumours that do not arise from APUD cells and, apart from their ability to secrete hormones, no single distinctive property has been shown to be common to all non-endocrine tumours associated with these syndromes.

Hormone secretion by tumours does not always cause an endocrine syndrome. This may be because insufficient is secreted to cause a persistently raised plasma concentration (particularly since normal secretion of the hormone may be suppressed) or because the principal secretory product is an inactive precursor of the hormone.

Some tumours associated with aberrant hormone secretion are shown in *Fig. 18.1*. The most frequently encountered paraneoplastic endocrine syndromes are dilutional hyponatraemia, hypercalcaemia and Cushing's

Some non-endocrine tumours associated with hormone secretion		
Tumour	**Hormone**	**Syndrome**
small cell carcinoma of bronchus	ACTH (and precursors) vasopressin hCG	Cushing's syndrome dilutional hyponatraemia gynaecomastia
squamous cell carcinoma of bronchus	PTHrP	hypercalcaemia
breast carcinoma	calcitonin	none
carcinoid tumours*	ACTH vasopressin	Cushing's syndrome dilutional hyponatraemia
renal adenocarcinoma	PTHrP	hypercalcaemia
mesenchymal tumours	insulin-like growth factors	hypoglycaemia

Fig. 18.1 Non-endocrine tumours frequently associated with aberrant hormone secretion. Renal adenocarcinomas may also secrete erythropoietin, causing polycythaemia, but this is not ectopic secretion since this hormone is a normal product of the kidney. PTHrP = PTH-related peptide.
*Carcinoid tumours also secrete vasoactive amines (*see p. 325*).

syndrome. Calcitonin secretion is thought to be common, but is clinically silent.

Cushing's syndrome

Cushing's syndrome is the condition that results when tissues are exposed to supraphysiological concentrations of glucocorticoids. It is discussed in detail in *Chapter 8*.

Ectopic secretion of ACTH by non-endocrine tumours is common. Evidence of it has been found in up to 50% of patients with small cell bronchial carcinomas, though massive secretion, giving rise to the typical features as shown by *Case History 18.1*, is uncommon. ACTH is produced by post-translational modification of the precursor, pro-opiomelanocortin (POMC), and both this precursor, and other products of the POMC gene (*see p. 125*), may be secreted in some cases.

With bronchial carcinomas, the prognosis is usually very poor unless the tumour is suitable for surgical excision. As discussed on *p. 153*, medical treatment may provide symptomatic relief.

Ectopic antidiuretic hormone (ADH) secretion

A case of this syndrome is described in *Case History 2.3*. The secretion of ADH (vasopressin) by the tumour is

uncontrolled and thus likely to be greater than the body's normal requirements, resulting in water retention with dilutional hyponatraemia. When this is mild and develops slowly, it is often asymptomatic; however, severe hyponatraemia is associated with water intoxication, which can be fatal. The symptoms (drowsiness, confusion, fits and coma) may mimic those of cerebral metastases. Ectopic ADH secretion is most commonly seen with small cell carcinomas of the bronchus but other tumours may be responsible (e.g. carcinoid tumours and pancreatic adenocarcinomas). A similar syndrome results from the inappropriate secretion of ADH that can occur in a variety of non-malignant diseases (*see p. 27*).

Tumour-associated hypercalcaemia

Hypercalcaemia is common in malignant disease. When bony metastases are present, dissolution of calcium from bone by the metastases themselves may contribute to hypercalcaemia. However, there is in general a poor correlation between the extent of metastatic bone involvement and the severity of any hypercalcaemia; also, hypercalcaemia can occur in the absence of detectable metastasis. Although hypercalcaemia can affect renal function adversely and decrease calcium excretion, it should suppress parathyroid hormone secretion by the

Case history 18.1

A retired warehouseman presented with muscle weakness and back pain. He had also lost 5 kg in weight in the previous two months and had recently been passing more urine than usual. He had smoked 25–30 cigarettes a day for many years but had generally enjoyed good health. On examination, in addition to the weakness and signs of weight loss, he was found to have glycosuria and was hypertensive, but his appearance was otherwise normal and no abnormal physical signs were elicited.

Investigations

serum:	sodium	144 mmol/L
	potassium	2.2 mmol/L
	bicarbonate	39 mmol/L
blood:	glucose	10.2 mmol/L
plasma (0900 h):		
	cortisol	1520 nmol/L
	ACTH	460 ng/L (normal <80 ng/L)

High-dose dexamethasone suppression test: 0900 h plasma cortisol after dexamethasone 2 mg, 4 times daily
for 2 days   1500 nmol/L

A discrete mass was present in the left lower zone on chest radiography.

Comment

The greatly elevated plasma cortisol and ACTH concentrations are typical of ectopic ACTH secretion. Plasma ACTH concentrations are generally much higher than those seen in Cushing's disease, except when a carcinoid or thymic tumour is responsible. Since ACTH secretion is not under normal feedback control, the hypercortisolaemia is not suppressed by dexamethasone.

With ectopic ACTH secretion, the clinical presentation is typically dominated by the metabolic sequelae of excessive cortisol secretion, as in this case. These include hypokalaemia with alkalosis, which exacerbates the physical weakness due to steroid-induced myopathy, glucose intolerance, sometimes sufficient to cause frank diabetes, and hypertension. Osteoporosis predisposes to crush fractures of the vertebrae and the presence of secondary tumour deposits may also give rise to back pain. The classic somatic manifestations of Cushing's syndrome are often absent, a reflection of the very rapid progression of the condition in most cases. ACTH-secreting carcinoid and thymic tumours are an exception: the clinical syndrome in these cases may closely resemble Cushing's disease even to the extent that ACTH secretion, and hence that of cortisol, is suppressible by dexamethasone.

parathyroid glands. This would be expected to decrease renal tubular calcium reabsorption, and allow excretion of calcium mobilized from bone. These observations argue strongly in favour of the involvement of humoral factors in the hypercalcaemia of malignancy. Parathyroid hormone-related peptide (PTHrP) is most frequently responsible.

Hypercalcaemia is common in haematological malignancies, particularly myeloma, and is due to the release of osteoclast-activating cytokines [e.g. interleukin-1, tumour necrosis factor (TNFβ)] by the tumours. Osteoclasts may also be activated by prostaglandins produced by tumour metastases in bone, for example metastases from breast carcinoma.

Case history 18.2

An elderly man presented with loin pain and increasing thirst. Examination of the urine showed haematuria but no glycosuria.

Investigations

serum:
calcium	3.2 mmol/L
phosphate	0.7 mmol/L
alkaline phosphatase	80 U/L
parathyroid hormone	below detection limit of the assay

An intravenous urogram showed an irregularly enlarged left kidney with a distorted pelvicalyceal system.

Arteriography demonstrated an abnormal circulation in the left kidney, strongly suggestive of a tumour.

Skeletal survey and isotopic bone scan showed no evidence of metastatic disease and a chest radiograph was normal.

At operation, a tumour was seen in the upper part of the left kidney. The patient underwent nephrectomy and made an uneventful recovery. Following the operation his plasma calcium concentration decreased and subsequently remained normal.

Comment

The combination of hypercalcaemia and hypophosphataemia is compatible with excessive PTH secretion, although the plasma phosphate may be normal or even raised if there is renal impairment. The absence of detectable PTH suggests that secretion of the hormone by the parathyroid glands is suppressed, as would be expected were the hypercalcaemia to be due to some agent other than PTH. True ectopic secretion of PTH is very rare. In most cases, hypercalcaemia of malignancy is due to the secretion of PTHrP by tumours. This substance, which has some N-terminal amino acid sequence homology with PTH, binds to PTH receptors and has similar actions to PTH itself but is not measured in most assays for PTH.

Tumour-associated hypoglycaemia

This condition is discussed in detail in *Chapter 11*. It is only rarely due to ectopic insulin secretion by non-β-cell tumours. Tumour-associated hypoglycaemia is usually associated with large mesenchymal tumours and is probably due to the secretion of insulin-like growth factors (somatomedins) by the tumours.

Other paraneoplastic endocrine syndromes

Gynaecomastia may occur in patients with bronchial carcinomas, due to secretion of human chorionic gonadotrophin (hCG). Precocious puberty may develop in male children with hepatic tumours secreting hCG, but this is very rare. Secretion of erythropoietin is responsible for the polycythaemia that can occur in association with uterine fibromyomata and the rare tumour cerebellar haemangioblastoma. Secretion of erythropoietin by adenocarcinomas of the kidney can cause polycythaemia but this is not ectopic secretion, since the kidneys are the normal source of this hormone.

Paraneoplastic syndromes are common, but it must be remembered that an endocrine syndrome in a patient with a tumour may be due to coexistent endocrine disease and not necessarily to the secretion of a hormone or other factor by the tumour.

OTHER METABOLIC COMPLICATIONS OF MALIGNANT DISEASE

Metabolic complications in patients with malignant disease are not always due to aberrant hormone secretion. They may be due to some other effect of the tumour, or develop as a consequence of treatment.

Renal failure can occur for many possible reasons. Causes include obstruction of the urinary tract, hypercalcaemia, direct infiltration of the kidneys (e.g. by lymphoma), Bence Jones proteinuria (in myeloma), antibiotics, cytotoxic drugs and the tumour lysis syndrome. This latter is the result of massive necrosis of tumour cells during the treatment of tumours with cytotoxic drugs. Features include hyperkalaemia, hyper-uricaemia, hyperphosphataemia and hypocalcaemia. It is particularly likely to occur with large, chemosensitive tumours such as some lymphomas, and with leukaemias, and can cause acute renal failure. Preventative measures include the maintenance of adequate hydration, giving allopurinol to inhibit uric acid synthesis and careful monitoring of fluid and electrolyte status.

Hypomagnesaemia (often accompanied by hypokalaemia) is a particular complication of treatment with cisplatin, a cytotoxic drug. Massive renal loss of potassium can occur in patients requiring treatment with amphotericin for fungal infections, which can develop as a result of the immunosuppressive effect of some tumours and cytotoxic drugs.

CANCER CACHEXIA

Cachexia, a syndrome of weakness and generalized wasting, is a common feature of malignant disease. Its characteristics are summarized in *Fig. 18.2*. Its causes are imperfectly understood. Deficient food intake, due either to mechanical obstruction of the alimentary tract

Cancer cachexia	
Characteristics	**Pathogenic factors**
anorexia and early satiety	anorexia, obstruction, causing decreased food intake
weight loss	loss of protein (e.g. from ulcerated mucosa)
muscle weakness	
	malabsorption
non-specific anaemia	infection
pyrexia	consumption of nutrients by tumour
	abnormal metabolism by tumour
	secretion of cachectin, causing increase in metabolic rate
	treatment with cytotoxic drugs

Fig. 18.2 Characteristics and pathogenesis of cancer cachexia.

or to the anorexia that is often present in malignant disease, may be partly responsible, and there may also be loss of protein from ulcerated mucosa or due to blood loss.

The tumour itself requires nitrogen and energy for growth, and this will be met from body stores if intake is inadequate. Associated infection or products of the tumour itself may cause pyrexia, and increase energy requirements.

The metabolism of many tumours is primarily anaerobic: lactate is produced which is converted back to glucose in the liver and kidney. This represents a waste of energy, since glycolysis results in the net formation of only two molecules of ATP per molecule of glucose, while gluconeogenesis, the reverse process, consumes six.

Cachexia can be seen in patients both with large or widespread tumours and with small tumours. Indeed, it may be the presenting feature of malignancy. In many cases, production of cytokines (particularly TNFα, also known as cachectin) may be in part responsible. TNFα is a normal product of macrophages and may be produced by activated macrophages within tumour tissue or possibly by tumour cells themselves. Among many other effects, TNFα increases the body's energy expenditure.

In the majority of cases, the pathogenesis of cancer cachexia is probably multifactorial; contributory factors are indicated in *Fig. 18.2*. Management is difficult. Nutritional support may be beneficial, but the condition is rarely completely reversible unless the underlying tumour can be treated successfully.

CARCINOID TUMOURS

Carcinoid tumours arise from the enterochromaffin cells of the gut, cells of the APUD series; 90% of these tumours are found in the appendix and ileocaecal region but they also occur elsewhere in the gut, gallbladder, biliary and pancreatic ducts, and in the bronchi. They are of low-grade malignancy: while they frequently invade local tissue, distant metastases are rare.

The carcinoid syndrome is a result of the liberation of vasoactive amines, such as serotonin, and peptides from the tumour into the circulation. It is usually only seen with bronchial tumours, which liberate their products directly into the systemic circulation, or when tumours in the gut have metastasized to the liver. Since the greater part of the gut is drained by the portal circulation, the secreted products of tumours in the gut pass to the liver, where they are inactivated. However, the secreted products of hepatic metastases reach the systemic circulation via the hepatic veins.

Serotonin (5-hydroxytryptamine, 5-HT) is synthesized from tryptophan (*Fig. 18.3*). In patients with carcinoid syndrome, 50% of dietary tryptophan (rather than the usual 1%) may be metabolized by this pathway, diverting tryptophan away from protein and nicotinic acid synthesis. (Pellagra-like skin lesions due to nicotinic acid deficiency are an occasional feature of the carcinoid syndrome.) The major amine secreted by intestinal carcinoid tumours (derived from embryonic midgut) is 5-hydroxytryptamine. Bronchial carcinoids (derived from foregut) tend to produce 5-hydroxytryptophan since they often lack the decarboxylase enzyme. All carcinoid tumours may also produce histamine and kinins, which are important in the symptomatology of the carcinoid syndrome. Furthermore, the secretion of peptide hormones (e.g. ACTH) is often demonstrable and may contribute to the clinical presentation.

Management

Carcinoid tumours are difficult to manage. Once metastases have developed, surgical removal is usually not possible though partial resection may be palliative since the tumours are usually slow growing. Symptomatic relief may be obtained with simple anti-diarrhoeal agents (e.g. codeine phosphate or loperamide), but the most effective medical treatment is with octreotide, a somatostatin analogue: this causes symptomatic relief and may cause some tumour regression. Interferon has also been used with some success. Hepatic metastases may be destroyed by hepatic arterial embolization.

MULTIPLE ENDOCRINE NEOPLASIA

The syndromes of multiple endocrine neoplasia (MEN) are familial disorders with an autosomal dominant inheritance in which tumours (benign or malignant) or hyperplasia develop in two or more endocrine glands. They are uncommon, but it is important to recognize that a patient presenting with certain endocrinopathies could have one of these syndromes. The glands affected are shown in *Fig. 18.5*. Although the syndromes are inherited, the predominant features

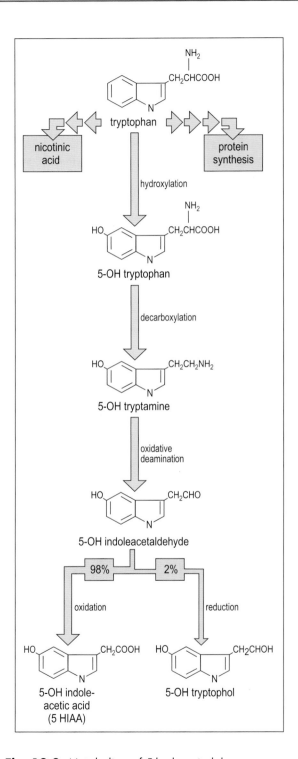

Fig. 18.3 Metabolism of 5-hydroxyindoles.

Case history 18.3

A 50-year-old woman presented with a history of episodic facial flushing and dizziness, sometimes accompanied by wheezing respiration. These attacks could occur at any time but she was frequently embarrassed by them at meal times.

Investigations

urinary 5-hydroxyindoleacetic acid excretion
   270 µmol/24 h (normal 10–50 µmol/24 h)

An isotopic scan of the liver revealed multiple filling defects suggestive of tumour deposits.

A distorted hepatic vasculature with evidence of tumour circulation was demonstrated on arteriography, but the primary tumour could not be located.

Comment

Facial flushing is the commonest clinical feature of carcinoid syndrome and may be provoked by the ingestion of food or alcohol, or by emotional stimuli. It may become continuous and spread to other parts of the body. The vasodilatation causes transient hypotension and patients may complain of dizziness. Other clinical features are listed in *Fig. 18.4* and include intermittent abdominal discomfort, diarrhoea and bronchospasm with wheezing. Right-sided valvular lesions of the heart, particularly pulmonary stenosis, may lead to cardiac failure.

The diagnosis is confirmed by demonstrating an increase in the urinary excretion of 5-hydroxyindoleacetic acid. This is usually more than twice the upper limit of normal and may be much greater. Foodstuffs containing serotonin (including bananas, various other fruits and some nuts) and drugs such as reserpine, which stimulate endogenous serotonin release must be avoided during collection.

Clinical features of the carcinoid syndrome

Gastrointestinal
discomfort, hyperperistalsis and borborygmi
diarrhoea
nausea and vomiting
colicky pain

Cardiovascular
flushing
pulmonary stenosis (may lead to right heart failure and occasionally mitral stenosis)

Respiratory
bronchospasm
variable rate and depth of breathing

Other
pellagra
manifestations of secretion of other hormones

Fig. 18.4 Clinical features of the carcinoid syndrome.

---

vary in different members of the same family: thus one person may present with recurrent peptic ulceration due to a gastrinoma (Zollinger–Ellison syndrome), while a sibling may have urinary calculi as a result of hyperparathyroidism.

TUMOUR MARKERS

Tumour markers are substances that can reflect the presence or progress of a tumour. They include substances, including enzymes, other proteins and smaller peptides, which are secreted into body fluids by tumours, and antigens expressed on cell surfaces. Clinical chemistry laboratories are usually only involved in the measurement of tumour markers falling into the first category.

An ideal secreted tumour marker could be used for:

- screening
- diagnosis
- prognosis
- monitoring treatment
- follow-up to detect recurrence.

Glands affected in multiple endocrine neoplasia
MEN type 1*
parathyroids
pancreatic islets
anterior pituitary
MEN type 2a
thyroid (medullary cell carcinoma)
adrenal medulla (phaeochromocytoma)
parathyroids
MEN type 2b
thyroid (medullary cell carcinoma)
adrenal medulla (phaeochromocytoma)
parathyroids (rarely)
various somatic abnormalities:
Marfanoid habitus
mucosal neuromata
pigmentation

Fig.18.5 Glands affected in multiple endocrine neoplasia (MEN).
*Other tumours, e.g of adrenal cortex and thyroid, are sometimes present, but much less frequently than those listed.

Although some markers are reliable for some of these purposes, probably only one (chorionic gonadotrophin, a marker for choriocarcinoma) is widely used for all. The development of monoclonal antibody techniques has led to the discovery and subsequent investigation of many new tumour markers in recent years but, overall, the number of markers that are of proven clinical value remains small.

α-Fetoprotein

α-Fetoprotein is a glycoprotein of molecular weight 67 kDa. It is synthesized by the yolk sac and the fetal liver and gut. In the fetus, it is a major plasma protein; in adults, the normal concentration is less than 10 μg/L. Increased plasma concentrations of α-fetoprotein are seen in normal pregnancy. Its use in the diagnosis of neural tube defects is discussed in *Chapter 16*.

α-Fetoprotein is a valuable marker for hepatocellular carcinomas (HCC) and testicular teratomas. Overall, primary liver cancer is uncommon in the UK, and therefore population screening for the condition cannot

Case history 18.4

A two-year-old boy presented with progressive abdominal swelling. On examination, the liver was found to be massively enlarged. Ultrasound and radiological examinations suggested the presence of a tumour, and histological examination of tissue obtained by percutaneous needle biopsy showed this to be a hepatoblastoma.

Investigations

serum α-fetoprotein   42 000 μg/L

A partial hepatectomy was performed but complete removal of the tumour was not possible because of its extent. The child was therefore started on a course of cytotoxic therapy.

Comment

Such a massively elevated concentration of α-fetoprotein in a child of this age is effectively diagnostic of hepatoblastoma (though it should be noted that infants normally have higher concentrations than adults, particularly during the first month of life). The change in serum α-fetoprotein is shown in *Fig. 18.6*. Partial hepatectomy produced a temporary fall in α-fetoprotein but continued growth of the tumour resulted in a further increase. Cytotoxic treatment produced a sustained decline in α-fetoprotein concentrations, and this corresponded to clinical remission.

be justified. However, some groups of patients – notably those with cirrhosis, persistence of hepatitis B virus and haemochromatosis – are at particularly high risk, and selective screening (e.g. at six-monthly intervals) using α-fetoprotein measurement may be of value. α-Fetoprotein concentrations are elevated in the majority of patients with cirrhosis and HCC, although in only about half those with tumours in the absence of cirrhosis. A concentration of >500 μg/L in a patient with cirrhosis is virtually diagnostic of HCC. The finding of concentrations in the range 50–500 μg/L warrants further investigation. As a tumour marker in this

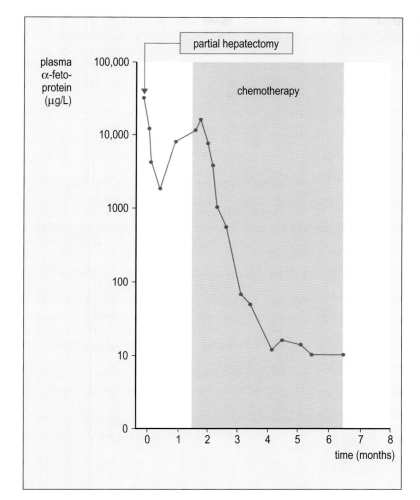

Fig. 18.6 α-Fetoprotein concentration in a patient with hepatoblastoma.

context, α-fetoprotein lacks specificity: concentrations of up to 100 μg/L can occur in cirrhosis in the absence of malignancy. α-Fetoprotein does not appear to be of value prognostically. However, in histologically confirmed liver cancer, serial measurements of α-fetoprotein are of considerable value in monitoring the response of the patient to treatment. The normal hepatic regeneration that occurs following partial hepatic resection may cause an increase in α-fetoprotein concentration, but this is only transient.

In patients with testicular teratomas, α-fetoprotein measurements are valuable in assessing prognosis, in staging and in monitoring therapy. A very high concentration indicates a massive tumour load and a poor prognosis (a mortality rate greater than 40% if α-fetoprotein concentration is greater than 1.26 mg/L). A rapid fall to normal after orchidectomy implies that the disease was limited to the testis. Remission is achieved in 80% of patients with metastatic teratoma of the testis, using a combination of surgery and chemotherapy.

The efficacy of treatment can be assessed from the decline in plasma α-fetoprotein concentration, which reflects the decrease in tumour mass. Once a patient is in remission, repeated measurements are essential; a rise in concentration will be due to recurrence of the tumour and indicates the need for further treatment or a change in the chemotherapeutic regimen. It should be appreciated that plasma concentrations of α-fetoprotein within the 'normal' range are compatible with the presence of tumour; a rise in concentration, even if within this range, should raise the suspicion of tumour recurrence. On the other hand, tumours may lose the ability to secrete α-fetoprotein, so vigorous clinical assessment remains an important part of the follow-up of these patients.

Teratomas comprise some 32% of all testicular tumours. More common are seminomas (40%) but these rarely secrete either α-fetoprotein or βhCG, another marker for teratomas (*see below*).

Carcinoembryonic antigen (CEA)

This tumour marker is present in elevated concentrations in the plasma of 60% of patients with colorectal cancer, more commonly so with advanced disease (80–100% if hepatic metastases are present) than with tumours confined to the colon. However, elevated concentrations are also found in a variety of non-malignant conditions, including liver disease of various types, pancreatitis and inflammatory bowel disease, and in some people who smoke heavily.

CEA is neither sufficiently specific nor sensitive to be used in screening for colorectal carcinoma. CEA concentrations in plasma correlate poorly with tumour bulk, which limits the usefulness of measurements in monitoring treatment. Following surgical resection of a tumour, plasma CEA concentration can be expected to fall. However, while a subsequent rise suggests a recurrence, recurrence is not always heralded by such a rise and, even when it is, it may not affect the clinical outcome since further treatment may not be feasible.

Paraproteins

Paraproteins (*see p. 244*) are detectable in either serum or urine in 98–99% of patients with myeloma. Not only is their detection valuable in the diagnosis of this condition, but also paraprotein concentrations correlate well with tumour bulk, with the result that the reduction in the amount of paraprotein is a good indicator of the efficacy of treatment.

Human chorionic gonadotrophin (hCG)

hCG is a hormone produced by the normal placenta, reaching a maximum concentration in plasma by the eighth week of pregnancy. hCG is composed of an α- and a β-subunit: the α-subunit is identical to that of luteinizing hormone (LH), follicle stimulating hormone (FSH) and thyroid stimulating hormone (TSH); the β-subunit, however, is specific to hCG and is therefore measured in assays for the hormone. The presence of hCG in the plasma at other times indicates the presence of abnormal trophoblastic tissue or a tumour secreting the hormone ectopically.

βhCG is an almost ideal tumour marker for choriocarcinoma, a malignant proliferation of chorionic villi that may develop from hydatidiform mole, itself a potentially malignant proliferation of this tissue, which occurs in approximately 1 in 2000 pregnancies in the UK. Hydatidiform mole is treated by uterine curettage, but the patient is at risk of developing choriocarcinoma if removal is incomplete. βhCG is an extremely sensitive tumour marker; tumours weighing only 1 mg (corresponding to 10^5 cells) may be detectable. All patients who have had hydatidiform moles must be followed up with regular checks of plasma βhCG concentration. Should a tumour develop, the marker can be used as an indicator of the response to treatment and, if this is successful, in long-term follow-up thereafter.

hCG is also secreted by approximately 50% of testicular teratomas and should be measured together with α-fetoprotein in the follow-up of patients after treatment of the tumour. Since LH concentrations rise after orchidectomy, it is important that an assay specific to the β-chain of hCG is employed, to avoid cross-reaction causing an apparent increase in hCG.

Other hormones as tumour markers

Hormones secreted both eutopically and ectopically can provide useful tumour markers. The measurement, for example, of catecholamines in phaeochromocytomas and of metabolites of serotonin in the diagnosis of carcinoid syndrome is discussed elsewhere (*pp 158, 327*). Calcitonin is a valuable marker, particularly for medullary cell carcinoma of the thyroid (eutopic secretion) and occasionally in carcinoma of the breast (ectopic secretion). Medullary cell carcinoma of thyroid is frequently familial and can be part of a pluriglandular syndrome. Calcitonin measurements can be used to screen for this tumour in the families of affected patients. Although basal plasma concentrations of calcitonin may be normal, an excessive rise following provocation, for example with alcohol, pentagastrin or calcium infusion, is typical in patients with medullary carcinoma.

Ectopic hormonal markers of other tumours, for example bronchial carcinomas, are of little practical use in the management of patients. They are not present sufficiently frequently to be of use in screening, and the response to treatment is, in general, so poor that their measurement provides no practical support to the clinician.

Markers of prostatic cancer

Prostatic cancer is the second most common cancer in males. Prostate specific antigen (PSA) is a marker for this tumour. PSA is a 33 kDa glycoprotein serine protease. It is normally secreted into the prostatic duct system but small amounts diffuse into the plasma. This diffusion, and in consequence plasma PSA concentrations, tends to be increased in prostatic cancer but the sensitivity and specificity of PSA as a marker are limited by the fact that PSA is detectable in the plasma of normal men, and because its concentration increases both with increasing age and in benign prostatic hypertrophy, a very common affliction of elderly men. Using a cut-off of 4 µg/L, specificity is 97% in men over the age of 40, and sensitivity for stage I disease, 67%. The likelihood of cancer increases significantly at concentrations >10 µg/L. The finding of an elevated concentration of PSA in a patient with prostatism is thus not diagnostic of prostatic cancer but should prompt the patient's referral to a urologist for consideration for biopsy and histological diagnosis. Digital rectal examination may increase plasma PSA concentration slightly and transiently, but significant increases can occur in acute urinary retention and prostatitis.

Considerable effort has been expended in trying to improve the sensitivity and specificity of PSA measurements as a marker for cancer. Approaches have included: the development of age-related reference ranges; relating PSA concentration to prostatic volume as estimated by ultrasound; determining the rate of change of concentration with time, and measuring free and bound PSA. This last approach appears the most promising. It is based on the observation that, while most PSA in the plasma of normal men is protein bound, the bound proportion is higher in the presence of prostatic cancer. However, prostatic cancer is an unusual tumour. In many cases it progresses relatively slowly, and many men die with prostatic cancer rather than of it; in some cases it spreads rapidly and has a poor outcome, even with treatment. Major trials are presently under way to determine if screening for prostatic cancer using PSA alters the clinical outcome in a significant proportion of men.

Before the introduction of PSA as a marker for prostatic cancer, prostate-specific acid phosphatase was widely used for this purpose, but it has been superseded and is now obsolete.

Enzymes as tumour markers

Plasma enzyme activities are often increased in patients with cancer, but this is usually tumour related rather than tumour derived; that is, it is a secondary effect of the tumour rather than a result of secretion of an enzyme by the tumour. Examples include the increases in alkaline phosphatase activity seen in patients with biliary obstruction or bony metastases.

Alkaline phosphatase has several isoenzymes, and an increase in the plasma activity of the placental type in plasma occurs in many patients with testicular seminomas and is tumour derived. Measurement of placental alkaline phosphatase is of value in monitoring the response of such patients to treatment.

Neuron-specific enolase is an isoenzyme of enolase present in nerve and neuroendocrine cells. Small cell carcinomas of bronchus, which are neuroendocrine in origin, frequently secrete this enzyme and when this occurs, patients' response to treatment can be monitored by serial measurements.

Carbohydrate antigen (CA) markers

These are tumour markers that have been identified as a result of attempts to develop monoclonal antibodies against tumour extracts or tumour-derived cell lines. They are high molecular weight glycoproteins. Many CA markers have been identified and investigated; none has yet been identified which is specific for a particular tumour, or even tissue, and, in general, those that are in use clinically are used for monitoring rather than for screening or diagnosis. An exception is CA 125, a marker for ovarian cancer. There is some evidence that population screening for ovarian cancer based initially on measurement of CA 125, followed, if the concentration is above a specified cut-off (30 U/mL), by ultrasonography and then gynaecological referral can detect tumours before they are apparent clinically, albeit with a significant false-positive rate. Whether early detection affects mortality from ovarian cancer has yet to be determined. Neither test is sufficiently sensitive or specific on its own. CA 125 can be increased in benign conditions (e.g. endometriosis) and in non-ovarian malignancies. The CA 125 concentration at the time of diagnosis is of little prognostic significance, but serial measurements are valuable in monitoring patients following surgical resection of a tumour. An inadequate fall in concentration during chemotherapy suggests that treatment is being unsuccessful and may prompt a change in treatment to palliative treatment only.

Other tumour markers of this category that are of potential value in monitoring the response of patients to treatment include CA 19-9 for adenocarcinoma of pancreas and possibly colorectal and gastric carcinomas, CA 50 for colorectal carcinoma and CA 15-3 for carcinoma of breast. Plasma CA 19-9 concentrations are elevated in more than 80% of patients with carcinoma of the exocrine pancreas, but only occasionally in benign disease. However, its potential value as a marker is diminished by the fact that pancreatic cancer tends to present late, when no effective treatment is available.

Plasma CA 19-9 also increases in patients with primary sclerosing cholangitis, a non-malignant inflammatory condition of the bile ducts of autoimmune origin, and can be used to monitor disease activity. Patients with this condition are at risk of developing cholangiocarcinoma. If this occurs, there is usually a rapid increase in CA 19-9 to very high concentrations. Measurement of CA 19-9 can be combined with CEA: CEA tends not to be elevated in sclerosing cholangitis but does increase in cholangiocarcinoma.

In carcinoma of the breast, both CA 15-3 and mucin-like carcinoma associated antigen (MCA) may help to identify patients who have metastases at the time of diagnosis.

Other tumour markers

New tumour markers are continually being developed and their use investigated. Their clinical utility remains to be proven. They include S-100 for melanoma, and CYFRA-21 and SCC in bronchial carcinoma.

CONCLUSION

The clinical usefulness of secreted tumour markers for screening and diagnosis is limited to a small number of markers (*Fig. 18.7*) and relatively uncommon tumours.

Some clinically useful tumour markers

Marker	Tumour	Uses
α-fetoprotein	hepatoma germ cell	SDMF DPMF
β-human chorionic gonadotrophin	germ cell choriocarcinoma	DPMF SDPMF
carcinoembryonic antigen	colorectal carcinoma	MF
paraproteins	myeloma	DMF
calcitonin	medullary thyroid carcinoma	SDMF
prostate specific antigen	prostatic carcinoma	MF
CA 125	ovarian carcinoma	SPM

S = screening (only in individuals at high risk)
D = diagnosis
P = prognosis
M = monitoring treatment
F = follow-up

Fig. 18.7 Some clinically useful tumour markers.

Other markers are of use in monitoring the response of patients to treatment and there is considerable research in progress in this field. Antibodies developed against tumour cell-surface antigens are of considerable value in the differential diagnosis of lymphomas and leukaemias, although their measurement is not usually the responsibility of the clinical biochemist.

It should be appreciated that the existence of a marker for a cancer, however sensitive and specific (and most are not), does not on its own imply clinical utility. The aim of using markers, whether for screening, diagnosis or monitoring the response to treatment, should be to improve outcome. This depends not only on the properties of the marker, but on the availability of safe and effective treatment. It can be argued that tumour markers, like drugs, should only be introduced into routine use when they have been shown to be of proven benefit. In practice, markers are often measured when there is little evidence that this can benefit the patient and without a full understanding of their limitations.

SUMMARY

- Patients with malignant disease frequently suffer from disorders not directly attributable to the physical presence of the tumour. These 'paraneoplastic' syndromes include metabolic disorders, notably those in which **ectopic hormone secretion** occurs. This term refers to the secretion of a known hormone (or a substance with hormone-like activity) by a non-endocrine tumour. The clinical features produced can closely resemble those seen when a hormone is secreted in excess by its normal tissue of origin (eutopic secretion). Examples include: **Cushing's syndrome** and the **syndrome of inappropriate antidiuretic hormone secretion** caused by the production of adrenocorticotrophin and antidiuretic hormone (vasopressin), respectively, by small cell carcinomas of bronchus and various other tumours; **hypercalcaemia**, particularly in some patients with squamous cell carcinomas of bronchus and renal adenocarcinomas, and **hypoglycaemia**, which may occur in patients with large mesenchymal tumours, though is not due to insulin. Other hormones that have been shown to be secreted by non-endocrine tumours include chorionic gonadotrophin, growth hormone releasing hormone, calcitonin and erythropoietin. The mechanism of ectopic hormone secretion is unclear but it is presumed that selective derepression of the appropriate genes occurs in the tumour cells.

- **Cancer cachexia**, a non-specific syndrome of weight loss, anorexia and weakness, is common in patients with cancer. It is probably multifactorial in origin but the secretion of a humoral substance by the tumour may be partly responsible.

- **Carcinoid tumours** are derived from argentaffin cells, members of the APUD family (cells of neuroectodermal origin characterized by their ability to take up and decarboxylate amines). These tumours are mainly found in the gut; they are of low-grade malignancy and may go unnoticed unless metastasis occurs. They tend to secrete 5-hydroxytryptamine (5-HT); this is released into the portal circulation and usually metabolized by the liver but, when hepatic metastases are present, 5-HT reaches the systemic circulation and may produce the **carcinoid syndrome**. The diagnosis is made by demonstrating an increased urinary excretion of the 5-HT metabolite, 5-hydroxyindoleacetic acid.

- Some tumours occur in association and this tendency is often inherited. There are several **syndromes of multiple endocrine neoplasia**. Tumours that may be present in these syndromes include parathyroid adenomas, medullary cell carcinomas, phaeochromocytomas and pancreatic endocrine tumours.

- **Tumour markers** are substances that can be measured in body fluids in patients with cancer. They include hormones secreted by tumours but in general the fact that any particular hormone is also being produced by its normal source and is usually not consistently secreted by a particular tumour vitiates their measurement for this purpose. Some tumours, however, regularly secrete substances that are not usually detectable in the plasma and these may be useful markers both for diagnosis and for following the progress of a malignancy. The best-established examples of such tumour markers are α-**fetoprotein** (for testicular teratoma and hepatocellular carcinoma), β-**human chorionic gonadotrophin** (choriocarcinoma), **prostate specific antigen** (carcinoma of prostate), **carcinoembryonic antigen** (colorectal carcinoma) and **paraproteins** (myeloma).

- Many **newer tumour markers** are currently being evaluated. They include **CA 125**, which is in established use in the management of ovarian cancer and may prove to be of value in screening for this disease.

19 Therapeutic drug monitoring and chemical aspects of toxicology

INTRODUCTION

Clinical chemistry laboratories are called upon to measure drugs in body fluids for three main purposes:

- to provide information relevant to the diagnosis and management of patients suspected to have taken drug overdoses
- to provide such information in patients taking drugs therapeutically
- to screen for the presence of drugs of abuse.

This chapter covers these topics and discusses the metabolic sequelae of some common poisonings.

THERAPEUTIC DRUG MONITORING

The questions that should be addressed when prescribing a drug are summarized in *Fig. 19.1*. All patients treated with drugs should be monitored clinically to assess the efficacy of treatment and to detect any adverse effects; laboratory assessment may also be helpful for these

Prescribing a drug

What effect is it hoped to achieve?

Is the drug chosen capable of producing the desired effect?

What are the side-effects of the drug and, if they are predictable, do the likely benefits of using the drug outweigh the disadvantages?

Are there any special factors in the patient which increase the likelihood of an abnormal response to the drug?

How should the effect of the drug be monitored?

If the drug is not effective, or produces undesirable effects, why does this happen?

Fig. 19.1 Questions that must be addressed when prescribing a drug.

purposes. Thus, it may be possible to measure a particular index of therapeutic response, for example the blood glucose concentration in a patient with diabetes treated with insulin, or thyroid function tests in a patient with thyrotoxicosis treated with carbimazole. Additionally, the laboratory may also be asked to monitor for possible toxic effects: for example, proteinuria in patients treated with penicillamine, or abnormalities of thyroid function in patients treated with the iodine-containing anti-arrhythmic drug, amiodarone.

An individual's response to a particular drug is dependent upon many factors, for example age, sex, renal function and the concurrent administration of other drugs. These factors should be borne in mind when deciding what dose of drug to prescribe, but in many cases the optimum dosage can be arrived at by commencing treatment with a standard dose and modifying this as necessary in the light of the observed response.

This approach is suitable for the many drugs whose effects can be assessed reliably, such as hypotensive agents, anticoagulants, insulin and oral hypoglycaemics, but it is not universally applicable. Obviously, optimization of drug dosage in this way is impossible when the effect of treatment is not easily ascertainable. An example is the use of anticonvulsants as prophylaxis in epilepsy. The incidence of seizures prior to treatment is unpredictable in many patients, making it difficult to assess the effect of the drug in preventing them. It is also difficult to adjust dosage on the basis of the therapeutic effect when a drug has a low therapeutic ratio (that is, the dose required to produce a therapeutic effect is close to that at which features of toxicity are seen, as is the case, for example, with lithium) especially if the adverse effects are hard to recognize. In such cases, measurement of the concentration of the drug in the plasma may provide valuable objective information.

It is outside the scope of this chapter to discuss in detail the many factors that can influence the relationship between the dose of a drug and the intensity of its effects. Some of these are listed in *Fig. 19.2*. It is reasonable to assume that there will be a greater correlation between the intensity of a drug's effect and its plasma concentration than with the dose of the drug that the patient takes. Despite this, plasma concentrations and tissue effects may

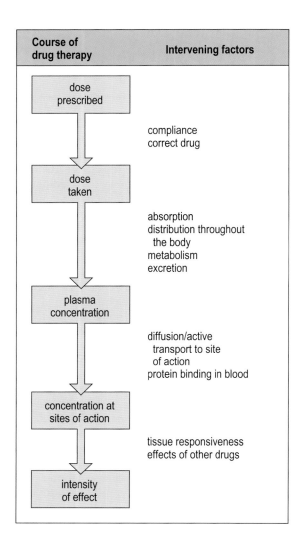

Course of drug therapy	Intervening factors
dose prescribed	
	compliance correct drug
dose taken	
	absorption distribution throughout the body metabolism excretion
plasma concentration	
	diffusion/active transport to site of action protein binding in blood
concentration at sites of action	
	tissue responsiveness effects of other drugs
intensity of effect	

Fig. 19.2 Factors influencing the relationship between drug usage and the intensity of its effect; the latter is not necessarily directly related to the plasma concentration but may be more closely related to it than the dose prescribed.

correlate poorly, since the drug must first travel from the plasma to its site of action and, once there, the responsiveness of the tissues may not be constant or predictable. Additionally, there may be no correlation at all when a drug is itself inactive (but is metabolized to an active substance in the body) or when it acts irreversibly.

Nevertheless, the correlation between the plasma concentration and pharmacological effect is surprisingly strong for many drugs and provides the rationale for the use of concentration measurement in therapeutic drug monitoring (TDM). It is important that any experimentally determined relationship between plasma drug concentration and the effect of a drug is confirmed in a clinical setting, and that plasma drug concentrations are interpreted in the particular clinical context. The time of sampling in relation to the time of dosage may be critical and the sensitivity of the target organ may vary, being influenced, for example, by genetic factors, nutritional status, the presence of other drugs and the health of the patient.

Even if there is good evidence that measuring the plasma concentration of a particular drug can provide useful information, in individual cases there should always be a rational reason for the request (i.e. a specific question should be asked, the answer to which will influence management); the right specimen (particularly with regard to timing) must be provided, and the analysis must be accurate and its result interpreted correctly. Finally, appropriate action should ensue.

In addition to individualizing the drug therapy, measurements of plasma concentrations of drugs can be useful in the diagnosis of suspected toxicity and in the assessment of compliance.

Although TDM is based mainly on serum or plasma measurements, there has been some interest in developing assays using saliva. These should reflect the plasma concentration of the non-protein bound drug, i.e. free drug that is directly available to the tissues; the advantage of this technique is that venepuncture is not required, but there are considerable technical problems with the assays and they are not in general routine use.

Measuring plasma concentration

The most frequently used assays measure total plasma concentration of a drug. With drugs that are protein bound, changes in plasma protein concentration may have a disproportionate effect on the total drug concentration relative to the amount free in the plasma and thus available to tissues. The assay chosen must be specific for the drug itself (or its active metabolite where appropriate) and should not measure inactive metabolites or be affected by other drugs that the patient may be taking.

As with other biochemical measurements, plasma concentrations of drugs are compared with standard data. The term 'reference range' is inappropriate in this context, since healthy people will not be taking the drug. The term 'therapeutic' or 'target' range is used instead. This is the range between the minimum effective concentration of the drug and the maximum safe concentration. Often, only the upper limit is stated, since a drug may be efficacious in some individuals at concentrations below the generally accepted minimum effective concentration. On the other hand, optimum management may sometimes require that a drug's concentration is maintained above the upper limit of the therapeutic/target range. Such ranges are not absolute: for example, hypokalaemia increases sensitivity to digoxin and effectively lowers the upper limit.

Readers should be aware that drug concentrations in body fluids may be reported in some laboratories in mass units (e.g. mg/L) but by others in molar units (e.g. µmol/L). In the UK, and in many other countries, the mole is used as the unit of substance concentration for the majority of analytes. The action of drugs is related to their molar concentrations rather than their mass concentrations. However, drugs are usually prescribed using mass units (e.g. mg), although it may be noted that the use of molar units would obviate the problems that can occur when drugs may be given in different molecular forms (e.g. different salts). It is therefore important, when making clinical use of drug concentrations (whether measured in the context of TDM or for other purposes), to be aware of the units used, and the appropriate ranges to aim for, or toxic concentrations that should determine intervention.

When a drug is first taken, the plasma concentration rises relatively rapidly as it is absorbed, and then falls, more slowly, as it is taken up into tissues, metabolized and excreted. Many drugs are taken in doses and at intervals such that a steady-state plasma concentration is achieved. This occurs after a period equivalent to five half-lives, and is often the most relevant concentration to measure. For some drugs with short half-lives, significant fluctuations in plasma concentration occur and it is the peak and trough concentrations, achieved shortly after and immediately before the drug is taken, respectively, that are measured.

In the following section, the use of plasma measurements of a few representative and commonly used drugs is discussed to illustrate the general principles of therapeutic drug monitoring.

MONITORING OF SPECIFIC DRUGS

Phenytoin

The therapeutic effectiveness of this frequently prescribed anticonvulsant drug is difficult to assess without monitoring. It has a low therapeutic ratio and the signs of toxicity may mimic the neurological diseases that can be associated with epilepsy. Furthermore, phenytoin has unusual pharmacokinetic properties: the enzyme responsible for the elimination of the drug becomes saturated within the therapeutic range of plasma concentrations. This phenomenon has several important implications. In particular, the relationship between plasma concentration and dose is non-linear (*Fig. 19.3*);

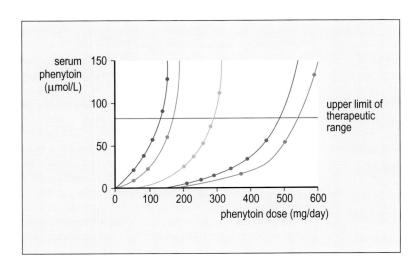

Fig. 19.3 Relationship between the steady-state serum concentration of phenytoin and dose; 80 µmol/L is the upper limit of the therapeutic range. Data for five patients are shown. Redrawn from Richens, A. and Dunlop, A. (1975) Serum phenytoin levels in the management of epilepsy. *Lancet*, **2**, 247–248.

Case history 19.1

A young woman developed idiopathic epilepsy at the age of 19 and had three generalized convulsions in 10 days before being started on phenytoin, 150 mg/day. She had a further fit two days after the first dose but thereafter remained fit-free.

Investigations

plasma phenytoin (4 weeks after
    starting treatment)   30 µmol/L

Comment

Phenytoin has a long plasma half-life, and steady-state plasma concentrations may not be reached for 3–4 weeks. The upper limit of the therapeutic range is 80 µmol/L. The usual procedure when commencing treatment is to give a standard dose of 150–200 mg/day (in adults) and to measure the plasma concentration after 3–4 weeks. If the patient is well controlled and there are no features of toxicity the same dose may be continued even if, as in this case, the plasma concentration is low in the therapeutic range. A dose increment is not indicated if the patient is fit-free just on the basis of the plasma concentration of the drug. In the well-controlled patient, this initial plasma concentration may be useful later to help ascertain the cause (for example, poor compliance, drug interaction) should seizures recur.

If the patient is not well controlled, increments in dose can be made, guided by measurement of plasma concentrations, to produce a steady-state concentration in the therapeutic range. Because of its long half-life, plasma concentrations of phenytoin during chronic administration remain relatively constant throughout the day. For this reason (unusually in therapeutic drug monitoring) the time of sampling in relation to the time the drug is taken is not critical. However, it is essential to leave sufficient time after changing the dose to allow a new steady state to develop. This takes approximately five times the plasma half-life of the drug.

thus small increments in dose may lead to disproportionate increases in steady-state plasma concentrations. On the other hand, even if the dose is unchanged, a small decrease in drug-metabolizing enzyme activity, or the presence of other drugs that inhibit phenytoin metabolism, could transform a therapeutic plasma concentration to a toxic concentration. *Fig. 19.3* also indicates the wide variation of doses required to achieve therapeutic plasma concentrations in different individuals.

The measurement of plasma phenytoin concentration is also useful if adverse effects occur, if there is an unexplained deterioration in the patient's control, and if a drug known to interact with phenytoin has to be prescribed. It is of particular value in children and during pregnancy, when dramatic fluctuations in plasma concentrations and in epileptic control may occur. As mentioned above, however, measurements should be interpreted in the light of clinical circumstances: some patients only achieve effective control of seizures at plasma concentrations greater than the upper limit of the target range, yet do not experience toxicity, while others, particularly older patients, may achieve good control at relatively low concentrations. Decisions on dosage should not be based on measurements of plasma concentrations alone.

Other anticonvulsants

The value of measuring the plasma concentrations of some other anticonvulsant drugs is shown in *Fig. 19.4*. For carbamazepine, TDM is useful to identify potentially subtherapeutic concentrations of the drug, although, for other purposes, the issue is complicated by the drug's having active metabolites, which are not measured in the standard assay. The dosage of ethosuximide can often be adjusted on clinical grounds, as toxicity is easily recognizable when it is being used alone. With sodium valproate there is no clear safe maximum concentration, there is a poor correlation between plasma concentration and efficacy, and hepatotoxicity, which is anyway rare, cannot be predicted from plasma concentration. Vigabatrin and lamotrigine are newer anticonvulsant drugs. TDM of vigabatrin is unlikely to be of value. Plasma concentrations show little relationship to clinical effect, probably because the drug binds irreversibly to its target enzyme (γ-aminobutyric acid transferase) in the brain. Its measurement may, however, be helpful in assessing recent compliance with

Therapeutic monitoring for anticonvulsant drugs		
Drug	**Therapeutic range**	**Monitoring**
phenytoin	<80 µmol/L	essential
carbamazepine	<42 µmol/L	useful but not essential
ethosuximide	<700 µmol/L	useful but not essential
phenobarbital	<170 µmol/L	tolerance makes upper limit imprecise
primidone		metabolized to phenobarbital (which should be monitored) primidone concentrations not useful
sodium valproate	>700 µmol/L ?	not proven to be useful
clonazepam	<285 µmol/L	not proven to be useful
lamotrigine	4–16 µmol/L	probably useful
vigabatrin		not useful

Fig. 19.4 Therapeutic monitoring of anticonvulsant drugs.

treatment. TDM for lamotrigine may be useful, particularly when the drug is used with phenytoin or carbamazepine (which reduces its plasma half-life) or valproate (which prolongs it).

Digoxin

Digoxin is frequently used in the management of cardiac failure with atrial fibrillation, a common problem in the elderly. Plasma digoxin measurements are valuable not only in the assessment of the appropriate dose to prescribe, but also in the diagnosis of digoxin toxicity and in assessing patient compliance. Failure to take a prescribed medication (non-compliance) is a common cause of failure to achieve a therapeutic response.

The therapeutic range for plasma digoxin concentration is generally taken as 1.0–2.6 nmol/L. There is a significant increase in plasma concentration following a dose of the drug and a minimum period of 6 h should elapse before blood is drawn for assessment of the mean steady-state concentration. In practice it is often simplest, and satisfactory for clinical purposes, if a blood sample is taken shortly before a dose is due.

While the therapeutic effect is minimal when plasma concentration is below 1 nmol/L and toxicity becomes more common at concentrations above 2.6 nmol/L and is almost invariable if they exceed 3.8 nmol/L, there is in general a rather poor correlation between plasma concentration of digoxin and therapeutic effect. Furthermore, evidence of toxicity may sometimes be seen in patients whose plasma concentration is below 2.6 nmol/L while others may tolerate concentrations 50% higher than this without ill effect.

This phenomenon is partly a result of the existence of various factors which alter either the therapeutic response to a given plasma concentration of digoxin or the plasma concentration achieved on a particular dose (*Fig. 19.5*). Hypokalaemia is a particular problem since many patients treated with digoxin are also receiving diuretics, which may cause this (*see Case History 21.2*); also, renal impairment may be a consequence of congestive cardiac failure. It is thus very important to consider the clinical setting when assessing the significance of plasma digoxin concentrations.

Digoxin concentrations are also useful in the diagnosis of digoxin toxicity. This is important because some of the features of toxicity are relatively non-specific (for

Sensitivity to digoxin	
Stimulatory factors	**Inhibitory factors**
hypokalaemia	hypocalcaemia
hypercalcaemia	hyperthyroidism
hypomagnesaemia	
hypoxia	
hypothyroidism	

Fig. 19.5 Factors affecting sensitivity to digoxin. In addition, renal impairment and hypothyroidism may increase the plasma concentration of digoxin in relation to the dose taken; hyperthyroidism may decrease the concentration.

example, nausea and vomiting), while others include dysrhythmias that could possibly be a complication of the underlying heart disease. It is important that the possible influence of pathological and physiological factors is considered (*see Fig. 19.5*).

If a patient taking digoxin is symptom-free yet has a plasma concentration less than 1 nmol/L, it is likely that the drug is not required, and it may be withdrawn, although under supervision.

Antidysrhythmics

Methods are available for the measurement of many other drugs used in patients with heart disease, in particular antidysrhythmics. The arguments relating to the value of plasma concentrations in monitoring treatment are complex and the place of therapeutic drug monitoring is debatable. It may be useful under some circumstances in patients treated with lidocaine (lignocaine) or amiodarone.

Lithium

Lithium is widely used in the management of acute mania and for prophylaxis in manic-depressive psychosis. The optimum therapeutic plasma concentration varies from patient to patient with an overall range of 0.3–1.3 mmol/L 12 h after the last dose. Higher concentrations are required to produce a satisfactory effect in acute illness than when the drug is used for prophylaxis. Lithium has a low therapeutic ratio and there are wide interindividual differences in dose require-

ments; monitoring of plasma concentration is vital to the management of patients on lithium therapy.

Lithium is nephrotoxic and is excreted by the kidneys, and consequently toxicity may be self-perpetuating. Renal handling of lithium is also related to sodium balance and diuretics may cause lithium retention.

Plasma concentrations >1.5 mmol/L should be avoided. In lithium toxicity, dialysis may be required to remove the drug if the concentration exceeds 3.5 mmol/L. Its efficacy can be monitored by plasma lithium measurements.

Blood samples for monitoring lithium treatment should be taken 12 h after the previous dose; up to a week may be needed after dosage is changed before a new steady state is attained.

Theophylline

This is a bronchodilator, used in the treatment of asthma and neonatal apnoea. Response to theophylline in different patients varies considerably in relation to dosage but correlates well with plasma concentration. The therapeutic range is 55–100 μmol/L (25–80 μmol/L in infants, *see below*); toxicity (principally cardiac dysrhythmias) may occur at higher concentrations. Because patients requiring intravenous theophylline for severe asthma may already be being treated with an oral preparation and thus have the drug in their blood, there may be a requirement to measure concentrations rapidly. In infants, in whom the drug is used as a respiratory stimulant, significant metabolism to caffeine occurs; this metabolite is also pharmacologically active and ideally its concentration should be measured as well as that of theophylline.

Immunosuppressive drugs

TDM is of proven value for ciclosporin and tacrolimus, drugs that are widely used following transplant surgery to prevent graft rejection. Ciclosporin is nephrotoxic but toxicity should be avoidable if plasma concentrations are monitored. Measurements may also help to distinguish between drug toxicity and incipient rejection of a grafted kidney, both of which can cause an increase in plasma creatinine concentration.

Tacrolimus is chemically dissimilar to ciclosporin but has a similar mode of action and is also nephrotoxic. In addition, it is neurotoxic and can cause hyperglycaemia.

Aminoglycoside antibiotics

These agents (for example, gentamicin) are nephro- and ototoxic, but relatively high concentrations are needed for bactericidal effects. They have a short plasma half-life. Toxicity appears to relate to the trough concentration (i.e. that found immediately before a dose); bactericidal action requires a sufficient peak concentration (achieved shortly after a dose has been given), although too high a peak concentration should be avoided. The peak and trough concentrations can be manipulated independently to some extent by altering the dose and the frequency of dosage. Thus, increasing the dose will increase both concentrations but, if the peak concentration is satisfactory and the trough too low, the same dose may be given, but at more frequent intervals.

Other drugs

Methotrexate

The use of high doses of methotrexate (a cytotoxic drug) is made safer by the use of TDM. Methotrexate inhibits dihydrofolate reductase and depletes intracellular stores of reduced folate. At high concentrations, this depletion may become potentially harmful to the host as well as the tumour by causing bone marrow suppression. Marrow damage becomes maximal later than the effect on tumour cells, and can be prevented by the use of leucovorin (folinic acid) 'rescue' treatment if a high plasma concentration of methotrexate suggests that there is a significant risk of its occurring.

Erythropoietin

Erythropoietin is used to stimulate the production of red blood cells, for example in patients with chronic renal failure on dialysis. Although erythropoietin produces an easily measurable response (an increase in haemoglobin), there is a delay before this occurs and TDM can prevent wasteful over-treatment with this expensive drug.

CHEMICAL TOXICOLOGY

Poisoning is a common reason for hospital admission. In most cases, the patient has taken an overdose of a prescribed or over-the-counter drug, but poisoning may also be the result of accident (common in children), suicide or homicide; the range of toxic substances is vast, including industrial and domestic chemicals, plants and fungi as well as drugs.

Metabolic abnormalities (particularly acid–base disturbances, hypokalaemia and hypoglycaemia) are common in poisoned patients. They may be due to direct toxic effects of the poison, or to non-specific effects on vital function. The drugs most frequently taken in overdose include ethanol, paracetamol and salicylates (each of which causes significant, specific metabolic derangements), and benzodiazepines and tricyclic antidepressants (which do not). Other relatively frequent causes of poisoning include carbon monoxide (*see p. 310*), ethylene glycol and heavy metals.

Management

There are no specific antidotes for most poisons. Management is therefore primarily directed towards the support of vital functions. This may be supplemented by measures to prevent further absorption (e.g. oral activated charcoal, for most organic poisons) or to remove the drug from the body. In severe cases, the laboratory has an important role in monitoring vital functions, for example measuring arterial blood gases. Measurement of the plasma concentration of the poison may indicate the need to take steps to increase its elimination and is valuable in monitoring such treatment. For some poisons, specific treatments are available but these may themselves not be without risk to the patient. Plasma concentrations can be used to indicate whether such treatment is likely to be of value.

Few poisons produce specific physical signs: patients' histories, if available, may not be reliable and mixed drug overdoses are common. There is, therefore, a need for an analytical service to identify what poisons may have been ingested, particularly if a patient does not respond to conventional management. This presents an entirely different problem for the laboratory since what is required is a screening service capable of identifying any of a large number of toxins, rather than providing quantitative data on a small number (*see p. 348*).

POISONING WITH SPECIFIC AGENTS

Paracetamol

A specific antidote is available for paracetamol, the metabolism of which is summarized in *Fig. 19.6*. The

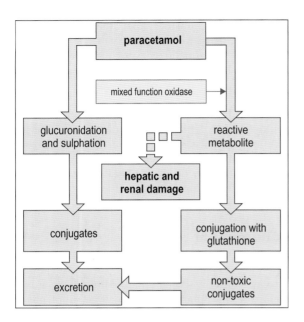

Fig. 19.6 The metabolism of paracetamol. When the drug is taken in therapeutic doses, the toxic metabolite formed, *N*-acetyl-*p*-benzoquinoneimine (NAPQI), is detoxified by conjugation with glutathione; when taken in overdose, glutathione supplies are rapidly exhausted and NAPQI accumulates, causing cell damage.

Signs and symptoms of paracetamol poisoning
<24 h anorexia, nausea and vomiting
24–48 h abdominal pain, hepatic tenderness, prolonged prothrombin time, elevated plasma aminotransferases and bilirubin
>48 h jaundice, encephalopathy, renal and hepatic failure

Fig. 19.7 Signs and symptoms of paracetamol poisoning.

major products of its metabolism are harmless glucuronide and sulphate conjugates, which are excreted in the urine together with a small amount of the unchanged drug. Small quantities of a highly hepatotoxic metabolite (*N*-acetyl *p*-benzoquinoneimine, NAPQI) are also formed through the action of the mixed function oxidase (cytochrome P450) enzyme system: this is normally detoxified by conjugation with glutathione. However, the glucuronidation and sulphation pathways are saturable so that, when an overdose of the drug is taken, a greater proportion is converted to NAPQI. Glutathione supplies are limited, and if they are insufficient to detoxify this metabolite, liver damage will result. In addition, depletion of glutathione reduces the liver's defence mechanisms against oxidizing damage. NAPQI is also nephrotoxic, and its generation in the kidneys can cause renal failure in paracetamol poisoning.

Clinical features

Paracetamol is an insidious poison since there may be no clinical disturbance during the first 24 h after taking an overdose, except anorexia, nausea and vomiting (*Fig. 19.7*). The conscious state is normal unless a sedative drug has been taken concurrently (compound preparations containing paracetamol and a sedative, such as dextropropoxyphene, are common). If liver damage occurs, abdominal pain with hepatic tenderness will develop and liver function tests become abnormal (prolonged prothrombin time, elevated plasma aminotransferase activity and bilirubin concentration). The prothrombin time is the best marker of severity. With massive overdoses, patients may develop hepatic failure (*see p. 92*). If renal failure occurs, plasma creatinine concentration is a better indicator of renal function than that of urea, since hepatic urea synthesis may be decreased. An increase in plasma creatinine concentration and the development of systemic acidosis more than 24 h after overdose are both indicators of a poor prognosis.

It is possible to predict the likelihood of liver damage from the plasma concentration of paracetamol. The blood sample must be taken at least 4 h after ingestion of the drug. The plasma concentration can be used as a guide to patient management, that is, whether or not to treat the patient with an antidote (*Fig. 19.8*). Unfortunately, the time at which the drug was taken may not be known and it is then wisest to treat the patient actively if the concentration falls within the treatment zone. Patients on treatment with enzyme inducing drugs (e.g. phenytoin) with a high habitual alcohol intake, eating disorders or pre-existing liver disease are at greater risk of developing liver damage. Even if patients present more than 15 h after ingestion of paracetamol, its

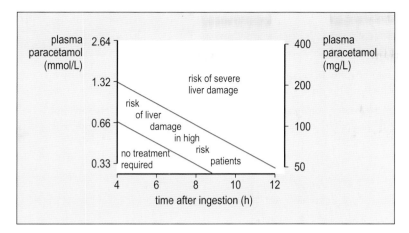

Fig. 19.8 Plasma paracetamol concentrations and prognosis in paracetamol poisoning. Specific treatment is indicated if the concentration is above the line joining concentrations of 1.32 mmol/L at 4 h and 0.33 mmol/L at 12 h. For patients at high risk (*see text*), a lower treatment line is applicable.

measurement is valuable to confirm the diagnosis and, together with the prothrombin time, plasma amino-transferase activities and acid–base status, to assess the need for treatment.

Management

The antidote of choice is *N*-acetylcysteine. This is given by intravenous infusion, initially at a high dose and then at a lower dose over a period of 20 h. Plasma creatinine concentration and the prothrombin time should be checked before starting and at the end of treatment. *N*-Acetylcysteine acts by promoting hepatic glutathione synthesis, thereby increasing the capacity of the liver to detoxify the active metabolite. *N*-Acetylcysteine may also repair oxidative damage, and there is evidence of benefit from its continued use even once liver damage has occurred. Methionine, which can be given orally, also promotes glutathione synthesis, but *N*-acetylcysteine is generally preferred, particularly if a patient is vomiting or unconscious. Methionine can, however, be compounded into tablets with paracetamol, and its addition reduces the risk of toxicity if an overdose is taken.

In treating paracetamol poisoning, general emergency measures must not be forgotten. Administration of activated charcoal is only of proven value if given in the first hour after an overdose. The patient must be kept hydrated, preferably using 5% dextrose since there may be a tendency to hypoglycaemia with hepatic damage. Vitamin K can be given prophylactically. Should liver failure develop, close clinical and laboratory monitoring are vital. Liver transplantation may be appropriate in the most severe cases.

Salicylates

Salicylate poisoning, usually with aspirin (acetylsalicylic acid) is common. It can produce profound metabolic disturbances and although there is no specific antidote, measures can be taken to increase the excretion of the drug that, though effective, are not without hazard in themselves. The upper limit of the therapeutic range of plasma salicylate concentration is approximately 2.5 mmol/L (350 mg/L), but tinnitus, an early symptom of toxicity, may become apparent at lower concentrations.

The effects of salicylates that lead to metabolic disturbances are summarized in *Fig. 19.9*, and include stimulation of the respiratory centre, a non-respiratory acidosis, uncoupling of oxidative phosphorylation and a central emetic effect.

Management

There is no specific antidote to aspirin. It is metabolized by hydrolysis to salicylic acid, the active form of the drug, which is excreted unchanged in the urine; other metabolites include various inactive conjugates. The conjugation pathways are saturable, and once they are saturated, urinary excretion becomes the major route for elimination of the drug. If the urine is acidic, salicylic acid is not ionized and, though filtered by the glomeruli, is reabsorbed by the tubules. If the urine is alkaline, salicylic acid ionizes: its tubular reabsorption is decreased and urinary excretion is enhanced. This is the rationale for alkalinization using sodium bicarbonate infusions in the treatment of salicylate poisoning. However, this

Case history 19.2

A 20-year-old male student was brought into hospital in a confused state, having been found at home by his flatmate with an empty bottle of aspirin tablets on his desk.

On admission, he was hyperventilating and sweating profusely. He was pale but not anaemic. He was not grossly dehydrated but the inside of his mouth was dry and there was a smell of ketones on his breath. His pulse was 112/min, blood pressure 110/60 mmHg and temperature 39.5°C.

Investigations

serum:		
	sodium	131 mmol/L
	potassium	3.2 mmol/L
	bicarbonate	10 mmol/L
	urea	10 mmol/L
	glucose	3.2 mmol/L
	salicylate	3.9 mmol/L

arterial blood:

hydrogen ion	62 nmol/L (pH 7.20)
P_{CO_2}	3.5 kPa (26 mmHg)
prothrombin time	18 s (control 14 s)

Comment

The results are consistent with the metabolic effects of salicylates described above. There is an acidosis, compensated to some extent by hyperventilation (*see Chapter 3*). The initial acid–base disturbance (in adults, but usually not in children) is a respiratory alkalosis due to direct stimulation of the respiratory centre. This is often overwhelmed by the developing acidosis, but during the alkalotic phase any compensatory renal excretion of bicarbonate will deplete the capacity of the body to buffer excess hydrogen ions, thus making the acidosis more dangerous.

Patients who have taken overdoses of salicylates are rarely comatose; irritability is an early feature and later hallucination and delirium may occur. Tinnitus may be a prominent feature. Hyperpyrexia is thought to reflect the uncoupling of oxidative phosphorylation that occurs with toxic doses. The prothrombin time may be prolonged, as in this case, due to decreased hepatic activation of clotting factors. Salicylates also inhibit platelet aggregation. However, although gastric erosions may occur, due directly to the action of salicylate on the gastric mucosa, severe bleeding is uncommon in aspirin overdosage. Nevertheless, prophylactic vitamin K is often administered.

process is in itself potentially dangerous and requires careful monitoring. It should not be attempted if the patient already has a systemic alkalosis or if the urine pH exceeds 8, the aim being to maintain a urine pH greater than 7.5 during treatment. Potassium supplements are required (hypokalaemia may hinder effective alkalinization of the urine); dehydration and hypoglycaemia must be corrected, and fluid balance, blood glucose, arterial hydrogen ion concentration and urine pH must be monitored. It is often advocated that a high intravenous fluid input is maintained to promote a diuresis, but fluid overload must be avoided. It is far more important to ensure adequate alkalinization of the urine.

Aspirin is absorbed only slowly from the gut and activated charcoal is widely used to reduce absorption of the drug. The decision whether or not to embark on active treatment should be based on clinical grounds but be guided by laboratory data. Maintenance of adequate hydration and general supportive measures are important

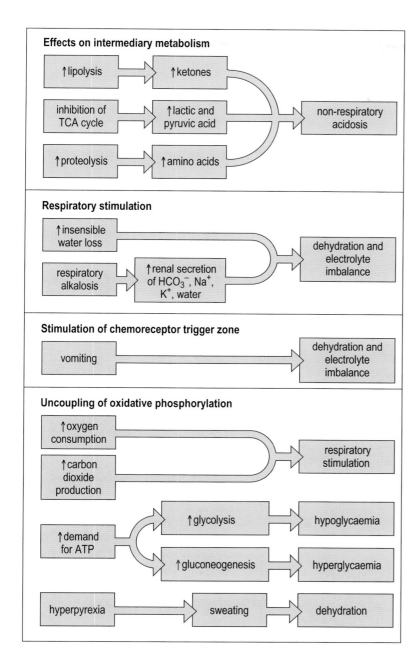

Fig. 19.9 Pathophysiology of salicylate poisoning.

for all patients. Alkalinization should be considered if plasma salicylate concentration exceeds 3.6 mmol/L (500 mg/L) in adults and 2.2 mmol/L (300 mg/L) in children more than 6 h after the overdose. If the initial concentration exceeds 5.1 mmol/L (900 mg/L) and if there is renal impairment or if other therapeutic measures fail, haemoperfusion or haemodialysis will usually be necessary. Plasma salicylate concentrations should be measured during treatment as an indication of its efficacy.

Iron

Iron poisoning, although much less common now than in the past, still occurs and can cause severe illness, especially in young children. Iron causes necrosis of the gastrointestinal mucosa with resultant haemorrhage and fluid and electrolyte loss. Patients may develop encephalopathy and renal failure with circulatory collapse, and acute liver necrosis may develop in those who survive these complications.

Severe poisoning is indicated by plasma iron concentrations in excess of 90 µmol/L in a child, or 145 µmol/L in adults. Management involves the use of desferrioxamine, an iron-chelating agent, to promote iron excretion, together with appropriate supportive measures.

Lead

Acute lead poisoning is very uncommon but chronic poisoning occurs more frequently. In children, the source may be old paint or toys, and cosmetics and patent medicines imported from the Indian subcontinent. In adults, most cases are associated with occupational exposure (e.g. battery manufacture, smelting, ship-breaking), and lead poisoning is a notifiable industrial disease. Lead is concentrated in erythrocytes and, in persons who are not occupationally exposed to the metal, a blood concentration of greater than 1.2 µmol/L should be followed up. In lead workers, the presently accepted upper limit for blood lead is 2.9 µmol/L. Symptomatic lead poisoning is usually associated with concentrations in excess of 5 µmol/L, but in children, symptoms may be present at lower concentrations.

Tests

Although blood lead measurement is the screening method of choice for excessive exposure, other tests may sometimes be useful. Lead interferes with several steps in porphyrin synthesis (*see p. 314*) and porphyrinuria (due mainly to coproporphyrin III) may be present in lead poisoning although this is not a very sensitive test. An excess of δ-aminolaevulinic acid in the urine is also characteristic but not specific. An excess of proto-porphyrin in erythrocytes is a more sensitive indicator of excessive exposure to lead but again is not specific, also occurring in iron deficiency. However, the results of these tests may indicate a need to measure blood lead concentration itself, which may involve sending the blood sample to a specialized laboratory if the assay is not available locally.

Chemical pathology laboratories are becoming increasingly involved in screening for other industrial toxins, especially heavy metals. Specialized laboratories should be able to provide an analytical service for cadmium and mercury as well as lead.

Clinical features and management

Lead poisoning causes nausea, vomiting and severe abdominal colic. In the nervous system, encephalopathy with convulsions and impairment of consciousness may lead to coma and death. In severe cases, usually due to acute lead poisoning, treatment is with a chelating agent, e.g. oral dimercaptosuccinic acid (DMSA) or intravenous sodium calcium edetate, to promote lead excretion. For asymptomatic persons whose blood concentration indicates excessive exposure to lead, the source of lead should be identified and removed or the exposed person removed from the source.

Alcohol

Although there is no specific antidote to ethanol, drug overdose is often complicated by the simultaneous ingestion of alcohol. It potentiates the action of many drugs and measurement of blood alcohol concentration may provide the explanation for an unexpected delay in a patient's recovery from drug overdose.

Blood alcohol measurements may also be of value in the management of patients with head injuries. The effects of alcohol may make it difficult to assess the clinical effect of the injury, but a low alcohol concentration should suggest that the head injury, rather than the alcohol, is the cause of any neurological deficit.

Clinical features and effects

Chronic alcoholism is now a major health problem in many areas of the world. In addition to its well-known harmful effects on the liver, chronic alcohol ingestion can damage many organs and tissues in the body. Metabolic sequelae include hypertriglyceridaemia, hypoglycaemia, hypogonadism, hyperuricaemia, a form of Cushing's syndrome, thiamin deficiency and cutaneous hepatic porphyria. Measurement of blood alcohol concentration may be of value in establishing a diagnosis of alcoholism.

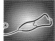 **Case history 19.3**

A garage mechanic was admitted to the emergency room unconscious, having been found in this state at home by his flatmate. He had been acutely depressed since the death of his girlfriend in a road traffic accident two weeks before. On examination, he was unrousable. Temperature, blood pressure and pulse were normal but he was hyperventilating.

Investigations

serum: (multi-channel auto-analyzer 'profile')

sodium	138 mmol/L
potassium	5.2 mmol/L
bicarbonate	4 mmol/L
urea	7.0 mmol/L
creatinine	110 μmol/L
glucose	4.5 mmol/L
calcium	1.5 mmol/L
osmolality	326 mmol/kg

(phosphate, protein, 'liver function' tests were within reference limits)

paracetamol, salicylate: not detected

blood: hydrogen ion   104 nmol/L

    P_{CO_2} 2.0 kPa

urine: negative for glucose and ketones

Comment

There is a severe non-respiratory acidosis; diabetic ketoacidosis is excluded by the normal glucose and lack of ketonuria. The calculated osmolarity is approximately 288 mmol/L, giving an 'osmotic gap' of 38 mmol/L, suggesting the presence of some other osmotically active substance(s) in the blood. A lactate concentration this high in lactic acidosis would be exceptional. The substance could be ethanol (although the acidosis of ethanol poisoning is usually a ketoacidosis) or some other alcohol. The clue to the diagnosis is provided by the low calcium concentration. The combination of severe acidosis and hypocalcaemia is characteristic of ethylene glycol poisoning. This substance is metabolized to various organic acids, including oxalic acid, which combines with calcium to form insoluble calcium oxalate. This can precipitate in tissues and in the renal tubules and urine. Renal failure may occur.

Ethylene glycol poisoning is treated by giving a competitive inhibitor of alcohol dehydrogenase to block the metabolism of ethylene glycol to toxic organic acids. Ethanol was formerly used for this purpose, but 4-methyl pyrazole is now preferred. Hypocalcaemia and acidosis may require correction. Haemodialysis may be required in severe cases.

It has been suggested that the finding of an ethanol concentration of greater than 65 mmol/L (3 g/L) at any time is diagnostic; in a patient who is asymptomatic, the concentration suggested is 33 mmol/L (1.5 g/L). The combination of a raised plasma γ-glutamyl transferase and increased mean red cell volume is a characteristic and sensitive index of excessive alcohol intake, although not an entirely specific one. Measurement of carbohydrate-deficient transferrin (plasma concentration increased in alcohol abuse) has been promoted as a useful test in this context, but, as with other tests, significant numbers of false-negative results occur.

Other poisons

The possibility of poisoning should always be investigated in a comatose patient when no cause is obvious. Measurement of plasma osmolality and comparison with the calculated value may sometimes reveal the presence of a foreign substance in the blood, as demonstrated in *Case History 19.3*.

Carbon monoxide poisoning is diagnosed by measurement of carboxyhaemoglobin (*see p. 310*).

SCREENING FOR DRUGS

It has been pointed out that when a toxin does not have a specific antidote, precise knowledge of its plasma concentration does not contribute to patient management. Nevertheless, qualitative rather than quantitative measurement of a toxic agent may be desirable. If a patient is admitted to hospital unconscious for no readily discernible reason, identification of a drug may help to eliminate other possible causes. It may also draw attention to possible specific complications or suggest treatment (e.g. haemofiltration or dialysis) to remove the drug from the body.

Screening for drugs is also necessary in cases of suspected brain death. Symptoms of apparent brain death may be due to the presence of CNS-depressant drugs and it is vital that this possibility is eliminated before true brain death is diagnosed. When drug measurements are made for medicolegal reasons, it is essential that secure evidence of a chain of custody is maintained, so that there is no doubt about the identity of the specimens subjected to analysis.

In cases of suspected homicide, the identification of any poisons present is vital and must be carried out by suitably qualified personnel whose testimony would be accepted in court if they were to be called upon as witnesses.

It is not practical for all laboratories to provide facilities for screening for all possible toxins. In the UK, there is a network of poisons reference laboratories providing advice and an analytical service for such purposes. It is also often more efficient to concentrate screening for drugs of abuse in specialized laboratories. Such screening may be required for medicolegal reasons but is also important to confirm what drugs are being taken when dependent patients are to be prescribed drugs, and to monitor compliance with treatment for drug dependency.

Samples for drug screening should be collected after consultation with the nearest laboratory. Urine is in general more useful for screening than blood, as many drugs and their metabolites are cleared rapidly from the blood but will be present in high concentration in the urine. Urine and blood samples, stomach contents and any tablets or material that may have been ingested should be collected, carefully labelled and, if analysis is not going to be performed immediately, stored in a refrigerator or deep-frozen.

Patterns of usage both of therapeutic drugs, 'recreational' drugs and drugs of abuse are always changing. As a result, laboratories must keep their repertoire of drug tests under constant review, so that they are able to offer an appropriate analytical service.

SUMMARY

- **Therapeutic drug monitoring** is the measurement of the concentration of drugs, usually in plasma, to provide a guide to the dose to prescribe. It is valuable for drugs that have a low therapeutic ratio (i.e. when the range of plasma concentrations over which the maximum beneficial effect is seen is only a little less than that at which it becomes toxic) and when it is difficult to assess their effects clinically.

- Drugs for which therapeutic drug monitoring is useful include **phenytoin**, **lithium**, **digoxin**, **aminoglycoside antibiotics**, **aminophylline**, **ciclosporin** and **tacrolimus**.

SUMMARY (*cont'd*)

- Therapeutic drug monitoring is **not required** for drugs whose effects can readily be assessed clinically or by clinical or laboratory measurements, or when a drug of low toxicity has a virtually guaranteed effect when given in a standard dose. It is of no value when the effect of a drug is due to a metabolite, unless the concentration of the metabolite can be measured.

- Measurements of drug concentrations in body fluids are also valuable in the investigation and management of patients who have taken **overdoses of drugs** or been **poisoned**. Whilst the management of many forms of poisoning and drug overdosage is essentially conservative, so that identification of the substance is of little direct use in management, for those drugs for which specific antidotes exist, or for which it is possible to take measures to promote their excretion, measurement of plasma concentrations may be very helpful. Examples include **paracetamol**, for which the value of treatment with N-acetylcysteine to prevent hepatic damage can be predicted from the plasma paracetamol concentration, and **aspirin**, for which the plasma salicylate concentration provides a guide to the use of alkaline diuresis to accelerate excretion of the drug.

- Other toxins for which measurement of plasma concentrations can be valuable in management include **iron** and **lead**.

- Many drugs and poisons cause **metabolic disturbances**, particularly in acid–base, glucose and sodium, water and potassium homoeostasis, and clinical chemistry laboratories have an important role in the management of patients who develop such disturbances.

- A further role is in relation to the detection of **drugs of abuse**, and the monitoring of patients on treatment programmes for drug dependency.

INTRODUCTION

An adequate intake of nutrients is essential for normal growth and development and for the maintenance of health. These nutrients include proteins, to supply amino acids, energy substrates (carbohydrates and fat), inorganic salts, vitamins, and other essential nutrients such as essential fatty acids. The daily requirements for these nutrients are determined by many factors, including age, sex, physical activity and the presence of disease; if an individual's requirements are not met, a clinical deficiency syndrome may develop.

This chapter discusses the pathology of some specific deficiency syndromes, with particular reference to the role of the laboratory in their diagnosis and management. This role is also discussed in relation to patients suffering from, or at the risk of, generalized malnutrition. Nutritional support for these patients can be provided enterally (that is, into the alimentary tract, either by mouth or through a feeding tube) or parenterally (intravenously, bypassing the gut). Such treatment requires close co-operation between the clinician and the laboratory, particularly when the patients are also acutely ill, and when such support is required in the long term.

Excessive intake of nutrients can also be harmful. Obesity is a common condition in the developed world, and its prevalence is increasing. Its ultimate cause is an intake of energy substrates in excess of requirements, although the factors that contribute to this are complex and not fully understood. There is much evidence linking several common diseases, including coronary heart disease, hypertension and some cancers, with a relative excess or insufficiency of one or more components of the diet.

VITAMIN DEFICIENCIES

Vitamin deficiency states can arise as a result of:

- inadequate intake (with normal requirements)
- impaired absorption
- impaired metabolism (if metabolism is necessary for function)
- increased requirements
- increased losses.

The biochemical functions of most vitamins are well understood, but while the deficiency syndrome may obviously relate to the known function (e.g. osteomalacia in vitamin D deficiency) this is not always the case (e.g. beriberi and Wernicke's encephalopathy in thiamin deficiency). Although the clinical presentation of individual vitamin deficiency states is usually characteristic, in generalized malnutrition, multiple deficiencies can occur and cause a complex clinical presentation.

The classical deficiency syndromes are the end result of a process in which deficiency of a vitamin leads first to mobilization of body stores, then to tissue depletion, biochemical impairment (subclinical deficiency) and eventually to frank deficiency. The functions of vitamins are almost entirely intracellular, and their plasma concentrations do not necessarily reflect intracellular concentrations and thus functional availability.

It follows that plasma concentrations of vitamins may be unreliable as indicators of the body's vitamin status. In deficiency states, plasma concentrations tend to fall before tissue concentrations. On the other hand, if a vitamin is administered to a deficient patient, a rise in plasma concentration to normal is not necessarily indicative of adequate replacement.

In practice, the best means of assessing a patient's vitamin status depends upon the vitamin in question. The range of techniques that can be used is illustrated by the examples given in the following sections.

WATER-SOLUBLE VITAMINS

Vitamin B$_1$ (thiamin)

Thiamin pyrophosphate is a cofactor in the metabolism of pyruvate and 2-oxoglutarate to acetyl CoA and succinyl CoA respectively, and in a reaction of the pentose shunt pathway catalyzed by the enzyme transketolase. The body contains only about 30 times the daily requirement of this vitamin. Subclinical thiamin deficiency may be unmasked in malnourished

Case history 20.1

An elderly lady, resident in a private nursing home, complained of difficulty in walking, with paraesthesiae and numbness in her legs. The physical signs were consistent with a peripheral neuropathy.

There had been suggestions that residents were not fed adequately and the doctor took a blood sample for measurement of transketolase before giving his patient vitamin supplements.

Investigations
red cell transketolase activity:
    without added thiamin pyrophosphate
                        2.0 mmol/h/10^9 red cells
    with added thiamin pyrophosphate
                        2.4 mmol/h/10^9 red cells

Comment
The patient's symptoms showed some improvement with the vitamin supplements. Red cell transketolase activity (measured by the decrease in substrate concentration as it is metabolized) was at the lower limit of normal and increased by 20% in the presence of thiamin pyrophosphate. This is consistent with mild thiamin deficiency: an increase of up to 14% is considered normal, while an increase of greater than 25% is clear evidence of deficiency. Peripheral neuropathy is a common clinical problem: thiamin deficiency is but one of many causes.

patients given glucose intravenously, which increases the metabolic requirement for the vitamin.

Deficiency of vitamin B_1 causes a primarily sensory polyneuropathy (dry beriberi), cardiac failure (wet beriberi), Wernicke's encephalopathy, characterized by ophthalmoplegia and ataxia and which may progress rapidly to stupor and death, and Korsakoff's psychosis, of which memory loss is usually the most obvious feature. These can occur alone or in combination. In the UK, the most frequent manifestation is encephalopathy, seen chiefly in chronic alcoholics whose diet is poor.

Wernicke's encephalopathy responds rapidly to thiamin and since the vitamin is cheap and non-toxic this therapeutic response can be used to make the diagnosis. Laboratory tests for deficiency are seldom necessary.

It may, however, be necessary formally to document deficiency in nutritional research. One method involves administration of a glucose load and measurement of the plasma pyruvate concentration. An excessive rise is seen in thiamin deficiency because the vitamin is a cofactor for the conversion of pyruvate to acetyl CoA. However, the most sensitive method, which will detect subclinical deficiency, is measurement of transketolase in a red cell haemolysate, the enzyme activity being measured both with and without the addition of thiamin pyrophosphate to the reaction mixture. Enzyme activity may be normal in subclinical deficiency but is increased by the addition of the coenzyme. If the deficiency is clinically obvious, the basal enzyme activity will be low.

An analogous technique can be used for assessing riboflavin status (by measurement of the red cell enzyme glutathione reductase with and without the vitamin) and pyridoxine (using red cell alanine or aspartate aminotransferases). Deficiency of each of these vitamins (manifest in both cases principally by angular stomatitis, cheilosis and dermatitis) is uncommon in developed countries but may sometimes be seen in alcoholics and grossly malnourished individuals.

Nicotinic acid

Nicotinic acid is the precursor of nicotinamide. This is a constituent of the coenzymes nicotinamide adenine dinucleotide (NAD) and its phosphate (NADP), which are essential to glycolysis and oxidative phosphorylation.

Part of the body's nicotinic acid requirement is met by endogenous synthesis from tryptophan. The deficiency syndrome, pellagra (comprising an erythematous skin rash that leads to desquamation, gastrointestinal disturbance, particularly diarrhoea, and dementia), can result from either an inadequate dietary intake of nicotinic acid or decreased synthesis. The latter may be a feature of the carcinoid syndrome, in which there is increased metabolism of tryptophan to hydroxyindoles with consequently less available for nicotinic acid synthesis, and of Hartnup disease, a rare inherited disorder of the epithelial transport of neutral amino acids, due to decreased intestinal absorption of tryptophan from the gut.

Nicotinic acid status can be assessed either by a microbiological assay of the vitamin in plasma or by measurement of its urinary metabolites.

Folic acid

A derivative of folic acid is vital to purine and pyrimidine (and hence nucleic acid) synthesis. Folic acid deficiency is relatively common; its most usual manifestation is as a macrocytic anaemia with megaloblastic marrow changes. Folic acid is usually measured by immunoassay, although microbiological assays were widely used in the past. The concentration in red cells reflects the body's folate status more accurately than that in plasma.

It is essential to diagnose the cause of megaloblastic anaemia before it is treated. Giving folate alone to patients with vitamin B_{12} deficiency risks precipitating or exacerbating the neurological manifestations of vitamin B_{12} deficiency.

The use of folate supplements in pregnancy to reduce the risk of neural tube defects is discussed in a later section.

Vitamin B_{12}

Vitamin B_{12} comprises a number of closely related substances called cobalamins, which are essential to nucleic acid synthesis. Deficiency can cause megaloblastic anaemia and neurological manifestations, either alone or together. The neurological features are caused by demyelination and include peripheral neuropathy, subacute combined degeneration of the spinal cord, dementia and optic atrophy.

Dietary deficiency of this vitamin is rare except in strict vegetarians (vegans): considerable amounts are stored in the liver, with the result that deficiency is not common even with severe malabsorption (unless very long-standing). Vitamin B_{12} deficiency is most commonly seen in pernicious anaemia. This is an autoimmune disease, in most cases of which there is a lack of intrinsic factor essential for the absorption of the vitamin from the gut.

Vitamin B_{12} is measured in plasma by immunoassay. Tests of vitamin B_{12} absorption are discussed in *Chapter 6*.

Vitamin C (ascorbic acid)

Ascorbic acid is essential for the hydroxylation of proline residues in collagen and thus for the normal structure and function of this protein. It acts by maintaining the iron in the hydroxylating enzyme in the reduced (Fe^{2+}) state, i.e. acting as an antioxidant. It also facilitates

the intestinal absorption of dietary non-haem iron by keeping it in the Fe^{2+} state. Subclinical deficiency of ascorbic acid is quite often present in elderly housebound people. The concentration of ascorbate in plasma reflects recent dietary intake and is a poor index of tissue stores of the vitamin. These are better assessed by determination of ascorbate concentration in leucocytes. In practice, this is seldom necessary, since ascorbic acid is cheap and non-toxic, so a therapeutic trial of vitamin supplementation is the simplest procedure to confirm suspected vitamin C deficiency.

FAT-SOLUBLE VITAMINS

Vitamin A

This vitamin is a constituent of the retinal pigment rhodopsin. It is also essential for the normal synthesis of mucopolysaccharides and growth of epithelial tissue.

Mild deficiency causes night blindness while in more severe cases, degenerative changes in the eye may lead to complete loss of vision. The normal liver contains considerable stores of the vitamin and deficiency is rarely seen in affluent societies. It is, however, an important cause of blindness in many areas of the world.

Vitamin A is present in the diet and can also be synthesized from dietary carotenes. It can be measured in plasma, in which it is transported bound to prealbumin and a specific retinol-binding globulin. A low binding protein concentration can cause the plasma concentration of vitamin A to be low and impair its delivery to tissues even when hepatic stores of the vitamin are adequate. Measurements of vitamin A status are rarely required in practice, since deficiency is rare in the western world. In areas where deficiency is endemic, the diagnosis is usually obvious clinically and the facilities required to provide laboratory confirmation of the diagnosis are often not available.

Vitamin D

Vitamin D is obtained from endogenous synthesis, by the action of ultraviolet light on 7-dehydrocholesterol in the skin to form cholecalciferol (vitamin D_3), and from the diet. Dietary vitamin D is largely vitamin D_2 (ergocalciferol); the only important dietary sources are fish and some margarines, which are artificially fortified with vitamin D. Vitamins D_2 and D_3 undergo the same metabolic changes in the body and have identical physiological actions. For this reason, the terms cholecalciferol and vitamin D are frequently used to refer to both forms of the vitamin.

In most individuals, endogenous synthesis is the major source of vitamin D. Privational (dietary) vitamin D deficiency is seen most frequently in people who also have decreased endogenous synthesis, such as the elderly housebound. It is also seen in the UK in people of Southern Asian origin, particularly women, in whom the effects of low intake may be exacerbated by decreased exposure to sunlight due to their traditional clothing. Binding of calcium in the gut by dietary phytates may also contribute to the osteomalacia to which they are prone. Breast milk contains relatively little vitamin D and infants are at risk of vitamin D deficiency particularly if premature (the vitamin is transported across the placenta mainly in the last trimester of pregnancy) or if the mother is vitamin D deficient.

Cholecalciferol itself has little physiological activity. It is hydroxylated first in the liver to 25-hydroxycholecalciferol (25-HCC, calcidiol) and then in the kidney to 1,25-dihydroxycholecalciferol (1,25-DHCC, calcitriol). These metabolites are transported in the circulation by a specific binding protein. Calcitriol is a hormone of vital importance in calcium homoeostasis; its actions and the control of its production are discussed in *Chapter 12*.

Vitamin D status can be assessed in the laboratory by measurement of the plasma concentration of calcidiol, the major circulating metabolite. This undergoes seasonal variation, being higher in the summer than in the winter.

Decreased synthesis or dietary deficiency of vitamin D causes rickets in children and osteomalacia in adults. Other causes include disordered metabolism of chole-calciferol and malabsorption. The clinical biochemistry of rickets and osteomalacia is considered in more detail in *Chapter 15*.

Vitamin K

Vitamin K is required for the γ-carboxylation of glutamate residues in coagulation factors II (prothrombin), VII, IX and X. This process confers physiological activity by permitting the binding of calcium to the proteins. Vitamin K deficiency results in an increase in the prothrombin time, a functional assay of relevant coagulation factor activity. These factors are synthesized in the liver and the prothrombin time is also used as a test of liver function. Its most frequent use is in the monitoring of patients on anticoagulant treatment with antagonists of vitamin K (e.g. warfarin).

Vitamin E

Vitamin E (tocopherol) is an important antioxidant, particularly in cell membranes, protecting unsaturated fatty acid residues against free radical attack. Clinical deficiency may occur in severe malabsorption, particularly in infants. Manifestations include haemolytic anaemia and neurological dysfunction.

VITAMINS AS DRUGS

In addition to their long-appreciated role as essential micronutrients, there is evidence that taking some vitamins in supra-physiological amounts may be beneficial. The term 'nutraceuticals' has been used to describe nutrients used pharmacologically. For example, folic acid supplements taken very early in pregnancy have been proven to reduce (though not abolish) the risk of the fetus having a neural tube defect.

Vitamin E is an antioxidant. It is known that the atherogenicity of LDL cholesterol is increased by oxidation and there has been considerable interest in the possibility that supplementation of the diet with vitamin E might reduce the risk of coronary heart disease but this has not been borne out in clinical trials. Nevertheless, the possibility that vitamin E and other antioxidants (e.g. vitamin C, selenium, β-carotene and dietary flavonoids) may help protect against a variety of other diseases continues to be the subject of much research. However, a high intake of vitamins may not be without risk: vitamins A and D are toxic in excess and even water-soluble vitamins (an excess of which can be excreted in the urine) may be harmful in high amounts. For example, pyridoxine, which has been used in the prophylaxis of premenstrual tension, can be neurotoxic when taken in excess.

High intakes of certain vitamins are used in the management of some inherited metabolic diseases, as discussed in *Chapter 16*.

TRACE ELEMENTS

The maintenance of normal health requires provision in the diet not only of adequate protein, energy substrates and vitamins, but also of various inorganic salts and trace elements. Trace elements in the body are by definition present in concentrations less than 100 parts per million (ppm); they are shown in *Fig. 20.1*. None is required in more than milligram quantities per day while the daily requirement for some is measurable in micrograms. Consequently the 'essential' status of some of these trace elements is difficult to confirm.

Trace element deficiency

Deficiencies of trace elements can occur for the same general reasons as vitamin deficiencies.

The commonest trace element deficiency is that of iron; it is common even in affluent societies, particularly in women during the reproductive years. Iodine deficiency causes goitre and, if severe, hypothyroidism; it is now uncommon in the developed world but is still a problem in some areas. Deficiency of other trace elements is uncommon except under special circum-

Trace elements in the human body	
Element	**Function**
chromium	deficiency causes glucose intolerance
cobalt	component of vitamin B_{12}
copper	cofactor for cytochrome oxidase
fluorine*	present in bone and teeth
iodine	component of thyroid hormones
iron	component of haem pigments
manganese	cofactor for several enzymes
molybdenum	cofactor for xanthine oxidase
selenium	cofactor for glutathione peroxidase
silicon*	present in cartilage
tin*	?
zinc	cofactor for many enzymes

Fig. 20.1 Trace elements in the human body. * Indicates elements which are present, but are not known to be essential.

stances. These include severe malnutrition, artificial feeding (especially if prolonged), prematurity and the presence of excessive losses (such as with enterocutaneous fistulae or severe diarrhoea). Multiple deficiencies may occur in these conditions, confusing the clinical picture and making diagnosis difficult.

Laboratory assessment

Unfortunately, the laboratory assessment of the body's trace element status is difficult, as specialized equipment and considerable technical expertise are required. Measurements are often made in plasma, but these may not accurately reflect the concentration of a trace element at its (usually intracellular) site of action. Although a low plasma concentration may not indicate deficiency in the tissues, such deficiency is usually accompanied by a low plasma concentration, with the result that if a low concentration is found, it is reasonable to provide appropriate supplementation. Trace element deficiency should be anticipated in patients at risk and steps taken to prevent the occurrence of a deficiency syndrome.

Zinc

Zinc is a trace element of particular importance. It is essential for the activity of many enzymes, including several involved in nucleic acid and protein synthesis. The clinical manifestations of zinc deficiency include dermatitis and delayed wound healing; there is, however, no evidence that zinc supplementation accelerates wound healing in patients who are not deficient. Zinc deficiency is a well-recognized potential complication of artificial (particularly parenteral) nutrition if in-sufficient supplementation is provided. Patients who are catabolic, for example following trauma or major surgery, lose large amounts of zinc in the urine and are at risk of becoming depleted. Severe deficiency is seen in the condition acrodermatitis enteropathica, in which there is an inherited defect in intestinal zinc absorption.

Plasma zinc concentrations must be interpreted with caution: blood should be collected in the fasting state since zinc concentrations may fall by up to 20% following a meal. Low plasma concentrations are not exclusive to zinc deficiency: they are also seen in conditions such as malignant disease and chronic liver disease without associated clinical evidence of tissue deficiency. Plasma zinc concentrations fall during an acute phase response, as a result of uptake by the liver. Measurement of C-reactive protein (CRP, see p. 241) as an indicator of the acute phase response may help with the interpretation of plasma zinc concentrations. Finally, because zinc is extensively bound to albumin, plasma zinc concentration should be considered in relation to that of albumin.

Copper

Copper is also essential for the activity of certain enzymes, notably cytochrome oxidase and superoxide dismutase. In the blood, 80–90% of copper is present in caeruloplasmin. Copper deficiency is uncommon: mani-festations include anaemia and leucopenia. Wilson's disease, a disorder characterized by excessive tissue deposition of copper, is discussed in *Chapter 5*.

Selenium

Selenium is required as a prosthetic group for the enzyme glutathione peroxidase. This, together with the tocopherols (vitamin E), is part of the antioxidant system that protects membranes and other vulnerable structures from oxidative attack by free radicals. These highly reactive species can be generated, for example, as a result of the activation of phagocytic cells or exposure to ionizing radiation. Selenium deficiency is usually only seen as a result of a low intake (it is endemic in some parts of China that have a low soil selenium content) and has been reported in patients on long-term parenteral nutrition. The most obvious clinical feature is myopathy (especially cardiomyopathy). Selenium can be measured in plasma but measurement of red cell glutathione peroxidase activity provides a better measure of tissue selenium status.

PROVISION OF NUTRITIONAL SUPPORT

Patients who have, or are at risk of developing, nutritional deficiencies, require nutritional support. In the case of specific deficiencies, for example of vitamin D, dietary supplementation may be all that is required. Generalized undernutrition, usually encompassing an inadequate intake of protein, energy substrates and micronutrients, requires generalized nutritional support. This should be provided enterally (using the gut) wherever possible, but in patients with intestinal failure (*see Chapter 6*), parenteral (intravenous) nutrition is required.

Undernutrition increases the morbidity and mortality of patients in hospitals yet is a relatively frequent finding. Nutritional assessment should be a routine part of any medical examination, and nutritional support considered for any patient who cannot eat normally.

All forms of nutritional support require close cooperation between the laboratory and the clinical team. Laboratory data may contribute to the decision to initiate nutritional support, and are essential to the assessment of requirements and monitoring to ensure adequate provision and avoidance of metabolic compli-cations. There is good evidence to indicate that nutri-tional support is best provided by a multidisciplinary nutritional team, including, for example, a clinician, pharmacist, dietitian, specialist nurse and often a member of the laboratory staff. Such teams can be involved in the care of patients receiving nutritional support in the community as well as in hospital.

Nutritional assessment

Various techniques are available for nutritional assessment, including analysis of recent food intake, anthropometric measurements (body height and weight, skinfold thicknesses, mid-arm muscle bulk), functional measurements (e.g. grip strength) and laboratory measurements, particularly of plasma protein concentrations.

The diagnosis of severe malnutrition does not require laboratory tests since it is clinically obvious. Neither are they required to confirm a need for nutritional support in patients at risk, for example, following massive small intestinal resection. A plasma albumin concentration of less than 30 g/L is often taken as evidence of malnutrition, but plasma albumin concentrations are affected by many pathological processes, and this is a non-specific finding and an insensitive test. In simple starvation, plasma albumin concentrations may remain within reference limits for several weeks (decreased synthesis is accompanied by a decrease in the rate of catabolism) whereas in septic or catabolic patients, plasma albumin concentrations can fall rapidly, as a result of increased breakdown and redistribution out of the vascular compartment. Other plasma proteins (e.g. transferrin, retinol-binding protein) show no advantage over albumin as indices of nutritional status. Even combinations of biochemical and anthropometric measurements in 'prognostic nutritional indices' have not been shown to be superior to careful, informed, clinical assessment in determining which patients are likely to benefit from nutritional support.

Techniques for generalized nutritional support

Enteral nutrition is safer, cheaper and usually more convenient for the patient than parenteral feeding. It is more physiological, since nutrients are absorbed into the portal circulation and not delivered directly into the systemic circulation, and appears to have a role in maintaining the barrier function of the gut and preventing the translocation of intestinal bacteria into the circulation. If patients are unable to eat (e.g. owing to loss of the ability to swallow as a result of stroke or neurological disease), nutritionally complete liquid feeds can be administered either through a nasogastric tube or, when enteral feeding is likely to be required other than in the short term (days or a few weeks), through a gastrostomy or jejunostomy.

If a patient's complete nutritional requirements cannot be met enterally, parenteral supplementation will be required, and patients with intestinal failure will require total parenteral nutrition (TPN), in which all nutritional requirements are met using an intravenously administered admixture of amino acids, glucose, fat, vitamins and minerals.

The causes of intestinal failure are summarized in *Chapter 6*. In a patient who has previously been well nourished, short-lived loss of intestinal function (for example, due to ileus following abdominal surgery) is not an indication for parenteral nutritional support, but, in general, nutritional support should be instituted if a patient has been unable to eat normally for a period of more than five days. Pre-operative parenteral nutrition in nutritionally depleted patients (for example, prior to surgery for carcinoma of the oesophagus) should be for at least 8–10 days if it is to improve outcome. However, each patient must be assessed individually. Patients with irreversible intestinal failure require lifelong nutritional support, and although this will be initiated in hospital, it can be continued in the patient's home.

Parenteral nutrition

In total parenteral nutrition, all a patient's nutritional requirements are compounded together under sterile conditions in a single container, and infused at a steady rate, preferably controlled by a pump. The high osmolality of feeds containing high concentrations of glucose as the major source of energy results in their being irritant to the vascular endothelium, and they are often infused into a dedicated catheter placed in a central vein, to allow rapid dilution of the feed with a large volume of blood. This technique is certainly preferred for long-term TPN, but parenteral supplementation of enteral feeding, and short-term TPN, can be provided through a peripheral vein, particularly if the feed can be compounded using a fat emulsion (these are isotonic) as the major energy source. Feeds are usually infused over 24 h, but patients' mobility is improved if shorter periods are used; patients on TPN at home typically infuse their feeds overnight. If this is done, the rate of administration should be decreased gradually over the last hour, to avoid rebound hypo-glycaemia (*see below*).

Patients' nutritional requirements must be assessed individually. Energy requirements can be based on an assessment of basal requirements (e.g. as given by the Harris–Benedict equation) modified to take into account such factors as whether the patient is mobile, pyrexial, catabolic, etc. (all these increase energy expenditure). In practice, clinical assessment is usually adequate. Energy is usually provided as a mixture of glucose solution and fat emulsion: the latter also provides essential fatty acids. Nitrogen requirements are provided as a balanced mixture of essential and non-essential L-amino acids: maintenance requirements are typically 0.15 g/kg body weight but more is often appropriate to replace pre-existing deficiencies. However, the provision of large quantities of amino acids cannot itself reverse a catabolic state, and may be harmful, increasing the amount of nitrogen that has to be excreted by the kidneys and causing an increase in plasma urea concentration. Typical requirements for the major minerals are indicated in *Fig. 20.2*, but many of these can be affected by numerous factors. For example, patients with significant nasogastric aspirates, diarrhoea or fistulae will have increased sodium requirements, whereas these may be decreased in patients with liver disease or renal failure. Micronutrients are usually provided using commercially prepared 'cocktails' containing adequate quantities, but these may require supplementation, e.g. with thiamin, zinc, etc., according to the needs of the individual patient.

Complications of parenteral feeding can be divided into catheter-related and metabolic complications. Catheter-related complications include damage to nearby

Daily composition of a typical parenteral feed for a 60 kg adult	
energy	1800 kcal (1000 mL 20% dextrose, 500 mL 20% fat emulsion)
nitrogen	12 g (as amino acids)
sodium	60–100 mmol
potassium	60–100 mmol
calcium	5–10 mmol
magnesium	5–10 mmol
phosphate	30 mmol
water (total volume)	2.5 L

Fig. 20.2 Daily composition of a typical parenteral feed for a 60 kg adult. Precise requirements must be determined individually, on the basis of clinical assessment and laboratory tests. Sodium is usually given as sodium chloride, potassium as acid phosphate. Vitamins and trace elements are usually given in standard quantities.

 Case history 20.3

A 30-year-old woman with Crohn's disease was admitted to hospital with severe diarrhoea and weight loss of 7 kg over the preceding month. Her weight on admission was 36 kg. She was prescribed loperamide and prednisolone and a tunnelled subclavian catheter was inserted for parenteral feeding. She was started on a standard TPN regimen.

Investigations

		on admission	after 24 h TPN
serum:	sodium	136 mmol/L	132 mmol/L
	potassium	4.2 mmol/L	2.9 mmol/L
	phosphate	0.9 mmol/L	0.32 mmol/L
	creatinine	58 μmol/L	56 μmol/L
	glucose	4.6 mmol/L	9.2 mmol/L

Comment

Falls in potassium and phosphate concentrations despite apparently adequate provision in the feed (60 mmol and 30 mmol respectively) are often seen when TPN is started, and are a result of rapid intracellular uptake of these ions, the former in part stimulated by insulin secreted in response to the glucose load and the latter by repletion of cellular high-energy phosphate compounds. Daily biochemical monitoring is essential when patients are first started on TPN, both to ensure the adequacy of provision and to detect complications. Glucose intolerance is frequent in catabolic patients and those treated with corticosteroids, and insulin may need to be given to prevent hyperglycaemia. Note also the low–normal creatinine concentration, a reflection of her low muscle bulk.

structures during placement, infection, venous thrombosis and catheter blockage. Scrupulous adherence to sterile technique is essential during catheter placement and when the feed is changed. Metabolic complications are summarized in *Fig. 20.3*. They include hypo- and hyperkalaemia, hyperglycaemia, etc. Rebound hypoglycaemia may occur if a feed is stopped suddenly. Mild hyponatraemia (sodium concentration 125–135 mmol/L) is frequent in patients receiving TPN. It is often multifactorial and is not on its own an indication for increasing the amount of sodium in the feed. Sodium depletion is confirmed by finding a low urine sodium concentration (provided that renal function is normal). Spurious hyponatraemia (*see p. 24*) may occur if lipid is not being cleared adequately. The plasma will appear lipaemic: if lipid is being cleared normally from the plasma, it will only be faintly opalescent. Measurement of plasma triglyceride concentration will resolve the issue if there is doubt. Liver function tests may become abnormal, exhibiting a cholestatic pattern: contributory factors may include hepatic steatosis, due to provision of energy in excess of requirements, and biliary stasis. This is a reversible finding in adults but occasionally children on TPN develop irreversible liver damage.

Laboratory monitoring

Careful clinical monitoring, especially of weight, fluid status and temperature, is essential during parenteral nutrition. The frequency of laboratory monitoring will depend on individual circumstances, including the patient's illness as well as the requirement to monitor the provision of TPN. Given the widespread use of multichannel auto-analyzers, analytes may be measured more frequently than is strictly required. Monitoring will need to be more frequent during the first few days of TPN, if major deficiencies are identified and if a patient's clinical condition is unstable. In stable patients, monitoring can be less frequent; patients on home TPN require monitoring only every 6–8 weeks. A guide to the frequency of monitoring is given in *Fig. 20.4*.

If patients are being fed adequately, they will be in neutral (if previously adequately nourished) or positive (if undernourished) nitrogen balance. Plasma protein concentrations respond to nitrogen status but must be interpreted with caution as they can be affected by other factors. Albumin has a long half-life and its concentration increases only slowly in response to improved nutrient intake. Measurement of 24 h urine nitrogen excretion to assess nitrogen balance is technically demanding. Since the majority of nitrogen excreted in the urine is in the form of urea, measurement of 24 h urea excretion (assuming that the patient's renal function is stable) provides a crude estimate of nitrogen excretion (500 mmol urea contains 14 g nitrogen). However, the proportion of urinary nitrogen excreted as urea can vary considerably and some nitrogen is always

Metabolic complications of parenteral nutrition
hyperglycaemia
hypokalaemia/hyperkalaemia
hyponatraemia/hypernatraemia
hypophosphataemia
abnormal liver function tests
acidosis
hypoglycaemia (rebound)
long-term parenteral nutrition
metabolic bone disease
deficiency states

Fig. 20.3 Metabolic complications of parenteral nutrition, listed in approximate order of frequency.

Frequency of monitoring in patients receiving parenteral nutrition	
Analyte (in plasma/blood)	**Frequency**
sodium, potassium, glucose,* phosphate, urea, creatinine	daily
liver function tests, calcium, albumin	twice weekly
magnesium, full blood count, red cell indices	weekly
zinc, copper	two weekly
selenium	monthly

Fig. 20.4 Frequency of laboratory monitoring in patients receiving TPN. All analytes (with the exception of copper and selenium, unless there is longstanding undernutrition) should be measured before TPN is started, as a guide to the formulation of the feed. *In patients with hyperglycaemia, more frequent measurement of glucose is required.

lost in other forms. Furthermore, there may be additional losses (e.g. protein in the urine or from mucosal surfaces). In practice, most patients requiring parenteral nutrition require it for relatively short periods (12–14 days) and accurate assessment of nitrogen balance is unnecessary. In patients fed over longer periods, anthropometric measurements can be used and, since urine creatinine excretion is related to muscle bulk, muscle protein status can be assessed by measurement of 24 h urine creatinine excretion.

Measurements of urine sodium and potassium excretion are sometimes recommended on a routine basis for patients on TPN, but in the authors' experience are of little practical value. They must be interpreted with regard to intake and the clinical circumstances. For example, potassium balance is usually negative in patients who are catabolic, but becomes positive if they become anabolic.

OBESITY

Contrary to a widely held belief among lay people, obesity [defined as a body mass index (BMI) (weight/height^2) exceeding 30 kg/m^2, the ideal BMI being 20–25 kg/m^2] is rarely a consequence of a specific endocrine disorder. Rare hypothalamic disorders can cause hyperphagia as a result of interference with the satiety and appetite centres, but although patients with Cushing's syndrome, hypothyroidism and sometimes hypogonadism tend to be overweight, they are not usually obese. Obesity is a common disorder in developed countries (prevalence over 20% in adults in the UK). Its prevalence is increasing in developed and (particularly among children) developing countries.

Overweight and obesity are a consequence of an intake of energy substrates in excess of requirements, and numerous factors, including genetic, socio-economic and behavioural, may contribute to this. Elucidation of the mechanisms responsible for controlling food intake may help in our understanding of this common clinical problem and allow the development of acceptable pharmacological approaches to management where dietary and lifestyle intervention fails. Counselling regarding modification of the diet and of eating habits, and encouragement of an appropriate level of aerobic exercise, are central to the management of obesity. Such modification must be long term: weight lost rapidly is almost invariably regained. A high degree of personal motivation on the patient's part is essential. Successful lifestyle management requires a multidisciplinary approach, for example involving physicians, dietitians, psychologists and nurses. Many patients need a continuing high level of support and the financial implications are considerable.

Two drugs are currently licensed for the treatment of obesity in the UK. These are orlistat, an inhibitor of pancreatic lipase, which decreases the digestion and hence the absorption of dietary fat, and sibutramine, a centrally acting drug that enhances satiety. Replacement treatment with leptin, a peptide produced by fat cells that is involved in appetite control, has proved to be effective in a few obese children with leptin deficiency, but the majority of obese people have high leptin concentrations (reflecting their high fat mass), to which they appear to be resistant, and do not respond to leptin treatment. Surgical intervention may be effective in patients with severe obesity: procedures are of two types, purely restrictive procedures to reduce the size of the stomach and restrictive procedures that also cause a degree of malabsorption (e.g. gastric by-pass). Intestinal by-pass procedures to produce malabsorption have been abandoned because of unacceptable side-effects.

Patients with obesity frequently have mild hepatic steatosis with slightly abnormal liver function tests (especially an increase in aminotransferases, *see p. 95*). Other associated abnormalities include hyperuricaemia, hyperlipidaemia and glucose intolerance. Obesity (particularly visceral or abdominal) is a major risk factor for the development of type 2 diabetes mellitus. Obesity causes insulin resistance, probably through multiple and incompletely understood mechanisms, including a direct effect of high plasma non-esterified fatty acid concentrations on pancreatic β-cell function. There is a clear association between insulin resistance, fasting hypertriglyceridaemia (mainly in very low density lipoproteins), low plasma HDL cholesterol concentration and hypertension. This clustering is known variously as 'syndrome X', the metabolic syndrome and Reaven's syndrome, and is a major risk factor for coronary heart disease.

SUMMARY

- **Nutritional deficiency syndromes** include those due to the lack of a single nutrient and those in which there is generalized deficiency.

- Specific laboratory methods are available for the diagnosis of **deficiencies of individual water-soluble vitamins** but, with the exception of those for folic acid and vitamin B_{12}, they are rarely required in clinical practice. Among the **fat-soluble vitamins**, vitamin A deficiency is rare in the developed world, but vitamin D deficiency, leading to rickets and osteomalacia, occurs relatively frequently, particularly in the elderly, premature infants, patients with malabsorption and in certain racial groups. Vitamin K deficiency leads to impairment of blood clotting with prolongation of the prothrombin time.

- **Deficiencies of minerals** required in large amounts by the body (for example, sodium, potassium, calcium and magnesium) can usually be inferred from clinical observation and measurement of their plasma concentrations. It is more difficult to diagnose **deficiencies of trace elements**, such as zinc, manganese and copper, since plasma concentrations may not accurately reflect the body's status with regard to these elements.

- Patients with **generalized malnutrition** show characteristic, though not specific, biochemical abnormalities, for example low plasma concentrations of albumin, transferrin and certain other proteins and decreased urinary creatinine excretion. There may also be evidence of specific deficiencies of vitamins or minerals. These patients require **nutritional support**. This should be enteral wherever possible, that is using the gut, either by supplementation of the diet or by tube feeding.

- In patients with **intestinal failure**, feeding must be parenteral. This entails the infusion of nutrients intravenously and is a potentially hazardous procedure. There is a risk of metabolic complications, for example hyperglycaemia, hypophosphataemia and hypo- or hyperkalaemia, but these should be preventable by frequent biochemical monitoring. Biochemical and clinical monitoring are also necessary to follow the patient's response to treatment.

- Some essential nutrients can be harmful if taken in excess; if an individual's total energy intake is greater than requirements, **obesity** will develop. Obesity can cause hepatic steatosis and hyperlipidaemia and is a major risk factor for the development of type 2 diabetes.

21 Clinical chemistry at the extremes of age

OLD AGE: INTRODUCTION

The investigation and management of illness in the elderly poses a number of special problems, for both the physician and the clinical biochemist. These include:

- different patterns of disease
- different presentation of disease
- decline in normal functions with age
- different reference ranges.

There is no precise definition of what constitutes 'elderly': the changes in physiological function that occur in older people correlate only loosely with chronological age and can occur much earlier in individuals with conditions characterized by premature ageing (e.g. progeria). Nevertheless, many conditions are more common in the elderly than in younger adults; examples of such conditions of particular relevance to clinical biochemistry include diabetes mellitus (*see Chapter 11*), Paget's disease of bone (*see p. 281*) and thyroid diseases (*see p. 175*). Further, the presentation of diseases in the elderly may be different from that normally seen in younger people. Thus myocardial infarction may present with confusion, consequent on a reduction in cerebral blood flow, rather than chest pain; the presenting feature of diabetes mellitus may be one of its complications, for example ischaemic ulceration, rather than polyuria and thirst. *Case Histories 21.1–21.4* provide more detailed examples of these problems.

The functions of some organs decline with age; although this may not be apparent in healthy individuals, the consequent decreased reserve capacity may become apparent in even mild disease. In addition, functional decline may be accelerated by even mild disease. For example, the glomerular filtration rate decreases with age and so does the creatinine clearance. However, plasma creatinine concentration changes little because creatinine production also falls with age; this reflects a decrease in muscle mass and often also in meat consumption. Despite the fall in the glomerular filtration rate, renal function remains sufficient for normal homoeostasis although it may not be adequate to allow complete excretion of a drug or to sustain any further decrease in glomerular filtration without a failure of homoeostasis.

Elderly people, particularly if they have impaired mobility or live alone, may have poor nutrition. Also, they are more likely than younger people to be taking medication, often multiple, which may have adverse effects in addition to the expected therapeutic effects.

REFERENCE RANGES

Such changes in normal function mean that the reference ranges applicable to healthy adults may not be applicable to the elderly, while the increased incidence of many diseases with increasing age makes it difficult to obtain data on normal people. Ideally, laboratories should construct age-related reference ranges for age-dependent analytes (where appropriate: it is not, for example, for glucose) (*Fig. 21.1*), but in practice this is not always done.

Plasma constituents showing age-dependent changes in concentration	
cholesterol	increases progressively during adult life
glucose	increases (glucose tolerance decreases with age)
alkaline phosphatase	increases
urate	increases
total protein	decreases (slight decrease probably related to decreased protein intake)
albumin	decreases (as total protein)

Fig. 21.1 Plasma constituents showing age-dependent changes in concentration.

This problem is exemplified by the enzyme alkaline phosphatase. Common causes of raised activity of this enzyme in the plasma in the elderly include malignant disease with metastasis to bone or liver, osteomalacia and Paget's disease of bone. In the UK, the prevalence of Paget's disease exceeds 5% in people aged over 60. Many cases are mild and clinically silent, being discovered only after a raised plasma alkaline phosphatase has been found, often as part of a biochemical screening test. Asymptomatic patients with Paget's disease do not require treatment, but screening programmes are only worthwhile if abnormal results are followed up. How extensively this can be done may be governed by economic factors. The practice in many laboratories is to assume that, in the absence of any clinical or other laboratory evidence of disease, an alkaline phosphatase of up to one and a half times the upper limit of normal for young adults does not justify further investigation in an elderly subject.

SCREENING

The higher prevalence of many diseases in the elderly provides some of the justification for screening programmes. If a condition has a high prevalence in a population, the predictive value of a positive test is much higher than if it is low (*see Chapter 1*). Such screening may be carried out in general practice, at over-60s clinics, in geriatric assessment centres or on admission to hospital. The biochemical tests which should form part of such a screen (*Fig. 21.2*) reflect the diseases that are of particular concern in this age group, some of which have been mentioned above. Plasma potassium is included since diuretics are frequently prescribed in the elderly and, according to the type used, may cause hypokalaemia or hyperkalaemia. The possible influence of intercurrent disease on tests of thyroid status must be borne in mind. The results of such tests may erroneously suggest thyroid disease in a patient who is ill for some other reason (sick euthyroid syndrome) and it is best to avoid doing these tests at such a time.

CHILDHOOD: INTRODUCTION

Just as the elderly present particular problems for the clinical biochemist, so too do children. The most obvious of these relates to the size of the blood sample. For the very young it is essential to employ analytical methods that will use the smallest possible amount of

Biochemical tests used to screen for disease in the elderly	
Analyte	**Common abnormalities**
plasma potassium	hypokalaemia (diuretic and purgative-induced) hyperkalaemia (potassium-sparing diuretic with poor renal function)
plasma creatinine	increased (renal impairment)
plasma calcium	hypercalcaemia (hyperparathyroidism) hypocalcaemia (osteomalacia)
plasma alkaline phosphatase	increased (osteomalacia, Paget's disease and malignancy)
plasma glucose*	increased (diabetes mellitus)
plasma TSH and fT4	hypothyroidism and hyperthyroidism
faecal occult blood	carcinoma of the large bowel

Fig. 21.2 Biochemical tests used to screen for disease in the elderly.
*The sensitivity of glycosuria as an indication of possible diabetes is lower in the elderly because the renal threshold for glucose is usually higher than in younger people.

plasma and this usually means using special equipment. Small quantities of capillary blood can be conveniently collected by pricking the heel, but this should be done by experienced personnel and the results obtained may be affected by haemolysis or by contamination with tissue fluid.

Complete, accurately timed collections of urine are difficult to obtain in children. It may be more reliable to relate the concentrations of urinary constituents to urine creatinine concentration.

In the immediate neonatal period, the concentration of metabolites in infants may still reflect maternal

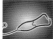 **Case history 21.1**

A GP was called to see a previously fit man in an old people's home. The patient had become acutely short of breath 2 h before, soon after his breakfast, and developed a cough with frothy white sputum. He also complained of dizziness, but denied chest pain.

On examination, he had widespread crepitations throughout his lung fields; his blood pressure was 120/70 mmHg but had been 150/90 mmHg when checked by the doctor two months previously.

He was given a diuretic, with considerable symptomatic relief ensuing. An ECG showed changes consistent with a very recent myocardial infarct. The doctor took a blood sample for measurement of creatine kinase activity and was surprised when the laboratory telephoned him to say that this was normal.

Comment

The breathlessness, cough and crepitations are classic features of left ventricular failure. A likely cause of this, and the fall in blood pressure, was myocardial infarction: chest pain does not always occur, particularly in the elderly. The GP should not have been surprised that the creatine kinase was normal: the blood had been taken too soon after the presumed infarction. He was advised by the clinical biochemist to take a further blood sample: this was timed at 26 h after the onset of symptoms and the creatine kinase was clearly raised at 280 U/L.

 Case history 21.2

An elderly woman presented with an exacerbation of congestive cardiac failure. She was being treated with digoxin and a thiazide diuretic.

Investigations

serum:	digoxin (12 h after previous dose)	3.2 nmol/L
	potassium	3.0 mmol/L
	urea	11.2 mmol/L
	creatinine	160 µmol/L

Comment

Drug interactions are an important cause of ill-health at all ages, but particularly in the elderly. An exacerbation of cardiac failure in a patient treated with digoxin should raise the suspicion of digoxin toxicity. The serum concentration here is compatible with this and digoxin toxicity is enhanced by hypokalaemia: thiazide diuretics are an important cause of this. The elevated serum creatinine concentration indicates impaired renal function; this can impair the excretion of digoxin and lead to its accumulation in the plasma (*see also Case History 2.7*).

Loop diuretics, and excessive use of purgatives, are also relatively frequent causes of hypokalaemia in the elderly.

metabolism, and may be affected by the function of organs that are relatively immature. Pharmacokinetics can also be different in neonates in comparison with older children or adults. Many conditions present exclusively, or predominantly, in the neonatal period: examples include many congenital diseases and inherited metabolic disorders (*see Chapter 16*). Other disorders may become apparent at any time during childhood, in particular disorders of growth and of sexual differentiation and development.

Paediatric medicine no longer begins with the birth of the child. It is now becoming possible to treat some fetal disorders *in utero*, and clinical biochemistry laboratories will be required to provide an appropriate service to support this.

In a book of this size, it is possible only to outline some of the more important areas where paediatric medicine and clinical biochemistry interact. The reader seeking more detailed information should consult more specialized textbooks.

REFERENCE RANGES

The reference ranges for certain analytes are different in the newborn from the adult (*Fig. 21.3*) and may vary

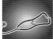

Case history 21.3

A 70-year-old woman presented with a painful ulcer on the sole of her left foot. On examination her foot felt cold and appeared ischaemic: no pulses were palpable below the femorals on either side.

Her urine contained a trace of glucose and a biochemical screen revealed a random plasma glucose concentration of 15 mmol/L although she denied any thirst or polyuria. A repeat (fasting) glucose concentration was 9.2 mmol/L.

Comment
The patient's random plasma glucose concentration is highly suggestive of diabetes mellitus and the diagnosis was confirmed by the second measurement.

It should be noted that, if classic symptoms are not present, the diagnosis of diabetes requires the demonstration of abnormally high blood glucose concentrations on two separate occasions (see p. 197).

The classic thirst and polyuria of diabetes may not always be present, particularly in the elderly, in whom the renal threshold for glucose is often elevated as a result of a decreased glomerular filtration rate. This may just be a feature of declining renal function with age, but can be exacerbated by renal disease, which can develop as a complication of diabetes.

through childhood; the concentrations of some analytes, in particular phosphate and calcium, are affected by the diet. A result should always be interpreted in the light of the reference range appropriate to the child's age. The age-related changes in plasma alkaline phosphatase and immunoglobulins are discussed in *Chapter 13*. Creatinine clearance must be corrected for surface area in a child, since it increases as the child grows.

SCREENING

The well-established programmes for neonatal screening for phenylketonuria and congenital hypothyroidism are discussed in *Chapter 16*. The rapid increase in the identification of mutations responsible for many inherited metabolic diseases, together with the development of techniques for obtaining and analyzing fetal DNA, is increasing the availability of reliable antenatal screening, particularly in high-risk pregnancies (i.e. where there is a strong family history of a particular disorder).

CHILDHOOD DISORDERS

Neonatal hypoglycaemia

This important condition is discussed in *Chapter 11*. It is particularly likely to occur in low birth weight infants, both premature and 'small-for-dates', babies born to diabetic mothers, and babies who are ill or who have feeding problems. In such babies, blood glucose measurements should be made every 4 h for the first 48 h and at appropriate intervals thereafter to monitor treatment if hypoglycaemia has occurred. Persistent hypoglycaemia or requirement for glucose infusion at a rate exceeding 10 mg/kg body weight/min to prevent hypoglycaemia should prompt a search for metabolic and endocrine causes (*see Fig. 11.14*).

Neonatal hypocalcaemia and hypomagnesaemia

The clinical signs of hypoglycaemia include irritability, twitching and convulsions. If the baby's blood glucose concentration is not low, hypocalcaemia, which presents with similar signs, should be suspected.

Plasma calcium concentration, which at birth is higher (up to 3.00 mmol/L) than in normal adults, falls rapidly, then rises to reach adult values by the third or fourth day of life. The transient, physiological hypocalcaemia is rarely symptomatic but tends to be exaggerated, and may be symptomatic, in pre-term infants, infants born to diabetic mothers and following birth asphyxia. It can be prevented by giving adequate calcium; if the baby is not feeding normally, intravenous calcium may be required.

Hypocalcaemia occurring after the first 2–3 days of life is uncommon. Causes are shown in *Fig. 21.4*. Most of these conditions are discussed in *Chapter 12*. Hypocalcaemia is a potential complication of exchange blood transfusion (clotting of donor blood is prevented by chelating calcium ions) and can be prevented by giving calcium during a transfusion.

Case history 21.4

An elderly woman was admitted to hospital after she had fallen at home and fractured her femur. She was a recluse and rarely went out, depending on a home help to do her shopping.

In addition to the fracture a radiograph showed typical features of osteomalacia.

Investigations

serum: calcium	1.75 mmol/L
phosphate	0.70 mmol/L
alkaline phosphatase	440 U/L
albumin	30 g/L

Her fracture was treated by replacement arthroplasty. After her operation, a medical student took a detailed history from the patient and discovered that she had recently developed constipation and had passed some fresh blood *per rectum*. He found her liver to be enlarged and a barium enema revealed a stenosing carcinoma of the sigmoid colon. A laparotomy was performed and the tumour was resected, but the liver was seen to contain several metastatic tumour deposits. Measurement of alkaline phosphatase isoenzymes showed an increase in both the bone and the liver isoenzymes.

Comment

The low serum calcium (even when the low albumin is taken into account), slightly reduced phosphate (a reflection of secondary hyperparathyroidism) and raised alkaline phosphatase (reflecting increased osteoblastic activity) are typical of osteomalacia. This is more common in the elderly and both poor nutrition (the low albumin would be consistent with this) and decreased endogenous synthesis of vitamin D (due to lack of exposure to sunlight) may be important in its pathogenesis. The plasma 25-hydroxycholecalciferol concentration is usually low. Typical radiological features are not always present: the definitive technique for making the diagnosis is histological examination of a bone biopsy, but this is a specialized, invasive procedure and in practice the diagnosis is often confirmed by the response to a therapeutic trial of vitamin D. Any patient may be suffering from more than one disease, but such an occurrence is more common in the elderly.

Other case histories of particular relevance may be found on *pp. 26, 58* and *168*.

Hypocalcaemia is often accompanied by hypomagnesaemia, and magnesium supplements should be given together with calcium in treating hypocalcaemia. If magnesium is not given, hypocalcaemia is often resistant to treatment. Isolated hypomagnesaemia is rare; it most frequently occurs in the infants of diabetic mothers.

Jaundice

Most babies become mildly jaundiced shortly after birth. This 'physiological' jaundice is due to immaturity of the hepatic conjugating enzymes, normal postnatal haemolysis and enterohepatic circulation of bilirubin (conversion of bilirubin to urobilinogen in the gut cannot occur until the gut becomes colonized with bacteria). In physiological jaundice, the bilirubin is primarily unconjugated and its plasma concentration rarely exceeds 100 µmol/L; the jaundice is never present at birth and does not persist beyond 14 days of life. Physiological jaundice can be exacerbated by various factors, including dehydration, hypoxia, prematurity and birth trauma leading to bruising or a cephalohaematoma.

At high concentrations of unconjugated bilirubin (>350 µmol/L) there is a risk of brain damage (kernicterus) developing. Since unconjugated bilirubin is bound to albumin, the risk is greater if the plasma

Common analytes having different reference ranges in children

Analyte	Difference
plasma potassium	mean and upper limit higher in newborn
plasma calcium	higher at birth; normal adult concentrations by 72 h
plasma phosphate	higher at birth, then falls but remains higher than adult concentrations throughout childhood; rises at puberty then falls to adult concentration
plasma alkaline phosphatase	as phosphate

Fig. 21.3 Common analytes with different reference ranges in children.

Causes of hypocalcaemia in infancy

high phosphate intake (unmodified cows' milk)
vitamin D deficiency
hypoparathyroidism
DiGeorge syndrome
pseudohypoparathyroidism
blood transfusion (exchange transfusion)
hypomagnesaemia

Fig. 21.4 Causes of hypocalcaemia in infancy, excluding transient neonatal hypocalcaemia.

When to investigate neonatal jaundice

present at birth or appears during first 24 h of life
persists beyond 14 days of life
total plasma bilirubin concentration >250 μmol/L
conjugated hyperbilirubinaemia
jaundice associated with other signs or symptoms of disease

Fig. 21.5 Circumstances in which neonatal jaundice should be investigated.

Causes of unconjugated hyperbilirubinaemia in the newborn

Increased haemolysis
rhesus blood group incompatibility
ABO blood group incompatibility
red cell enzyme defects:
　　glucose 6-phosphate dehydrogenase deficiency
　　pyruvate kinase deficiency

Decreased conjugation
Crigler–Najjar syndrome
hypothyroidism
breast milk jaundice (a benign condition seen in some breast-fed infants and thought to be due to interference with bilirubin conjugation by free fatty acids)

Fig. 21.6 Causes of unconjugated hyperbilirubinaemia in the newborn.

Causes of conjugated hyperbilirubinaemia in the newborn

haemolytic conditions (enterohepatic circulation of bilirubin)
hepatic dysfunction ('neonatal hepatitis') due to:
　　infection:
　　　　congenital, e.g. rubella, cytomegalovirus, syphilis
　　　　acquired, e.g. urinary tract infection, septicaemia, hepatitis
　　metabolic disorders:
　　　　α_1-antitrypsin deficiency
　　　　galactosaemia
　　　　tyrosinaemia
　　congenital abnormality:
　　　　biliary atresia

Fig. 21.7 Causes of conjugated hyperbilirubinaemia in the newborn.

albumin concentration is decreased or bilirubin is displaced from albumin, for example by hydrogen ions in acidosis, by certain drugs or by high concentrations of free fatty acids. Unconjugated hyperbilirubinaemia can be treated by increasing water intake, phototherapy or exchange transfusion as appropriate, and of course by treatment of the underlying cause if this can be ascertained and treatment is feasible. Circumstances

Case history 21.5

A female baby was born at 38 weeks' gestation by spontaneous vaginal delivery to a primigravid woman. The baby appeared normal at birth but was slow to feed and frequently vomited after feeds. On the third day after birth, she was noticed to be jaundiced. On examination, she was found to have an enlarged liver and bilateral cataracts.

Investigations

serum:	bilirubin (total)	168 µmol/L
	(direct)	45 µmol/L
	aspartate aminotransferase	122 IU/L
	alkaline phosphatase	244 IU/L
urine:	Clinitest	positive

Comment

Direct-reacting bilirubin is conjugated bilirubin, and its presence in the plasma is always pathological. The elevated aminotransferase activity with normal (for age) alkaline phosphatase is typical of 'neonatal hepatitis' – a term used to denote hepatic inflammation with patent bile ducts – the causes of which include infection (congenital and acquired) and various metabolic disorders. The presence of cataracts and the presence of a reducing substance in the urine suggest a diagnosis of galactosaemia (see p. 298). The child was started on a galactose-free feed and improved clinically. The diagnosis was confirmed by the finding of a low erythrocyte galactose 1-phosphate uridyl transferase activity.

Biochemical tests do not always reliably distinguish between neonatal hepatitis and extrahepatic biliary atresia. Ultrasonography or an isotopic excretion test may be required.

Screening tests for metabolic causes of illness in the newborn	
Urine	
reducing substances	bilirubin
glucose	sugar and amino acid chromatography
ketones	organic acids
Blood	
glucose	hydrogen ion
Plasma	
sodium	magnesium
potassium	conjugated bilirubin
urea	ammonia
creatinine	chromatography for amino acids
calcium	
phosphate	lactate

Fig. 21.8 Screening tests for metabolic causes of illness in the newborn.

Some of the more important causes are listed in *Fig. 21.7*.

Metabolic disorders

Although inherited metabolic diseases are individually rare, they are collectively an important cause of illness in the neonatal period. Conditions that may present at this time include, *inter alia*, disorders of amino acid, organic acid and carbohydrate metabolism, and urea cycle disorders. If an inherited metabolic disease is suspected, accurate diagnosis is essential. This applies even if there is a fatal outcome as there may be consequences for subsequent pregnancies and parents can be offered genetic counselling or possibly the option of prenatal diagnosis.

The clinical features of metabolic disorders are rarely specific to any one condition; the salt loss and virilization of female infants with steroid 21-hydroxylase deficiency (*see p. 157*) are exceptional in this respect. Some clinical features, such as severe acidosis and coma (*see p. 296*), suggest that a metabolic disorder may be present, but in many cases they are non-specific, babies afflicted by such disorders presenting, for example, with vomiting or 'failure to thrive'.

which should prompt investigation of neonatal jaundice are given in *Fig. 21.5*.

Other causes of unconjugated hyperbilirubinaemia in the newborn are given in *Fig. 21.6*.

There are also many causes of conjugated hyper-bilirubinaemia in infants: this is always pathological.

Case history 21.6

Thirty-six hours after birth, a male infant started vomiting, developed grunting respiration and rapidly became lethargic and unresponsive. He appeared physically normal and was born at term after a normal pregnancy. The parents were first cousins; it was the woman's first pregnancy. A metabolic screen revealed a very high plasma ammonia concentration (>1000 µmol/L) but the infant was not acidotic. The plasma urea was at the lower end of the reference range and plasma amino acid chromatography showed an excess of glutamine and alanine. Despite intensive treatment, including peritoneal dialysis, the baby died 72 h after birth.

Comment

Hyperammonaemia is an important cause of both morbidity and mortality in infants. This was a typical presentation of hyperammonaemia; toxic encephalopathy is usually a prominent feature. Although there are many causes of hyperammonaemia (see Fig. 21.9), a case as severe as this, without any suggestion of liver disease, and in a child born of a first cousin marriage, should raise the suspicion of an inherited metabolic disorder of the urea cycle. The excess plasma amino acids, low–normal urea and lack of acidosis are consistent with this. Patients with organic acidaemias and hyperammonaemia are usually acidotic: patients with urea cycle disorders are usually not. This child's urine was found to contain a high concentration of orotic acid. This pattern of abnormalities suggests ornithine transcarbamoylase (OTC) deficiency and this was confirmed by enzyme analysis of a post-mortem biopsy of the liver.

Deficiencies of all five enzymes of the urea cycle occur. The plasma amino acid profile is specific in citrullinaemia (arginosuccinic acid synthetase deficiency), arginosuccinic aciduria (arginosuccinase deficiency) and arginase deficiency but may be normal or non-specifically abnormal in OTC deficiency and carbamoyl phosphate synthetase deficiency; of these two, orotic aciduria only occurs with OTC deficiency. All five disorders can be diagnosed by measurement of enzyme activity in a liver biopsy.

Consanguineous parents, or a history of a previous neonatal death, should increase one's suspicion that an inherited metabolic disease may be responsible for a child's illness.

The determination of the precise diagnosis of a metabolic disorder may require complex and lengthy investigation, so it is important to be able to carry out some simple screening tests to indicate whether a metabolic disorder may be the cause of a baby's illness. An appropriate selection of tests is shown in *Fig. 21.8*. If the results of these are all normal, a metabolic disorder is unlikely; if there are abnormalities, the pattern of these may suggest a possible diagnosis or indicate what further investigations would be appropriate. It is important that the child should, if at all possible, be on a normal diet when these tests are done: potential abnormalities may otherwise be masked. Thus, disorders associated with an abnormal pattern of amino acid secretion may be missed if the infant does not have a normal protein intake.

If a baby suspected of having an inherited metabolic disease appears likely to die before a diagnosis has been established, it is essential that samples of blood, urine and skin (for fibroblast culture) are taken during life or immediately post mortem. Making a diagnosis after death will be valuable in counselling and management should another pregnancy be contemplated. Samples of liver and muscle may also be helpful for this purpose.

Failure to thrive

This is a common paediatric problem and some of the causes are shown in *Fig. 21.10*. Where there are no suggestive clinical features, either in the history or on examination, the results of tests listed in *Fig. 21.8*, together with simple haematological tests and a screen for infectious disease, will in many cases provide a starting point for definitive investigation.

Some causes of hyperammonaemia in infancy

transient neonatal hyperammonaemia*
inherited disorders of the urea cycle*
other inherited metabolic disorders*
    such as organic acidaemias
liver disease (including Reye's syndrome)
severe systemic illness* (asphyxia, infection,
    sepsis)
parenteral nutrition (excessive amino acid
    input)
sodium valproate therapy

*Important causes in the newborn.

Fig. 21.9 Some causes of hyperammonaemia in infancy. Reye's syndrome is a cause of encephalopathy in children, associated with fatty infiltration of the liver and hyperammonaemia; the cause is not known but there is an association with aspirin treatment.

Some causes of failure to thrive

malnutrition
malabsorption
inherited metabolic diseases
infection
chronic diseases:
    renal
    hepatic
    pulmonary
    cardiac
psychosocial deprivation
hypothyroidism
hypopituitarism

Fig. 21.10 Some causes of failure to thrive.

Disorders of sexual differentiation and abnormal puberty

Precocious sexual development, which may become apparent shortly after birth, is rare: some causes are given in *Fig. 21.11*. True precocious puberty, in which the gonads are fully developed and contain gametes, should be distinguished from pseudoprecocious puberty in which they are not. Pseudoprecocious puberty is often

Causes of precocious puberty and pseudoprecocious puberty

Precocious puberty
idiopathic
pineal tumours, hypothalamic hamartomas
post meningitis or encephalitis
hypothyroidism

Pseudoprecocious puberty
gonadotrophin-secreting tumours
congenital adrenal hyperplasia
adrenal tumours
ovarian and testicular tumours

Fig. 21.11 Causes of precocious puberty and pseudoprecocious puberty.

Causes of abnormal sexual differentiation

Male pseudohermaphroditism
(genotypic males with incomplete
    masculinization)
decreased testosterone production:
    various inherited enzyme abnormalities
impaired testosterone metabolism:
    5α-reductase deficiency
    androgen insensitivity syndromes
congenital anomalies

Female pseudohermaphroditism
(genotypic female with virilization)
adrenal tumours
congenital adrenal hyperplasia
Cushing's syndrome
premature adrenarche
androgen-secreting ovarian tumours

**Syndromes of abnormal gonadal
    differentiation**
Turner's syndrome (45XO karyotype)
Klinefelter's syndrome (47XXY karyotype)
other chromosomal abnormalities
true hermaphroditism

Fig. 21.12 Causes of abnormal sexual differentiation.

amenable to treatment, albeit palliative, whereas true precocity is often not. Delayed puberty is much more common: it is discussed in detail in *Chapter 10*. Virilization of females is also discussed in that chapter. It is rare in children: causes include congenital adrenal hyperplasia, Cushing's syndrome, adrenal tumours and premature adrenarche (in all of which the adrenals are the source of the excess androgens), and ovarian tumours. Disorders of sexual differentiation can be very complex: some examples are shown in *Fig. 21.12*. Although also rare, all these conditions are of immense importance to the patients and their parents, and laboratory investigations are vital in their diagnosis and management.

Disorders of growth

Many conditions can cause retardation of growth in childhood, including the causes of failure to thrive in infancy (*see Fig. 21.10*). A significant increase in growth rate occurs during puberty, and delayed puberty may be diagnosed (particularly in boys) because of short stature. Accurate clinical and anthropometric assessment is essential for diagnosis but simple laboratory tests can also provide valuable information. Growth hormone deficiency is rare: its diagnosis is discussed in *Chapter 7*. It can be treated by hormone replacement. The effects and diagnosis of growth hormone excess are also considered in *Chapter 7*.

SUMMARY

- **Many biochemical and physiological functions change with age**; some of these are related to specific events, in particular puberty and the menopause, but for others the change is more gradual, for example a decrease in the glomerular filtration rate in the elderly. This must be borne in mind when interpreting the results of biochemical tests in the elderly and ideally such results should, where appropriate, be compared with **age-related reference ranges**.

- **The presentation of certain diseases may be different** in the elderly; for this reason, and because of the frequency of multiple pathology, laboratory investigations may assume a greater importance in diagnosis.

- **It may be appropriate to screen elderly people** for conditions whose prevalence increases with increasing age, for example thyroid disease and diabetes mellitus.

- **In children** too, the reference ranges for some biochemical variables are different from those in adults. Examples include plasma phosphate concentration and alkaline phosphatase activity (both higher) and cholesterol and urate (both lower). Many conditions present more frequently, or even exclusively, in childhood; thus many inherited metabolic diseases characteristically present at or soon after birth.

- **Metabolic problems** that occur particularly frequently in the newborn include hypoglycaemia, hypocalcaemia and hypomagnesaemia.

- **Jaundice** occurs frequently in the first few days of life but in most cases this is benign. This 'physiological' jaundice is due to an increase in unconjugated bilirubin. Conjugated hyperbilirubinaemia is always pathological.

- The clinical features of **inherited metabolic disorders** presenting in infancy and childhood are often non-specific. For children who, for example, fail to thrive or show unusual irritability or lethargy, simple screening tests on urine and plasma should be performed to identify any abnormality that might be due to an inherited metabolic disease.

SUMMARY (cont'd)

- **Disorders of sexual differentiation** are uncommon but, following clinical assessment, the results of simple laboratory tests (for example, measurement of the concentrations of adrenal and gonadal hormones, and gonadotrophins) are often of vital importance in formulating a differential diagnosis and indicating the course of further investigations. This is also true of **delayed puberty**, a much more common complaint.

- There are many causes of **growth failure**, including systemic disease, social deprivation and malabsorption; relatively few cases are due to growth hormone deficiency. Again, the results of accurate clinical assessment, combined with simple laboratory tests, will often indicate the diagnosis and thus the appropriate mode of treatment.

Appendix: Adult reference ranges

These reference ranges, from the first author's laboratory, are provided for the interpretation of data presented in the case histories. Readers should note that reference ranges may differ between different laboratories; this applies particularly to hormones and enzymes. All values are for concentrations (activities in the case of enzymes) in serum or plasma, except where indicated otherwise.

adrenocorticotrophic hormone (ACTH): at 0900 h	<50 ng/L
albumin	35–50 g/L
aldosterone: recumbent	100–450 pmol/L
alkaline phosphatase	30–150 U/L
ammonia	10–47 µmol/L
amylase	<300 U/L
aspartate aminotransferase (AST)	10–50 U/L
bicarbonate total (CO_2)	22–30 mmol/L
bilirubin: total	3–20 µmol/L
calcium	2.2–2.6 mmol/L
carbon dioxide (P_{CO_2}) (arterial blood)	4.5–6.0 kPa (35–46 mmHg)
cholesterol: total	<5.0 mmol/L*
high density lipoprotein (HDL)	>1.2 mmol/L*
low density protein (LDL)	<3.0 mmol/L*

*indicates ideal values, see p. 269

copper	12–19 µmol/L
cortisol: at 0900 h	140–690 nmol/L
at 2400 h	<100 nmol/L
creatine kinase (total)	<90 U/L
creatinine	60–120 µmol/L
α-fetoprotein (AFP)	<10 µg/L

follicle-stimulating hormone (FSH):	
adult males	2–10 U/L
females: follicular phase	2–8 U/L
post-menopausal	>15 U/L
glucose fasting	2.8–6.0 mmol/L
γ-glutamyl transferase (γGT)	<60 U/L
growth hormone:	
following glucose load	<2 mU/L
following stress	>20 mU/L
haemoglobin: males	13–18 g/dL
females	12–16 g/dL
hydrogen ion: arterial blood	35–46 nmol/L (pH 7.36–7.44)
insulin: in hypoglycaemia	<20 pmol/L
luteinizing hormone (LH):	
adult males	2.0–10 U/L
adult females:	
follicular phase	2.0–10 U/L
post-menopausal	>20 U/L
magnesium	0.7–1.0 mmol/L
osmolality	282–295 mmol/L
oxygen (P_{O_2}) (arterial blood)	11–15 kPa (85–105 mmHg)
parathyroid hormone	10–65 g/L
phosphate	0.8–1.4 mmol/L
potassium	3.6–5.0 mmol/L

prolactin	50–400 mU/L
protein: total	60–80 g/L
renin (plasma renin activity, PRA): recumbent	1.1–2.7 pmol/L/h
sodium	135–145 mmol/L
testosterone: adult males adult females	9–30 nmol/L 0.5–2.5 nmol/L
thyroid-stimulating hormone (TSH, thyrotrophin)	0.3–4.0 mU/L

thyroxine (T4): total free	60–150 nmol/L 9–26 pmol/L
triglyceride: fasting	0.4–1.8 mmol/L
triiodothyronine (T3): total free	1.2–2.9 nmol/L 3.0–8.8 pmol/L
urea	3.3–6.7 mmol/L
uric acid	0.1–0.4 mmol/L
zinc	12–20 µmol/L

Self-assessment questions

These questions are based on clinical information and biochemical results. They are designed to test both knowledge and understanding. They are of three types: multiple determinate questions, each with a stem and five responses, any number of which may be correct; single best answer questions, comprising a stem and five responses, of which the most appropriate should be chosen; and extended matching questions (EMQs), based on a specified topic, for which the correct answers to five questions should be chosen from the list of possible responses. In the EMQs, any response may be used more than once or not at all.

MULTIPLE DETERMINATE QUESTIONS

1. An overnight dexamethasone suppression test is performed on a middle-aged man. Serum cortisol concentration at 0900 h next morning is 180 nmol/L. With which of the following is this result compatible?
   A. Alcoholism
   B. Cortisol-secreting adrenal adenoma
   C. Cushing's disease
   D. Depression
   E. Severe stress

2. A fasting plasma sample is observed to be lipaemic. Which of the following is/are possible causes?
   A. Chylomicronaemia
   B. High triglyceride concentration
   C. Increased HDL cholesterol concentration
   D. Increased LDL cholesterol concentration
   E. Untreated diabetes mellitus

3. An elderly man is admitted to hospital with retention of urine. Serum urea concentration is 48 mmol/L, serum creatinine 520 μmol/L. Which of the following additional findings would suggest that he has underlying chronic renal failure?
   A. Anaemia
   B. High serum alkaline phosphatase activity
   C. Hyperphosphataemia
   D. Hyponatraemia
   E. Small kidneys on ultrasound examination

4. A middle-aged man presents with renal colic. Which of the following findings would suggest a possible cause?
   A. Tendon xanthomata
   B. Evidence of malabsorption
   C. History of acute arthritis affecting the big toe one year previously
   D. Serum calcium concentration of 2.82 mmol/L
   E. Unconjugated hyperbilirubinaemia

5. A child aged 6 is investigated for short stature. The results of which of the following investigations might suggest a possible cause?
   A. Measurement of serum growth hormone concentration during a glucose tolerance test
   B. Serum creatinine concentration
   C. Serum TSH concentration
   D. Sweat chloride concentration
   E. Testing urine for reducing substances

6. An elderly patient with atrial fibrillation and congestive cardiac failure is symptom-free on treatment with digoxin and a thiazide diuretic. Serum digoxin concentration, ten hours after the previous dose, is 2.9 nmol/L. Which of the following statements is/are true?
   A. Plasma potassium concentration should be measured.
   B. The concentration should be checked three hours after the next dose.
   C. The drug is probably unnecessary and could be withdrawn without detriment to the patient.
   D. The dose of digoxin should be reduced.
   E. There is a risk of imminent renal failure.

ANSWERS AND EXPLANATIONS: MULTIPLE DETERMINATE QUESTIONS

1. A, B, C, D, E
Dexamethasone normally suppresses ACTH, and hence cortisol, secretion. A failure of suppression is characteristic of Cushing's syndrome whatever the cause but can occur in the other conditions, too.

2. A, B, E
Of the various lipoproteins only chylomicrons and VLDL (both of which transport triglycerides) are sufficiently large to scatter light, and thus cause the plasma to appear lipaemic. Both may be present in excess in untreated diabetes mellitus (both types 1 and 2).

3. A, B, E
Hyperphosphataemia and hyponatraemia occur in both acute and chronic renal failure. The kidneys are usually small in chronic renal failure (unless caused by polycystic disease or amyloid). Patients with chronic renal failure are usually anaemic (decreased erythropoietin synthesis) and often have renal osteodystrophy, causing elevated plasma alkaline phosphatase activity.

4. B, C, D
Tendon xanthomata are associated with hyper-cholesterolaemia, which does not cause renal calculi. Neither does hyperbilirubinaemia (unconjugated hyperbilirubinaemia is a cause of gallstones). Hyper-calcaemia usually causes increased urinary calcium excretion; malabsorption can cause increased urinary oxalate excretion; both predispose to calculus formation. Monoarticular arthritis affecting the big toe is suggestive of gout, in which hyperuricaemia can lead to increased urinary urate excretion and the formation of urate calculi.

5. B, C, D, E
Growth hormone secretion is normally suppressed during a glucose tolerance test; this is used to diagnose excessive growth hormone secretion. The other tests might identify renal failure, hypothyroidism, cystic fibrosis and diabetes, respectively, all of which can cause growth retardation.

6. A
The blood has been drawn at an appropriate time after the last dose. The concentration is slightly above the therapeutic range but, if the patient is well, that is not on its own an indication to reduce the dose. Digoxin toxicity is potentiated by hypokalaemia. Renal failure is not a feature of digoxin toxicity; the patient is clearly taking the drug and there is no reason to suspect that it is not required.

7. A young woman takes an overdose of paracetamol. She is discovered and admitted to hospital, approximately 36 hours after the overdose. Which of the following findings at that time would be unlikely to be due to the effects of paracetamol alone?
A. Arterial P_{CO_2} 7.8 kPa
B. Blood glucose concentration 34 mmol/L
C. Prolonged prothrombin time
D. Serum aspartate aminotransferase (AST) activity 450 IU/L
E. Serum creatine kinase (CK) activity 320 IU/L

8. A patient with chronic renal failure secondary to diabetic nephropathy is being monitored regularly but does not yet require dialysis. His serum concentrations of creatinine and urea are 252 µmol/L and 28 mmol/L, respectively. At his previous clinic attendance, four weeks before, creatinine was 248 µmol/L and urea 18.2 mmol/L. These findings could be due to:
A. Dehydration
B. Gastrointestinal haemorrhage
C. Improvement in renal function
D. Increased dietary protein intake
E. Treatment with an angiotensin-converting enzyme (ACE) inhibitor

9. A newborn infant has ambiguous genitalia; chromosomal studies show the karyotype to be 46XX. Which of the following statements is/are correct?
A. Congenital adrenal hyperplasia is a possible diagnosis.
B. Measurement of serum 17-hydroxyprogesterone is indicated.
C. The infant is at risk of developing hypoglycaemia.
D. The infant is genotypically female.
E. Turner's syndrome is a likely diagnosis.

10. A 26-year-old man is investigated for infertility associated with a low sperm count. Plasma FSH 18 U/L, LH 19 U/L, testosterone 4 nmol/L. Which of the following statements is/are correct?
A. A history of mumps may be relevant to his problem.
B. Testosterone concentration would be expected to increase in response to administration of clomiphene.
C. The data are consistent with primary testicular failure.
D. The presence of a pituitary tumour secreting gonadotrophins would explain these data.
E. Treatment with testosterone would be likely to restore fertility.

11. A patient develops a pancreatic fistula following surgery for a pancreatic pseudocyst. Results of serum analysis are: sodium 134 mmol/L, potassium 3.5 mmol/L, bicarbonate 14 mmol/L, urea 10 mmol/L, creatinine 90 µmol/L. Which of the following statements is/are correct?
A. A normal anion gap would be expected.
B. He is likely to have a non-respiratory acidosis.
C. Intravenous infusion of isotonic aqueous sodium chloride would be expected to restore his acid–base status to normal.
D. Loss of bicarbonate-rich fluid would explain these results.
E. The serum creatinine concentration indicates a normal glomerular filtration rate.

12. A young woman is admitted to the accident and emergency department. She had been found semiconscious at home by her flatmate in the evening, but had been well that morning. On examination she is dehydrated, pyrexial and hyperventilating. Arterial blood [H^+] 50 nmol/L (pH 7.30), P_{CO_2} 3.0 kPa, bicarbonate 10 mmol/L; blood glucose concentration 6.5 mmol/L; urine negative for ketones. Which of the following statements is/are correct?
A. Acute alcohol poisoning is a likely diagnosis.
B. Salicylate poisoning would explain these results.
C. The diagnosis is diabetic ketoacidosis.
D. There is evidence of a non-respiratory acidosis.
E. There is evidence of a respiratory alkalosis.

7. A, B, E

Paracetamol poisoning alone does not cause carbon dioxide retention nor such severe hyperglycaemia; respiratory alkalosis and hypokalaemia are more likely if hepatic failure develops. Liver damage causes release of aspartate aminotransferase (AST), and functional impairment causes prolongation of the prothrombin time. Muscle damage is not a feature of paracetamol poisoning, so that there is no increase in creatine kinase (CK).

8. A, B, D

An increase in urea concentration with no change in creatinine can occur in dehydration (due to increased back-diffusion of urea from the tubular fluid), and with increased urea synthesis from dietary protein, blood in the gut or as a result of endogenous protein breakdown. Loss of renal function is irreversible in chronic renal failure and an improvement would anyway be expected to decrease both urea and creatinine. Treatment with an ACE inhibitor can cause a rapid decrease in renal function in patients with renal artery stenosis; this would be expected to lead to an increase in both urea and creatinine concentrations.

9. A, B, C, D

The infant is genotypically female. The usual genotype in Turner's syndrome is 45XO; ambiguous genitalia are not a feature of this condition. Congenital adrenal hyperplasia can cause virilization of female infants: serum 17-hydroxyprogesterone is elevated in the majority of cases. There is a risk of hypoglycaemia from cortisol deficiency.

10. A, C

The low testosterone with elevated gonadotrophins suggests primary testicular failure; mumps orchitis is a recognized cause of this. Stimulation of gonadotrophin secretion with clomiphene has no effect on testosterone secretion in primary testicular failure. Gonadotrophin-secreting tumours are extremely rare and should not cause a low testosterone. Testosterone does not restore fertility in primary gonadal failure.

11. A, B, D

Non-respiratory acidosis can occur as a result of loss of bicarbonate from a pancreatic fistula. The acidosis is not due to increased production of organic acids and the anion gap should be normal. Plasma creatinine concentration is an insensitive test of renal impairment and can be normal even if the glomerular filtration rate (GFR) is moderately decreased.

12. B, D, E

She is acidotic: the low P_{CO_2} precludes this being of respiratory origin, and indicates that she also has a respiratory alkalosis. This could be compensatory, but the combination of respiratory alkalosis and non-respiratory acidosis is typical of salicylate poisoning. Alcohol can cause ketoacidosis but she is not ketotic.

13. A 38-year-old man is screened for hypercholesterolaemia after his elder brother suffered a myocardial infarction and is found to have hypercholesterolaemia. Serum cholesterol concentration (non-fasting) is 13.0 mmol/L, triglycerides 1.9 mmol/L. Which of the following statements is/are correct?
    A. A high HDL cholesterol concentration would be expected.
    B. Lipid-lowering treatment is indicated if there are no other risk factors for coronary artery disease.
    C. The molecular basis of this disorder is increased apoliprotein B synthesis.
    D. The most likely diagnosis is familial hypercholesterolaemia.
    E. The serum cholesterol concentration is unreliable since he was not fasting.

14. A patient on parenteral feeding is having continuous 24-hourly collections of urine made to assess nitrogen excretion. On a constant input of 14 g daily, values for urea excretion on successive days are 400 mmol, 480 mmol, 390 mmol, 50 mmol. Serum urea is unchanged over this period, and urine volume is appropriate for fluid input. Which of the following is/are true?
    A. Acute renal failure is the probable cause of the decreased urea excretion.
    B. Bacterial contamination of the urine could explain the result on the fourth day.
    C. Laboratory error could explain the result on the fourth day.
    D. The approximate nitrogen excretion (as urea) on the first three days is 7.5 g/24 h.
    E. The data for the first three days suggest that she is in positive nitrogen balance.

15. A baby boy, born at term by normal vaginal delivery and initially well, develops tachypnoea on the third day of life. Arterial blood [H^+] 50 nmol/L (pH 7.30), P_{CO_2} 3.3 kPa. Urine is negative for reducing substances. He becomes progressively more acidotic, and next day plasma ammonia concentration is measured and found to be very high. Which of the following diagnoses should be considered?
    A. Congenital hypothyroidism
    B. Galactosaemia
    C. Organic acidaemia
    D. Respiratory distress syndrome
    E. Urea cycle defect

16. An elderly woman is brought to hospital by ambulance, having been found at home by a neighbour in an unrousable state. On examination, she is very dehydrated. Respiration is normal; her urine is positive for glucose, negative for ketones. Biochemical analysis shows serum sodium concentration 150 mmol/L, potassium 4.8 mmol/L, bicarbonate 20 mmol/L, urea 45 mmol/L, creatinine 180 µmol/L, blood glucose 62 mmolL. Which of the following is/are true?
    A. A plasma osmolality of approximately 400 mmol/kg would be expected.
    B. She is severely acidotic.
    C. The most likely diagnosis is hyperosmolar, non-ketotic hyperglycaemia.
    D. The results for urea and creatinine suggest that she has been consuming a high protein diet.
    E. The sodium concentration suggests a high habitual salt intake.

17. The following measurements are made for the calculation of an elderly female diabetic patient's creatinine clearance: 24 h urine volume 1.44 L; serum creatinine concentration 100 µmol/L; urine creatinine concentration 6.6 mmol/L. Which of the following is/are true?
    A. Clinical features of renal impairment would be expected.
    B. Serum creatinine alone indicates impaired renal function.
    C. Serum potassium concentration should be measured urgently.
    D. The data suggest renal impairment.
    E. There is reason to suspect an incomplete urine collection.

13. B, D

The presence of hypercholesterolaemia with normal triglycerides, together with hypercholesterolaemia in a first-degree relative, is effectively diagnostic of familial hypercholesterolaemia. In this disorder, there is decreased expression of LDL receptors, leading to increased plasma LDL concentrations. There is often little response to dietary changes and the increased risk of coronary heart disease is such that lipid-lowering treatment is invariably recommended. Plasma cholesterol concentration is not significantly affected by recent food intake.

14. B, C, E

The unchanged serum urea concentration effectively excludes renal failure. One mole of urea [$CO(NH_2)_2$] contains one mole of nitrogen (N_2, molecular weight 28). Approximate nitrogen excretion is at least equal to the nitrogen excreted as urea [$(390/1000) \times 28 = 10.9$ g]. Allowing 2 g for non-urea losses, the data suggest that she is in positive nitrogen balance (input 14 g, output 13 g). Bacteria can metabolize urea to ammonia. When a result is unexpected, a laboratory error should be considered, but never assumed.

15. C

Hyperammonaemia can occur in urea cycle enzyme defects, organic acidaemias, hypoxia and liver disease (which can be a consequence of galactosaemia) but not congenital hypothyroidism. However, a positive urine test for reducing substances would be expected in galactosaemia, a respiratory or mixed acidosis in respiratory distress syndrome (the acidosis here is non-respiratory) and patients with urea cycle disorders are usually not acidotic.

16. A, C

The calculated osmolarity is as given: bicarbonate concentration is only slightly low, suggesting only a mild disturbance of acid–base homoeostasis. These results are typical of hyperosmolar, non-ketotic hyperglycaemia: excessive water loss causes hyper-natraemia and dehydration causes renal impairment, the increase in urea concentration often being relatively much greater than that in creatinine because of diffusion from the tubular lumen back into the extracellular fluid.

17. D

Creatinine clearance is $(6600 \times 1440/1440)/100 = 66$ mL/min. This suggests renal impairment. Plasma creatinine concentration is normal and does not suggest (though clearly does not exclude) the presence of impaired renal function: plasma creatinine concentration is an insensitive index of renal impairment. Clinical evidence of renal impairment is unlikely to be present with a glomerular filtration rate this high and significant hyperkalaemia is also unlikely. The urine volume is within normal limits: the patient is an elderly woman who might be expected to have a small muscle bulk and thus low endogenous creatinine production and excretion.

18. A patient with type 1 diabetes mellitus is admitted to hospital after collapsing during a 50-mile cycle race, which he had entered to raise money for charity. His blood glucose concentration is 0.5 mmol/L. He is given 50% dextrose intravenously and makes a rapid recovery. Plasma creatine kinase activity is normal on admission but 12 hours later is reported as 280 IU/L. A urine sample taken on admission is positive for glucose and protein. Which of the following is/are true?
    A. A very low glycated haemoglobin (HbA$_{1c}$) level would be expected.
    B. Exercise is known to decrease insulin requirements.
    C. Since he was hypoglycaemic on admission, the positive test for glucose in the urine at this time must be an error.
    D. The creatine kinase result could be a direct result of exercise.
    E. The proteinuria indicates that he has diabetic nephropathy.

19. A male infant is born at term to parents who are first cousins. He refuses feeds, and 12 hours after birth is noticed to be 'jittery'; blood glucose concentration measured by reagent stick is 1.0 mmol/L. Before any action can be taken, he develops focal seizures. Investigations reveal: arterial blood [H$^+$] 50 nmol/L (pH 7.30), PCO$_2$ 3.4 kPa; urine negative for reducing substances, positive for ketones. Which of the following is/are true?
    A. Glycogen storage disease type I is a possible diagnosis.
    B. Hereditary fructose intolerance is a likely diagnosis.
    C. Measurement of plasma lactate concentration would be diagnostically useful.
    D. The acidosis is respiratory in origin.
    E. The presence of an elevated plasma urate concentration would suggest a specific diagnosis.

20. Which of the following pairs of nutrients and clinical features is/are correctly linked with regard to the effects of nutrient deficiency?
    A. Ascorbic acid: prolonged prothrombin time
    B. Folic acid: macrocytic anaemia
    C. Iron: microcytic anaemia
    D. Vitamin B$_{12}$: peripheral neuropathy
    E. Zinc: skin rash

18. B, D

Glycated haemoglobin is stable once formed: it does not fall as a result of a short-lived episode of hypoglycaemia. Exercise increases glucose uptake into muscle and decreases insulin requirements. Exercise can cause an increase in plasma creatine kinase activity, and can also cause transient proteinuria. The presence or absence of glucose in the urine reflects blood glucose concentration since the bladder was last emptied: the cyclist may have started the race with a relatively high blood glucose that was greater than his renal threshold.

19. A, C, E

He is hypoglycaemic and ketotic with a partially compensated non-respiratory acidosis; this is typical of glycogen storage disease type I (the acidosis is a lactic acidosis), in which hyperuricaemia is often present. Hereditary fructose intolerance causes hypoglycaemia on exposure to fructose (and sucrose) and is associated with fructosuria, causing a positive test for reducing substances.

20. B, C, D, E

Ascorbic acid (vitamin C) deficiency causes peri-follicular haemorrhage, due to impaired collagen synthesis. Prolongation of the prothrombin time is a feature of vitamin K deficiency: this vitamin is required for the activation of coagulation factors II, VII, IX and X.

SINGLE BEST ANSWER QUESTIONS

1. An obese 19-year-old man has a free health screen arranged by his employer. Apart from fairly frequent headaches, he is well. The results of 'liver function tests' include a serum aspartate aminotransferase activity of 72 U/L; total bilirubin concentration, and alkaline phosphatase and γ-glutamyl transferase activities are within normal limits. Which one of the following is the most likely cause of this abnormality?
   A. Early viral hepatitis
   B. Excessive alcohol ingestion
   C. Gallstones
   D. Non-alcoholic steatohepatitis
   E. Therapeutic use of paracetamol

2. An elderly woman presents with back pain: serum total protein concentration is 90 g/L; albumin, 35 g/L. Her serum creatinine concentration is 150 μmol/L and she appears anaemic. Which one of the following conditions would explain all these abnormalities?
   A. Multiple myeloma
   B. Osteoarthritis
   C. Osteoporosis
   D. Paget's disease of bone
   E. Renal osteodystrophy

3. A 40-year-old journalist with a history of excessive alcohol ingestion undergoes an 'executive health screen'. Which one of the following laboratory results is unlikely to be related to alcohol?
   A. Early morning plasma cortisol concentration 720 nmol/L
   B. Mean red cell volume 105 fL (normal 88–98)
   C. Plasma cholesterol concentration 9.6 mmol/L
   D. Plasma triglyceride concentration (fasting) 4.2 mmol/L
   E. Plasma urate concentration 0.48 mmol/L

4. A 54-year-old man with a history of excessive alcohol consumption is referred to a dermatologist with a blistering rash on the face and hands. Porphyrin analysis shows a massively elevated urinary uroporphyrin excretion; no porphobilinogen is detectable in the urine. What is the most likely diagnosis?
   A. Acute intermittent porphyria
   B. Congenital erythropoietic porphyria
   C. Cutaneous hepatic porphyria
   D. Hereditary coproporphyria
   E. Lead poisoning

5. Three days after an abdominal operation, biochemical analysis of a patient's serum reveals: urea 9.6 mmol/L, creatinine 90 μmol/L, calcium 2.72 mmol/L, phosphate 1.25 mmol/L, albumin 51 g/L. No biochemical abnormality had been present pre-operatively. Which one of the following is the most likely explanation for these results?
   A. Acute phase response
   B. Acute tubular necrosis
   C. Dehydration
   D. Administration of parenteral feed with high amino acid content
   E. Primary hyperparathyroidism

6. Which one of the following is an accepted criterion for generalized biochemical screening for a condition in the neonatal period?
   A. Early treatment improves the prognosis.
   B. It has an incidence more frequent than 1 in 10,000 live births.
   C. It is fatal if untreated.
   D. Screening can be done using a dried blood spot.
   E. The screening test has 100% specificity.

7. Which one of the following findings in a patient with acute pancreatitis would suggest that another condition is also present?
   A. Methaemalbuminaemia
   B. Plasma amylase activity eight times the upper limit of normal
   C. Plasma aspartate aminotransferase (AST) activity twice the upper limit of normal
   D. Plasma calcium concentration 2.93 mmol/L
   E. Plasma urea concentration 12 mmol/L

ANSWERS: SINGLE BEST ANSWERS

1. D

The commonest cause of an isolated increase in aspartate aminotransferase (AST) activity is probably non-alcoholic steatohepatitis associated with obesity. Excessive alcohol ingestion can also cause an elevated AST, but the γ-glutamyl transferase activity is usually elevated as well. Patients with early hepatitis usually feel unwell and may have an increase in serum bilirubin concentration. Paracetamol does not cause liver damage in therapeutic doses. Asymptomatic gallstones do not cause liver function tests to be abnormal.

2. A

All these conditions can cause back pain. The high total protein concentration with slightly low albumin implies a high globulin concentration. Chronic inflammation (e.g. osteomyelitis) can cause a polyclonal increase in immunoglobulins; multiple myeloma causes a monoclonal increase. Complications of myeloma include renal impairment and anaemia. Renal osteodystrophy is not associated with an increased total plasma protein concentration. Neither osteoarthritis nor osteoporosis is associated with any of these laboratory abnormalities. A low plasma albumin concentration is a common non-specific finding in chronic illness.

3. C

Hyperuricaemia, hypertriglyceridaemia, elevated cortisol concentration (pseudo-Cushing's syndrome) and an increased red cell volume are all recognized features of excessive alcohol ingestion. While hyper-cholesterolaemia can occur in cirrhosis (of which alcohol is an important cause) it is not a feature of milder forms of alcoholic liver disease.

4. C

Acute intermittent porphyria (AIP) is not a photo-sensitizing condition; porphobilinogen is present in the urine during an acute attack. Lead poisoning can mimic AIP. Uroporphyrin is not excreted in the urine in hereditary coproporphyria. Uroporphyrin is excreted in the urine in cutaneous hepatic and congenital erythropoietic porphyria (CEP); the former can be inherited, but, unlike CEP, can also develop in patients with alcoholic liver disease.

5. C

'Corrected' calcium is normal, effectively excluding primary hyperparathyroidism. Plasma albumin concentration decreases during the acute phase response but can be increased by dehydration. The slightly elevated urea and normal creatinine are compatible with dehydration: much higher concentrations would be expected in acute tubular necrosis (in which a high albumin concentration would not be expected). A high amino acid input could account for the high urea concentration, but not the high albumin.

6. A

The incidence of a condition will have a bearing on the economics of any screening programme, but a high incidence is not a criterion for screening. The outcome, untreated, should be harmful, and the prognosis should be improved by early detection but the condition need not be fatal. Screening for phenylketonuria is based on dried blood spots, but screening programmes could be based on other samples. High specificity (no false positive results) is desirable, but high sensitivity (no cases are missed) is usually regarded as more important.

7. D

Hypercalcaemia is a rare cause of pancreatitis but is not a consequence: patients with acute pancreatitis frequently develop hypocalcaemia. The other findings are all typical of acute pancreatitis: a high urea concentration may be due to both renal impairment and accelerated protein catabolism. Methaemalbumin is formed when albumin binds free haem, and can give plasma a brown colour.

8. Which one of the following findings in a patient with primary hypothyroidism could not be explained by this condition?
   A. Hyponatraemia
   B. Increased mean red cell volume
   C. Plasma cholesterol concentration 7.2 mmol/L
   D. Plasma alkaline phosphatase activity twice the upper limit of normal
   E. Plasma creatine kinase activity twice the upper limit of normal

9. An elderly woman presents with tiredness and exertional dyspnoea. She is clinically anaemic. Which one of the following findings is inconsistent with iron deficiency being the cause of her anaemia?
   A. Low mean red cell volume (microcytosis)
   B. Low mean red cell haemoglobin (hypochromasia)
   C. Low plasma concentration of soluble transferrin receptors
   D. Low plasma iron concentration
   E. Normal plasma ferritin concentration

10. A patient is brought into the accident and emergency department having been found unconscious in the street. His breath smells strongly of alcohol. Which one of the following findings would be most suggestive of recent alcohol ingestion?
    A. Blood glucose concentration 11.2 mmol/L
    B. Increased mean red cell volume
    C. Plasma aspartate aminotransferase activity twice the upper limit of normal
    D. Plasma γ-glutamyl transferase activity three times the upper limit of normal
    E. Plasma osmolality 322 mmol/kg

11. Consecutive repeat measurements of blood glucose concentration (all values in mmol/L) in a single blood sample, using the same point of care analyser, are: 5.1, 4.9, 5.0, 5.0, 5.1, 5.0, 5.2, 5.1, 5.0, 5.1. On the basis of these data, which one of the following statements about the analyser/method is most applicable?
    A. It has high accuracy.
    B. It has high precision.
    C. It is specific for glucose.
    D. It is suitable for use by patients with diabetes to monitor their blood glucose concentrations.
    E. It should be capable of detecting hypoglycaemia in patients even if they are asymptomatic.

12. A young woman undergoes investigation for Cushing's syndrome having presented with acne and oligomenorrhoea. Early morning plasma cortisol concentration is 824 nmol/L; plasma ACTH concentration is at the upper limit of the normal range. Early morning plasma cortisol concentration after taking dexamethasone 1 mg at midnight is 766 nmol/L. After taking dexamethasone 2 mg six-hourly for 48 hours, plasma cortisol concentration is 40 nmol/L. Which of the following is the most likely diagnosis?
    A. Adrenal adenoma
    B. Adrenal carcinoma
    C. Cushing's disease (pituitary tumour secreting ACTH)
    D. Depression
    E. Ectopic secretion of ACTH by small cell carcinoma of bronchus

13. Which one of the following is the most important in the pathogenesis of obesity?
    A. An energy intake in excess of expenditure
    B. Genetic predisposition
    C. Insulin resistance
    D. Leptin deficiency
    E. Intrauterine under-nutrition

14. Which one of the following is most frequently the cause of hypercalcaemia in patients with malignant disease?
    A. Calcitonin
    B. Calcitriol
    C. Parathyroid hormone
    D. Parathyroid hormone-related peptide
    E. Tumour necrosis factor-alpha (TNFα)

15. Which one of the following hormones is most frequently secreted in excess in patients with pituitary tumours?
    A. Corticotrophin (ACTH)
    B. Follicle-stimulating hormone (FSH)
    C. Growth hormone
    D. Prolactin
    E. Thyroid stimulating hormone (TSH)

8. D

Hyponatraemia (due to inappropriate secretion of vasopressin), macrocytosis (there is an association between hypothyroidism and macrocytosis; autoimmune hypothyroidism is associated with pernicious anaemia), hypercholesterolaemia (due to decreased expression of LDL receptors) and myopathy (causing an increase in plasma creatine kinase activity) are all recognized features of primary hypothyroidism. Plasma alkaline phosphatase activity is increased in bone diseases associated with increased osteoblastic activity and in cholestatic hepatobiliary disease, but neither is associated with primary hypothyroidism.

9. C

The anaemia of iron deficiency is typically microcytic and hypochromic. Plasma iron concentration may be low but is a poor indicator of iron status. Although plasma ferritin concentration is typically low in iron deficiency, it is an acute phase protein, and normal values can occur during an acute phase reaction. An increased plasma concentration of soluble transferrin receptors is a more reliable indicator of iron deficiency.

10. E

Acutely, alcohol ingestion can cause hypoglycaemia. Increased mean red cell volume and aspartate aminotransferase and γ-glutamyl transferase activities suggest a habitual high alcohol intake: the plasma activity of the latter can remain elevated for several weeks after stopping alcohol. Normal plasma osmolality is approximately 285–295 mmol/kg: a high value can be due to high concentrations of normal low molecular weight constituents of plasma or the presence of a foreign substance. A concentration of ethanol of 80 mg/dL (the upper legal limit for driving in the UK) contributes 17 mmol/kg to osmolality.

11. B

The method appears precise (values are clustered in a small range) but there is no information to judge accuracy (the result of analysis by a reference method) or specificity for glucose (the results of measurements made in the presence of known concentrations of glucose and possible cross-reacting substances), nor on the performance of the method in practice (ease of use, sensitivity to low concentrations of glucose).

12. C

ACTH secretion is suppressed by the increased cortisol secretion in patients with adrenal adenomas or carcinomas, leading to low plasma concentrations. Plasma ACTH concentrations are typically significantly elevated in ectopic ACTH secretion by carcinomas (less so with carcinoid tumours). Although exceptions occur, plasma cortisol concentrations in patients with depression tend to be suppressed by dexamethasone; failure of suppression at low dose but suppression by a high dose of dexamethasone is typical of Cushing's disease.

13. A

Genetic predisposition (frequently) and leptin deficiency (rarely) are well-documented factors of importance in the pathogenesis of obesity. There is considerable evidence linking intrauterine under-nutrition with obesity in adult life. Insulin resistance appears to be a consequence of obesity. The essential pathogenetic factor, however, is an energy intake in excess of expenditure, whatever its cause.

14. D

Excessive calcitonin secretion (as occurs, for example, in medullary cell carcinoma of thyroid) does not affect calcium concentration. True ectopic secretion of parathyroid hormone (PTH) is rare, as is secretion of calcitriol by tumours. TNFα is responsible for the hypercalcaemia in some patients with myeloma but this is a relatively uncommon form of malignancy. Secretion of parathyroid hormone-related peptide, a peptide with N-terminal amino acid homology with PTH, is frequently present in patients with hypercalcaemia and malignancy, even when osseous metastases are present.

15. D

Secretion of TSH or FSH by pituitary tumours is rare. Secretion of ACTH (causing Cushing's disease) or growth hormone (causing acromegaly) are more common. Excessive secretion of prolactin is more frequent still, either from a tumour or from normal pituitary cells deprived of the inhibitory effect of dopamine by interruption of the hypothalamic–pituitary portal circulation by a tumour.

16. Which of the following is NOT a recognized feature of the carcinoid syndrome?
   A. Bronchospasm
   B. Diarrhoea
   C. Facial flushing
   D. Pellagra
   E. Syncope

17. Which one of the following is inconsistent with a diagnosis of cranial diabetes insipidus in a patient who complains of thirst and polyuria?
   A. Plasma sodium concentration 152 mmol/L
   B. Plasma urea concentration 8.9 mmol/L
   C. Plasma total protein concentration 85 g/L
   D. Urine osmolality 822 mmol/kg following eight hours without fluid intake
   E. Weight loss of 2% initial body weight following eight hours without fluid intake

18. A 68-year-old man presents with back pain, and has tenderness over the lumbar vertebrae. He also has symptoms of prostatism. Results of investigations: plasma calcium concentration 2.52 mmol/L, phosphate 1.22 mmol/L, alkaline phosphatase 622 U/L, creatinine 82 μmol/L, prostate specific antigen (PSA) 6 ng/L. Which of the following is the most likely cause of the high alkaline phosphatase activity?
   A. Hyperparathyroid bone disease
   B. Metastatic prostatic carcinoma
   C. Osteoporosis
   D. Osteomalacia
   E. Paget's disease

19. A 22-year-old woman is investigated for infertility. On examination, she is overweight and has severe acne. Which one of the following suggests a diagnosis other than polycystic ovary syndrome?
   A. Fasting blood glucose concentration 8.2 mmol/L
   B. Plasma gonadotrophin concentrations: LH 14.2 U/L, FSH 3.6 U/L five days after end of last period
   C. Plasma progesterone concentration 15 nmol/L seven days before the expected date of the next period
   D. Plasma prolactin concentration 300 nmol/L
   E. Plasma testosterone concentration 8.6 nmol/L

20. A 6-day-old male infant becomes acutely unwell, with hypotension and tachycardia. Plasma sodium concentration is 128 mmol/L, potassium 5.6 mmol/L, urea 6.2 mmol/L; blood glucose concentration is 1.8 mmol/L. Which one of the following investigations will be of most help in reaching a definitive diagnosis?
   A. Plasma cortisol
   B. Plasma 17-hydroxyprogesterone
   C. Plasma insulin
   D. Plasma osmolality
   E. Plasma renin activity

16. E

The release of vasoactive amines by carcinoid tumours can cause bronchospasm (hence wheezing respiration), diarrhoea and facial flushing, but not syncope. Pellagra can be a feature of carcinoid syndrome, as a result of decreased formation of nicotinic acid.

17. D

High plasma concentrations of sodium, urea and protein may occur in water loss from any cause. Weight loss (due to uncontrolled water loss) is typical of untreated diabetes insipidus if patients are denied fluid. A urine osmolality of 822 mmol/kg is a normal response to fluid deprivation, and excludes diabetes insipidus.

18. E

Plasma alkaline phosphatase is normal in uncomplicated osteoporosis. The marginally elevated PSA makes metastatic prostatic cancer unlikely (although it does not exclude it). Patients with hyperparathyroidism are typically hypercalcaemic (and such a high alkaline phosphatase would be exceptional) whereas most patients with osteomalacia are hypocalcaemic. Disease activity in Paget's disease correlates well with plasma alkaline phosphatase activity.

19. E

Impaired glucose tolerance is frequently present in patients with polycystic ovary syndrome (PCOS) and the high ratio of LH to FSH is typical of (though not invariably present in) this condition. The low plasma progesterone at day 21 merely suggests an anovulatory cycle, without indicating a possible cause. Plasma prolactin concentration is normal. Plasma testosterone concentration is typically slightly elevated in PCOS, but a value this high is suggestive of an adrenal or ovarian tumour secreting testosterone.

20. B

The clinical diagnosis is congenital adrenal hyperplasia (CAH). Measurement of plasma cortisol and 17-hydroxyprogesterone would be essential but the finding of a high 17-hydroxyprogesterone concentration is diagnostically more useful. The results should be available rapidly and allow appropriate treatment to be given. Steroid profiling, involving analysis of the pattern of steroids and metabolites in urine is recommended for confirmation and to indicate the likely enzyme abnormality (most frequently steroid 21-hydroxylase, but there are several others). Plasma osmolality would be expected to be low in any patient with hyponatraemia. An increase in plasma renin activity would be expected but not diagnostically useful. Hypoglycaemia is a recognized finding in most types of CAH, so measurement of insulin is not indicated.

EXTENDED MATCHING QUESTIONS

Acid-base disorders

A. Acute hypoventilation

B. Anxiety-induced hyperventilation

C. Chronic obstructive pulmonary disease

D. Comatose patient with raised intracranial pressure five days after a head injury

E. Diabetic ketoacidosis

F. Ethylene glycol poisoning

G. Lactic acidosis

H. Resuscitation following cardiopulmonary arrest

I. Salicylate poisoning

J. Vomiting with pyloric stenosis

For each of the following sets of results of arterial blood gas analysis, select one diagnosis from the list above that you consider the most appropriate.

1. $[H^+]$ 30 nmol/L (pH 7.52), P_{CO_2} 3.6 kPa, P_{O_2} 14.0 kPa, $[HCO_3^-]$ 23 mmol/L

2. $[H^+]$ 30 nmol/L (pH 7.52), P_{CO_2} 7.0 kPa, P_{O_2} 12.2 kPa, $[HCO_3^-]$ 42 mmol/L

3. $[H^+]$ 48 nmol/L (pH 7.32), P_{CO_2} 8.1 kPa, P_{O_2} 8.7 kPa, $[HCO_3^-]$ 30 mmol/L

4. $[H^+]$ 60 nmol/L (pH 7.22), P_{CO_2} 9.0 kPa, P_{O_2} 6.2 kPa, $[HCO_3^-]$ 27 mmol/L

5. $[H^+]$ 80 nmol/L (pH 7.10), P_{CO_2} 8.0 kPa, P_{O_2} 24.2 kPa, $[HCO_3^-]$ 17 mmol/L

Hypercalcaemia

A. Familial hypocalciuric hypercalcaemia

B. Milk–alkali syndrome

C. Myeloma

D. Paget's disease

E. Primary hyperparathyroidism

F. Sarcoidosis

G. Squamous cell carcinoma of bronchus

H. Tertiary hyperparathyroidism

I. Treatment with thiazides

J. Thyrotoxicosis

For each of the following clinical scenarios concerning a patient with hypercalcaemia, select one diagnosis from the above list that you consider the most appropriate.

1. An elderly man with a short history of back pain and who has a normochromic, normocytic anaemia.

2. A 45-year-old man who has had two episodes of renal colic during the past year but has otherwise been well.

3. A 58-year-old woman who has recently undergone successful renal transplantation for end-stage renal failure.

4. A 38-year-old man whose plasma calcium concentration has not fallen following parathyroidectomy.

5. A 36-year-old man with a history of cough and shortness of breath, who now complains of painful, red eyes.

Hyperkalaemia

A. Acute renal failure

B. Addison's disease

C. Chronic renal failure

D. Diabetic ketoacidosis

E. Excessive oral potassium intake

F. Steroid 21-hydroxylase deficiency

G. Treatment with an ACE inhibitor

H. Treatment with a potassium-sparing diuretic

I. Type 4 renal tubular acidosis

For each of the following hyperkalaemic patients, select one diagnosis from the above list that you consider the most appropriate.

1. A male infant with signs of severe fluid depletion and coexistent hyponatraemia.

2. A 13-year-old boy with a recent history of polyuria and polydipsia, who now presents in a drowsy condition, with deep, sighing respiration and his breath smelling of acetone.

3. A 23-year-old man who recently underwent a splenectomy following a road traffic accident, and now appears fluid-depleted with a plasma creatinine concentration of 225 μmol/L.

4. A 52-year-old man with treated hypertension, who did not tolerate treatment with thiazides or β-blockers.

5. A 58-year-old man with cystinuria and a long history of recurrent renal stones, in spite of treatment with penicillamine.

Hypocalcaemia

A. Acute pancreatitis

B. Acute rhabdomyolysis

C. Chronic renal failure

D. Hungry bone syndrome

E. Hypomagnesaemia

F. Hypoparathyroidism

G Malabsorption

H. Pseudohypoparathyroidism

I. Vitamin D-dependent rickets

J. Vitamin D deficiency

For each of the following scenarios involving patients with hypocalcaemia, select one diagnosis from the above list that you consider the most appropriate.

1. A 52-year-old man with newly diagnosed hypertension, a history of feeling generally unwell for at least a year, who is clinically anaemic. Serum calcium concentration 1.92 mmol/L, albumin 36 g/L, phosphate 2.4 mmol/L, alkaline phosphatase 224 U/L.

2. A 19-year-old man, previously in good health, who sustains abdominal trauma in a street fight and undergoes resection of part of the distal small intestine with fashioning of an ileostomy. Serum calcium concentration 2.02 mmol/L, albumin 44 g/L, phosphate 1.2 mmol/L, alkaline phosphatase 96 U/L.

3. A 6-year-old child whose parents are concerned about his frequent episodes of diarrhoea and abdominal discomfort. Serum calcium concentration 1.94 mmol/L, albumin 36 g/L, phosphate 0.8 mmol/L, alkaline phosphatase 452 U/L.

4. A housebound elderly woman with proximal muscle weakness. Serum calcium concentration 1.84 mmol/L, albumin 32 g/L, phosphate 0.6 mmol/L, alkaline phosphatase 254 U/L.

5. A 'jittery' three-week-old infant with muscle spasms who sustains a generalized convulsion. Serum calcium 1.72 mmol/L, albumin 41 g/L, phosphate 3.2 mmol/L, alkaline phosphatase 200 U/L.

Hypokalaemia

A. Conn's syndrome

B. Cushing's syndrome

C. Decreased oral potassium intake

D. Diuretic phase of acute renal failure

E. Purgative abuse

F. Pyloric stenosis

G. Secondary aldosteronism

H. Transcellular potassium movement secondary to insulin administration

I. Treatment with diuretics

J. Villous adenoma of the rectum

For each of the following hypokalaemic patients, select one diagnosis from the above list that you consider the most appropriate.

1. A two-week-old male infant with intractable vomiting, who is found to have an arterial hydrogen ion concentration ($[H^+]$) of 28 nmol/L (pH 7.56).

2. A 23-year-old man, who begins to produce large volumes of urine while he is recovering from an episode of prerenal uraemia.

3. A 45-year-old hypertensive woman with an obese abdomen but thin arms and legs, who is found to have a 0900 h plasma cortisol concentration of 286 nmol/L after taking 1 mg dexamethasone the previous evening.

4. A 49-year-old man with hypertension, who is found to have a plasma potassium concentration of 2.5 mmol/L, plasma bicarbonate of 35 mmol/L and a high plasma aldosterone:renin ratio.

5. A 52-year-old woman with alcoholic cirrhosis and ascites.

Hyponatraemia

A. Addison's disease

B. Analgesic nephropathy

C. Cerebral salt wasting

D. Compulsive water drinking

E. Hypothyroidism

F. Intravenous infusion of copious amounts of 'dextrose–saline'

G. Secondary aldosteronism

H. Steroid 21-hydroxylase deficiency

I. Syndrome of inappropriate antidiuresis

J. Treatment with diuretics

For each of the following hyponatraemic patients, select one diagnosis from the above list that you consider the most appropriate.

1. A 72-year-old woman on longstanding treatment for essential hypertension.

2. A 64-year-old woman with recent-onset ankle oedema, who is found to have a plasma albumin concentration of 24 g/L and a 24-h urine protein excretion of 3.6 g.

3. A 54-year-old male smoker complaining of weight loss and haemoptysis, who is found to have a plasma sodium concentration of 114 mmol/L.

4. A 32-year-old woman complaining of excessive thirst, who is found to have a plasma osmolality of 272 mmol/kg and a urine osmolality of 186 mmol/kg.

5. A 23-year-old man with increasing lethargy, who is found to have postural hypotension, increased skin pigmentation and the following plasma results: sodium 121 mmol/L, potassium 5.7 mmol/L.

Jaundice in adults

A. Alcoholic cirrhosis

B. Autoimmune chronic hepatitis

C. Carcinoma of head of pancreas

D. Chronic haemolytic anaemia

E. Cirrhosis secondary to haemochromatosis

F. Early viral hepatitis

G. Gilbert's syndrome

H. Hepatic metastases from carcinoma of colon

I. Primary biliary cirrhosis

J. Sclerosing cholangitis

For each of the following scenarios, select one diagnosis from the above list that you consider the most appropriate.

1. An elderly woman with weight loss and abdominal pain radiating to the back. Serum bilirubin 225 µmol/L, albumin 36 g/L, total protein 68 g/L, aspartate aminotransferase (AST) 42 U/L, alkaline phosphatase 455 U/L, γ-glutamyl transaminase (GGT) 72 U/L. Urine positive for bilirubin.

2. A 55-year-old woman who has had pruritus for several months and recently became jaundiced. Serum bilirubin 235 µmol/L, albumin 34 g/L, total protein 86 g/L, AST 50 U/L, alkaline phosphatase 412 U/L, GGT 102 U/L. Urine positive for bilirubin.

3. A 45-year-old man who presented with a haematemesis from oesophageal varices. Serum bilirubin 196 µmol/L, albumin 22 g/L, total protein 55 g/L, AST 122 U/L, alkaline phosphatase 420 U/L, GGT 510 U/L. Urine positive for bilirubin.

4. A 19-year-old man noticed to be jaundiced following a bout of gastroenteritis, who is otherwise well. Serum bilirubin 68 µmol/L, albumin 45 g/L, total protein 74 g/L, AST 20 U/L, alkaline phosphatase 81 U/L, GGT 30 U/L. Urine negative for bilirubin.

5. A 16-year-old girl who has been feeling unwell for a week, with nausea and pain in the right upper quadrant of the abdomen. Serum bilirubin 122 µmol/L, albumin 44 g/L, total protein 72 g/L, AST 412 U/L, alkaline phosphatase 98 U/L, GGT 65 U/L. Urine positive for bilirubin.

Malabsorption

A. Bacterial overgrowth

B. Chronic pancreatitis

C. Coeliac disease

D. Crohn's disease

E. Cystic fibrosis

F. Intestinal disaccharidase deficiency

G. Pernicious anaemia

H. Zollinger–Ellison syndrome

For each of the following patients, select one diagnosis from the above list that you consider the most appropriate.

1. A three-year-old boy who is failing to thrive, who has a positive test for antibodies to tissue transglutaminase in his plasma.

2. A four-year-old boy with a history of recurrent respiratory tract infections, who now presents with diarrhoea.

3. A 34-year-old woman with intermittent abdominal discomfort and diarrhoea, whose symptoms are reproduced by ingesting a 50 g dose of lactose dissolved in water.

4. A 46-year-old male publican with symptoms suggestive of steatorrhoea, who has recently developed diabetes mellitus.

5. A 62-year-old woman on treatment with thyroxine, who is found to have macrocytic anaemia.

Neonatal jaundice

A. α_1-Antitrypsin deficiency

B. Biliary atresia

C. Breast milk jaundice

D. Congenital rubella infection

E. Galactosaemia

F. Glucose 6-phosphate dehydrogenase deficiency

G. Hypothyroidism

H. Physiological jaundice

I. Rhesus blood group incompatibility

J. Tyrosinaemia

For each of the following jaundiced neonates, select one diagnosis from the above list that you consider the most appropriate.

1. A full-term male infant who develops unconjugated hyperbilirubinaemia at three days old. The plasma bilirubin peaks at 76 μmol/L and is normal again by the time he is two weeks old.

2. A full-term female infant who is found to have a conjugated hyperbilirubinaemia, together with an enlarged liver, bilateral cataracts and urine that tests positive for reducing substances.

3. The second child of a rhesus D negative mother, who has unconjugated hyperbilirubinaemia and anaemia at birth.

4. The pre-term son of Greek parents.

5. A full-term, male, breast-fed infant who appeared normal at birth, but who developed an unconjugated hyperbilirubinaemia that has persisted until he is 15 weeks old.

Thyroid disorders

A. Compensated primary hypothyroidism

B. Early hyperthyroidism

C. Erratic compliance with thyroxine replacement

D. Established hyperthyroidism

E. Established primary hypothyroidism

F. Medullary cell carcinoma of thyroid

G. Mild sick euthyroid syndrome

H. Over-treatment of hypothyroidism with thyroxine

I. Physiological goitre

J. Secondary hypothyroidism

For each of the following sets of data, select one diagnosis from the above list that you consider to be the most appropriate.

1. Serum [TSH] <0.01 mU/L, free thyroxine 34 pmol/L, free triiodothyronine 2.1 pmol/L

2. Serum [TSH] <0.01 mU/L, free thyroxine 34 pmol/L, free triiodothyronine 6.2 pmol/L

3. Serum [TSH] 2.2 mU/L, free thyroxine 7.2 pmol/L, free triiodothyronine 1.6 pmol/L

4. Serum [TSH] 3.2 mU/L, free thyroxine 14.2 pmol/L, free triiodothyronine 1.1 pmol/L

5. Serum [TSH] 12.2 mU/L, free thyroxine 11.4 pmol/L, free triiodothyronine 1.8 pmol/L

ANSWERS AND EXPLANATIONS: EXTENDED MATCHING QUESTIONS

Acid–base disorders

Answers: 1B, 2J, 3C, 4A, 5H

Explanation

The results in both 1 and 2 indicate an alkalosis. The low P_{CO_2} in 1 indicates that this is respiratory in origin, and must be the result of hyperventilation leading to carbon dioxide being excreted at a rate greater than its production. In 2, P_{CO_2} is elevated: the alkalosis must therefore be non-respiratory in origin, and the elevated P_{CO_2} is a result of compensatory hypoventilation (though not sufficient to cause significant hypoxaemia; *see p. 53*). The results in 3, 4 and 5 indicate an acidosis, and the elevated P_{CO_2} in each case indicates a respiratory component. Knowing that in an acute (uncompensated) respiratory acidosis, [H^+] increases by approximately 6 nmol/L for each 1 kPa rise in P_{CO_2}, it can be seen that the data in 4 indicate an acute respiratory acidosis; those in 3, where the [H^+] is lower, a compensated respiratory acidosis, while, in 5, the acidosis is more severe than expected so that there must also be a non-respiratory component. The high P_{O_2} reflects the administration of oxygen during the resuscitation: since oxyhaemoglobin is normally fully saturated when breathing air at sea level, a high arterial P_{O_2} can only result when the percentage of oxygen in the inspired gas is higher than the normal of approximately 20%.

Hypercalcaemia

Answers: 1C, 2E, 3H, 4A, 5F

Explanation

Back pain and anaemia are both common in the elderly and both are frequently present in myeloma, as also is hypercalcaemia. Hypercalcaemia in a patient with renal colic is most likely to be due to primary hyperparathyroidism; this condition is sometimes confused with familial hypocalciuric hypercalcaemia (FHH) as plasma PTH can be within the reference range in both (though usually only elevated in hyperparathyroidism), but renal colic is rare in FHH. Tertiary hyperparathyroidism typically presents in patients with longstanding chronic renal disease following successful transplantation. Cough, exertional dyspnoea and uveitis are frequently features of sarcoidosis, in which hypercalcaemia is caused by increased formation of calcitriol.

Hyperkalaemia

Answers: 1F, 2D, 3A, 4G, 5C

Explanation

Steroid 21-hydroxylase deficiency can present in a number of ways (e.g. ambiguous genitalia, pseudoprecocious puberty). However, neonates with complete deficiency of the enzyme present shortly after birth with a life-threatening salt-losing state accompanied by hyponatraemia and hyperkalaemia. Diabetic ketoacidosis may be the first presentation of type 1 diabetes mellitus, although in this patient the polyuria and polydipsia do suggest hyperglycaemia had been present previously. A raised plasma creatinine concentration generally indicates a markedly reduced glomerular filtration rate, and the recent history of a road traffic accident and clinical evidence of fluid depletion suggest that this is an acute rather than a chronic condition. Angiotensin-converting enzyme (ACE) inhibitors are one of several groups of drugs that may be considered for the treatment of hypertension when thiazides and β-blockers are not tolerated. They occasionally cause hyperkalaemia. The renal stone disease caused by cystinuria can usually be controlled by appropriate medical and surgical interventions, but some patients do progress to chronic renal failure.

Hypocalcaemia

Answers: 1C, 2E, 3G, 4J, 5F

Explanation

If serum total calcium concentration is decreased, the possibility of this being secondary to a low albumin concentration (resulting in a decrease in protein-bound calcium) should always be considered. In the scenarios above, even where the albumin concentration is low, the 'corrected calcium' (*see p. 221*) is also low. An elevated alkaline phosphatase activity in a hypocalcaemic patient (bearing in mind that normal levels in children are higher than in adults) suggests active bone disease (although the possibility of hepatobiliary disease should also be borne in mind). This is seen in renal osteodystrophy and osteomalacia/rickets. A high phosphate concentration suggests either decreased parathyroid hormone secretion (or insensitivity to its actions) or renal impairment; the physiological response to hypocalcaemia is for parathyroid hormone secretion to increase (secondary hypoparathyroidism), which tends to reduce plasma phosphate concentration.

The data in scenario 1 would be compatible with hypoparathyroidism except that alkaline phosphatase is usually normal in this condition: the other features are typical of chronic renal failure. The normal alkaline phosphatase in scenario 2 suggests that the hypocalcaemia is acute: considerable amounts of magnesium can be lost in ileostomy fluid. Malabsorption from any cause can lead to impaired absorption of vitamin D and hypocalcaemia with rickets/osteomalacia. The elderly housebound are at particular risk of vitamin D deficiency because of their decreased exposure to sunlight and, in some cases, poor diet. The high plasma phosphate concentration and relatively low alkaline phosphatase in scenario 5 favour hypoparathyroidism over a vitamin D-related cause of hypocalcaemia.

Hypokalaemia

Answers: 1F, 2D, 3B, 4A, 5G

Explanation

Pyloric stenosis is more common in male infants and is not usually manifest until the second or third week of life. The loss of gastric secretions through projectile vomiting produces a systemic alkalosis, as seen here. Prerenal uraemia may progress to acute tubular necrosis, in which the oliguric phase is followed by a diuretic phase and then a recovery phase. The diuretic phase reflects an improvement in the glomerular filtration rate before tubular function recovers, and large volumes of urine with a composition similar to protein-free plasma are produced. Plasma cortisol should suppress to below 50 nmol/L in an overnight dexamethasone suppression test. Failure to suppress is not always due to Cushing's syndrome, but the clinical picture here (truncal obesity, muscle wasting, hypertension) makes this the likely diagnosis. Hypertension with hypokalaemia should trigger suspicion of Conn's syndrome, particularly when, as here, there is an associated alkalosis. The high aldosterone:renin ratio confirms the diagnosis. Cirrhosis (from any cause) with ascites is one of several conditions where there is sodium and water excess but continued secretion of aldosterone, a syndrome known as secondary aldosteronism.

Hyponatraemia

Answers: 1J, 2G, 3I, 4D, 5A

Explanation

Diuretics (in particular, thiazides) remain part of the standard treatment of essential hypertension and may sometimes cause hyponatraemia (*p. 25*). The presence of proteinuria, hypoalbuminaemia and oedema constitutes the nephrotic syndrome, a recognized cause of secondary aldosteronism. Weight loss and haemoptysis in a smoker suggest a diagnosis of bronchial carcinoma, and the associated hyponatraemia is most likely due to ectopic (and inappropriate) secretion of antidiuretic hormone (ADH) by the tumour. Dilute urine in association with excessive thirst might be due to diabetes insipidus, or it might be an appropriate response to compulsive water drinking. The fact that the plasma osmolality is slightly low, rather than high–normal, suggests that the latter is the case. Lethargy, postural hypotension and the associated hyponatraemia and hyperkalaemia all point to adrenal insufficiency; increased skin pigmentation suggests a high plasma concentration of ACTH, so this is primary (Addison's disease) rather than secondary adrenal insufficiency.

Jaundice in adults

Answers: 1C, 2I, 3A, 4G, 5F

Explanation

Both patients 1 and 2 have cholestatic jaundice. The high total protein in patient 2 suggests a high globulin concentration: this is typical of autoimmune liver disease (in primary biliary cirrhosis it is IgM, antimitochondrial antibody). In autoimmune chronic hepatitis (which usually presents at a younger age), there is usually an increase in AST. The history of patient 1 is typical of pancreatic carcinoma, a cause of extrahepatic biliary obstruction. Serum GGT activity can be elevated in both hepatocellular and cholestatic jaundice, but the very high activity in patient 3, whose presentation and other liver function tests (LFTs) suggests cirrhosis, is typical of alcohol-related disease. In Gilbert's syndrome, jaundice is always mild, occurs sporadically and is unconjugated (hence no bilirubinuria), while the other LFTs are typically normal. The hyperbilirubinaemia of chronic haemolysis is also unconjugated, but tends to be persistent. The presentation of patient 5 is typical of viral hepatitis, in which serum AST activity tends to be greatly elevated early in the course of the illness, although alkaline phosphatase may increase later.

Malabsorption

Answers: 1C, 2E, 3F, 4B, 5G

Explanation
'Failure to thrive' is a common reason for children to be referred for investigation. In this case the positive antibodies to tissue transglutaminase strongly suggest that coeliac disease is the cause. Children with cystic fibrosis develop recurrent respiratory infections leading to irreversible lung disease, and pancreatic insufficiency leading to malabsorption. Symptoms that are reproduced by ingestion of lactose suggest lactase deficiency, although formal assessment of the plasma glucose response to lactose, or measurement of lactase in a biopsy, may be performed for confirmation. The combination of steatorrhoea and diabetes mellitus suggests that pancreatic damage may have resulted in a loss of both exocrine and endocrine pancreatic function. In a publican, the suspicion must be of chronic pancreatitis secondary to prolonged alcohol excess. There is an association between autoimmune thyroid disease and other forms of autoimmune disease. Pernicious anaemia is one such disease, which results in a macrocytic anaemia (with a megaloblastic bone marrow).

Neonatal jaundice

Answers: 1H, 2E, 3I, 4F, 5C

Explanation
In physiological jaundice, the jaundice is never present at birth and does not persist beyond 14 days of life. It is due mainly to unconjugated bilirubin and the plasma concentration rarely exceeds 100 µmol/L. Conjugated hyperbilirubinaemia in an infant is always pathological: in this instance, the other findings are typical of galactosaemia. Rhesus haemolytic disease of the newborn occurs in a rhesus D negative mother who is sensitized by a rhesus D positive pregnancy and who then has a further rhesus D positive child. The incidence has been dramatically reduced by the prophylactic use of IgG anti-D antibodies in rhesus D negative mothers. Glucose 6-phosphate deficiency is sex-linked, affecting males, and particularly affects certain races, including those from around the Mediterranean. Breast milk jaundice is an unconjugated hyperbilirubinaemia that can persist in breast-fed infants for 2–16 weeks. It is benign, and if breast feeding is discontinued for 24–48 h, the plasma bilirubin falls.

Thyroid disorders

Answers: 1H, 2D, 3J, 4G, 5A

Explanation

A very low [TSH] is characteristic of hyperthyroidism or over-treatment of hypothyroidism; in the latter, [fT4] is elevated, but [fT3] is normal or low, since the only source of T3 is peripheral deiodination. In hyperthyroidism, the overactive gland usually produces an excess of both thyroid hormones. In secondary hypothyroidism, the concentrations of both thyroid hormones and of TSH tend to be low; similar results can be found in sick euthyroid patients, but in milder cases, [fT3] tends to fall before [fT4]. Except in the very rare instances where hyperthyroidism is TSH-dependent, and sometimes in patients recovering from illness, an elevated [TSH] is indicative of primary hypothyroidism, but in early or compensated hypothyroid states, the increased TSH drive may maintain normal (albeit usually low–normal) concentrations of fT4.

Subject Index